WITHDRAWN
WRIGHT STATE UNIVERSITY LIBRARIES

Serotonin, the Cerebellum, and Ataxia

Serotonin, the Cerebellum, and Ataxia

Editors

Paul Trouillas, M.D.
*Professor of Neurology
Alexis Carrel Faculty of Medicine
Neurological Hospital and
Claude Bernard University
Lyon, France*

Kjell Fuxe, M.D.
*Professor of Histology
Departments of Histology
and Neurobiology
Karolinska Institute
Stockholm, Sweden*

Raven Press ⚡ New York

Raven Press, Ltd., 1185 Avenue of the Americas, New York, New York 10036

© 1993 by Raven Press, Ltd. All rights reserved. This book is protected by copyright. No part of it may be reproduced, stored in a retrieval system, or transmitted, in any form or by any means, electronic, mechanical, photocopy, or recording, or otherwise, without the prior written permission of the publisher.

Made in the United States of America

Library of Congress Cataloging-in-Publication Data
Serotonin, the cerebellum, and ataxia / editors, Paul Trouillas,
  Kjell Fuxe.
      p. cm.
  Includes bibliographical references and index.
  ISBN 0-88167-957-7
  1. Cerebellar ataxia—Pathophysiology. 2. Cerebellar ataxia—Chemotherapy.
  3. Serotoninergic mechanisms. I. Trouillas, Paul. II. Fuxe, Kjell.
    [DNLM: 1. Ataxia—drug therapy. 2. Ataxia—etiology. 3. Cerebellum—
  drug effects. 4. Cerebellum—physiology. 5. Serotonin—pharmacology. WL
  320 S486]
  RC394.C44S47   1993
  616.8′38—dc20
  DNLM/DLC
  for Library of Congress   92-49910
                                                                             CIP

   The material contained in this volume was submitted as previously unpublished material, except in the instances in which credit has been given to the source from which some of the illustrative material was derived.
   Great care has been taken to maintain the accuracy of the information contained in the volume. However, neither Raven Press nor the editors can be held responsible for errors or for any consequences arising from the use of the information contained herein.
   Materials appearing in this book prepared by individuals as part of their official duties as U.S. Government employees are not covered by the above-mentioned copyright.

9 8 7 6 5 4 3 2 1

Contents

Contributing Authors ix

Preface xix

1. Novel Aspects on Central 5-Hydroxytryptamine
   Neurotransmission: Focus on the Cerebellum 1
   *Kjell Fuxe, L. F. Agnati, B. Bjelke, P. Hedlund, A. Ueki,
   B. Tinner, B. Bunnemann, H. Steinbusch, D. Ganten, and
   A. Cintra*

Raphe

2. A Quantitative Study of the Raphe Serotonin Neurons in the
   Normal Human Brain Stem 37
   *V. Chan-Palay, M. Höchli, B. Jentsch, R. G. H. Cotton, and
   T. Zetsche*

3. The Cerebellar Projection from the Neurons of the Raphe
   Nuclei and the Origin of the Serotoninergic Innervation of the
   Cerebellum 51
   C. Batini

4. Distribution of Tryptophan Hydroxylase Immunoreactive
   Neurons in the Human Brain Stem 63
   *Nicolas Kopp, Michèle Aguerra, Dominique Martin,
   Michel Maitre, and Marie-Françoise Belin*

5. Selective Organization of Tryptophan Hydroxylase Expression
   in the Raphe Dorsalis 81
   D. Weissmann, F. Richard, C. Rousset, and J. F. Pujol

Organization of Cerebellar Monoaminergic Systems

6. The Serotoninergic System in the Cerebellum: Origin,
   Ultrastructural Relationships, and Physiological Effects 91
   *Georgia A. Bishop, Christopher W. Kerr, Yi Fei Chen, and
   James S. King*

7. Serotonergic Innervation of the Inferior Olive and Tremor
   Generated in the Olivocerebellar Climbing Fiber System 113
   Leif Wiklund

8. A Small Population of Purkinje Cells in the Posterior Vermis Is Specifically Labeled by a Tyrosine Hydroxylase Antibody 121
   B. Berthie, H. Axelrad, C. Verney, and M. E. Marc

9. GABA Neurons and Innervation by Tryptophan Hydroxylase (PH8) and Monoamine Oxidase B Immunoreactive Axons in the Human Cerebellum 129
   T. Zetzsche and V. Chan-Palay

Morphogenesis of Serotonergic Neurons

10. The Brain Stem Origin and Development of Serotonin in the Opossum Cerebellum 137
    James S. King, James J. Walker, and Georgia A. Bishop

Serotonergic Receptors in the Cerebellum and Inferior Olive

11. Serotonergic Control of Glutamatergic Systems in the Cerebellum 155
    Maurizio Raiteri, Guido Maura, Pierpaola Lottero, and Licia Gastaldo

12. Visualization of 5-HT Receptors in the Cerebellum and Related Brain Stem Areas 167
    J. M. Palacios, M. Pompeiano, O. Pompeiano, and G. Mengod

13. 5-HT_{1A} Receptors in the Olivocerebellar Complex 179
    Daniel Vergé, Line Matthiessen, Hossein K. Kia, Henri Gozlan, Michel Hamon, Yannick Bailly, and Geneviève Daval

14. Effect of Chronic 5-HT Uptake Inhibition on Serotonergic Autoregulation 191
    Chantal Moret and Mike Briley

15. The Mouse 5-HT_{1B} Serotonin Receptor: Cloning, Functional Expression, and Localization in Motor Control Centers 201
    F. Saudou, L. Maroteaux, N. Amlaiky, U. Boschert, J. L. Plassat, and R. Hen

Neurophysiology of Cerebellar Serotonergic Transmission

16. Multiple Actions of Serotonin on the Electrophysiology of Purkinje Cells 211
    Howard K. Strahlendorf and Jean C. Strahlendorf

17. Differential Modulation by Serotonin of the Responses Induced by Excitatory Amino Acids in Cerebellar Nuclei Neurons and Purkinje Cells 225
    Robert Gardette and Francis Crepel

18. Modulation of Locus Coeruleus Activity by Serotoninergic Afferents 237
    Michel Buda, Hideo Akaoka, Gary Aston-Jones, Paul Charléty, Karima Chergui, Guy Chouvet, and Pierre-Hervé Luppi

19. Effects of Harmaline on Serotonergic Neurotransmission 255
    M. Weiss, P. Blier, and C. de Montigny

Models of Ataxia and Neurotransmitter Metabolism

20. 3-Acetylpyridine and Thiamine Deficiency-Induced Cerebellar Models and the Pathophysiology of Ataxia 269
    Andreas Plaitakis

21. Collateral Sprouting of Cerebellar Climbing Fibers After Subtotal Lesions of the Inferior Olive 291
    L. Wiklund, F. Rossi, P. Strata, and J. J. L. van der Want

22. Cerebellar Monoamines in the "Purkinje Cell Degeneration" Mutant Mouse 297
    B. Ghetti, L. C. Triarhou, and R. W. Fuller

23. L-5-Hydroxytryptophan, Serotonin, and Brain Protein Synthesis 307
    Patrick Lepetit, Monique Touret, Eric Grange, Nadine Gay, and Pierre Bobillier

24. Serotonergic CSF Abnormalities in Human Acquired and Genetic Ataxias 311
    P. Trouillas, N. Charles, B. Renaud, N. Eynard, and P. Adeleine

Clinical Aspects: L-5-Hydroxytryptophan Treatment of Ataxia

25. The Serotonergic Hypothesis of Cerebellar Ataxia and Its Pharmacological Consequences 323
    Paul Trouillas

26. L-5-Hydroxytryptophan in Cerebellar Syndrome Treatment ... 335
    J. M. Senard, W. Delage, M. Clanet, O. Rascol, J. L. Montastruc, and A. Rascol

27. Treatment of Ataxia with 5-Hydroxytryptophan: Clinical
Studies 337
K. Wessel, G. P. Huss, K. Schimrigk, N. Mai, and D. Kömpf

28. Quantitative Assessment of Postural Asynergy in Cerebellar
Pathology 343
*François Viallet, Bernadette Bonnefoi-Kyriacou,
Jean Massion, Roselyne Aurenty, and Richard Khalil*

29. Interest in L-5-HTP Administration in the Rehabilitation
Course of Patients with Cerebellar Ataxia 357
D. Boisson, G. Rode, and C. Froment

30. Continuous Subcutaneous Lisuride Infusion in
Olivopontocerebellar Atrophies 363
*L. Schöls, A. Heinz, M. Langkafel, J. Wöhrle, and
H. Przuntek*

Subject Index 371

Contributing Authors

P. Adeleine
Biostatistical Unit
Faculté Alexis Carrel
Laboratoire d'Informatique
 des Hospices Civils de Lyon
162 Avenue Lacassagne
69003 Lyon, France

L. F. Agnati
Department of Human Physiology
University of Modena
Via Campi 287
41100 Modena, Italy

Michèle Aguerra
Laboratoire d'Anatomie Pathologique
Faculté de Médecine Alexis Carrel
Rue Guillaume Paradin
69372 Lyon, Cedex 08, France

Hideo Akaoka
INSERM U171
CNRS URA 1195
Centre Hospitalier Lyon Sud
F-69310 Pierre-Bénite, France

N. Amlaiky
Laboratoire de Génétique Moléculaire des
 Eucaryotes du CNRS
INSERM U184
 de Biologie Moléculaire et de Génie
 Génétique
Faculté de Médecine
11 Rue Humann
67085 Strasbourg, Cedex, France

Gary Aston-Jones
Division of Behavioral Neurobiology
Department of Mental Health Sciences
Hahnemann University
Philadelphia, Pennsylvania

Roselyne Aurenty
CNRS LNF 3
31 Chemin Joseph Aiguier
13402 Marseille, Cedex 09, France

H. Axelrad
Laboratoire de Neurophysiologie
Faculté de Médecine Pitié-Salpêtrière
91 Boulevard de l'Hôpital
75013 Paris, France

Yannick Bailly
Developmental Neurobiology Laboratory
Institut des Neurosciences
CNRS UA 1199
Université Pierre et Marie Curie
7 Quai Saint Bernard
75252 Paris, Cedex 05, France

C. Batini
Laboratoire de Physiologie de la Motricité
CNRS URA 385
Université Pierre et Marie Curie
Faculté de Médecine Pitié-Salpêtrière
91 Boulevard de l'Hôpital
75013 Paris, France

Marie-Françoise Belin
Laboratoire d'Anatomie Pathologique
Faculté de Médecine Alexis Carrel
Rue Guillaume Paradin
69372 Lyon, Cedex 08, France

CONTRIBUTING AUTHORS

B. Berthie
Laboratoire de Neurophysiologie
Faculté de Médecine Pitié-Salpêtrière
91 Boulevard de l'Hôpital
75013 Paris, France

Georgia A. Bishop
Department of Cell Biology,
  Neurobiology, and Anatomy
The Ohio State University
333 W. 10th Avenue
Columbus, Ohio 43210-1239

B. Bjelke
Departments of Histology and
  Neurobiology
Karolinska Institute
Box 60400
S-104 01 Stockholm, Sweden

P. Blier
Neurobiological Psychiatry Unit
Department of Psychiatry
McGill University
1033 Pine Avenue West
Montreal, Quebec, Canada H3A 1A1

Pierre Bobillier
Groupe de Neuroanatomie Fonctionnelle
CNRS URA 1195
Laboratoire d'Anatomie Pathologique
Faculté de Médecine Alexis Carrel
Rue Guillaume Paradin
69372 Lyon, Cedex 08, France

D. Boisson
Service de Rééducation Fonctionnelle
Hôpital Henry Gabrielle
Route de Vourles
69230 Saint Genis Laval, France

Bernadette Bonnefoi-Kyriacou
Service de Neurologie
CHU la Timone
Boulevard Jean Moulin
13005 Marseille, France

U. Boschert
Laboratoire de Génétique Moléculaire des
  Eucaryotes du CNRS
INSERM U184
  de Biologie Moléculaire et de Génie
  Génétique
Faculté de Médecine
11 Rue Humann
67085 Strasbourg, Cedex, France

Mike Briley
Neurobiology Division I
Pierre Fabre Research Center
17 Avenue Jean Moulin
81106 Castres, Cedex, France

Michel Buda
INSERM U171
CNRS URA 1195
Centre Hospitalier Lyon Sud
F-69310 Pierre-Bénite, France

B. Bunnemann
Departments of Histology and
  Neurobiology
Karolinska Institute
Box 60400
S-104 01 Stockholm, Sweden

V. Chan-Palay
Neurology Clinic
University Hospital
Frauenklinikstrasse 26
CH-8091 Zurich, Switzerland

N. Charles
Neurology Service and Ataxia Research
  Center
Alexis Carrel Faculty of Medicine
Neurological Hospital and Claude
  Bernard University
59 Boulevard Pinel
69003 Lyon, France

Paul Charléty
INSERM U171
CNRS URA 1195
Centre Hospitalier Lyon Sud
F-69310 Pierre-Bénite, France

CONTRIBUTING AUTHORS

Yi Fei Chen
Department of Cell Biology,
Neurobiology, and Anatomy
The Ohio State University
333 W. 10th Avenue
Columbus, Ohio 43210-1239

Karima Chergui
INSERM U171
CNRS URA 1195
Centre Hospitalier Lyon Sud
F-69310 Pierre-Bénite, France

Guy Chouvet
INSERM U171
CNRS URA 1195
Centre Hospitalier Lyon Sud
F-69310 Pierre-Bénite, France

A. Cintra
Departments of Histology and
Neurobiology
Karolinska Institute
Box 60400
S-104 01 Stockholm, Sweden

M. Clanet
Service de Neurologie
CHU Toulouse
Hôpital de Purpan
Place du Docteur Baylac
31059 Toulouse, Cedex, France

R. G. H. Cotton
The Murdoch Institute
Royal Children's Hospital
Flamington Road
Parkville 3052
Melbourne, Australia

Francis Crepel
CNRS URA 1121
Building 440
Université Paris Sud
91405 Orsay, France

Geneviève Daval
Department of Cytology
Institut des Neurosciences
CNRS UA 1199
Université Pierre et Marie Curie
7 Quai Saint Bernard
75252 Paris, Cedex 05, France

W. Delage
Service de Pharmacologie
CHU Toulouse
Hôpital de Purpan
Place du Docteur Baylac
31059 Toulouse, Cedex, France

N. Eynard
Laboratoire de Neuropharmacologie
Biochimique
Service de Biologie
Hôpital Neurologique
59 Boulevard Pinel
69003 Lyon, France

C. Froment
Service de Rééducation Fonctionnelle
Hôpital Henry Gabrielle
Route de Vourles
69230 Saint Genis Laval, France

R. W. Fuller
Laboratory of Cellular and Molecular
Neuropathology
Department of Pathology
Indiana University School of Medicine
and Eli Lilly Research Laboratories
Indianapolis, Indiana 46202-5120

Kjell Fuxe
Departments of Histology and
Neurobiology
Karolinska Institute
Box 60400
S-104 01 Stockholm, Sweden

D. Ganten
Max Delbrück Center for Molecular
Medicine, Berlin-Buch
Robert Rössle Strasse 10
O-1115 Berlin-Buch, Germany

Robert Gardette
INSERM U159
2ter rue d'Alésia
75014 Paris, France

Licia Gastaldo
Istituto di Farmacologia e Farmacognosia
Università degli Studi di Genova
Viale Cembrano 4
16148 Genova, Italy

Nadine Gay
Groupe de Neuroanatomie Fonctionnelle
CNRS URA 1195
Laboratoire d'Anatomie Pathologique
Faculté de Médecine Alexis Carrel
Rue Guillaume Paradin
69372 Lyon, Cedex 08, France

B. Ghetti
Laboratory of Cellular and Molecular
  Neuropathology
Department of Pathology
Indiana University School of Medicine
and Eli Lilly Research Laboratories
Indianapolis, Indiana 46202-5120

Henri Gozlan
Cellular and Functional Neurobiology
  Laboratory
INSERM U288
Faculté de Médecine Pitié-Salpêtrière
91 Boulevard de l'Hôpital
75013 Paris, France

Eric Grange
Groupe de Neuroanatomie Fonctionnelle
CNRS URA 1195
Laboratoire d'Anatomie Pathologique
Faculté de Médecine Alexis Carrel
Rue Guillaume Paradin
69372 Lyon, Cedex 08, France

Michel Hamon
Cellular and Functional Neurobiology
  Laboratory
INSERM U288
Faculté de Médecine Pitié-Salpêtrière
91 Boulevard de l'Hôpital
75013 Paris, France

P. Hedlund
Departments of Histology and
  Neurobiology
Karolinska Institute
Box 60400
S-104 01 Stockholm, Sweden

A. Heinz
Neurologische Universitätsklinik
  im St. Josef Hospital
Gudrunstrasse 56
D-4630 Bochum, Germany

R. Hen
Laboratoire de Génétique Moléculaire des
  Eucaryotes du CNRS
INSERM U184
  de Biologie Moléculaire et de Génie
  Génétique
Faculté de Médecine
11 Rue Humann
67085 Strasbourg, Cedex, France

M. Höchli
Neurology Clinic
University Hospital
Frauenklinikstrasse 26
CH-8091 Zurich, Switzerland

G. P. Huss
Department of Neurology
Medical University of Lübeck
Ratzeburger Allee 160
D-2400 Lübeck, Germany

B. Jentsch
Neurology Clinic
University Hospital
Frauenklinikstrasse 26
CH-8091 Zurich, Switzerland

Christopher W. Kerr
Department of Cell Biology,
  Neurobiology, and Anatomy
The Ohio State University
333 W. 10th Avenue
Columbus, Ohio 43210-1239

CONTRIBUTING AUTHORS

Richard Khalil
Service de Neurologie
CHU la Timone
Boulevard Jean Moulin
13005 Marseille, France

Hossein K. Kia
Department of Cytology
Institut des Neurosciences
CNRS UA 1199
Université Pierre et Marie Curie
7 Quai Saint Bernard
75252 Paris, Cedex 05, France

James S. King
Department of Cell Biology,
  Neurobiology, and Anatomy
The Ohio State University
333 W. 10th Avenue
Columbus, Ohio 43210-1239

D. Kömpf
Department of Neurology
Medical University of Lübeck
Ratzeburger Allee 160
D-2400 Lübeck, Germany

Nicolas Kopp
Laboratoire d'Anatomie Pathologique
Faculté de Médecine Alexis Carrel
Rue Guillaume Paradin
69372 Lyon, Cedex 08, France

M. Langkafel
Neurologische Universitätsklinik
  im St. Josef Hospital
Gudrunstrasse 56
D-4630 Bochum, Germany

Patrick Lepetit
Groupe de Neuroanatomie Fonctionnelle
CNRS URA 1195
Laboratoire d'Anatomie Pathologique
Faculté de Médecine Alexis Carrel
Rue Guillaume Paradin
69372 Lyon, Cedex 08, France

Pierpaola Lottero
Istituto di Farmacologia e Farmacognosia
Università degli Studi di Genova
Viale Cembrano 4
16148 Genova, Italy

Pierre-Hervé Luppi
Département de Médecine Expérimentale
INSERM U52
Université Claude Bernard
8 Avenue Rockefeller
69008 Lyon, France

N. Mai
Clinical Neuropsychology
Städtisches Krankenhaus
  München-Bogenhausen
Dachauer Strasse 164
D-8000 Munich 50, Germany

Michel Maitre
INSERM U44
5 Rue Blaise Pascal
67085 Strasbourg, France

M. E. Marc
Laboratoire de Neurophysiologie
Faculté de Médecine Pitié-Salpêtrière
91 Boulevard de l'Hôpital
75013 Paris, France

L. Maroteaux
Laboratoire de Génétique Moléculaire des
  Eucaryotes du CNRS
INSERM U184
  de Biologie Moléculaire et de Génie
  Génétique
Faculté de Médecine
11 Rue Humann
67085 Strasbourg, Cedex, France

Dominique Martin
Laboratoire d'Anatomie Pathologique
Faculté de Médecine Alexis Carrel
Rue Guillaume Paradin
69372 Lyon, Cedex 08, France

CONTRIBUTING AUTHORS

Jean Massion
CNRS LNF 3
31 Chemin Joseph Aiguier
13402 Marseille, Cedex 09, France

Line Matthiessen
Department of Cytology
Institut des Neurosciences
CNRS UA 1199
Université Pierre et Marie Curie
7 Quai Saint Bernard
75252 Paris, Cedex 05, France

Guido Maura
Istituto di Farmacologia e Farmacognosia
Università degli Studi di Genova
Viale Cembrano 4
16148 Genova, Italy

G. Mengod
Department of Neurochemistry
Centro Investigación y Desarrollo,
  Consejo Superior Investigaciones
  Científicas
Jordi Girona 18-26
08034 Barcelona, Spain

J. L. Montastruc
Service de Pharmacologie
CHU Toulouse
Hôpital de Purpan
Place du Docteur Baylac
31059 Toulouse, Cedex, France

C. de Montigny
Neurobiological Psychiatry Unit
Department of Psychiatry
McGill University
1033 Pine Avenue West
Montreal, Quebec, Canada H3A 1A1

Chantal Moret
Neurobiology Division I
Pierre Fabre Research Center
17 Avenue Jean Moulin
81106 Castres, Cedex, France

J. M. Palacios
Research Institute
Laboratorios Almirall
Cardener 68-74
08024 Barcelona, Spain
Department of Neurochemistry
Centro Investigación y Desarrollo,
  Consejo Superior Investigaciones
  Científicas
Jordi Girona 18-26
08034 Barcelona, Spain

Andreas Plaitakis
Department of Neurology
Mount Sinai School of Medicine
1 Gustave L. Levy Place
New York, New York 10029

J. L. Plassat
Laboratoire de Génétique Moléculaire des
  Eucaryotes du CNRS
INSERM U184
  de Biologie Moléculaire et de Génie
  Génétique
Faculté de Médecine
11 Rue Humann
67085 Strasbourg, Cedex, France

M. Pompeiano
Institute of Biological Chemistry
University of Pisa
Via Roma 55
I-56100 Pisa, Italy

O. Pompeiano
Department of Physiology and
  Biochemistry
University of Pisa
Via S. Zeno 31
I-56127 Pisa, Italy

H. Przuntek
Neurologische Universitätsklinik
  im St. Josef Hospital
Gudrunstrasse 56
D-4630 Bochum, Germany

CONTRIBUTING AUTHORS

J. F. Pujol
CNRS UMR 105
CERMEP
59 Boulevard Pinel
69003 Lyon, France

Maurizio Raiteri
Istituto di Farmacologia e Farmacognosia
Università degli Studi di Genova
Viale Cembrano 4
16148 Genova, Italy

A. Rascol
Service de Neurologie
CHU Toulouse
Hôpital de Purpan
Place du Docteur Baylac
31059 Toulouse, Cedex, France

O. Rascol
Service de Pharmacologie
CHU Toulouse
Hôpital de Purpan
Place du Docteur Baylac
31059 Toulouse, Cedex, France

B. Renaud
Laboratoire de Neuropharmacologie
   Biochimique
Service de Biologie
Hôpital Neurologique
59 Boulevard Pinel
69003 Lyon, France

F. Richard
CNRS UMR 105
CERMEP
59 Boulevard Pinel
69003 Lyon, France

G. Rode
Service de Rééducation Fonctionnelle
Hôpital Henry Gabrielle
Route de Vourles
69230 Saint Genis Laval, France

F. Rossi
Department of Human Anatomy and
   Physiology
C.so Raffaelo 30
10125 Turin, Italy

C. Rousset
CNRS UMR 105
CERMEP
59 Boulevard Pinel
69003 Lyon, France

F. Saudou
Laboratoire de Génétique Moléculaire des
   Eucaryotes du CNRS
INSERM U184
   de Biologie Moléculaire et de Génie
   Génétique
Faculté de Médecine
11 Rue Humann
67085 Strasbourg, Cedex, France

K. Schimrigk
Department of Neurology
University Homburg/Saar
D-6650 Homburg, Germany

L. Schöls
Neurologische Universitätsklinik
   im St. Josef Hospital
Gudrunstrasse 56
D-4630 Bochum, Germany

J. M. Senard
Service de Neurologie
CHU Toulouse
Hôpital de Purpan
Place du Docteur Baylac
31059 Toulouse, Cedex, France

H. Steinbusch
Department of Pharmacology
Free University Medical Faculty
Van der Boechorststraat 7
1081 BT Amsterdam, The Netherlands

Howard K. Strahlendorf
Departments of Neurology and Physiology
Texas Tech University
  Health Sciences Center
Lubbock, Texas 79430

Jean C. Strahlendorf
Departments of Neurology and Physiology
Texas Tech University
  Health Sciences Center
Lubbock, Texas 79430

P. Strata
Department of Human Anatomy and
  Physiology
C.so Raffaelo 30
10125 Turin, Italy

B. Tinner
Departments of Histology and
  Neurobiology
Karolinska Institute
Box 60400
S-104 01 Stockholm, Sweden

Monique Touret
INSERM U52
CNRS URA 1195
Département de Médecine Expérimentale
Université Claude Bernard
8 Avenue Rockefeller
69008 Lyon, France

L. C. Triarhou
Laboratory of Cellular and Molecular
  Neuropathology
Department of Pathology
Indiana University School of Medicine
and Eli Lilly Research Laboratories
Indianapolis, Indiana 46202-5120

Paul Trouillas
Neurology Service and Ataxia Research
  Center
Alexis Carrel Faculty of Medicine
Neurological Hospital and Claude
  Bernard University
59 Boulevard Pinel
69003 Lyon, France

A. Ueki
Departments of Histology and
  Neurobiology
Karolinska Institute
Box 60400
S-104 01 Stockholm, Sweden

J. J. L. van der Want
Netherlands Ophthalmic
  Research Institute
P.O. Box 12141
1100 AC Amsterdam, The Netherlands

Daniel Vergé
Department of Cytology
Institut des Neurosciences
CNRS UA 1199
Université Pierre et Marie Curie
7 Quai Saint Bernard
75252 Paris, Cedex 05, France

C. Verney
INSERM U106
Neuromorphologie
Hôpital Salpêtrière
75013 Paris, France

François Viallet
Service de Neurologie
CHG Aix-en-Provence
14 Avenue des Tamaris
13616 Aix-en-Provence, France

James J. Walker
Department of Cell Biology,
  Neurobiology, and Anatomy
The Ohio State University
333 W. 10th Avenue
Columbus, Ohio 43210-1239

M. Weiss
Neurobiological Psychiatry Unit
Department of Psychiatry
McGill University
1033 Pine Avenue West
Montreal, Quebec, Canada H3A 1A1
Laboratoire de Pharmacodynamie
Faculté de Pharmacie
27 Boulevard Jean Moulin
F-13385 Marseille, Cedex 05, France

D. Weissmann
CNRS UMR 105
CERMEP
59 Boulevard Pinel
69003 Lyon, France

K. Wessel
Department of Neurology
Medical University of Lübeck
Ratzeburger Allee 160
D-2400 Lübeck, Germany

Leif Wiklund
Laboratoire de Physiologie Nerveuse
CNRS
91190 Gif-sur-Yvette, France
Current address:
Mölndals Sjukhus
S-431 80 Mölndal, Sweden

J. Wöhrle
Neurologische Universitätsklinik
im St. Josef Hospital
Gudrunstrasse 56
D-4630 Bochum, Germany

T. Zetzsche
Neurology Clinic
University Hospital
Frauenklinikstrasse 26
CH-8091 Zurich, Switzerland

Preface

Nature has played the card of serotonin (5-HT) in multiple biological systems. 5-HT-containing nerve cells were first described in the lower brain stem in 1964. Subsequent studies of the physiology and pharmacology of these neuronal systems showed 5-HT to be involved in multiple brain functions including a key role in the regulation of mood. With the discovery of serotonergic nerve terminal networks in the cerebellar cortex and nuclei, a new focus of interest centered on the physiological and pathophysiological role of these afferents that were so differently organized compared with the parallel and mossy fiber system to the cerebellar cortex.

This volume provides the first complete survey on cerebellar 5-HT and its role in ataxia. Several chapters deal with the anatomy of the raphe systems and their afferents using 5-HT and tryptophan hydroxylase immunocytochemistry. The human raphe system is described in detail involving three-dimensional reconstructions of these systems. Ultrastructural features of cerebellar 5-HT innervation are also described, especially in relation to nonjunctional versus junctional 5-HT nerve terminals. The hypothesis of volume transmission is introduced that cerebellar 5-HT nerve terminal networks mainly operate via release of 5-HT into the extracellular fluid pathways to reach high-affinity 5-HT receptors. The ontogenesis and phylogenesis of the serotonergic systems to the cerebellar cortex are also described.

The postsynaptic features of the cerebellar 5-HT nerve terminal systems are covered extensively. The distribution of the 5-HT receptor subtypes in the cerebellum, $5-HT_{1A}$, $5-HT_{1B}$, $5-HT_{1C}$, $5-HT_2$, is summarized. In other chapters, the neurophysiological role of $5-HT_{1A}$-like receptors and their interactions with glutamate receptors in the regulation of the electrophysiology of Purkinje cells is discussed.

A number of experimental models of cerebellar ataxia are studied including the thiamine deficiency model and the mutant mouse model. In 1977, the first patient with pure cerebellar ataxia was treated with D-L-5-hydroxytryptophan and clearly showed improvement with the treatment. Further clinical progress in this pharmacological field is presented in several chapters confirming the original observations on the therapeutic effects of 5-hydroxytryptophan in cerebellar ataxia. Thus, the diffuse raphe-olivocerebellar serotonergic system may play a critical role in readjusting the activity of olivary neurons, Purkinje cells, and cerebellar nuclei. These clinical observations on the role of 5-hydroxytryptophan in the treatment of cerebellar ataxia can now be explained on the basis of novel aspects on central 5-HT transmission, especially volume transmission and receptor-receptor interactions.

This volume is unique because it summarizes for the first time what is known about the cerebellum and ataxia, covering in particular all the aspects of cerebellar serotonergic innervation with some clinical correlates. This volume should be of substantial interest to molecular biologists, neurobiologists, neurologists, and clinicians involved in medical rehabilitation.

Paul Trouillas
Kjell Fuxe

Acknowledgments

To summarize for the first time the knowledge about serotonin, the cerebellum, and ataxia, major scientists and clinicians in the field met in Lyon, France, in September 1991. The conference and this book were made possible by the following pharmaceutical companies and institutions.

Outstanding sponsors:
    Sandoz
    Pan Medica Laboratories
    UCB Pharma
    Roche
    Schering
    Sanofi-Winthrop
    Ipsen

Sponsors:
    Lipha Oberval
    Schering Plough
    Specia Laboratories
    Pierre Fabre Laboratories
    The French Friedreich Ataxia Association
    Crédit Commercial de France Banking Trust
    Servier

We wish to give our most sincere thanks for this support.

*Serotonin, the Cerebellum,
and Ataxia*, edited by
P. Trouillas and K. Fuxe.
Raven Press, Ltd., New York © 1993.

1

Novel Aspects on Central 5-Hydroxytryptamine Neurotransmission: Focus on the Cerebellum

Kjell Fuxe, *L. F. Agnati, B. Bjelke, P. Hedlund, A. Ueki, B. Tinner, B. Bunnemann, †H. Steinbusch, ‡D. Ganten, and A. Cintra

*Departments of Histology and Neurobiology, Karolinska Institute, S-104 01 Stockholm, Sweden; *Department of Human Physiology, University of Modena, 41100 Modena, Italy; †Department of Pharmacology, Free University Medical Faculty, 1081 BT Amsterdam, The Netherlands; ‡Max Delbrück Center for Molecular Medicine, Berlin-Buch, O-1115 Berlin-Buch, Germany*

In the 1960s the central 5-hydroxytryptamine (5-HT) neurons were mapped out (1,14,15,23). The 5-HT nerve cell groups are mainly located within the raphe nuclei of the lower brain stem, but are also in the adjacent reticular formation of the medulla oblongata, pons, and midbrain (59a). The 5-HT nerve cell groups give rise to long descending and ascending projections to the spinal cord and the tel- and diencephalon (3,15). There also exists a monosynaptic 5-HT innervation of the cerebellar cortex (4,6,11,26,42) that mainly enters the cerebellar cortex via the periventricular route passing through the cerebellar nuclei to reach the cerebellar cortex. The 5-HT nerve terminals form fine varicose nerve terminal plexa within all layers of the cerebral and cerebellar cortex (diffuse innervation). In the latter region 5-HT parallel-like fibers can also be found within the molecular layer (5,6,11,42, 61). There also exists substantial 5-HT innervation of the cerebellar nuclei, the major output from the cerebellum, and of the inferior olive, the origin of the climbing fibers to the cerebellar cortex (11,23,42,66). These morphological features demonstrate that 5-HT neurons can influence all levels of the cerebellar circuitry (the afferent level, the cortex itself, granular and Purkinje cells, and the efferent level), making it possible to favor a certain state of activity in the cerebellar output systems via multiple coordinated actions (see Figs. 1–4).

In this chapter we will present novel aspects of the plasticity of cerebellar 5-HT innervation as observed in neonatal 6-hydroxydopamine (6-OHDA) treatment and neonatal corticosterone treatment as well as after induction of cerebellar damage

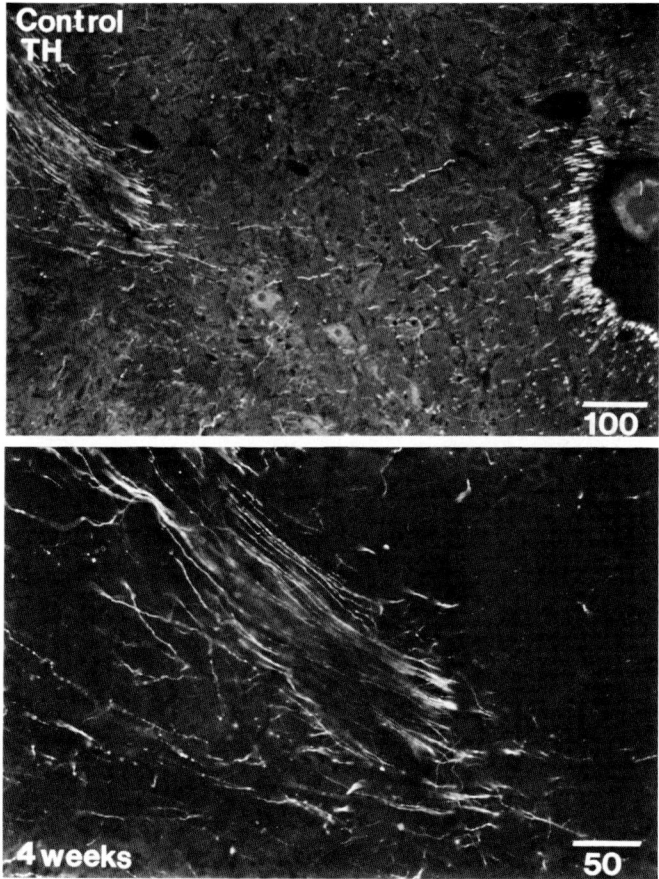

FIG. 1. 5-HT IR fibers running in a periventricular position close to the lateral wall of the fourth ventricle are seen to leave their position to cross laterally and dorsolaterally toward the cerebellum (4-week-old male rat). Indirect fluorescence was used with a rabbit 5-HT antiserum (1:400), with a secondary antibody, a FITC-conjugated sheep antirabbit immunoglobulin (1:20) (courtesy of Dr. H. M. Steinbusch). Coronal cryostate 14 μm thick section; bregma level: −13.30.

FIG. 2. 5-HT IR is demonstrated within all layers of the cerebellar cortex of the 2-month-old male rat. A rabbit 5-HT antiserum (1:400) was used. Indirect immunofluorescence was used involving as a secondary antibody a FITC-conjugated sheep antirabbit immunoglobulin (1:20). Coronal cryostate 14 μm thick sections. **A**: Nonhomogeneous distribution of the 5-HT IR nerve terminal plexa within the cerebellar cortex. Areas with few and many 5-HT nerve terminals are located adjacent to each other. The *lower panel* shows a higher magnification. **B**: 5-HT innervation of the granular cell layer (*upper and middle panels*). The 5-HT nerve terminals make no obvious associations with the Purkinje cell soma (*lower panel*).

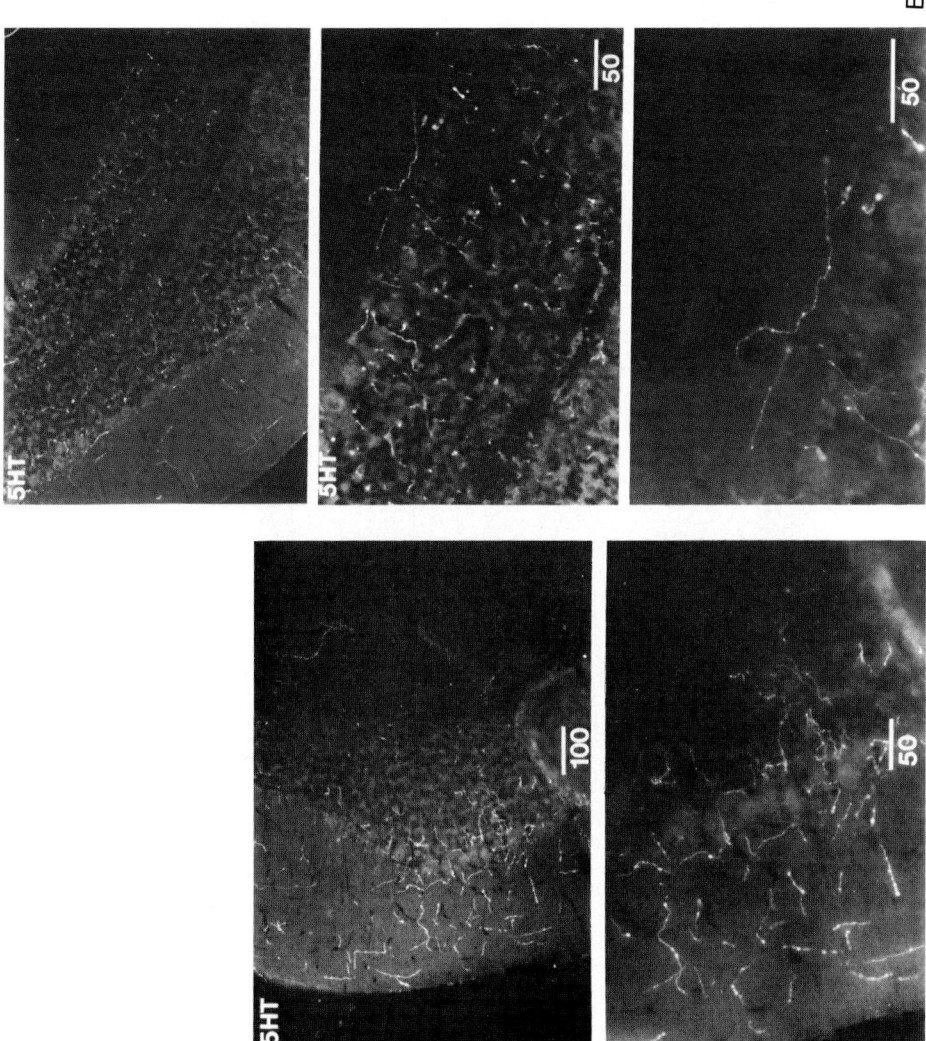

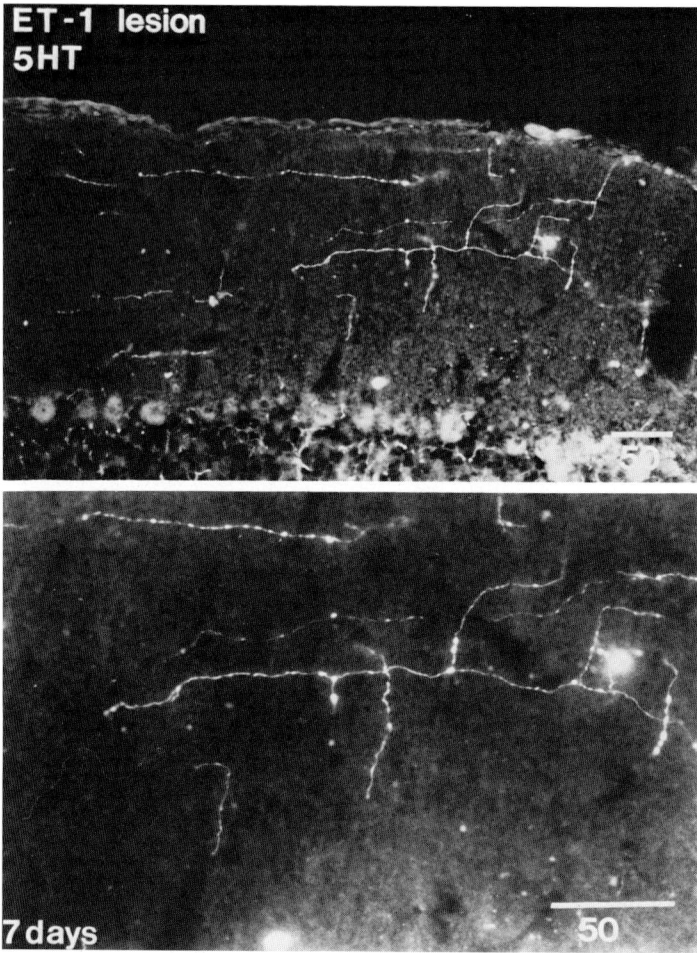

FIG. 3. 5-HT IR within the cerebellar cortex close to the ET-1-induced lesion in the dorsal vermis (1 μg/0.5 μl, 7 days after the lesion) in the 2-month-old male rat. Coronal cryostate 14 μm thick section. Primary rabbit 5-HT antiserum was used in a dilution of 1:400. Indirect immunofluorescence was used involving as a secondary antibody a sheep antirabbit FITC-conjugated IgG (1:20). Putatively sprouting 5-HT nerve terminals resembling parallel fibers are observed in the molecular layer having varicosities of various sizes. Some exhibit a very strong fluorescent intensity. 5-HT nerve terminals of this configuration within the molecular layer are rarely seen in the intact cerebellar cortex. The apparent 5-HT sprouts are given off perpendicular from the parallel-like 5-HT fiber.

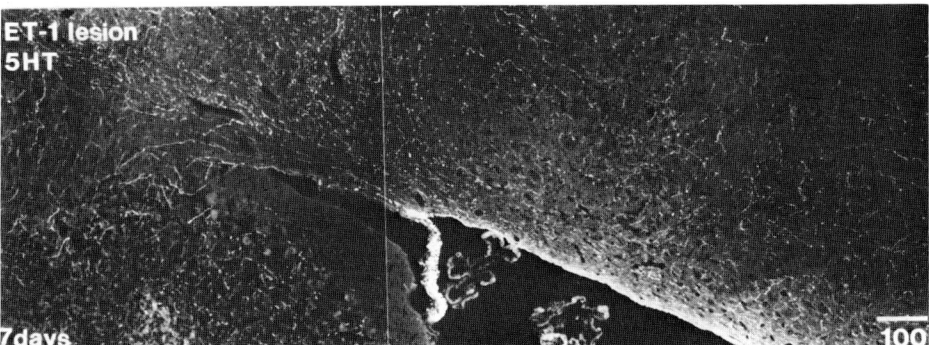

FIG. 4. 5-HT IR is demonstrated within the most ventral vermis and within the medial cerebellar nucleus following an ET-1-induced lesion (1 μg/0.5 μl) within the dorsal vermis. Primary rabbit 5-HT antiserum was used in a dilution of 1:400. Indirect immunofluorescence was used involving as a secondary antibody a sheep antirabbit FITC-conjugated IgG (1:20). The 5-HT IR nerve terminal plexus is observed having a low density and moderate intensity. A strong 5-HT IR is present within the ependymal cells due to the existence of the supraependymal 5-HT nerve terminal plexus, which cannot be clearly seen in this low magnification (see Fig. 18).

in adulthood via ischemic lesions produced by microinjections of endothelin-1 (ET-1) (32).

PLASTICITY OF 5-HT-MEDIATED INTERCELLULAR COMMUNICATION IN THE CEREBELLUM

Recently the concept has been introduced that there exist principally two modes of communication in the CNS: the classical synaptical wiring transmission (WT) (Fig. 5) and volume transmission (VT) (Fig. 6), which involves the brain extracellular fluid as a pathway for electrical and chemical communication. The main concept of VT is the conduction of the message along a leaking pathway. VT works and relies on the chemical characteristics of the message and the physical as well as structural features of the extracellular matrix. Segregation may be maintained by multiple messengers in the neurons matched by their corresponding high-affinity receptors. The VT includes very short-, short-, and long-distance diffusion of chemical signals, leading to long-term actions and thus also includes related phenomena, such as nonsynaptic (very short distance), paracrine (intermediate distance), and endocrine-like (long distance) events (31a). 5-HT and 5-HT cotransmitters are probably involved in both WT and VT transmission. Thus, upon pharmacological treatment with monoamine oxidase inhibitors and 5-HT uptake blocking agents, 5-HT was demonstrated to be present in the neuropil surrounding the 5-HT perikarya (10). Catecholamines (CA) and 5-HT were also shown to diffuse for long distances into the brain neuropil after intraventricular injections (24,25,35). Nonjunctional 5-HT nerve terminals have also been described within the cerebral as well as cerebellar

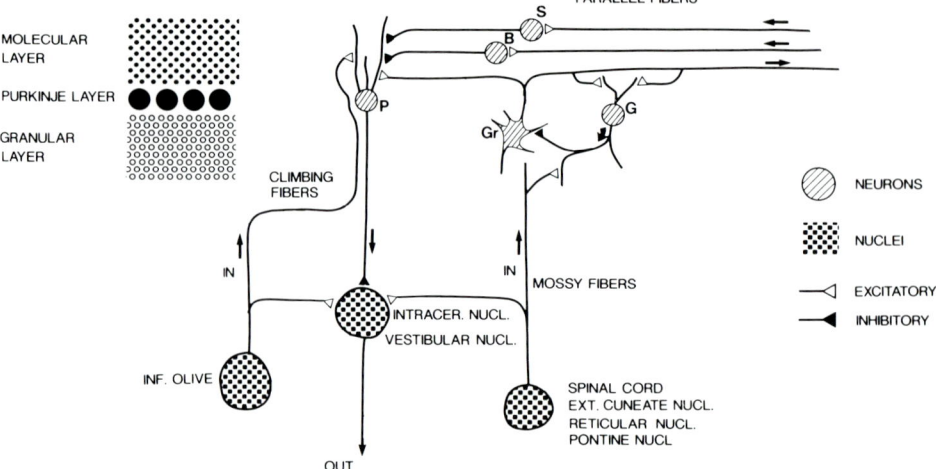

FIG. 5. Summary of the classical scheme of WT in the cerebellar cortex, including the afferent input and efferent output via the intracerebellar nuclei. S, stellate; B, basket; P, Purkinje; G, Golgi; Gr, granular.

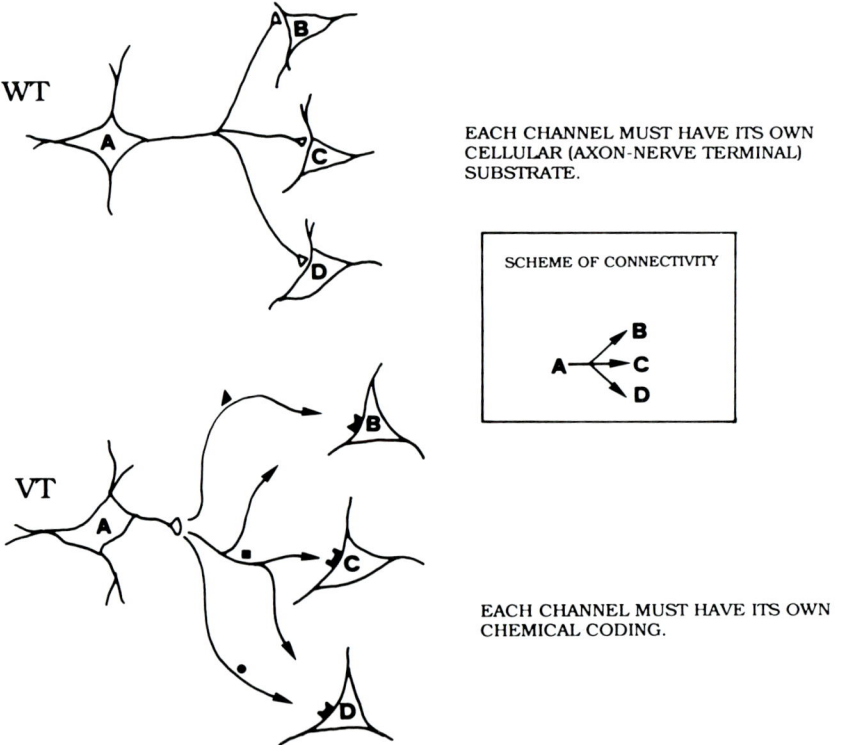

FIG. 6. Divergence and segregation in WT and VT modes of communication. In VT, segregation can be maintained by multiple transmitters, each having its corresponding high-affinity receptor.

cortex (12,20). 5-HT nerve terminal networks have been described within the ependyma, where they form supraependymal plexa of strongly 5-HT immunoreactive (IR) nerve terminals (Fig. 7) that can release 5-HT into the cerebrospinal fluid (CSF) to reach, e.g., the 5-HT$_{1C}$ receptors of the choroid plexus (Fig. 8). The 5-HT terminals can also participate to autocrine events by directly innervating 5-HT cell bodies and dendrites (Fig. 7).

5-HT may be a transmitter for VT, especially in the 5-HT networks that are less densely packed, so that the 5-HT membrane pump mechanism may not take it up as efficiently, but allows its diffusion to the high-affinity G protein-coupled 5-HT$_1$ receptors. Morphological observations are summarized in Fig. 9, supporting its presence in all layers of the cerebellar cortex. The 5-HT receptors for VT are probably of the 5-HT$_1$ type of receptors, having a high affinity for 5-HT (37,38). Thus, the 5-HT neuronal system, diffusely innervating the cerebellar and cerebral cortex, could, with VT, exert global regulation of the cortical networks via high-affinity 5-HT$_1$ receptors specifically modulating the efficacy of the transmission, e.g., at various synaptic receptors for GABA and glutamate (60; Chapters 6, 16–18, this volume). By this mode of communication it is easy to understand how 5-HT, within the cerebellar regions, could play a major role in modulating Purkinje cell activity via the high-affinity 5-HT$_{1A}$ receptors shown to suppress activity at non-NMDA receptors (see below). However, a synaptic mode of communication of 5-HT is probably also present (Fig. 10).

A sparse nonhomogeneous diffuse plexus of 5-HT nerve terminal networks is found within all the layers of the lobules of the cerebellar cortex, including the molecular layer, where the parallel fiber-like 5-HT nerve terminals are also found together with this diffuse plexus of 5-HT nerve terminals (Figs. 10 and 11). The 5-HT receptors so far demonstrated, which belong to these systems, have been mainly of the 5-HT$_{1A}$ type, that is, of the high-affinity G protein-coupled type, which may be predominantly linked to VT with higher densities being present within the molecular and Purkinje cell layers (65; Chapters 12 and 13, this volume). However, it must be emphasized that the overall number of binding sites of 5-HT receptors is very low within the cerebellar cortex, being somewhat higher within the cerebellar nuclei (Fig. 8) where they may be of the 5-HT$_{1D}$ type (Chapter 12). Thus, it must be assumed that the relatively few 5-HT$_1$ receptors present, which are known to be coupled to G proteins, have a critical location on the Purkinje cells and other parts of the networks of the cerebellar cortex. Only in this way may it be possible to explain the ability of 5-HT to modulate glutamate release (55,56) and Purkinje cell activity (16,44,60). The 5-HT terminals also control the Purkinje cells via effects on the granular cells, where a 5-HT$_2$ receptor subtype may dominate in the control of the glomeruli that regulate the excitation of the granular cells (Fig. 11) (47,48, 53,67).

Taken together, in view of the relatively sparse plexa of 5-HT nerve terminal networks in the three layers of the cerebellar cortex and the existence of high-affinity 5-HT$_1$ receptors mainly located on the rich plexus of Purkinje cell dendrites and Purkinje perikarya, it seems likely that cerebellar 5-HT and its cotransmitters

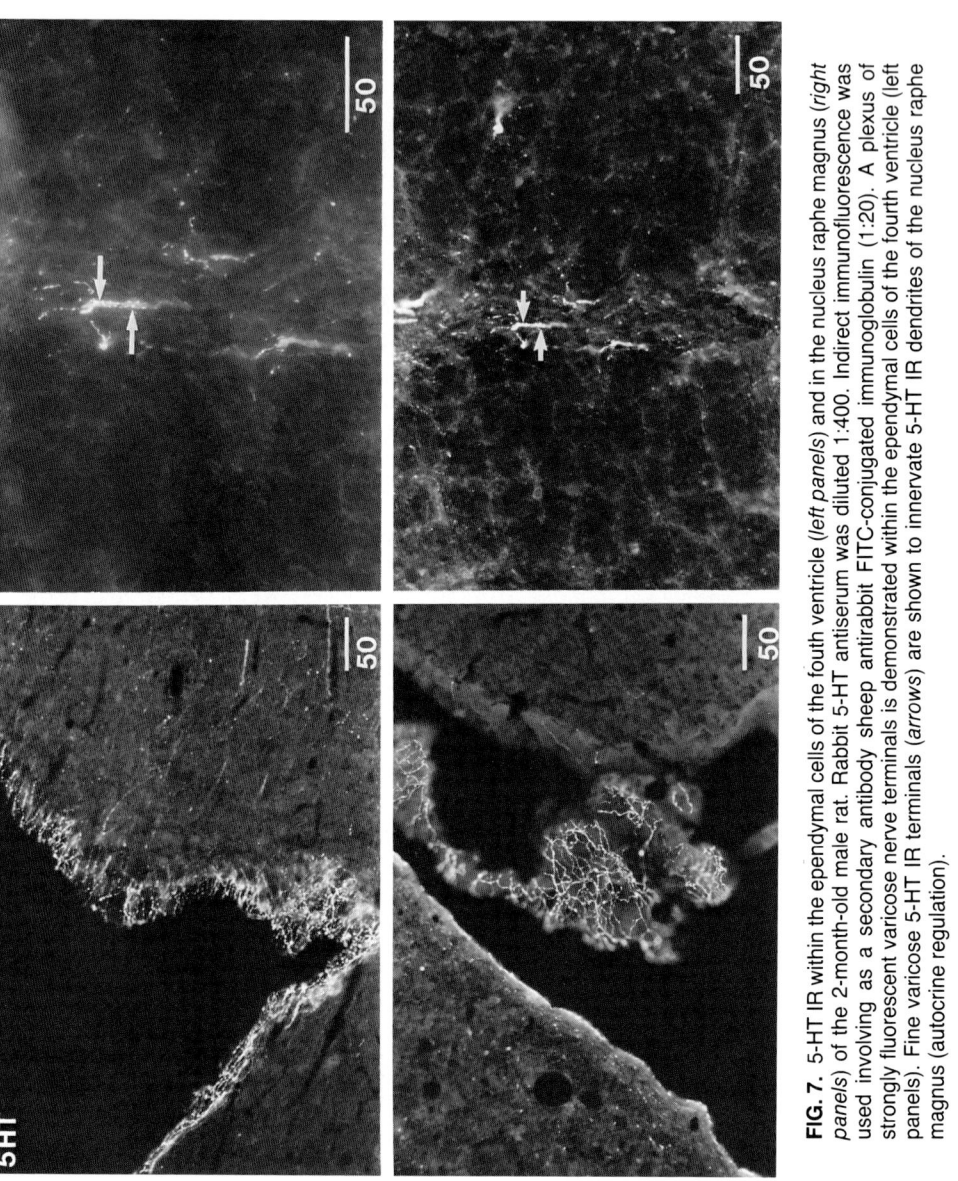

FIG. 7. 5-HT IR within the ependymal cells of the fouth ventricle (*left panels*) and in the nucleus raphe magnus (*right panels*) of the 2-month-old male rat. Rabbit 5-HT antiserum was diluted 1:400. Indirect immunofluorescence was used involving as a secondary antibody sheep antirabbit FITC-conjugated immunoglobulin (1:20). A plexus of strongly fluorescent varicose nerve terminals is demonstrated within the ependymal cells of the fourth ventricle (left panels). Fine varicose 5-HT IR terminals (*arrows*) are shown to innervate 5-HT IR dendrites of the nucleus raphe magnus (autocrine regulation).

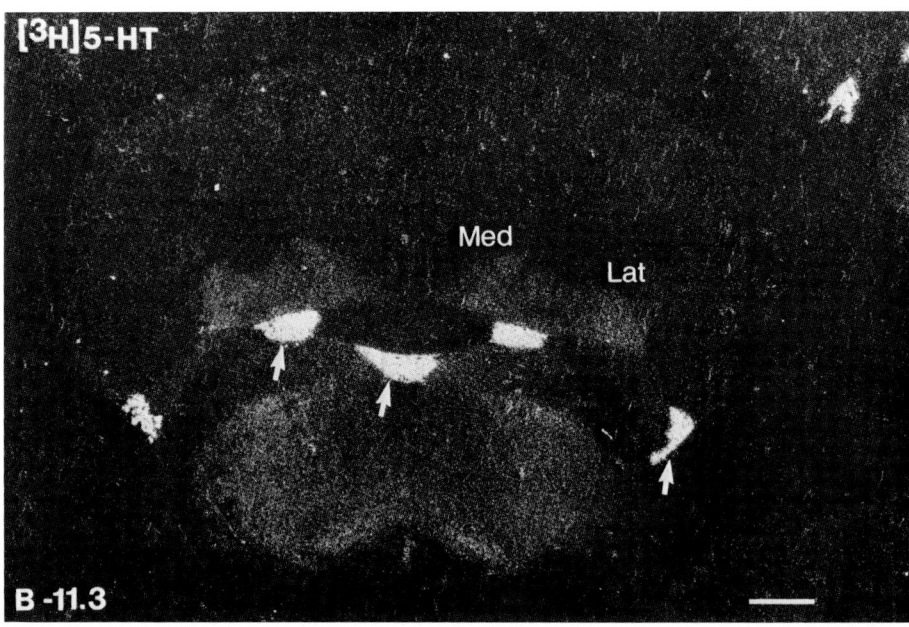

FIG. 8. Autoradiograph showing the distribution of [^{3}H]5-HT (2 nM; specific activity 28 Ci/mmol) binding sites in the rat cerebellum (bregma, −11.3 mm). With the present exposure time (6 weeks), labeling can only be observed in the deep cerebellar nuclei and not in the cortex due to the low density of receptors. Med, medial cerebellar nucleus; Lat, lateral cerebellar nucleus; *arrows* indicate the densely labeled choroidal plexus. Calibration bar = 1 mm.

		Presynaptic	Postsynaptic
Lamina Moleculare	5-HT NA DA	Nonjunctional terminals Low density	High affinity 5-HT receptors (5-HT$_{1A}$; 5-HT$_{1B}$)
Lamina Ganglionare	5-HT NA DA	Nonjunctional terminals Low density	High affinity 5-HT receptors (5-HT$_{1A}$; 5-HT$_{1B}$) High affinity D1 and ß adrenergic receptors
Lamina Granularis	5-HT NA	Nonjunctional terminals Low density	High affinity 5-HT receptors (5-HT$_{1A}$; 5-HT$_{1C}$)

FIG. 9. Summary of morphological observations supporting the VT mode of communication in the 5-HT, NE, and DA nerve terminal networks of the cerebellar cortex. It must be pointed out that in the granular layer there also exist low-affinity 5-HT$_2$ receptors inhibiting release of glutamate from the mossy fibers, suggesting a role of a synaptic transmission mode of communication in the 5-HT terminals innervating the glomeruli. Taken together, the morphological indications point to VT as a major mode of communication for monoamine systems within the cerebellar cortex.

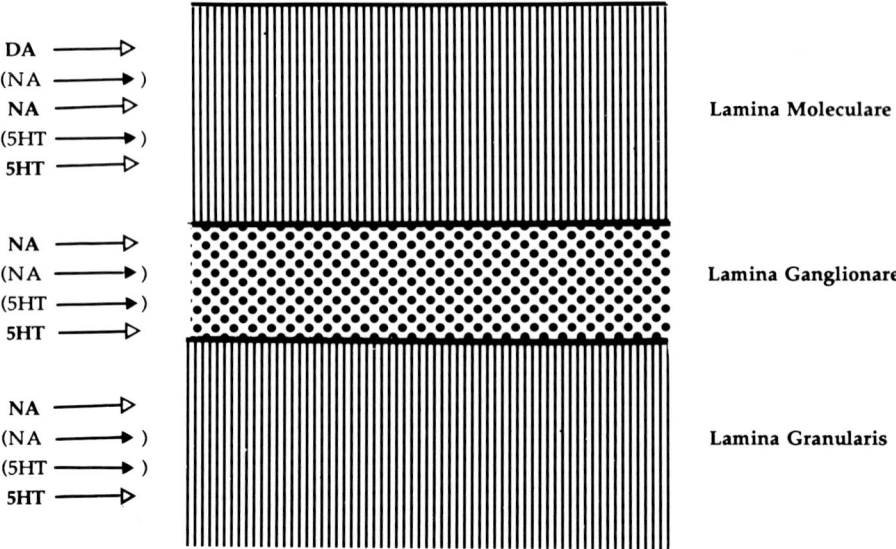

FIG. 10. Summary of the possible involvement of WT (→) (synaptic) and VT (-▷) modes of communication within the monoamine nerve terminal system of the cerebellar cortex. In all layers the major mode of communication seems to be VT. Therefore, the arrows for WT are in parentheses.

operate predominantly via the VT mode of communication to exert their biological actions (Figs. 9, 10, and 12). In support of this hypothesis double-immunolabeling experiments with DARPP-32 and 5-HT antisera have demonstrated the dramatic functional mismatch between the few 5-HT terminals and the large numbers of Purkinje cells with their rich dendritic plexa (Fig. 13). These results are most probably true also for the sparse plexa of dopamine (DA) nerve terminal networks (19) and norepinephrine (NE) nerve terminal networks in the cerebellar cortex (8,41, 51,68), since relatively few tyrosine hydroxylase (TH) IR nerve terminals, as demonstrated in double-immunolabeling procedures, are matched by a rich plexus of DARPP-32 IR Purkinje cell dendrites with no clear association of the CA nerve terminals with the cell bodies and dendrites (Fig. 14). The DA nerve terminals appear to operate via D_1 receptors, which have been demonstrated in the molecular layer (18,19), and the NE nerve terminals may mainly operate via β-adrenergic receptors (41), which, upon activation, can cause accumulation of cAMP within the Purkinje cells. With these high-affinity slow receptor systems coupled to G proteins and with a relatively low off rate, it seems possible for the diffusing DA and NE to induce modulatory actions on the Purkinje cell bodies and dendrites *inter alia*, especially since these monoamine receptor systems have a much lower off rate than the glutamate and gamma-aminobutyric acid (GABA) receptors, forming ion channels, allowing a prolonged modulation of the latter receptors. Again all the available observations support the view that the major mode of transmission involved is VT

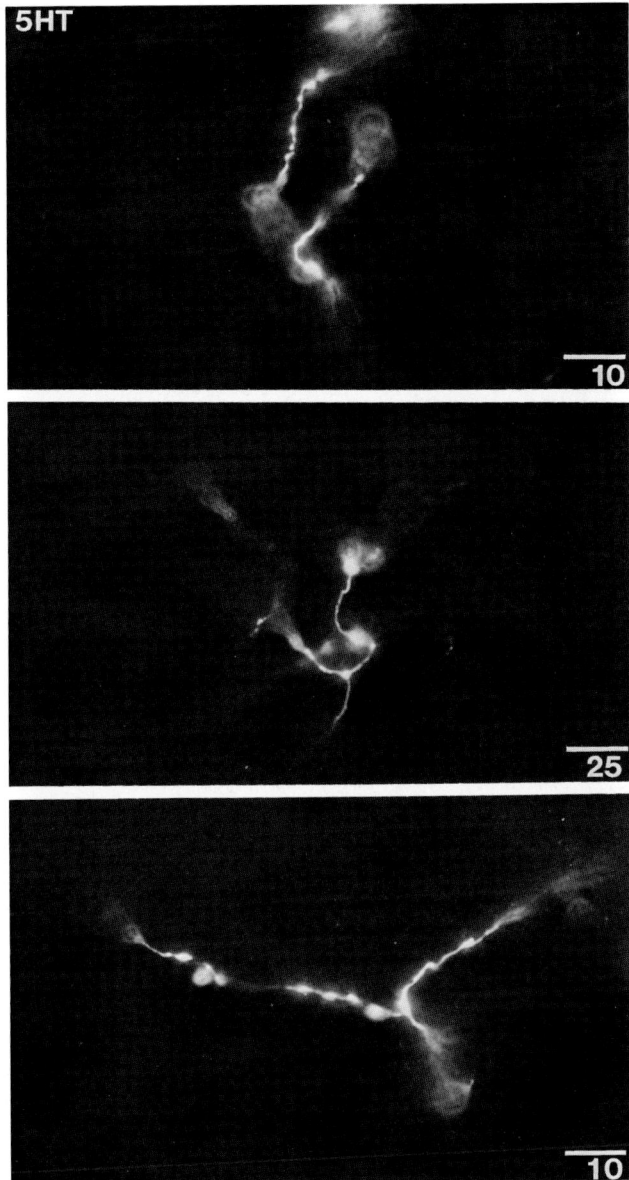

FIG. 11. 5-HT IR in the granular layer (see legend to Fig. 2). Details of the varicose 5-HT terminals in the granular layer are given. The variability of the size of the varicosities and of the intervaricose distance is illustrated.

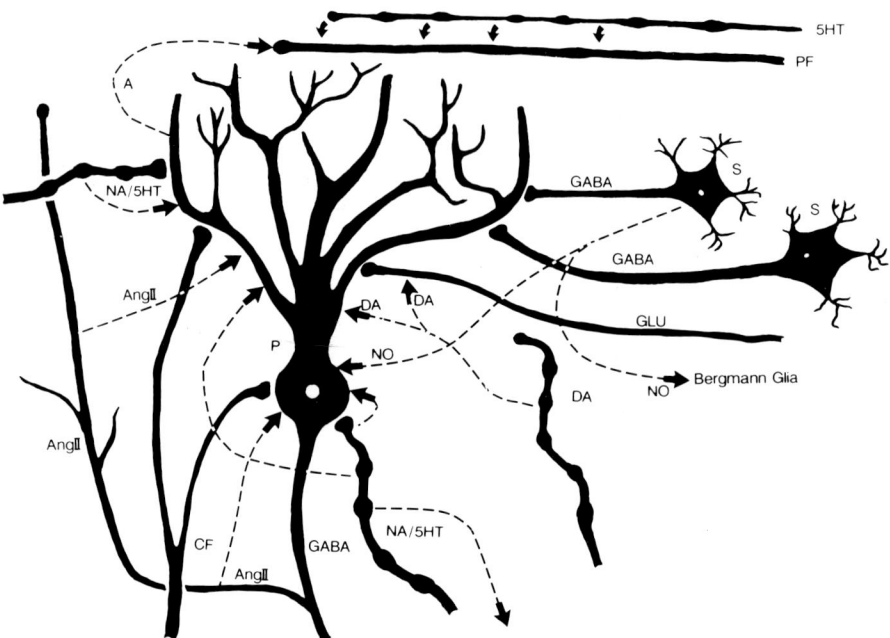

FIG. 12. Hypothesis of how Purkinje (P) cells can act as an integrator of WT and VT (- →) signals. The slow signals in VT are represented by monoamines and neuropeptides such as ANG peptides and adenosine (A). The rapid signals of VT are represented by nitric oxide (NO) arising, e.g., from stellate (S) GABA cells and activating guanylate cyclase in the Bergmann glia and Purkinje cells (33). The synaptic signals are represented by glutamate from parallel fibers (PF) and climbing fibers (CF) and by GABA from stellate cells.

for DA, NE, and 5-HT in the cerebellar cortex (Fig. 12). The Purkinje cell serves as an integrator of VT and WT signals.

When discussing the actions of 5-HT in relation to the cerebellar circuitry it should also be considered that the 5-HT nerve terminal networks act at multiple sites. Thus, at the afferent level they can control, for example, the activity in the climbing fibers by their innervation of the inferior olive as well (62), which is the major origin of the climbing fibers. It seems possible that the same 5-HT nerve cells may innervate both the inferior olive and cerebellar cortex (7). 5-HT nerve terminal networks can also regulate the efferent outflow from the cerebellum at the deep cerebellar nuclear level, probably by giving off collaterals from the ascending 5-HT axons to the cortex cerebelli. Finally, within the cerebellar cortex itself the 5-HT terminals appear to have the ability to directly influence the granular cells, parallel fibers, and Purkinje cells. Such multiple sites of action may act to strengthen the overall action of 5-HT on cerebellar function and may lead to the elicitation of a precise state of activity in the Purkinje cells and their associated nerve cells in the deep cerebellar nuclei.

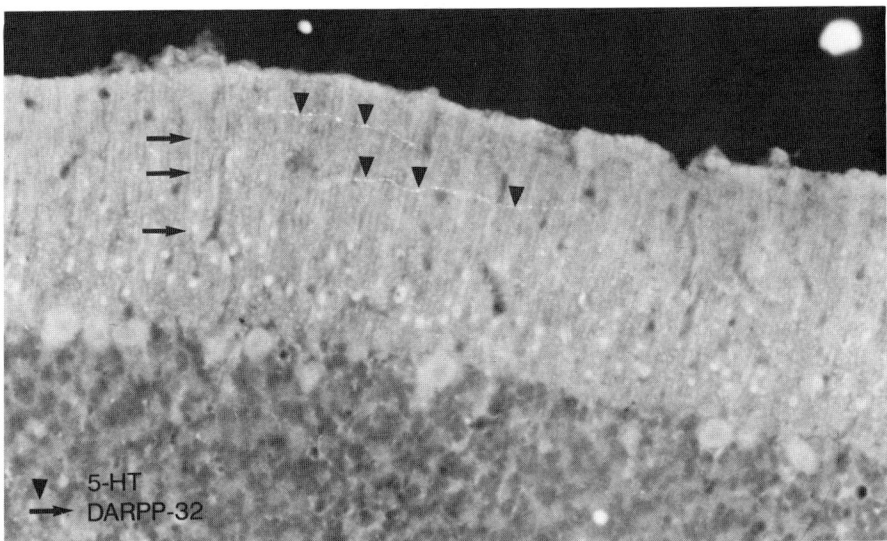

FIG. 13. DARPP-32 IR and 5-HT IR in the cerebellar cortex of the 2-month-old male rat. A coronal cryostate 14 μm thick section and a double-immunolabeling procedure were used. A monoclonal mouse DARPP-32 antiserum (1:500) and a rabbit 5-HT antiserum (1:400) were used (52). Biotinylated donkey antimouse IgG and FITC-conjugated sheep antirabbit IgG were used as secondary antibodies (Amersham 1:50 and 1:20, respectively). DARPP-32 IR was visualized by using streptavidin Texas red (1:100 Amersham). 5-HT IR nerve terminals are seen to run like parellel fibers within the molecular layer crossing the dendritic trees of a large number of Purkinje cells (dendritic trees are seen as lines in the transverse sections). 5-HT IR nerve terminals are few compared with the large numbers of Purkinje cells and their dendritic trees. No obvious associations are made with the Purkinje cell dendrites or soma.

PLASTICITY OF THE 5-HT DECODING SYSTEM

Recent evidence has indicated that interactions between receptors represent an important computational mechanism in the CNS (1,28,31). This interaction may take place at the intramembrane level with or without involvement of the G proteins (21,22), but could also involve second messenger cascades leading, for example, to altered phosphorylation of the receptors (36) (Fig. 15). We demonstrated earlier that [^{3}H]5-HT binding sites can be regulated by adjacent receptors, such as substance P (SP) receptors, in view of the ability of SP to reduce the affinity of 5-HT$_1$ binding sites (1,2). These results were obtained in biochemical experiments in membrane preparations, suggesting that an intramembrane interaction was involved. Thus, within the 5-HT terminals of the spinal cord it appears that SP receptors, probably belonging to the 5-HT/SP costoring terminal, upon activation can modulate the binding characteristics of adjacent 5-HT$_1$ receptors at the intrasynaptic level.

Other evidence suggests that galanin (GAL) receptors can be involved in controlling the 5-HT$_{1A}$ receptor subtype (29,59) (Fig. 16). Thus, using membrane preparations of the rat ventral limbic cortex GAL (10 nM) *in vitro* reduced the affinity of

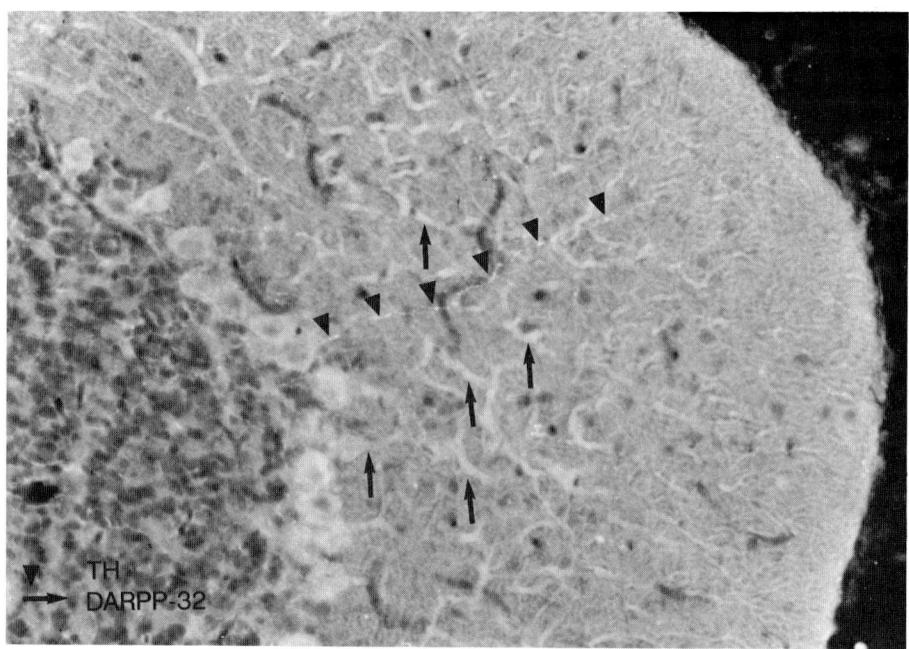

FIG. 14. DARPP-32 and TH IR in the cerebellar cortex of the 2-month-old male rat. Sagittal cryostate 14 μm thick sections and a mouse monoclonal DARPP-32 antiserum (1:500) and a rabbit TH antiserum (1:400) were used (46). Donkey antirabbit biotinylated IgG and sheep antimouse labeled IgG FITC (Amersham 1:50 and 1:20, respectively) were used as secondary antisera. Streptavidin Texas red (1:100) was used as a third compound. DARPP-32 IR is found exclusively within the Purkinje cell soma and dendrites. TH IR nerve terminals make no clear association with the dendritic tree of the Purkinje cells visualized from their contents of DARPP-32 IR.

the 5-HT_{1A} receptors by 40% using [^{3}H]8-hydroxy-2-(di-n-propylamino)tetralin ([^{3}H]8-OH-DPAT) as radioligand. It is of substantial interest that GAL could not affect the binding characteristics of 5-HT_2 nor 5-HT_{1B} receptors in this region. Thus, these results open up the possibility that GAL receptors, via a selective intramembrane interaction, can reduce the 5-HT_{1A} transmission line. This modulation has been shown also to take place in other areas including the raphe nuclei (40).

Histochemical analysis indicates that GAL IR terminals within the ventral limbic cortex are located independently of the 5-HT nerve terminals, and thus these results suggest that peptide receptors belonging to adjacent synapses but present on the same postsynaptic membrane can alter the 5-HT_{1A} receptors. It is of substantial interest that 8-OH-DPAT can in turn increase the affinity of [^{125}I]GAL binding sites, as studied both by quantitative receptor autoradiography and in membrane preparations (39,40). This increase in affinity by 8-OH-DPAT, that is, by 5-HT_{1A} receptor activation, appears to be G protein independent and could reflect an intramembrane reciprocal interaction between 5-HT_{1A} receptors and GAL receptors

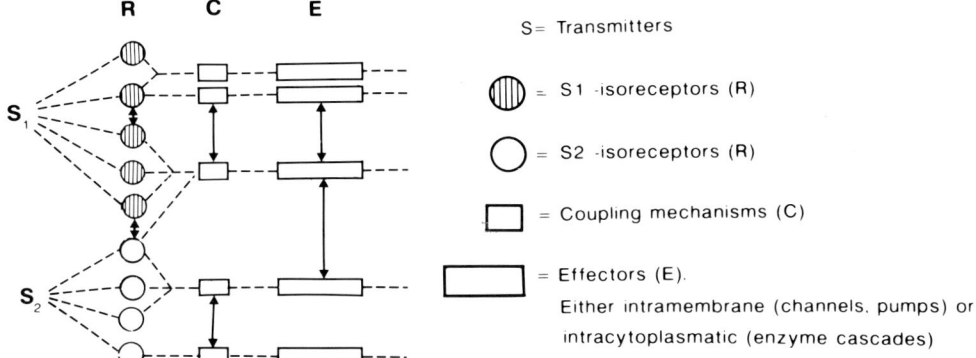

FIG. 15. Schematic overview of integrative mechanisms in the nerve cell membrane based on receptor-receptor interactions. Receptor-receptor interactions can take place at the receptor, G protein, and effector levels. The interactions can take place between isoreceptors (subtypes of receptors for the same transmitter) or receptor subtypes having different transmitters.

(Figs. 16 and 17). Thus, there may exist an intramembrane inhibitory feedback mechanism regulating 5-HT$_{1A}$ receptor transduction. It must be emphasized that the GAL receptor interacts exclusively with the 5-HT$_{1A}$ receptor subtype, suggesting that one reason for 5-HT receptor diversity is the need for selective interactions with adjacent receptor systems, such as the GAL receptors. Consequently, by activation of GAL receptors in some areas, it may become possible to produce a selective reduction of transduction at the 5-HT$_{1A}$ receptor subtype leading to a switch of

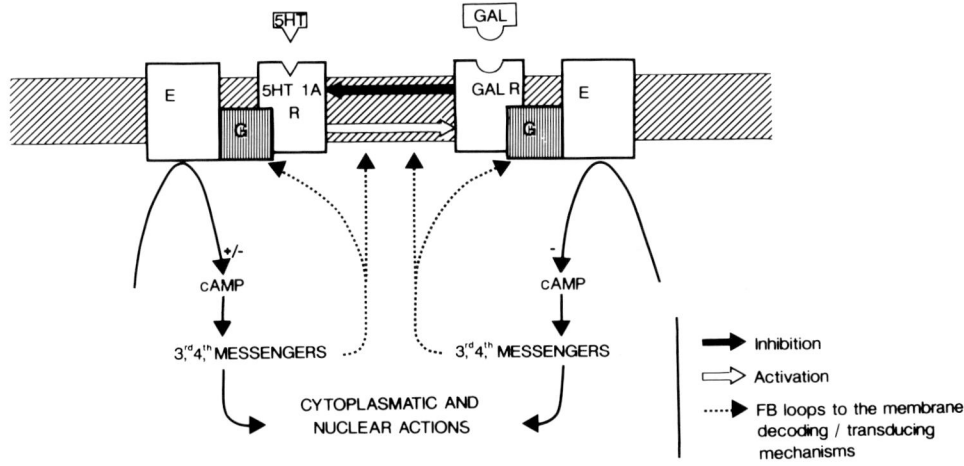

FIG. 16. 5-HT$_{1A}$/GAL receptor (R) interaction involving both intramembrane interactions and intracytoplasmic loops of second messengers that via, e.g., protein phosphorylation, may alter the decoding transduction mechanism of the adjacent receptor. FB, feedback loops; G, G protein; E, effector.

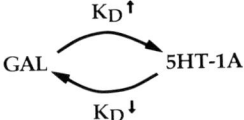

FIG. 17. A receptor can modulate and be modulated by another receptor. Bidirectional intramembrane interaction between 5-HT$_{1A}$ and GAL receptor, with the GAL receptor reducing the affinity of the 5-HT$_{1A}$ receptor (29) and the 5-HT$_{1A}$ receptors increasing the affinity of the GAL receptor (39).

5-HT transmission toward the other 5-HT receptor subtypes. This switch may be of particular relevance for VT, since the 5-HT$_{1A}$ receptor is a high-affinity receptor. Also, the increase in the affinity of GAL receptors produced by 8-OH-DPAT occurs not only in a number of tel- and diencephalic areas but in the 5-HT raphe nuclei and nucleus tractus solitarius as well, giving evidence that 5-HT$_{1A}$/GAL receptor interaction is a widespread phenomenon.

Recently we also obtained evidence for the existence of receptor-receptor interactions in the control of the 5-HT$_{1A}$ receptor binding characteristics in the cerebellum. Thus, as analyzed in cerebellar sections, NE in a concentration of 1 µM was found to substantially increase the binding at 5-HT$_{1A}$ receptors, suggesting that the activation of NE receptors may enhance the affinity of 5-HT$_{1A}$ receptors in the cerebellum (Fig. 18). The increased binding was demonstrated in both concentrations of 0.1 and 0.2 nM of [^{3}H]8-OH-DPAT. These results are the first indications that 5-HT$_{1A}$ receptors can be regulated by NE receptors, in this case belonging to the diffuse cerebellar NE innervation. Thus, NE and 5-HT may interact at the membrane level in the cerebellar cortex to synergistically inhibit Purkinje cell activity.

In our recent work we studied the plasticity of 5-HT and NE nerve terminal networks in response to neonatal and adult lesions as well as to neonatal corticosterone treatment.

PLASTICITY CHANGES IN THE 5-HT SYSTEMS AFTER NEONATAL 6-OHDA TREATMENT

As seen in Figs. 19 and 20 a 6-OHDA-induced (via a 50-µg i.c. injection) degeneration of CA nerve terminals on postnatal day 1 (45) led to inhibition of granular cell migration from the external layer into their adult position in the internal granular layer (43). This phenomenon was present independent of subsequent sprouting and regrowth of NE nerve terminals that took place in the cerebellar cortex after the lesion and led to a partial reinnervation of the islands of granular cells (Fig. 21). The formation of granular cell islands was a highly consistent finding demonstrated in all rats receiving 6-OHDA. It seems unlikely that the action was an unspecific toxic effect, since this inhibition of migration was predominantly demonstrated in certain lobules and deep within the fissures and thus far away from the fourth ventricle, into which 6-OHDA had been injected. It is of substantial interest that the islands, built of nonmigrating granular cells, became very strongly innervated by 5-HT nerve terminal networks and sprouting NE nerve terminals (Figs. 21 and 22). However, this reinnervation did not induce a migration of the abnormally located granular

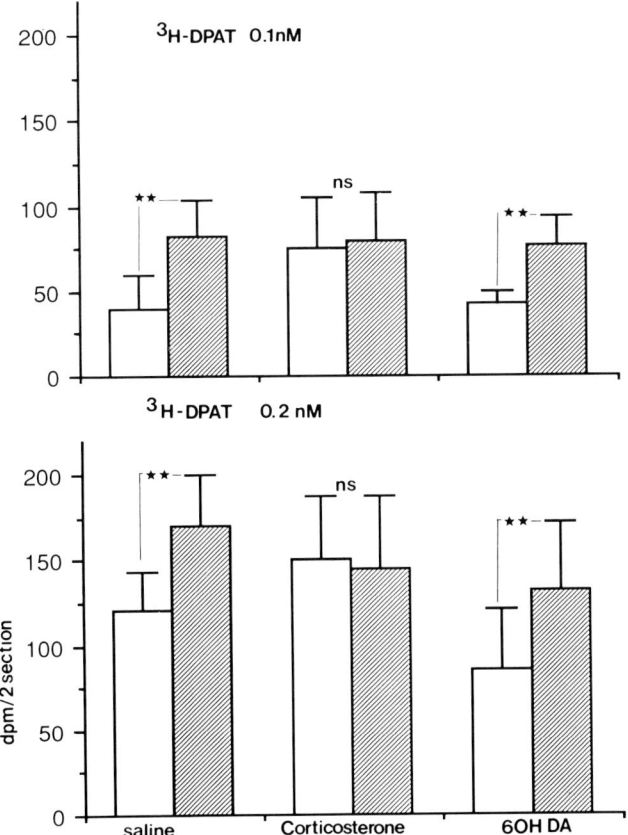

FIG. 18. Effects of NE on the binding of [^{3}H]8-OH-DPAT (specific activity 228 Ci/mmol) in transverse cerebellar rat sections in a pooled control group, a group treated with corticosterone neonatally (see text), and a group treated neonatally with 6-OH-DA (see legend to Fig. 26). The concentrations of [^{3}H]8-OH-DPAT used were 0.1 and 0.2 nM. The specific binding was defined as the binding in the presence of 8-OH-DPAT (1 μM). (For details on the binding procedure, see ref. 29.) NE was added in a concentration of 1 μM (▨). The radioactivity in two sections was determined by wiping the sections with filters followed by liquid scintillation spectroscopy. Means ± SEM are shown, $n = 7–8$ rats in the control group and 3–4 rats in the two experimental groups. Medium (□). Student's paired t test was used. **$p < 0.01$.

cells, indicating that the CA signal must be present at a critical time period in postnatal development in order for migration to take place.

These results also demonstrate that Purkinje cells are not essential for the innervation by 5-HT and NE terminals of the granular cells and may even inhibit their ingrowth, since hyperinnervation of the granular cell islands could be demonstrated (Figs. 21 and 22). The results underline an important role of 5-HT terminals in directly controlling granular cell activity. Corticosterone-releasing factor (CRF) IR mossy-like fibers were demonstrated in these islands of nonmigrated granular cells

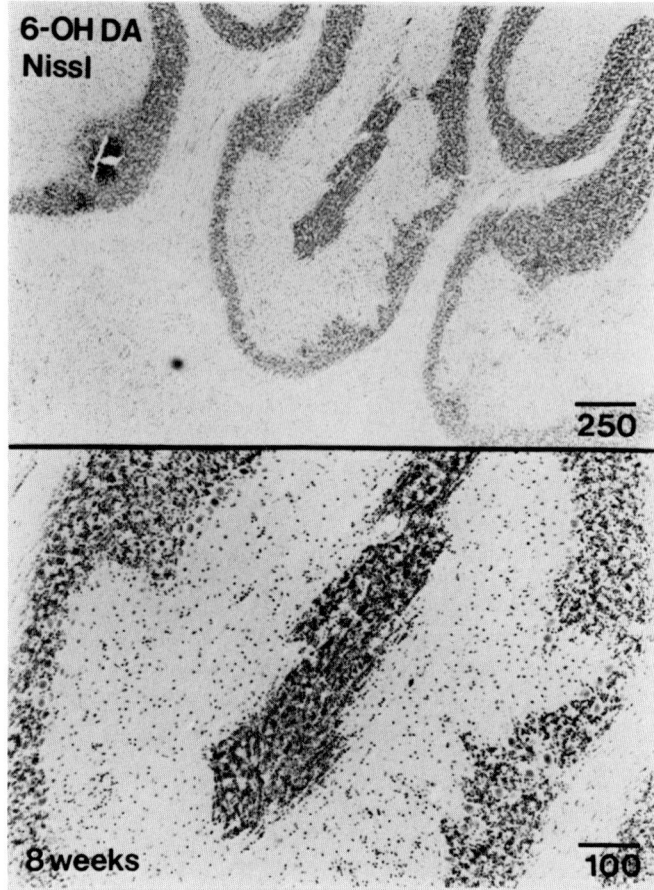

FIG. 19. Effects of neonatal i.c. 6-OHDA treatment (see legend to Fig. 26) on the nerve cell architecture within the cerebellar lobules in the 2-month-old male rat as revealed by Nissl staining (cresyl violet). Coronal cryostate sections (14 μm thick) were used. No association with Purkinje cells is demonstrated deep in several fissure islands of granular cells. These granular nerve cells have failed to migrate into the internal granular layer during postnatal development.

in a similar way, as observed in the adult granular layer. The islands of nonmigrated granular cells lacked DARPP-32 IR (Fig. 23), which was expected in view of the absence of Purkinje cell bodies and dendrites in these islands, as shown in Nissl stainings. Furthermore, DARPP-32 IR astroglia cells present within the internal granular layer of the adult type could not be demonstrated in these nonmigrated granular cell islands. With regard to glucocorticoid receptor (GR) IR within the granular cells of the islands, it was unaffected compared with the GR IR demonstrated in the granular cells of the adult granular layer. Of substantial interest, however, was the finding that the neonatal 6-OHDA treatment resulted in an increase in

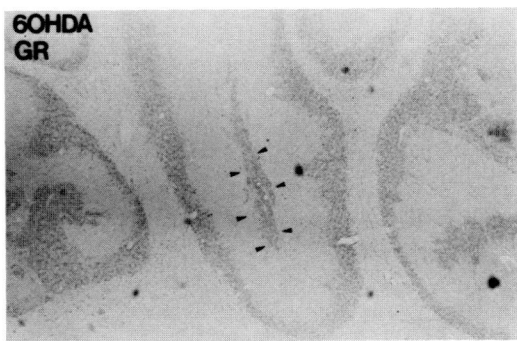
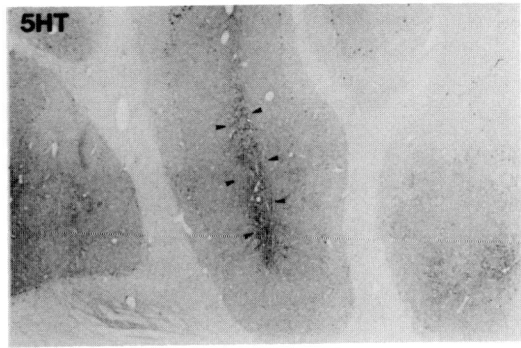
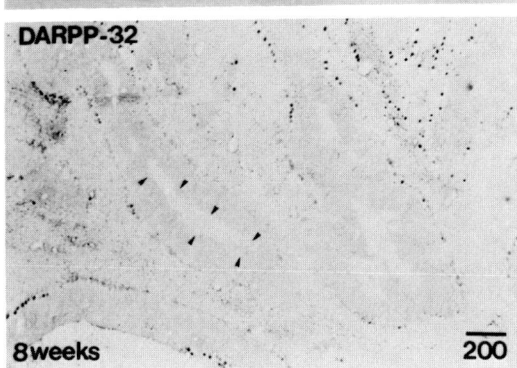

FIG. 20. Effects of neonatal intracisternal treatment with 6-OHDA on the GR IR, 5-HT IR, and DARPP-32 IR of the cerebellar cortex of the 2-month-old male rat. For details on 6-OHDA treatment, see legend to Fig. 26. Thin adjacent coronal cryostate sections (14 μm thick) were used. The primary antisera were diluted 1:750 (mouse antirat GR [50]), 1:1,000 (rabbit anti–5-HT), and 1:1,000 (monoclonal mouse anti–DARPP-32 antibody). The ABC technique was used with diaminobenzidine as a chromophore. The islands of granular cells (*arrowheads*) are shown to have unaltered GR IR, strongly increased 5-HT IR, and a lack of DARPP-32 IR.

the GR IR within all granular cells (Fig. 24). Thus, the CA nerve terminal networks in the postnatal period appear capable of regulating the degree of GR protein expressed in adulthood. Gene expression for GR, therefore, may be permanently altered by influencing the CA signal in the early postnatal period.

In the analysis of the granular islands, it was also noted that ornithine decarboxylase (ODC) IR fibers were completely absent. This is of considerable interest since the distribution of the ODC IR incoming fibers appears to be strictly linked to the axon hillock area of the Purkinje cells (Fig. 25). The fact that these ODC IR fibers

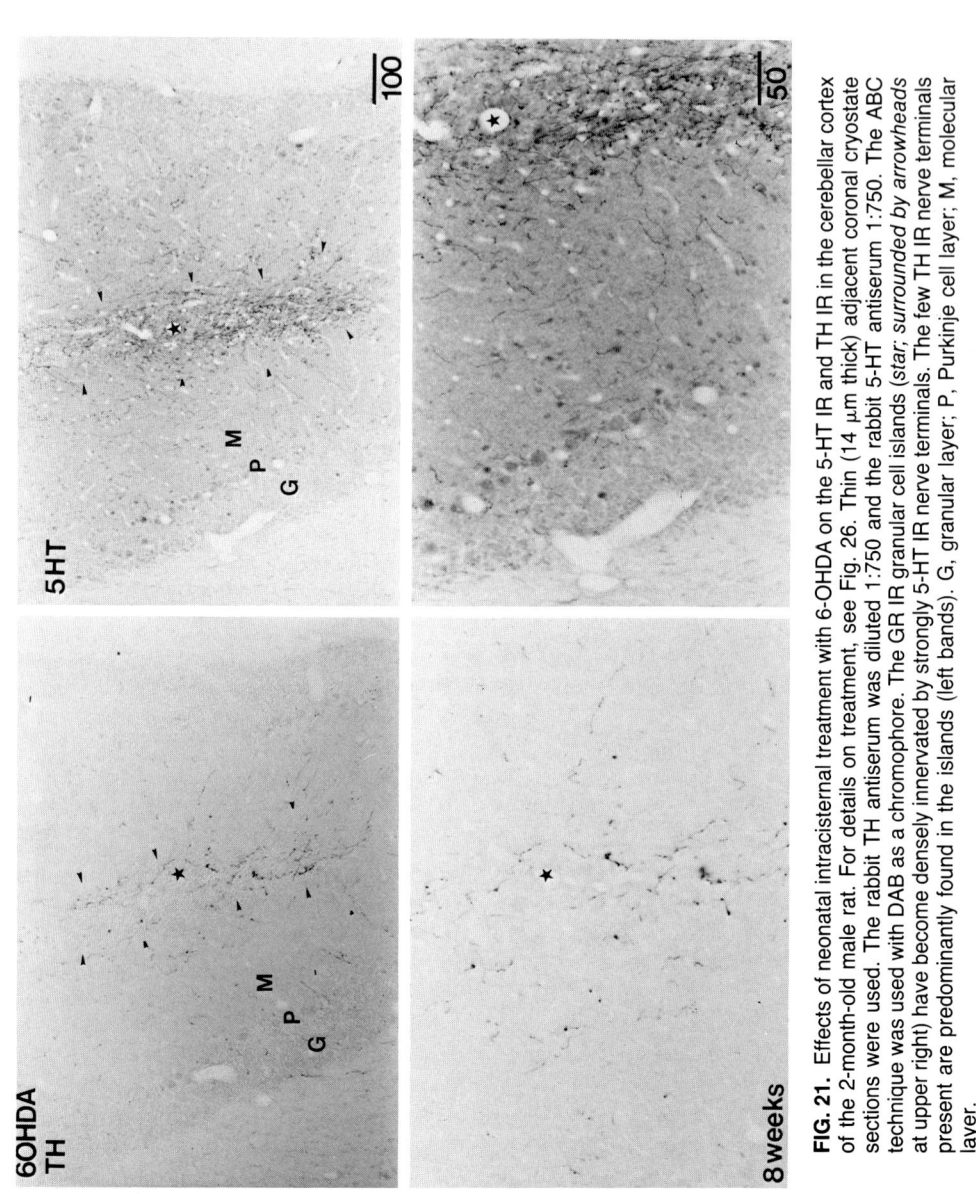

FIG. 21. Effects of neonatal intracisternal treatment with 6-OHDA on the 5-HT IR and TH IR in the cerebellar cortex of the 2-month-old male rat. For details on treatment, see Fig. 26. Thin (14 μm thick) adjacent coronal cryostate sections were used. The rabbit TH antiserum was diluted 1:750 and the rabbit 5-HT antiserum 1:750. The ABC technique was used with DAB as a chromophore. The GR IR granular cell islands (*star; surrounded by arrowheads at upper right*) have become densely innervated by strongly 5-HT IR nerve terminals. The few TH IR nerve terminals present are predominantly found in the islands (left bands). G, granular layer; P, Purkinje cell layer; M, molecular layer.

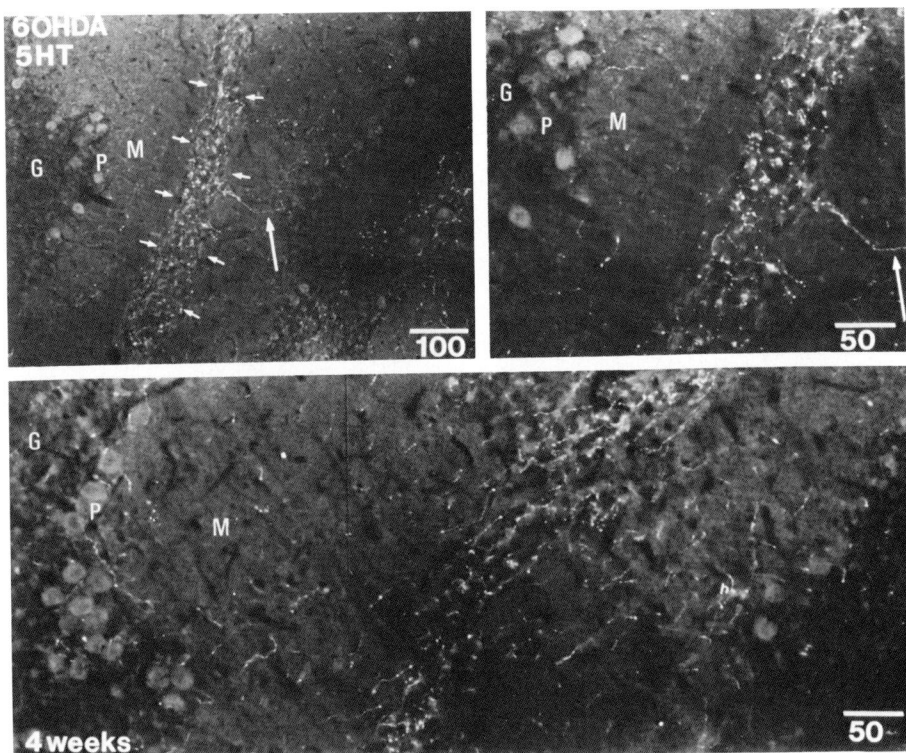

FIG. 22. Effects of neonatal intracisternal 6-OHDA treatment (see legend to Fig. 26) on 5-HT IR in the 4-week-old male rat, especially in relation to the islands of granular cells, which have failed to migrate into the internal granular layer. Coronal cryostate 14 μm thick sections were used. A rabbit 5-HT antiserum was used (1:400). Indirect immunofluorescence was used, involving as a secondary antibody a sheep antirabbit FITC conjugated IgG (1:20). The islands of granular cells that have failed to migrate are shown to have become hyperinnervated by strongly 5-HT IR nerve terminals. M, molecular layer; P, Purkinje cell layer; G, granular cell layer. *Small arrows* outline the cell island and *long arrow* points to incoming 5-HT terminals toward the island.

are absent within the islands of nonmigrated granular cells strongly underlines that this type of afference to the cerebellar cortex, which we have recently discovered, is truly linked to the Purkinje cells.

The biochemical studies demonstrated, in agreement with the histochemical analysis, a clear trend for an increase of 5-HT and 5-hydroxyindoleacetic acid (5-HIAA) levels in the cerebellar cortex, as evaluated 8 weeks later (Fig. 26), which is in line with the indications of sprouting of 5-HT terminal networks, as seen in the immunocytochemical analysis. The depletion of NE was significantly consistent with the presence of a reduced number of TH IR nerve terminals in the cerebellar cortex (Fig. 26). It was also found in the biochemical binding analysis that the [^{3}H]8-OH-DPAT binding (0.1 and 0.2 nM) was unaltered by the 6-OHDA treatment and that

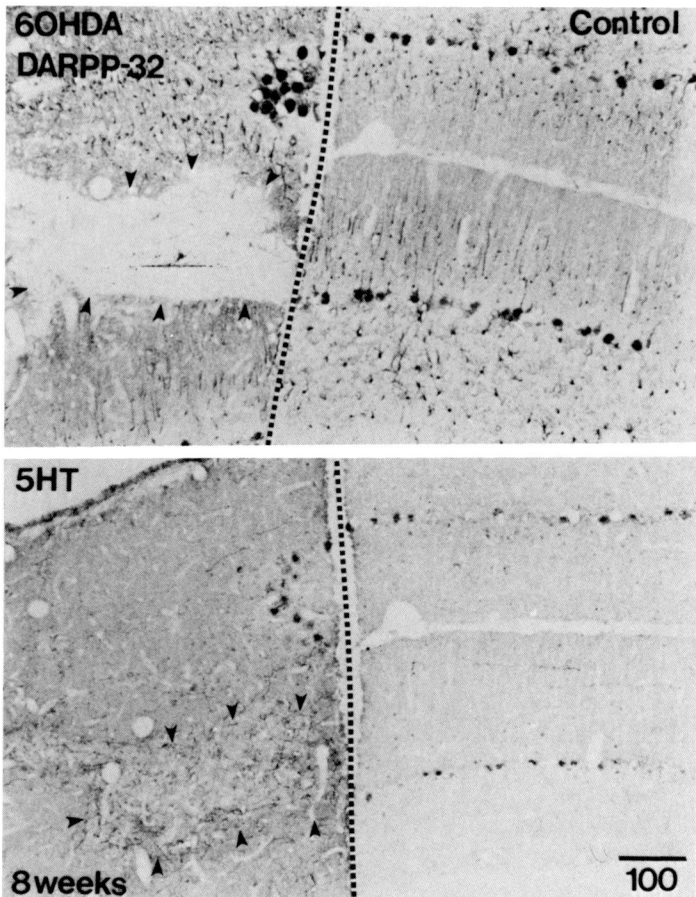

FIG. 23. DARPP-32 IR and 5-HT IR in adjacent coronal cryostate sections (14 μm thick) of the cerebellar cortex of control rats and rats after neonatal 6-OHDA treatment (see text), as analyzed in the 2-month-old male rat. The mouse monoclonal DARPP-32 antibody was diluted 1:3,000 and the rabbit 5-HT antiserum 1:1,000. The ABC technique was used. As secondary antisera donkey antimouse and goat antirabbit biotinylated IgGs (Vector) were used, diluted 1:200. Avidin and biotinylated peroxidase were used in a 1:100 dilution. The islands of granular cells are indicated by *arrowheads*. These islands are shown to lack DARPP-32 IR and to contain high densities of 5-HT IR nerve terminals. Corresponding control sections are shown in the right panels.

the NE could activate [^{3}H]8-OH-DPAT binding in a way similar to that in control rats (Fig. 18). Thus, this modulation by NE of [^{3}H]8-OH-DPAT binding was not clearly enhanced in spite of the presence of upregulated β-adrenergic receptors within the molecular layer in response to the CA denervation of the cerebellum (Fig. 27).

Taken together this analysis suggests that, in agreement with previous work (43),

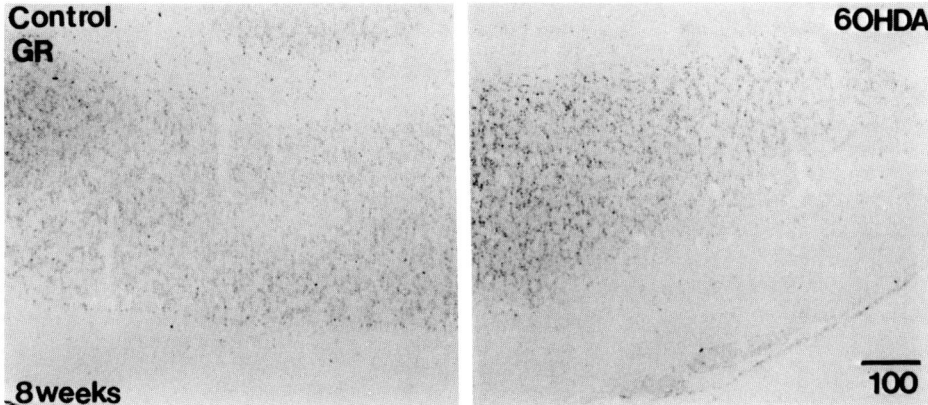

FIG. 24. Effects of neonatal intracisternal treatment with 6-OHDA on the GR IR in the granular layer of the cerebellar cortex of the 2-month-old male rat. The mouse monoclonal GR antibody (50) was diluted 1:750. The ABC technique was used, using DAB as a fluorophore. The neonatal 6-OHDA treatment produced an increase in the GR IR of the granular layer.

islands of nonmigrated granular cells exist in adulthood following 6-OHDA neonatal treatment. These islands maintain their position despite a collateral regrowth phenomenon in CA nerve terminals involving the entire cerebellar cortex, including a strong reinnervation of the granular cell islands. Thus, the results suggest that a possible absence of CA at a critical moment in the postnatal period will lead to a permanent failure of migration of the granular cells to their adult position. It should be mentioned that there exist indications for high densities of 5-HT_{1A} receptors, especially in the cerebellum, in the postnatal period, suggesting that 5-HT nerve terminal networks also are involved in the maturation of the cerebellar cortex (17,58). Demonstration of hyperinnervation of the granular cell islands by 5-HT nerve terminals in the absence of surrounding Golgi and Purkinje cells gives clear evidence for direct regulation also by 5-HT nerve terminals of granular cell activity (see Fig. 28).

PLASTICITY CHANGES IN THE CEREBELLAR 5-HT SYSTEM AFTER NEONATAL CORTICOSTERONE TREATMENT

Neonatal corticosterone treatment, as described by Agnati and colleagues (69), with 10 mg/kg injections on postnatal days 2, 4, 6, and 8 led to a transient reduction of TH IR terminals within various regions of the cerebellar cortex, as evaluated at the 4-week time interval. However, at the 8-week time interval, the densities of TH IR terminals appeared unchanged and no changes in cerebellar NE levels could be demonstrated, as determined biochemically (Fig. 26). Also, no clear alterations in GR IR existed within the granular cells of the cerebellar cortex upon neonatal corticosterone treatment, as evaluated 8 weeks later. The 5-HT IR nerve terminal net-

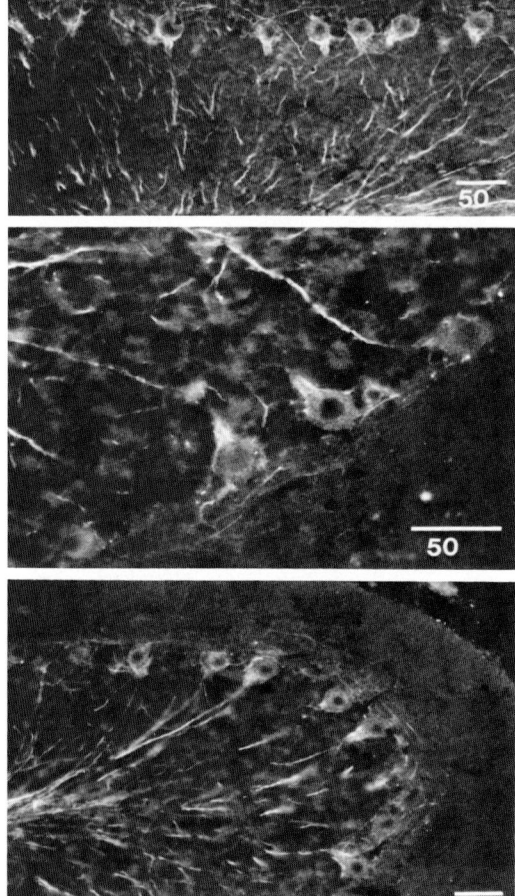

FIG. 25. ODC IR in a transverse 14 μm thick cryostate section of the cerebellar cortex of the 2-month-old male rat. The rabbit ODC antiserum (54) was diluted 1:500. Indirect immunofluorescence was used, involving as a secondary antibody a sheep antirabbit FITC conjugated IgG (1:30). The ODC IR fibers are shown to leave the medulla of the cerebellar cortex to almost exclusively innervate the axon hillock area of the Purkinje cells.

works were unaltered at both 4 and 8 weeks following neonatal corticosterone treatment.

The [^{3}H]8-OH-DPAT binding was not significantly altered by neonatal corticosterone treatment (Fig. 18). Instead, the major change induced by neonatal corticosterone treatment was the putative absence of interactions between the NE and 5-HT$_{1A}$ receptors, as seen in adulthood upon neonatal corticosterone treatment (Fig. 18). Thus, the increase in [^{3}H]8-OH-DPAT binding seen after NE incubation appeared to be absent in the animals treated neonatally with corticosterone. These

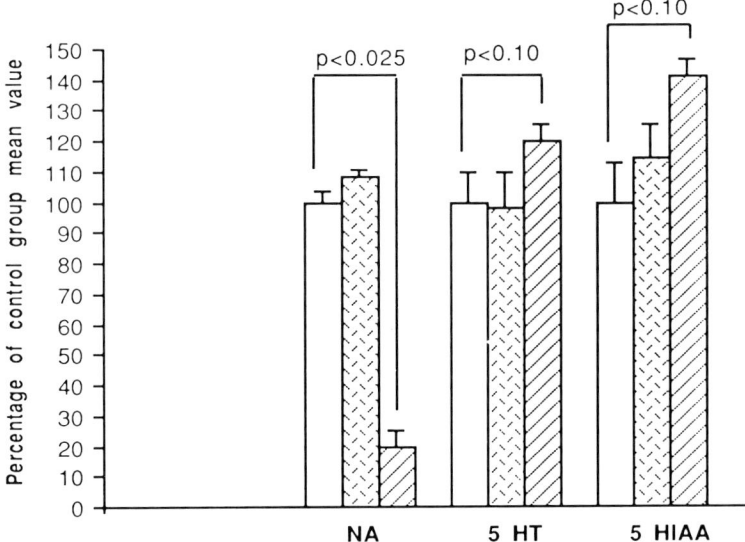

FIG. 26. Effects of neonatal corticosterone treatment and neonatal 6-OHDA treatment on the cerebellar NE 5-HT and 5-HIAA levels in the 2-month-old male rat. For treatment with neonatal corticosterone (▨), see text. The 6-OHDA treatment (▨) was performed on postnatal day 1 with an intracisternal injection of 50 μg/10 μl. Means ± SEM are shown in percentage of the respective control group (□) mean value; the common control group ($n = 8$) and the two other groups ($n = 4$). The absolute levels in the control group were, for NE, 330 ± 12; for 5-HT, 130 ± 16, and for 5-HIAA, 170 ± 16 nmol/g wet weight. Comparisons were made with respective control groups using Student's t test in combination with Bonferronis correction.

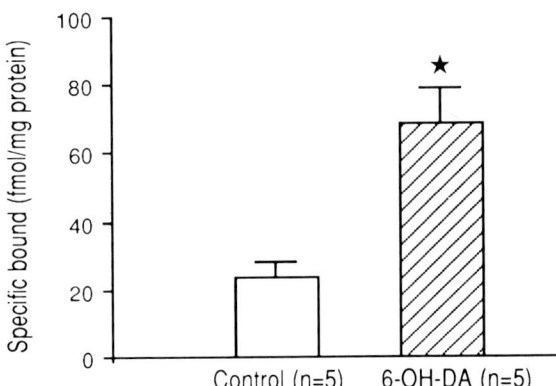

FIG. 27. Effects of postnatal treatment with 6-OHDA on the β-adrenergic antagonist binding in the cerebellar cortex of the 2-month-old male rat. For details of the 6-OHDA treatment, see legend to Fig. 26. As a radioligand was used the unselective β-adrenergic antagonist [^{125}I]-iodopindolol in a concentration of 2 nM. Quantitative receptor autoradiography was used. Unspecific binding was defined as the binding in the presence of 0.1 mM of L-NE. Binding was analyzed in the cerebellar lobules 5–6 as evaluated in sagittal sections. Means ± SEM are shown ($n = 5$). Statistical analysis was performed according to Student's t test. *$p < 0.05$.

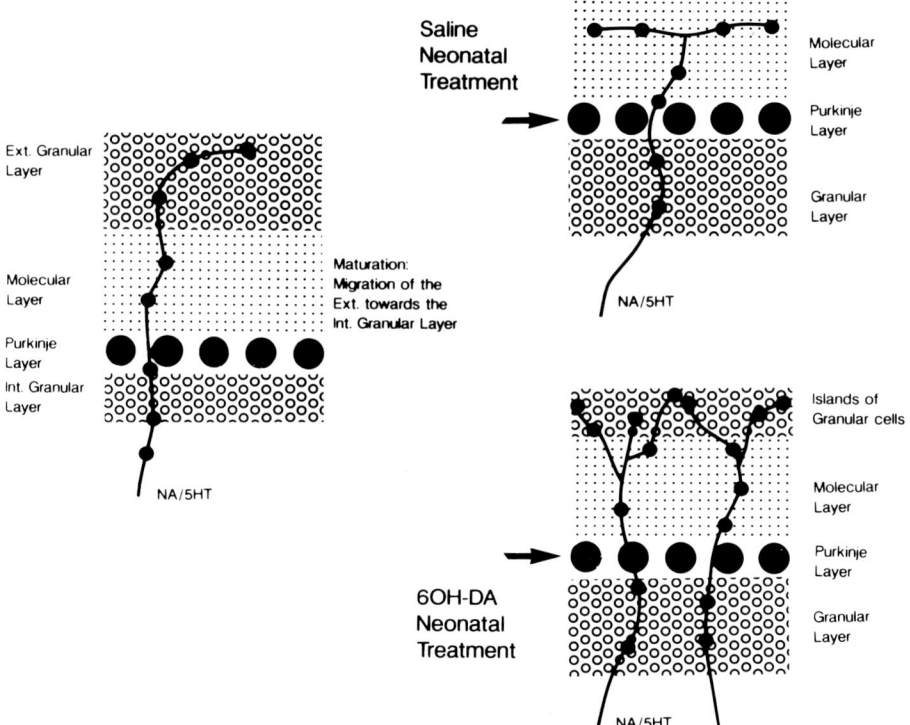

FIG. 28. Major morphological alterations demonstrated in this chapter within the cerebellar cortex upon neonatal 6-OHDA treatment. For details on the 6-OHDA treatment, see legend of Fig. 26. It is demonstrated that the 6-OHDA treatment neonatally leads to a blockade of the migration of the granular cells in the external granular layer to the internal granular layer. In the 2-month-old male rat this reduction of migration of external granular cells is associated with the presence of an increased number and intensity of 5-HT IR nerve terminals. Also the remaining NE nerve terminals are capable of remodeling, as shown by their ability to grow into these islands of granular cells and give rise to an increased density of NE nerve terminals compared to those found in the internal granular layer, where a highly reduced number of NE terminals is present compared with controls not treated with 6-OHDA.

results open up the possibility that stress, due to glucocorticoids in the postnatal period, may influence the development of appropriate interactions between receptor systems, in this case the NE and 5-HT$_{1A}$ receptors within the cerebellar cortex. It remains to be determined which NE receptor subtype is involved in this interaction. Such interactions will lead to altered information handling. Thus, stress in the neonatal period could lead to alterations in the learning of motor skills as well as the elaboration of other complex brain functions due to the demonstrated altered information handling within the cerebellar cortex and possibly other brain areas.

PLASTIC CHANGES IN THE 5-HT CEREBELLAR SYSTEM AFTER LOCAL ISCHEMIA INDUCED BY INTRACEREBELLAR MICROINJECTIONS OF ET-1

ET-1 (1 μg/0.5 μl) microinjected into a brain area leads to the loss of nerve and glial cells in the injected area due to probable ischemia, as demonstrated by Nissl staining and GFAP immunocytochemistry (Fig. 29) (30,31). As in the case of neonatal lesions with 6-OHDA, marked compensatory responses in terms of sprouting were demonstrated in the 5-HT nerve terminal networks, which also became strongly 5-HT IR (Fig. 30), even in areas far away from the lesion. Hyperinnervations by 5-HT terminals could be demonstrated, especially within the granular cells close to the lesioned area and often lacking association with Purkinje cells. Sprouting responses were also seen in the surrounding NE nerve terminal networks but to a

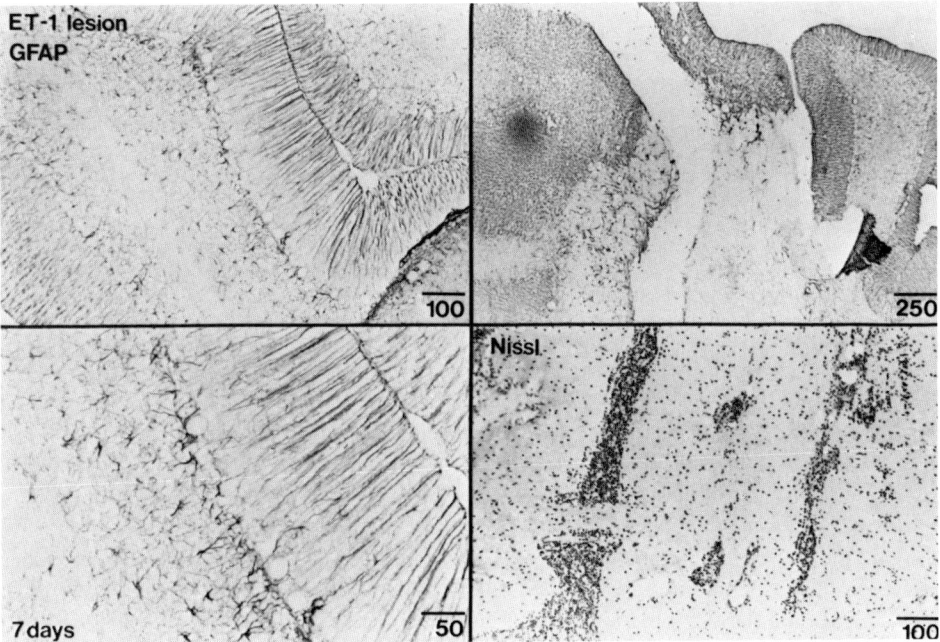

FIG. 29. Effects of ET-1-induced lesions within the vermis of the cerebellar cortex on GFAP IR and Nissl staining (cresyl violet) as evaluated in the male rat 7 days after an intracerebellar injection of ET-1 (1 μg/0.5 μl). For details, see refs. 30,32. The size of the lesion is on the order of 2 to 3 mm³. In the *upper right panel*, the size of the lesion can be evaluated from the absence of GFAP IR within the lesioned area. In the *lower right panel*, Nissl staining demonstrates strands of granular cells within the lesioned region, but the Purkinje cells have disappeared. The strands of granular cells located close to the lesion have become strongly hyperinnervated by 5-HT nerve terminal networks (see Fig. 30). In the *left panels*, a normal architecture of GFAP IR Bergmann glia and astrocytes in the granular layer is demonstrated in areas close to the lesion.

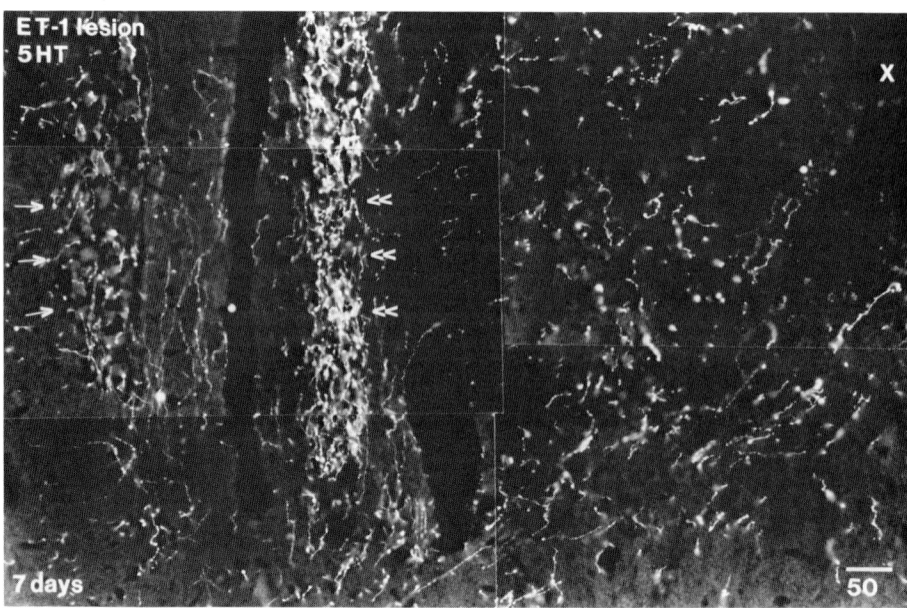

FIG. 30. Effects of ET-1-induced lesions in the cerebellar cortex on the 5-HT IR nerve terminal networks as evaluated 7 days after an intracerebellar injection of ET-1 (1 μg/0.5 μl) into the vermis using 5-HT immunocytochemistry. The lesion was on the order of 2–3 mm^3. Coronal cryostate 14 μm thick sections were used. Indirect immunofluorescence was used, involving as a secondary antibody a sheep antirabbit FITC conjugated IgG (1:20). The primary rabbit 5-HT antiserum was diluted 1:400. Strong 5-HT IR networks are seen close to the lesion area (X). Remaining granular cells in the lesioned area have become densely innervated by sprouting 5-HT nerve terminals (*arrowheads*), also having a strong fluorescent intensity, while granular cells further away from the lesion are less innervated by 5-HT terminals.

lesser degree. These results indicate that the diffuse 5-HT nerve terminal networks on lesions in the cerebellum could represent an important repair response by which the released 5-HT could act to counteract glutamate excitation on Purkinje cells close to the lesion (44). In this way malfunction in Purkinje cells could become silent and no longer disturb the flow of information from the deep cerebellar nuclei to brain areas. This action of 5-HT could also involve inhibition of glutamate release from the parallel fibers and inhibition of granular cell activity, in view of the dense 5-HT innervation by sprouting 5-HT terminals of the granular layer. Via this mechanism it would also be possible to postulate an increased survival of the Purkinje cells in the area surrounding the lesion, since fewer energy demands would be required in view of their inhibition by 5-HT. The surrounding NE nerve terminal networks could also enhance the action of 5-HT by increasing the affinity of the 5-HT$_{1A}$ receptors (besides their ability to inhibit Purkinje cells themselves) (41). Thus, plasticity responses in 5-HT afferents could be an important feature in the damaged cerebellum and probably involve not only regrowth phenomena but also increased 5-HT stores, both of which both will result in an increased diffusion of 5-HT toward distant high-affinity 5-HT_1 receptors. Thus, successful compensation responses may be elicited in the cerebellar 5-HT pathways to the cerebellum via increasing VT in the 5-HT systems, *inter alia*. The ability of L-5-hydroxytryptophan (L-5-HTP) treatment to improve cerebellar ataxias (64) may be related to its ability to enhance this endogenous mechanism that inhibits the exaggerated firing of the Purkinje cells in the lesioned regions. A new type of drug for the treatment of cerebellar ataxias may be indolpyruvate, which has been shown to increase 5-HT transmission in various brain areas, provided tryptophan-hydroxylase activity is intact in the cerebellum (57). This compound has also been shown to mimic the actions of 5-HT on food intake, corticosterone secretion, and the sleep/wakefulness cycle (57).

RESPONSES IN BASIC FIBROBLAST GROWTH FACTOR IR AND IN THE RENIN-ANGIOTENSIN SYSTEM

Recently it has been possible to demonstrate basic fibroblast growth factor (bFGF) IR within the DA neurons of the midbrain (13). This analysis has been continued and recent results indicate the existence of costorage of bFGF IR within the 5-HT perikarya of the nucleus raphe dorsalis. bFGF may therefore be a significant growth factor also within at least some of the 5-HT nerve cell systems. Also bFGF IR was recently demonstrated within the locus coeruleus, indicating that the bFGF may be a significant growth factor for both DA, NE, and 5-HT neurons. Large nerve cells in the deep cerebellar nuclei show that a strong bFGF IR and a weak bFGF IR exist in the Purkinje cells (Fig. 31). The Purkinje cells close to the ET-1 lesion react by forming increased amounts of bFGF IR, but no clear-cut increases of bFGF IR were demonstrated in the 5-HT nerve cells of the raphe nuclei.

Renin IR, but no angiotensinogen IR, exists in the Purkinje cells, which is exclusively located in the astroglia and especially the Bergmann glia surrounding the Purkinje cells (9,27). Angiotensin II (ANG II) IR is exclusively present in nerve terminals of the granular layer and especially of the Purkinje cell layer with fine varicose ANG II IR fibers ascending perpendicularly toward the surface of the molecular layer (Figs. 32 and 33). Their distribution pattern is thus entirely different from that of the 5-HT and CA terminals (Figs. 32 and 33). The ANG II IR terminals may belong to and represent collaterals of Purkinje and/or Golgi nerve cells.

ANG II IR is increased within these terminals surrounding the ET-1-induced lesion. Of substantial interest is that angiotensinogen IR appears in the Purkinje cell bodies close to the lesion, which may reflect an increased uptake of angiotensinogen released from the surrounding angiotensinogen-positive Bergmann glia cells. In view of the existence of renin IR in Purkinje cells, such a transport phenomenon may lead to an enhancement of ANG II synthesis within the Purkinje cells and thus increased release of ANG II. This interpretation of the results again underlines the importance of VT in plasticity responses, in this case within the renin-angiotensin

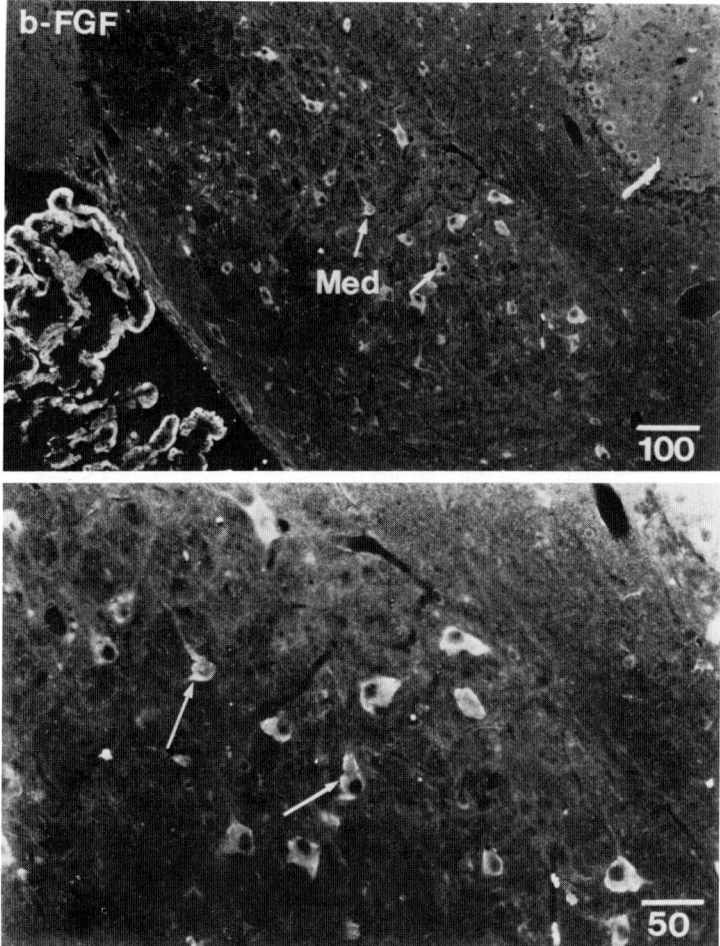

FIG. 31. Basic FGF-like IR is demonstrated in large nerve cells of the medial cerebellar nucleus in a coronal section from the 2-month-old male rat. The bFGF antiserum (courtesy of Dr. A. Baird) was used in a 1:500 concentration. As a secondary antibody, a sheep antirabbit FITC conjugated IgG (1:30) was employed. *Arrows* point to some examples of strongly bFGF IR nerve cell bodies in the medial cerebellar nucleus, and in most of these nerve cells, the bFGF IR is predominantly located in the cytoplasmic zone close to the nerve cell membrane. Only a weak bFGF IR is observed in the Purkinje cells, while a strong bFGF IR is present within the choroidal plexus.

system of the cerebellar cortex, and may indicate also a role of angiotensin peptides in the responses of the cerebellar cortex to lesions.

It is of special interest that the angiotensin peptides released may diffuse to reach the high-affinity ANG II receptors of the molecular layer, where they are probably located on the Purkinje cells (34,49). ANG II has been shown to depress Purkinje cell firing and to enhance the inhibitory actions of GABA (63). ANG II and 5-HT_{1A}

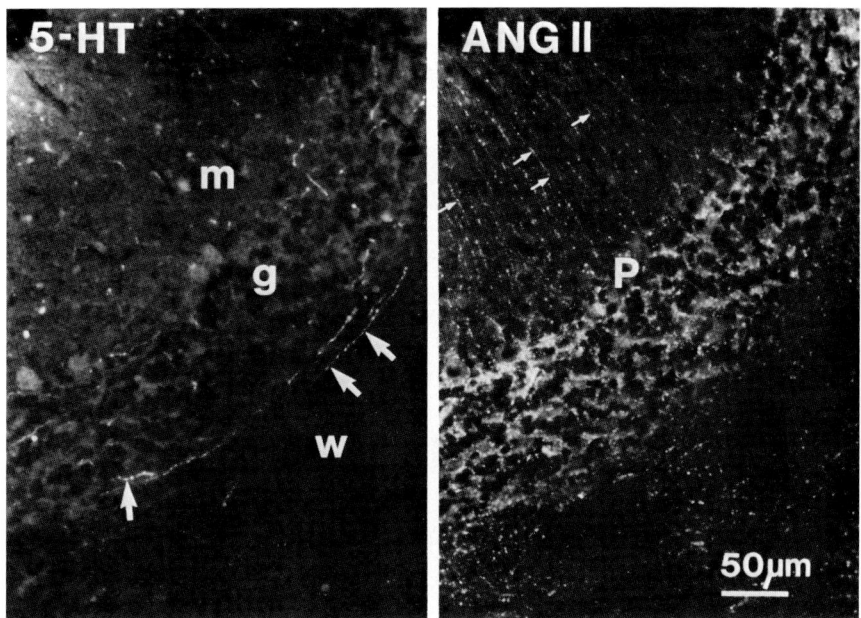

FIG. 32. 5-HT and ANG II IR in coronal cryostate 14 μm thick sections of the cerebellar cortex of the 2-month-old male rat. A double-immunolabeling procedure was used (see legend to Fig. 33). The rabbit 5-HT antiserum was diluted 1:400. The ANG II IR terminals are much more abundant than the 5-HT IR terminals, with no indications of coexistence as evaluated on the same section. ANG II IR is predominantly found in the Purkinje cell layer (P) with single varicose terminals sent regularly into the molecular layer (m). w, white matter of the folium; g, granular cell layer.

receptors may therefore act synergistically to inhibit Purkinje cell firing and thus possibly increase Purkinje cell survival and reduce the impact of dysfunctioning Purkinje cells on the deep cerebellar nuclei. Angiotensin peptides in the cerebellum could therefore be helpful in improving cerebellar ataxias, perhaps being released from recurrent collaterals of the Purkinje cells and acting in concert with the monoamine systems.

SUMMARY

These results provide morphological observations favoring the idea that VT is the major mode of transmission for the 5-HT, NE, and DA nerve terminal networks in the cerebellum (Fig. 12). These systems appear to operate via high-affinity, slow G protein-coupled receptors (5-HT_1 type) that can decode the VT signal in the extracellular fluid pathways of the cerebellar cortex and nuclei. There is little evidence for the existence of classical synapses (junctional 5-HT varicosities). These results emphasize a role of receptor-receptor interactions in the regulation of 5-HT_{1A} receptors within the cerebellar cortex. Thus, it has for the first time been demonstrated

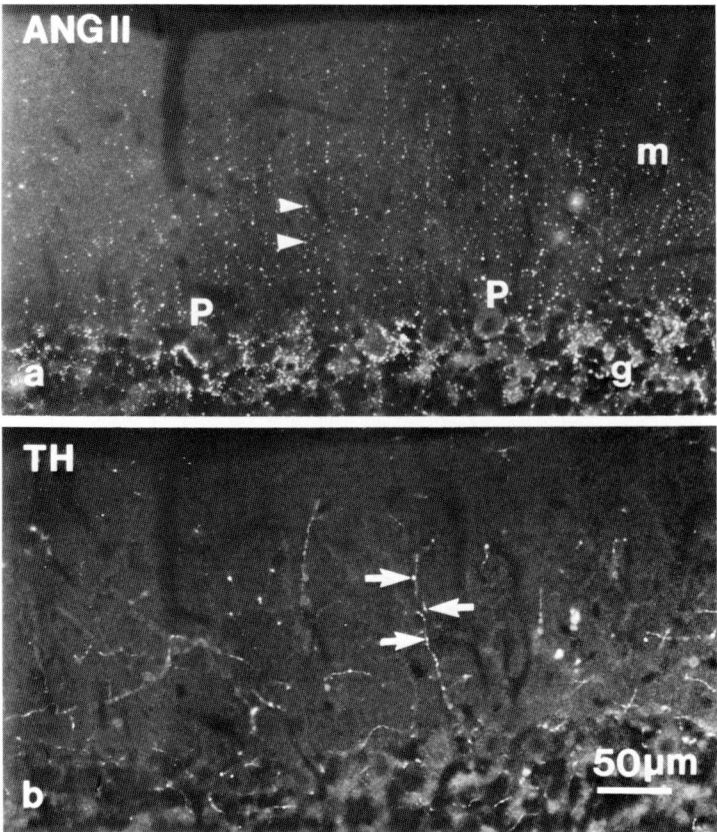

FIG. 33. ANG II IR (**a**) and TH IR (**b**) in the cerebellar cortex of the 2-month-old male rat. Double-immunolabeling procedure was used, involving a mouse monoclonal ANG II antibody (courtesy of Dr. D. Ganten) (1:750 dilution) together with a rabbit TH antiserum (1:750). As secondary antisera, a biotinylated donkey antirabbit IgG and a sheep antimouse FITC conjugated IgG (1:50 and 1:20, respectively, Amersham) were used. The ANG II IR was visualized using streptavidin Texas red (1:100). The angiotensin IR nerve terminals are much more abundant than the TH IR terminals (*arrows*), and there is no evidence for coexistence as evaluated in the same section. ANG II IR terminals predominantly innervate the Purkinje cell layer, but single fine varicose fibers are frequently sent at regular intervals perpendicularly across the molecular layer toward the surface (*arrowheads*). P, Purkinje cell layer; m, molecular layer; g, granular cell layer.

that NE receptors, upon activation, may increase the affinity of 5-HT$_{1A}$ receptors in the cerebellar cortex. Evidence has also been obtained in experiments with neonatal 6-OHDA treatment and with ET-1-induced cerebellar lesions in adulthood that 5-HT nerve terminal networks in the cerebellar cortex undergo highly plastic changes following such lesions. Thus, evidence has been provided for increased 5-HT content within the terminals as well as increases in its density after lesions. The outcome of these plastic responses will be greatly facilitated by the VT mode of communication for 5-HT, which will allow 5-HT to reach distant high-affinity 5-HT receptors regulating the fast receptors of synaptic transmission, i.e., the various glutamate and GABA receptors. We hypothesize that these plastic responses in 5-HT networks may be essential for repair mechanisms by, for example, allowing appropriate inhibition of surrounding dysfunctioning Purkinje cells close to a lesion, which probably are activated by excessive glutamate release from an activated parallel fiber system. It is proposed that the beneficial actions of L-5-HTP treatment of cerebellar ataxias may be related to its enhancement of the endogenous compensatory responses in 5-HT nerve terminal networks, the L-5-HTP being converted to 5-HT in the monoamine neurons and then released to diffuse via VT to reach the 5-HT receptors. In this way pathologically firing Purkinje cells can be inhibited, so that the output from the deep cerebellar nuclei is normalized and nerve cell survival may be increased. Indolpyruvate, by enhancing 5-HT synthesis and release in the brain, may possibly also have a beneficial role in the treatment of cerebellar ataxias. Based on the lesion-induced increases of cerebellar ANG II IR, it is postulated that increased levels and release of ANG peptides from recurrent collaterals of Purkinje cells may act synergistically with 5-HT in cerebellar pathology in view of their ability to, *inter alia*, depress Purkinje cell activity. On the basis of the indirect evidence for VT in the cerebellar cortex, the hypothesis is put forth that the Purkinje cell may act as an integrator of WT and VT signals.

ACKNOWLEDGMENT

This work was supported by grant 04X-715 from the Swedish Medical Research Council.

REFERENCES

1. Agnati L, Fuxe K, Zini I, Lenzi P, Hökfelt T. Aspects on receptor regulation and isoreceptor identification. *Med Biol* 1980;58:182–187.
2. Agnati L, Fuxe K, Benfenati F, Zini I, Hökfelt T. On the functional role of coexistence of 5-HT and substance P in bulbospinal 5-HT neurons. Substance P reduces affinity and increases density of 3H-5-HT binding sites. *Acta Physiol Scand* 1983;117:299–301.
3. Andén N-E, Dahlström A, Fuxe K, Larsson K, Olson L, Ungerstedt U. Ascending monoamine neurons to the telencephalon and diencephalon. *Acta Physiol Scand* 1966;67:313–326.
4. Beaudet A, Sotelo C. Synaptic remodeling of serotonin axon terminals in rat agranular cerebellum. *Brain Res* 1981;206:305–329.
5. Bishop G, Ho R, King J. Localization of serotonin immunoreactivity in the opossum cerebellum. *J Comp Neurol* 1985;235:301–321.
6. Bishop G, Ho R. The distribution and origin of serotonin immunoreactivity in the rat cerebellum. *Brain Res* 1985;331:195–207.
7. Bishop G, Ho R. Cell bodies of serotonin-immunoreactive afferents to the inferior olivary complex of the rat. *Brain Res* 1986;399:369–373.
8. Bloom F, Hoffer B, Siggins G. Studies on norepinephrine-containing afferents to Purkinje cells of rat cerebellum. *Brain Res* 1971;25:501–521.
9. Bunneman B, Fuxe K, Bjelke B, Ganten D. The brain renin-angiotensin system and its possible involvement in volume transmission. In: Fuxe K, Agnati LF, eds. *Volume transmission in the brain:*

novel mechanisms for neural transmission (*Advances in neuroscience*, vol 1). New York: Raven Press, 1991:131–158.
10. Carlsson A, Jonason J, Linqvist M, Fuxe K. Demonstration of extraneuronal 5-hydroxytryptamine accumulation in brain following membrane-pump blockade by chlorimipramine. *Brain Res* 1969;12:456–460.
11. Chan-Palay V. Fine structure of labelled axons in the cerebellar cortex and nuclei of rodents and primates after intraventricular infusions with tritiated serotonin. *Anat Embryol* 1975;148:234–265.
12. Chan-Palay V. The indoleamine afferent axons to the cerebellum. In: *Cerebellar dentate nucleus: organization, cytology and transmitters*. New York: Springer-Verlag, 1977:395–454.
13. Cintra A, Cao Y, Oellig C, et al. Basic FGF is present in dopaminergic neurons of the ventral midbrain of the rat. *Neuroreport (in press)*.
14. Dahlström A, Fuxe K. Evidence for the existence of monoamine containing neurons in the central nervous system. I. Demonstration of monoamines in the cell bodies of brainstem neurons. *Acta Physiol Scand* 1964;62:1–55.
15. Dahlström A, Fuxe K. Evidence for the existence of monoamine containing neurons in the central nervous system. II. Experimentally induced changes in the intra-neuronal amine levels. *Acta Physiol Scand* 1965;64:1–36.
16. Darrow E, Strahlendorf H, Strahlendorf J. Response of cerebellar Purkinje cells to serotonin and the 5-HT_{1A} agonists 8-OH-DPAT and ipsapirone in vitro. *Eur J Pharmacol* 1990;175:145–153.
17. Daval G, Vergé D, Becerril A, Gozlan H, Stampinato U, Hamon M. Transient expression of 5-HT_{1A} receptor binding sites in some areas of the rat CNS during postnatal development. *Int J Dev Neurosci* 1987;5:171–180.
18. Dawson T, Gehlert D, Wamsley J. Quantitative autoradiographic localization of the dopamine transport complex in the rat brain: use of a highly selective ligand: (^{3}H)GBR 12935. *Eur J Pharmacol* 1986;126:171–173.
19. Dawson T, Barone P, Sidhu A, Wamsley J, Chase T. The D1 dopamine receptor in the rat brain: quantitative autoradiographic localization using an iodinated liquid. *Neuroscience* 1988;26:83–100.
20. Descarries L, Séguéllá P, Watkins K. Nonjunctional relationships of monoamine axons terminals in the cerebral cortex of the adult rat. In: Fuxe K, Agnati LF, eds. *Volume transmission in the brain: Novel mechanisms for neural transmission* (*Advances in neuroscience*, vol 1). New York: Raven Press, 1991:53–62.
21. von Euler G, Fuxe K, van der Ploeg I, Fredholm B, Agnati L. Pertussis toxin treatment counteracts intramembrane interactions between neuropeptide Y receptors and alfa-2-adrenoceptors. *Eur J Pharmacol* 1989;172:435–441.
22. von Euler G, van der Ploeg I, Fredholm B, Fuxe K. Neurotensin decreases the affinity of dopamine D2 agonist binding by a G protein independent mechanism. *J Neurochem* 1991;56:178–183.
23. Fuxe K. Evidence for the existence of monoamine neurons in the central nervous system. IV. Distribution of monoamine nerve terminals in the central nervous system. *Acta Physiol Scand* 1965;64:39–85.
24. Fuxe K, Ungerstedt U. Localization of 5-hydroxytryptamine uptake in rat brain after intraventricular injection. *J Pharm Pharmacol* 1967;19:335–337.
25. Fuxe K, Ungerstedt U. Histochemical studies on the distribution of catecholamines and 5-hydroxytryptamine after intraventricular injections. *Histochemie* 1968;13:16–28.
26. Fuxe K, Jonsson G. Further mapping of central 5-hydroxytryptamine neurons: studies with the neurotoxic dihydroxytryptamines. In: Costa E, Gessa G, Sandler M, eds. *Serotonin—new vistas: histochemistry and pharmacology* (*Advances in biochemical psychopharmacology*, vol 10). New York: Raven Press, 1974:1–12.
27. Fuxe K, Ganten D, Locatelli V, et al. Renin-like immunocytochemical activity in the rat and mouse brain. *Neurosci Lett* 1980;18:245–250.
28. Fuxe K, Agnati L. Receptor-receptor interactions in the central nervous system. A new integrative mechanism in synapses. *Med Res Rev* 1985;5:441–482.
29. Fuxe K, vonEuler G, Agnati L, Ögren S-O. Galanin selectively modulates 5-hydroxytryptamine-1A receptors in the rat ventral limbic cortex. *Neurosci Lett* 1988;85:163–167.
30. Fuxe K, Cintra A, Andbjer B, Änggård E, Goldstein M, Agnati L. Centrally administered endothelin-1 produces lesions in the brain of the male rat. *Acta Physiol Scand* 1989;137:155–156.
31. Fuxe K, Agnati L, von Euler G, Benfenati F, Tanganelli S. Modulation of dopamine D1 and D2 transmission lines in the central nervous system. In: Osborne N, ed. *Current aspects of neurosciences*. London: Macmillan, 1990:203–243.
31a. Fuxe K, Agnati L, eds. *Volume transmission in the brain* (*Advances in neuroscience*, vol 1). New York: Raven Press, 1991.

32. Fuxe K, Kurosawa N, Cintra A, et al. Involvement of local ischemia in endothelin-1 induced lesions of the neostriatum of the anaesthetized rat. *Exp Brain Res (in press)*.
33. Garthwaite J. Glutamate, nitric oxide and cell-cell signalling in the nervous system. *Trends Neurosci* 1991;14.
34. Gehlert D, Speth R, Wamsley J. Distribution of ^{125}I-angiotensin binding sites in the rat brain: a quantitative autoradiographic study. 1986;18:837.
35. Glowinski J, Axelrod J, Iversen L. Regional studies of catecholamines in the rat brain. IV. Effects of drugs on the disposition and metabolism of ^{3}H-norepinephrine and ^{3}H-dopamine. *J Pharmacol Exp Ther* 1966;153:30–41.
36. Greengard P. Receptor-receptor interactions mediated by protein phosphorylation. In: Fuxe K, Agnati LF, eds. *Receptor-receptor interactions. A new intramembrane integrative mechanism.* London: Macmillan, 1987:444–453.
37. Hartig P. Molecular biology of 5-HT receptors. *Trends Pharmacol Sci Rev* 1989;10:64–69.
38. Hartig P. Molecular biology of the serotonin receptor family. In: Paoletti R, Vanhoutte P, Brunello N, Maggi F, eds. *Serotonin: from cell biology to pharmacology and therapeutics.* Dordrecht: Kluwer, 1990:7–10.
39. Hedlund P, von Euler G, Fuxe K. Activation of 5-hydroxytryptamine-1A receptors increases the affinity of galanin receptors in di- and telencephalic areas of the rat. *Brain Res* 1991;560:251–259.
40. Hedlund P, Aguirre J, Narvaez J, Fuxe K. Centrally coinjected galanin and a 5-HT$_{1A}$ agonist act synergistically to produce vasodepressor responses in the rat. *(in press)*.
41. Hoffer B, Siggins G, Oliver A, Bloom F. Activation of the pathway from locus coeruleus to rat cerebellar Purkinje neurons: pharmacological evidence for noradrenergic central inhibition. *J Pharmacol Exp Ther* 1973;184:553–569.
42. Hökfelt T, Fuxe K. Cerebellar monoamine nerve terminals, a new type of afferent fibers to the cortex cerebelli. *Exp Brain Res* 1969;9:63–72.
43. Lauder J. Hormonal and humoral influences on brain development. *Psychoneuroendocrinology* 1983;8:121–155.
44. Lee M, Strahlendorf J, Strahlendorf H. Modulatory action of serotonin on glutamate-induced excitation of cerebellar Purkinje cells. *Brain Res* 1986;361:107–113.
45. Luthman J, Fredriksson A, Sundström E, Jonsson G, Archer T. Selective lesion of central dopamine or noradrenaline neuron systems in the neonatal rat: motor behavior and monoamine alterations at adult stage. *Behav Brain Res* 1989;33:267–277.
46. Markey K, Kondo A, Schenkmann L, Goldstein M. Purification and characterization of tyrosine hydroxylase from a clonal chromocytoma cell line. *Mol Pharmacol* 1980;17:79–85.
47. Maura G, Bonando G, Pittaluga A, Ulivi M, Raiteri M. Serotonin-glutamate interaction in rat cerebellum: involvement of 5-hydroxytryptamine receptor subtypes. *Ann Ist Super Sanita* 1988;24:389–396.
48. Maura G, Roccatagliata E, Ulivi M, Raiteri M. Serotonin-glutamate interaction in rat cerebellum: involvement of 5-HT$_1$ and 5-HT$_2$ receptors. *Eur J Pharmacol* 1988;145:31–38.
49. Mendelsohn F, Quirion R, Saavedra J, Aguilera G, Katt K. Autoradiographic localization of angiotensin II receptors in rat brain. *Proc Natl Acad Sci USA* 1984;81:1575.
50. Okret S, Wikström A-C, Wrange Ö, Andersson B, Gustafsson J-Å. Monoclonal antibodies against the rat liver glucocorticoid receptor. *Proc Natl Acad Sci USA* 1984;81:1609–1613.
51. Olson L, Fuxe K. On the projection from the locus coeruleus noradrenaline neurons: the cerebellar innervation. *Brain Res* 1971;28:165–171.
52. Ouimet C, Miller P, Hemmings H, Walaas S, Greengard P. DARPP-32, a dopamine- and adenosine 3′: 5′-monophosphate-regulated phosphoprotein enriched in dopamine-innervated brain regions. III. Immunocytochemical localization. *J Neurosci* 1984;111–124.
53. Pazos A, Cortés R, Palacios J. Quantitative autoradiographic mapping of serotonin receptors in the rat brain. II. Serotonin-2 receptors. *Brain Res* 1985;346:231–249.
54. Persson L. Antibodies to ornithine decarboxylase. Immunochemical cross-reactivity. *Acta Chem Scand* 1982;36:685–688.
55. Raiteri M, Maura G, Bonnano G, Pittaluga A. Differential pharmacology and function of two 5-HT1 receptors modulating transmitter release in rat cerebellum. *J Pharmacol Exp Ther* 1986;237:644–648.
56. Raiteri M, Maura G, Barzizza A. Activation of presynaptic 5-hydroxytryptamine$_1$-like receptors on glutamatergic terminals inhibits N-methyl-D-aspartate-induced cyclic GMP production in rat cerebellar slices. *J Pharmacol Exp Ther* 1991;257:1184–1188.
57. Ruggeri M, Merlo-Pich E, Zini I, Fuxe K, Ungerstedt U, Agnati L. Indolepyruvic acid increases

5-hydroxyindoleacetic acid levels in the cerebrospinal fluid and frontoparietal cortex of the rat: a microdialysis study. *Acta Physiol Scand* 1990;138:97–98.
58. Seiger Å, Olson L. Late prenatal ontogeny of central monoamine neurons in the rat: fluorescence histochemical observations. *Z Anat Entwickl-Gesch* 1973;140:281–318.
59. Servin A, Amiranoff B, Rouyer-Fessard C, Tatemoto K, Laburthe M. Identification and molecular characterization of galanin receptor sites in rat brain. *Biochem Biophys Res Commun* 1987;144:298–306.
59a.Steinbusch HWM. Distribution of serotonin-immunoreactivity in the central nervous system of the rat cell bodies and terminals. *Neuroscience* 1981;6:557–618.
60. Strahlendorf J, Lee M, Strahlendorf H. Effects of serotonin on cerebellar Purkinje cells are dependent on the baseline firing rate. *Exp Brain Res* 1984;56:50–58.
61. Takeuchi Y, Kimura H, Sano Y. Immunohistochemical demonstration of serotonin-containing nerve fibers in the cerebellum. *Cell Tissue Res* 1982;226:1–12.
62. Takeuchi Y, Sano Y. Immunohistochemical demonstration of serotonin-containing nerve fibers in the inferior olivary complex of the rat, cat and monkey. *Cell Tissue Res* 1983;231:17–28.
63. Tongroach P, Sanguangrungsirikul S, Tantisira B, Kunluan P. Angiotensin II induced depression of Purkinje cell firing and possible modulatory action on GABA responses. *Neurosci Res* 1984;1:369–372.
64. Trouillas P, Brudon F, Adeleine P. Improvement of cerebellar ataxia with levorotatory form of 5-hydroxytryptophan. A double-blind study with quantified data processing. *Arch Neurol* 1988;45:1217–1222.
65. Waeber C, Dietl M, Hoyer D, Palacios J. 5-HT$_1$ receptors in the vertebrate brain. Regional distribution examined by autoradiography. *Naunyn Schmiedebergs Arch Pharmacol* 1989;340:486–494.
66. Wiklund L, Sjöland B, Björklund A. Morphological and functional studies on the serotonergic innervation of the inferior olive. *J Physiol (Paris)* 1981;77:183–186.
67. Xu J, Chuang D-M. Serotonergic, adrenergic and histaminergic receptors coupled to phospholipase C in cultured cerebellar granule cells of rats. *Biochem Pharmacol* 1987;36:2353–2358.
68. Yamamoto T, Ishikawa M, Tanaka C. Catecholaminergic terminals in the developing and adult cerebellum. *Brain Res* 1977;132:355–361.
69. Zoli M, Ferraguti F, Biagini G, Cintra A, Fuxe K, Agnati L. Corticosterone treatment counteracts lesions induced by neonatal treatment with monosodium glutamate in the mediobasal hypothalamus of the male rat. *Neurosci Lett* (*in press*).

*Serotonin, the Cerebellum,
and Ataxia*, edited by
P. Trouillas and K. Fuxe.
Raven Press, Ltd., New York © 1993.

2

A Quantitative Study of the Raphe Serotonin Neurons in the Normal Human Brain Stem

V. Chan-Palay, M. Höchli, B. Jentsch, *R.G.H. Cotton, and T. Zetzsche

*Neurology Clinic, University Hospital, CH-8091 Zurich, Switzerland;
The Murdoch Institute, Royal Children's Hospital, Parkville 3052, Melbourne, Australia

5-Hydroxytryptophan or serotonin (5-HT), a monoamine that has been detected peripherally and in the central nervous system of mammals (1) may act as a neurotransmitter or a neuromodulator (2,3). The morphological localization of 5-HT-containing structures was first made possible by a histofluorescence technique (4), by which it was shown that the majority of central 5-HT neurons are localized in the brain stem (5). Because 5-HT neurons form additional groups that do not fit completely into the classical nuclear division of the brain stem, a new nomenclature of these cell groups was designated as B1–B9. Some of these subgroups correspond to the raphe nuclei (6,7). This division was mostly confirmed and partially modified by subsequent studies that used autoradiography or immunohistochemical techniques to detect 5-HT (8–10). A similar nomenclature (A1–A10) was applied to the catecholaminergic brain stem neurons (5,11). Alterations of 5-HT and catecholamine-related structures and metabolism were reported for several neurological and psychiatric disorders including dementia, depression, and Parkinson's disease (12–25).

A reexamination of the raphe neurons in the human brain stem was recently performed using a monoclonal antibody (PH8), which was shown to crossreact with tryptophan hydroxylase (26) (the rate-limiting enzyme for the synthesis of 5-HT) (3) and which specifically labeled 5-HT neurons in the postmortem human brain (27–30). The study presented here was performed with the same antibody to quantify and three-dimensionally reconstruct 5-HT neurons in the brain stem of normal patients to provide a basis for later comparisons with the distribution of PH8 immunoreactivity in the brains of patients suffering from neurological disorders such as senile dementia of the Alzheimer type, multi-infarct dementia, and Parkinson's disease.

This study was expanded to obtain more information about monoamine-related structures in the human brain stem. Antibodies raised against tyrosine hydroxylase (TH), a key enzyme in catecholamine synthesis, were used to detect noradrenergic and dopaminergic neurons (21,22). Furthermore we applied monoclonal antibodies directed against human platelet monoamine oxidase (MAO) B (31) and human placental MAO A (32). These two MAO subtypes were originally defined according to their different substrate specificities and inhibition properties (33), and previous studies have shown that these antibodies specifically detect the cellular enzyme localization in postmortem human brains (34,35). It was demonstrated that the neurons of the serotoninergic raphe nuclei were immunoreactive for MAO B. On the other hand, MAO A was localized in noradrenergic neurons, for example, in the locus coeruleus (34,35). This part of our study was performed to provide additional data about the normal distribution of 5-HT and catecholamine-related structures in the normal human brain.

MATERIALS AND METHODS

The Zurich study on dementia is an interdisciplinary program that longitudinally follows a group of demented patients and age-matched controls in the chronic care hospitals of Zürich (22). The patients were entered into the study according to a diagnosis, based on clinical and apparative (electroencephalography, neuroradiology) evaluations. Every 6 months, the patients were reexamined neurologically and a set of psychological tests (e.g., Minimental status, Hamilton depression rating scale) performed by the responsible physicians in the hospitals. Only those controls without any signs of neurological or psychiatric disease were used for the part of the study presented here (three cases, ages 76–83 years, postmortem delay (pm): 4.5–7 hr). At autopsy the brains were perfused with 4% paraformaldehyde for 2 hr, after which approximately 8 mm thick blocks of different brain regions were cut according to a standardized protocol and fixed by immersion overnight (16 hr). In addition, as a special control for this study, two brain stems had been subjected to long-term fixation for up to several months in a preceding experiment. Because no differences in PH8 immunoreactivity were observed between tissues treated with the long-term or the standard overnight fixation times, the cases used for this study were fixed according to the standard procedure. Macroscopic and microscopic neuropathological examinations were performed, and counts of neuritic plaques and neurofibrillary tangles were made in Bodian silver-stained sections of the hippocampus (CA1) and in several neocortical areas (frontal, parietal, temporal, and occipital cortex) in 20 separate visual fields at $250\times$ magnification. Under the condition that no neuropathological abnormality was found, the brains of those patients were entered into this study. In each of these cases, the entire brain stem, which was sometimes as long as 10 cm, was sectioned with a freezing microtome in serial 70 μm thick coronal sections from the nucleus ruber to the decussation of the pyramidal tract. The sections were collected in groups of every fifth section. One series was stained with cresyl violet (Nissl) to reveal cytoarchitectonic boundaries and the others were used for free-floating immunostaining. The technical procedures of immunostaining are described elsewere (36). After preincubation sections were subjected to the following antibodies (for the description and specification of the antibodies, see text and references cited above): PH8 (dilution 1:6,000), TH (1:6,000), MAO A (1:20,000), and MAO B (1:500,000) in 1% normal goat serum for a 4-day incubation period at 4°C. The binding sites were visualized by the immunogold-silver staining method (IGSS). To study coexistence, immediately adjacent sections were reacted for different antibodies and compared. The technical procedures of immunostaining are fully described elsewhere (36). Every PH8-immunoreacted section was then subjected to computer-assisted cell counting and graphic reconstruction with the "cell-mate program" (Bioquant, Tennessee). The methods of the computer-assisted quantitative analysis are described in detail elsewhere (21). The atlas of Olszewski and Baxter (6) and the nomenclature of Törk and Hornung (30) were used for the division of the human raphe nuclei. Separate cell counts were performed in the following nuclei: dorsal raphe nucleus, median raphe, raphe magnus, raphe obscurus, and raphe pallidus. Color coding for the separation of the nuclei in graphic computer reconstructions was used.

RESULTS

PH8

In the human brain stem only neurons and their processes were specifically labeled with the PH8 antibody. The majority of neurons showed intensely immunoreactive somata and dendrites (including distal dendritic segments), but did not present a uniform morphology. Considerable differences regarding the somatic size, shape, and dendritic branching patterns could be detected. Most of the immunoreactive neurons were found in the midline portion and the bilaterally localized subgroups of the raphe nuclei in the mesencephalon, pons, and medulla oblongata. In addition, PH8-immunoreactive (PH8-i) neurons were found in groups or bands laterally to the median raphe or the caudal raphe nuclei in the pontine and medullary reticular formation. In this chapter we will limit our description of PH8-immunoreactivity to the neurons located in the raphe nuclei. The system of Törk and Hornung (30) for the division of the human raphe nuclei (dorsal raphe, median raphe, raphe magnus, raphe pallidus, raphe obscurus) could be confirmed, although the nuclei showed partial overlapping. Comparison of PH8-reacted sections with adjacent Nissl-stained sections revealed that the majority of the raphe neurons were immunoreactive, although more comprehensive quantitative studies would be necessary to define the exact proportion of immunoreactive to nonimmunoreactive neurons in each raphe nucleus. In the following section we will describe the morphology and distribution of PH8-i neurons in more detail.

Major assemblies of PH8-i neurons in the rostral brain stem were found in the nucleus centralis superior, the dorsal raphe nucleus, the median raphe nucleus, and the B9 group dorsally from the medial lemniscus. The immunoreactive neurons of the dorsal raphe nucleus were found in the central gray matter ventral to the cerebral aqueduct and the fourth ventricle. The nucleus extended from the midbrain at the level of the accessory oculomotor nucleus until the middle segments of the pons nearly reaching the motor trigeminal nucleus. The dorsal, medial, ventrolateral, and caudal subnuclei of the dorsal raphe nucleus could be distinguished according to differences in localization, neuronal morphology, and cell density. The majority of the dorsal raphe neurons were localized dorsal to the medial longitudinal fasciculi (Fig. 1a). Many of these neurons had elongated somata or a multipolar appearance. Their dendrites did not show a preferential orientation, but formed a more or less dense irregular network. Cell counting revealed that the total number of immunoreactive neurons in the dorsal raphe ranged between approximately 103,163 and 161,515 (Table 1).

The immunoreactive neurons of the median raphe were localized in the midline portion of the pons below the caudal subnucleus of the dorsal raphe (Fig. 1b). Rostrocaudally the nucleus extended from the decussation of the superior cerebellar peduncles to the motor trigeminal nucleus without sharp borders at either end. The neurons were arranged more or less symmetrically on both sides of the midline. No division into subnuclei was made in the case of the median raphe. Within this nucleus, spindle-shaped bipolar somata were a common finding, multipolar neurons were also detected, and both small and large neurons were immunoreactive. Especially in the ventral parts of the nucleus, the orientation of dendrites was often to the ventral or dorsal direction, but laterally or medially extending dendrites were not rare. A sagittal orientation of dendrites could result in a corkscrew-like appearance in the coronal plane. A total number of median raphe neurons between 68,550 and 77,460 was counted (Table 1).

Three raphe nuclei could be discriminated by the appearance of PH8-i neurons in the caudal parts of the brain stem: raphe magnus nucleus, raphe obscurus nucleus, and raphe pallidus nucleus. The raphe magnus nucleus extended from the caudal pons to the rostral part of the medulla oblongata with the largest part rostrally from the level of the inferior olivary nucleus. Most impressive were the large bipolar or multipolar neurons, which gave rise to long dendrites running parallel to the coronal plane and often arranged in bundles (Fig. 1c). The orientation of the dendrites was preferentially dorsoventral in the midline and mediolateral in the lateral aspects and included oblique oriented, laterally ascending dendrites. At the level of the caudal pons the rostral raphe obscurus nucleus began dorsally from the raphe magnus and reached caudally to the rostral spinal cord, with the greatest extension in the medulla oblongata at the level of the inferior olivary nucleus. Characteristically the obscurus neurons were arranged bilaterally on both sides of a midline zone, which contained only very few, mostly horizontally oriented, immunoreactive fibers (Fig. 1c). The orientation of the dendrites in both cellular columns was predominantly ventrodorsal. The immunoreactive neurons in the raphe pallidus constituted the smallest of the raphe nuclei, which was localized at the ventral part of the brain stem

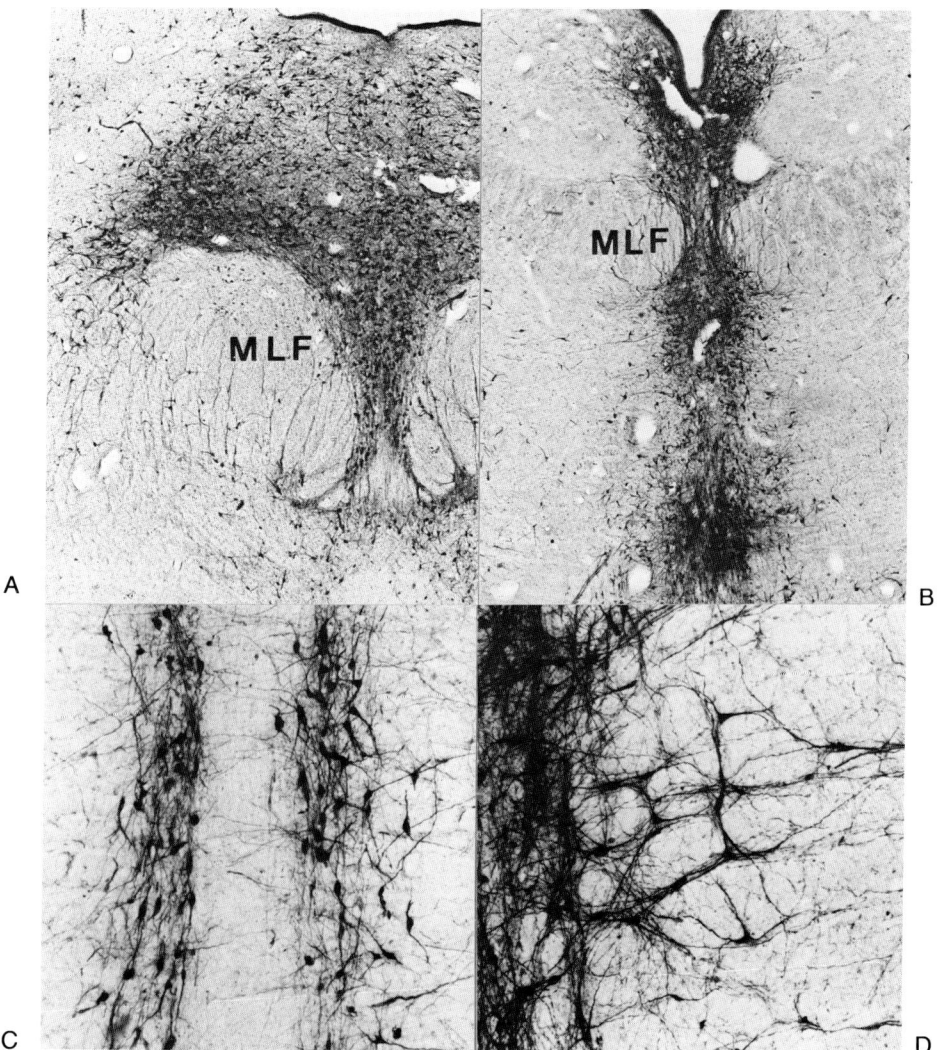

FIG. 1. PH8 immunoreactivity in the human brain stem. **A**: Dorsal raphe nucleus, most of the neurons are located dorsally of the medial longitudinal fasciculus (MLF). **B**: Median raphe nucleus, immunoreactive neurons are localized in the midline portion of the brain stem below the MLF. **C**: Raphe obscurus, immunoreactive neurons are arranged in two parallel bands bilaterally to the midline. **D**: Raphe magnus, immunoreactive dendrites form bundles in the lateral aspects of the nucleus (right side). IGSS. Magnification: A, B, ×13.13; C, D, ×43.5.

TABLE 1. *Numbers of PH8-neurons in the dorsal subnuclei and median raphe in the brain stem of control patients*

Case	Age	PM	Plaques/tangles	DD	DM	DVL	DC	DT	MT
1	83	4.5	0/0	48,530	28,350	51,435	33,200	161,515	68,550
2	78	7	0/0	38,950	26,020	39,175	22,470	126,615	77,460
3	76	5	0/0	37,530	20,663	26,385	18,545	103,163	77,210

Subgroups of the dorsal raphe: DD, dorsal; DM, medial; DVL, ventrolateral; DC, caudal. DT, total number of dorsal raphe; MT, total number of median raphe; PM, postmortem delay (hr); 0, minimum plaques or tangles (0–1) per visual field in temporal cortex (magnification ×250).

at the level of the caudal pons to the medulla oblongata. The total number of all caudal raphe nuclei ranged from 37,360 to 42,320 (Table 2).

Tyrosine Hydroxylase

Only the neurons and their processes, but not glia cells, were immunoreactive for the TH antibody. Assemblies of TH-immunoreactive (TH-i) neurons were ascribed to already known catecholaminergic nuclei in the human brain stem. The nuclei that contained the greatest numbers of TH-i neurons were the substantia nigra and the locus coeruleus and subcoeruleus. In addition immunoreactive neurons were found in the mesencephalon medially and dorsolaterally to the borders of the substantia nigra, the lateral tegmentum of the pons and the medulla oblongata, the solitary nucleus, and the dorsal motor vagal nucleus, all areas of the brain stem that were previously described as containing catecholaminergic neurons.

Monoamine Oxidase

MAO A and B immunoreactivity in the human brain stem was found in neuronal somata and dendrites, glia cells, glial and axonal processes and varicosities, and the walls of blood vessels.

In most cases immunoreactive neurons and glia cells could be readily distinguished according to their different size and morphology. Glia cells had very small

TABLE 2. *Numbers of PH8-neurons in the caudal raphe subnuclei in the brain stem of control patients*

Case	Age	PM	RM	RO	RP	RT
1	83	4.5	21,870	17,365	3,085	42,320
2	78	7	18,890	16,555	1,915	37,360
3	76	5	26,655	13,780	1,705	42,140

Subgroups of the caudal raphe: RM, raphe magnus; RO, raphe obscurus; RP, raphe pallidus; RT, total number of caudal raphe; PM, postmortem delay (hr).

somata and mostly a star-like arrangement of processes and were classified as astrocytes. These MAO-immunoreactive (MAO-i) astrocytes were found in many brain stem nuclei as well as in some fiber tracts. The total number of astrocytes that were immunoreactive for MAO B was consistently higher and the intracellular immunoreactivity was more intense compared to staining for MAO A. Some areas had only MAO B-i astrocytes or were strongly dominated by MAO B-i astrocytes (pyramidal tract). On the other hand, blood vessel walls generally showed a more prominent immunoreactivity to MAO A. This was most obvious in fiber tracts with a low density of MAO-i structures (e.g., superior cerebellar peduncle). In areas with densely immunoreactive neuropil it was often difficult to discriminate between isolated glial fibers and axonal processes solely on the basis of light microscopic criteria. But sometimes fine fibers with periodic enlarged varicosities running for long distances in the plane of section could be detected and identified as axonal processes. In those cases in which glial fibers and axonal processes could not be individually identified, the term "cellular processes" will be used in the following text. In general MAO A-i glia cells and cellular processes were concentrated in cell-dense areas, whereas MAO B-i glia cells and cellular processes were also found in the surrounding tissue. This was most clearly seen in some nuclei of cranial nerves. For example, dense cell "nests", which were formed in parts of the vestibular nuclei, had a high concentration of both MAO A-i and B-i cellular processes, whereas the immunoreactivity in the surrounding neuropil "matrix" was high only for MAO B and low for MAO A.

The highest density of MAO A or B immunoreactivity was found in the periaqueductal gray, the monoaminergic nuclei, the nuclei of some cranial nerves, the area postrema, and parts of the reticular formation. Four groups of MAO-i areas listed in Table 3 could be differentiated according to different compositions of immunoreactive structures, which will be described below. A dense immunoreactivity could be due mainly to MAO A (group Ia), MAO B (group Ib), or a mixed population of MAO A and B (group Ic) neuronal somata and dendrites that were surrounded more or less densely by glia and cellular processes. In other cases the staining was primarily due to glia and immunoreactive processes with a moderately high number of immunoreactive neurons (group IIa) or only with few scattered ones (group IIb). In other regions the immunoreactivity was found exclusively in glia and cellular processes and was missing in neuronal somata (group III). Low immunoreactivities for MAO were detected in some fiber tracts (group IV), where MAO A immunoreactivity was mainly restricted to the walls of blood vessels. Considerable differences existed in this group regarding the density of MAO B immunoreactivity, which was due to staining of astrocytes, cellular processes, and blood vessels. For example, MAO B immunoreactivity was exceptionally low in the superior cerebellar peduncle but high in the pyramidal tract because of the staining of numerous glia cells and cellular processes. In some fiber tracts groups of immunoreactive processes and cells were incorporated in between nonimmunoreactive fibers. This was the case in a part of the medial longitudinal fasciculus, which borders on the nucleus oculomotorius.

TABLE 3. Groups of MAO-immunoreactive areas in the human brain stem (for definition see text)

Group Ia	Locus coeruleus, oculomotor nucleus
Group Ib	Dorsal raphe nucleus, median raphe nucleus
Group Ic	Paranigral nucleus, nucleus subcoeruleus, solitary nucleus, dorsal motor vagal nucleus, abducens nucleus, lateral reticular formation of the medulla oblongata
Group IIa	Vestibular nuclei, inferior olivary nucleus, raphe obscurus
Group IIb	Substantia nigra
Group III	Superior colliculus, inferior colliculus, facial nucleus, motor trigeminal nucleus, trigeminal sensory nucleus, hypoglossal nucleus, trochlear nucleus, pontine gray matter
Group IV	Superior, middle, inferior cerebellar peduncle; medial lemniscus; medial longitudinal fasciculus; pontocerebellar fibers; pyramidal tract

In the following section a more detailed description of some selected MAO immunoreactive brain stem structures will be given. In the substantia nigra pars compacta, nonimmunoreactive neuronal somata were surrounded by an accumulation of MAO A and B-i astrocytes and cell processes, which were most clearly seen in the cell-dense layers of pigmented neurons. In addition, a high density of MAO B and a low density of MAO A-i processes were found in the pars reticulata. Only some scattered neurons inside and dorsal to the substantia nigra were MAO A-i or B-i. At the utmost medial and lateral borders of the substantia nigra, a high number of MAO A-i neurons were found. Numerous neurons were immunoreactive for MAO A in the medially adjacent paranigral nucleus and the interpeduncular region. This area, which is part of the catecholaminergic region A10, showed in addition intense immunoreactivity for TH in neuronal somata and dendrites and a dense accumulation of MAO B-i glia and cellular processes. In the nucleus centralis superior, which is localized rostral to the decussation of the superior cerebellar peduncles, assemblies of MAO B-i neurons were found in the same location as numerous PH8-i neurons.

In the locus coeruleus small- and large-sized bipolar or multipolar pigmented neurons were in most instances so strongly MAO A-i in their somata and dendrites that the cell nucleus could not be determined. Dendritic immunoreactivity often extended to distally located branches, although the dendritic staining was less complete compared to the TH immunoreactivity found in adjacent sections. Only occasionally nonpigmented small neurons inside or at the lower border of the locus coeruleus displayed MAO B immunoreactivity. Comparison with adjacent sections reacted for TH revealed a 1:1 coexistence of TH and MAO A. In the subcoeruleus most of the neurons were immunoreactive for MAO A, but, in contrast to the locus coeruleus proper, a higher portion of neurons also showed MAO B immunoreactivity.

In the raphe nuclei considerable differences in the staining intensity in neuronal somata and dendrites were encountered and often only the proximal parts of the dendrites were labeled. In some nuclei (e.g., median raphe, raphe obscurus) neuronal MAO B immunoreactivity, often restricted to the cytoplasmic rim around an unstained cell nucleus, could result in a racket-like appearance if a proximal dendrite was also stained. Raphe neurons were regularly surrounded by MAO B-i glial or axonal processes, with the highest density in the dorsal raphe. Only occasionally small neurons immunoreactive for MAO A were detected in the vicinity of raphe nuclei, for example, at the lateral borders of the rostral median raphe. Comparisons of adjacent sections that were stained for either MAO B or PH8 revealed that a different proportion of PH8-i raphe neurons were immunoreactive for MAO B in each of the raphe nuclei. In the rostrally localized nuclei a high proportion of neurons (e.g., nearly all of the neurons in the raphe dorsalis) were immunoreactive for MAO B. In contrast to these results only a small portion of neurons was MAO B-i in the caudal localized raphe obscurus. A higher portion was found in the median raphe and the raphe magnus.

Bilaterally to the median raphe numerous MAO B-i neurons were found in the oral reticular nucleus and the B9 group dorsally to the medial lemniscus. PH8-i neurons were detected in the same localization, but in distinctly greater number.

Neurons of the medullary reticular complex were part of a band of TH and MAO A-i neurons that could be traced from ventrolateral to the dorsomedial aspects of the medulla oblongata. The neurons often had elongated somata with dendrites emerging in the oblique axes. In the ventrolateral reticular formation, dorsal to the inferior olivary nucleus, numerous PH8-i neurons and a much smaller number of MAO B-i neurons were detected. In addition MAO A and B-i neuron populations overlap.

The wall of the fourth ventricle showed a high number of MAO B-i and fewer MAO A-i cellular processes. In adjacent sections axons and axonal varicosities were readily immunoreactive for TH and PH8.

In the solitary nucleus and the dorsal motor vagal nucleus, a subpopulation of neurons were MAO A-i and TH-i, although few scattered MAO B-i neurons were also found. This region corresponded to the catecholaminergic A2 group described for primates (11) and was localized at the dorsomedial end of the diagonal band of monoamine neurons described above.

The oculomotor nuclei contained a subpopulation of neurons that were immunoreactive for MAO A but not B. Considerable differences regarding the staining intensity were encountered, for example, some of the neurons were faintly immunoreactive or clearly nonimmunoreactive. Compared with the locus coeruleus most of the neurons in the oculomotor nuclei showed a less dense MAO A immunoreactivity and the dendritic immunoreactivity was restricted to the proximal segments. The density of MAO-i cellular processes that surrounded the neurons was, on the other hand, considerably higher than in the locus coeruleus. To study coexistence we used consecutive sections reacted with different antibodies. With this method it was obvious that in the oculomotor nucleus neuronal somata and dendrites were nonimmunoreactive for TH and PH8, but it was not possible to prove whether identical or separate cellular processes were immunoreactive for MAO A or B.

In the abducens nucleus a subpopulation of medium-sized multipolar and other types of neurons were MAO A-i and a fewer number of small bipolar or triangular neurons were MAO B-i. In the trochlear nucleus the immunoreactivity was due to labeled glia cells and cellular processes.

In the facial nucleus, motor trigeminal nucleus, and hypoglossal nucleus the nonimmunoreactive neuronal somata were surrounded by a dense accumulation of MAO A and B-i glia cells and cellular processes. In MAO A-immunoreacted sections the nuclei could be clearly discriminated due to their higher density of immunoreactive structures compared to the surrounding tissue.

In the periaqueductal gray the immunoreactivity of the glia and the cellular processes was extremely high for MAO B and considerably lower for MAO A. In the ventromedial aspects, which belong to the dorsal raphe nucleus, most neurons were immunoreactive for MAO B. More rostrally a far smaller number of MAO A-i small- and large-sized bipolar and multipolar neurons were found in the ventrolateral and medial aspects of the periaqueductal gray. The ventrolateral group of MAO A-i neurons did extend to the rostral tip of the locus coeruleus.

The gray matter of the inferior olivary nucleus and accessory olivary nuclei could be clearly discriminated because it contained a high density of MAO A-i and B-i glia and cellular processes compared to the surrounding tissue. Neuronal somata and dendrites were nonimmunoreactive for MAO A, but a subpopulation of neurons showed staining of perikarya and proximal dendrites for MAO B. The cell nuclei of these neurons were characteristically devoid of immunoreactivity.

DISCUSSION

Our results concerning PH8 immunoreactivity in the normal postmortem brain stem are in accordance with previous studies in humans (27–30), which have demonstrated that specifically labeled neurons are localized in areas already known to be serotoninergic, mainly in the raphe nuclei. The majority of raphe neurons were stained by the PH8 antibody, although some of these cells may be nonimmunoreactive. PH8 is crossreactive with TH (26). Because TH is the rate-limiting enzyme for the synthesis of 5-HT, these results indicate that most of the human raphe neurons may be capable of synthesizing this monoamine. The subdivisions of the human raphe nuclei into dorsal raphe, median raphe, raphe magnus, raphe pallidus, and raphe obscurus could be confirmed.

The distribution of MAO B immunoreactivity in the human brain stem has shown that many of the raphe neurons contained this monoamine degrading enzyme (34), although the percentage of immunoreactive neurons was considerably higher in the rostral raphe nuclei. Why MAO B could not be found in all PH8-i neurons especially in the caudal raphe is yet unknown. Many more brain stem structures were immunoreactive for MAO B than A and a major portion of MAO B was extraneuronally localized in glia cells. These data are supported by biochemical examinations that have demonstrated that in the human brain the vast majority of MAO enzyme activity (approximately 80%) occurs in the B form, which is the dominating type in glia cells (37). In contrast to this distribution MAO A was mostly found in neurons or the cellular processes that surrounded the neurons. In respect to the localization of MAO B in serotoninergic raphe neurons, it is interesting to note that

MAO B has a very low affinity for 5-HT (38). The hypothesis was formulated that MAO B in raphe neurons may serve primarily to degrade accumulated "foreign" amines and not 5-HT (34,35). On the other hand, MAO A, which is localized in the somata of the noradrenergic locus coeruleus neurons, has a higher affinity for both 5-HT and norepinephrine (39). The localization of MAO A in neurons of nuclei, which are known to be nonmonoaminergic (5,11) (e.g., the oculomotor nucleus), is somewhat astonishing. We could demonstrate that these neurons were not immunoreactive for TH or PH8, which indicates that they do not synthesize catecholamines or 5-HT. One possible function of MAO A in this localization could be to degrade monoamines from extrinsic sources, for example, from monoaminergic afferents. On the other hand, neurons of the substantia nigra did not contain either MAO A or B, although inhibitors of MAO B were shown to have beneficial therapeutic effects in Parkinson's disease (37). An explanation could be that these substances are effective in the target areas of the axons from the dopaminergic neurons in the substantia nigra. However, a similar immunohistochemical distribution of MAO was found by other groups (34).

The results of this study will provide a basis for further examination of 5-HT and catecholamine-related brain stem structures in neurodegenerative and dementing disorders.

ACKNOWLEDGMENTS

This work was supported in part by a grant from the Swiss National Foundation. We are grateful to Dr. C. W. Abell (University of Texas at Austin) for kindly providing the antibodies against human MAO A and B. Dr. B. Leonard was supported by an exchange postdoctoral fellowship 83NI-028031 from the NIH and Swiss National Foundation.

REFERENCES

1. Twarog BH, Page IH. Serotonin content of some mammalian tissues and urine and a method for its determination. *Am J Physiol* 1953;175:156–161.
2. McIlwain H, Bachelard HS. *Biochemistry and the central nervous system.* London: Livingstone, 1985.
3. Bradley PB. Serotonin: receptors and subtypes. In: Idzikowski C, Cowen PJ, eds. *Serotonin, sleep and mental disorders.* Petersfield: Wrightson, 1991:9–22.
4. Falck B, Hillarp NA, Thieme G, Torp A. Fluorescence of catecholamines and related compounds with formaldehyde. *J Histochem Cytochem* 1962;10:348–354.
5. Dahlström A, Fuxe K. Evidence for the existence of monoamine containing neurons in the central nervous system. I. Demonstration of monoamines in the cell bodies of brain stem neurons. *Acta Physiol Scand* 1964;232(suppl):1–55.
6. Olszewski J, Baxter D. *Cytoarchitecture of the human brain stem.* Basel: Karger, 1954.
7. Braak H. Ueber die Kerngebiete des menschlichen Hirnstammes II. Die Raphekerne. *Z Zellforsch* 1970;107:123–141.
8. Chan-Palay V. Indolamine neurons and their processes in the normal rat brain and in chronic diet-induced thiamine deficiency demonstrated by uptake of 3H-serotonin. *J Comp Neurol* 1977;176:467–494.

9. Steinbusch HW. Distribution of serotonin-immunoreactivity in the central nervous system of the rat—cell bodies and terminals. *Neuroscience* 1981;6:557–618.
10. Steinbusch HMW, Nieuwenhuys R. The raphe nuclei of the rat brainstem: a cytoarchitectonic and immunohistochemical study. In: Emson PC, ed. *Chemical neuroanatomy*. New York: Raven, 1983: 131–207.
11. Felten DL, Sladek JR. Monoamine distribution in primate brain V. Monoaminergic nuclei: anatomy, pathways and local organization. *Brain Res Bull* 1983;10:171–284.
12. Bowen DM, Allen SJ, Benton JS, et al. Biochemical assessment of serotonergic and cholinergic dysfunction and cerebral atrophy in Alzheimer's disease. *J Neurochem* 1983;41:266–272.
13. Curcio CA, Kemper T. Nucleus raphe dorsalis in dementia of the Alzheimer type: neurofibrillary changes and neuronal packing density. *J Neuropathol Exp Neurol* 1984;43:359–368.
14. Gottfries CG, Roos BE, Winblad B. Monoamine and monoamine metabolites in the human brain post mortem in senile dementia. *Aktuelle Gerontol* 1976;6:429–435.
15. Scatton B, Javoy-Agid F, Montfort JC, Agid Y. Neurochemistry of monoaminergic neurons in Parkinson's disease. In: Usdin E, ed. *Catecholamines: neuropharmacology and central nervous system—therapeutic aspects*. New York: Alan R Liss, 1984:43–52.
16. Tomlinson BE, Corsellis JAN. Ageing and the dementias. In: Adams JH, Corsellis JAN, Duchen LW, eds. *Greenfield's neuropathology*. London: Edward Arnold, 1984:951–1025.
17. Yamamoto T, Hirano A. Nucleus raphe dorsalis in Alzheimer's disease: neurofibrillary tangles and loss of large neurons. *Ann Neurol* 1985;17:573–577.
18. Jellinger K. Overview of morphological changes in Parkinson's disease. *Adv Neurol* 1986;45:1–18.
19. German DC, White CL, Sparkman DR. Alzheimer's disease: neurofibrillary tangles in nuclei that project to the cerebral cortex. *Neuroscience* 1987;21:305–312.
20. Elliott JM, Stephenson JD. Depression. In: Webster RA, Jordan CC, eds. *Neurotransmitters, drugs and disease*. London: Blackwell, 1989:355–393.
21. Chan-Palay V. Quantitation of catecholamine neurons in the locus coeruleus in human brains of normal young and older adults and in depression. *J Comp Neurol* 1989;287:357–372.
22. Chan-Palay V, Asan E. Alterations in catecholamine neurons of the locus coeruleus in senile dementia of the Alzheimer type and in Parkinson's disease with and without dementia and depression. *J Comp Neurol* 1989;287:373–392.
23. Chan-Palay V. Depression and senile dementia of the Alzheimer type: catecholamine changes in the locus coeruleus—basis for therapy. *Dementia* 1990;1:253–261.
24. Chan-Palay V. Depression and dementia in Parkinson's disease: catecholamine changes in the locus coeruleus: basis for therapy. *Dementia* 1991;2:7–17.
25. Idzikowski C, Cowen PJ. *Serotonin, sleep and mental disorder*. Petersfield: Wrightson, 1991.
26. Haan EA, Jennings IG, Cuello AC, et al. A monoclonal antibody recognizing all three aromatic amino acid hydroxylases allows identification of serotonergic neurons in human brain. *Brain Res* 1987;426:19–27.
27. Halliday GM, Li YW, Joh TH, et al. Distribution of monoamine-synthesizing neurons in the human medulla oblongata. *J Comp Neurol* 1988;273:301–317.
28. Baker KG, Halliday GM, Törk I. Cytoarchitecture of the human dorsal raphe nucleus. *J Comp Neurol* 1990;301:147–161.
29. Baker KG, Halliday GM, Halasz J-P, et al. Cytoarchitecture of serotonin-synthesizing neurons in the pontine tegmentum of the human brain. *Synapse* 1991;7:301–320.
30. Törk I, Hornung JP. Raphe nuclei and the serotonergic system. In: Paxinos G, ed. *The human nervous system*. New York: Academic Press, 1990:1001–1022.
31. Denney RM, Patel NT, Fritz NT, Abell CW. A monoclonal antibody elicited to human platelet monoamine oxidase. Isolation and specificity for human monoamine oxidase B but not A. *Molec Pharmacol* 1982;22:500–508.
32. Kochersperger LM, Waguespack A, Patterson JC, et al. Immunological uniqueness of human monoamine oxidase A and B. New evidence from studies with monoclonal antibodies to human MAO A. *J Neurosci* 5:2874–2881.
33. Johnston JP. Some observation upon a new inhibitor of monoamine oxidase in brain tissue. *Biochem Pharmacol* 1968;17:1285–1297.
34. Konradi CH, Svoma E, Jellinger K, Riederer P, Denney R, Thibault J. Topographic immunocytochemical mapping of monoamine oxidase-A, monoamine oxidase-B and tyrosine hydroxylase in human post mortem brain stem. *Neuroscience* 1988;26:791–802.
35. Westlund KN, Denney RM, Rose RM, Abell CW. Localization of distinct monoamine oxidase A and monoamine oxidase B cell populations in human brainstem. *Neuroscience* 1988;25:439–456.

36. Chan-Palay V. Somatostatin immunoreactive neurons in the human hippocampus and cortex shown by immunogold/silver intensification on vibratome sections: coexistence with neuropeptide Y neurons, and effects in Alzheimer-type dementia. *J Comp Neurol* 1987;260:201–223.
37. Riederer P, Konradi C, Schay V, et al. Localization of MAO-A and MAO-B in human brain: a step in understanding the therapeutic action of L-deprenyl. *Adv Neurol* 1986;45:111–116.
38. Goridis C, Neff N, Monoamine oxidase in sympathetic nerves: a transmitter specific enzyme type. *Br J Pharmacol* 1971;43:814–818.
39. Roth JA, Rivett AJ, Francis A, Pearce LB, Jeffrey D. Pathways of catecholamine metabolism: characterization, localization, and effects of reversible monoamine oxidase inhibitors. In: Tipton KF, Dostert P, Strolin-Benedetti M, eds. *Monoamine oxidase and disease: prospects for therapy with reversible inhibitors.* New York: Academic Press, 1984:459–468.

*Serotonin, the Cerebellum,
and Ataxia*, edited by
P. Trouillas and K. Fuxe.
Raven Press, Ltd., New York © 1993.

3

The Cerebellar Projection from the Neurons of the Raphe Nuclei and the Origin of the Serotoninergic Innervation of the Cerebellum

C. Batini

Laboratoire de Physiologie de la Motricité, CNRS URA 385, Université Pierre et Marie Curie, Faculté de Medicine Pitié-Salpêtrière, 75013 Paris, France

The classic afferent systems to the cerebellar cortex are the mossy fibers arising in multiple nuclei of the brain stem and the climbing fibers arising in the inferior olive (IO). A third category of afferents, the monoaminergic, later described by Hökfelt and Fuxe (15) includes fibers containing norepinephrine and serotonin (5-HT) (and, to a lesser extent, dopamine [23]). One question raised by this discovery is the location of the cell bodies giving rise to these specific afferents. We will try to describe in this chapter what is known about the origin of the 5-HT innervation of the cerebellum.

Most of the 5-HT neurons are located in the raphe nuclei. This was first shown by Dahlström and Fuxe (12) and confirmed by others, with histofluorescence, biochemical, and, more recently, immunohistochemical methods (24,25,27). Since Brodal et al. (9) demonstrated with the retrograde degeneration method that the neurons of the raphe nuclei project to the cerebellar cortex and the cerebellar nuclei, it was generally accepted that the 5-HT cerebellar afferents originate in these nuclei.

The connection of the raphe nuclei with the cerebellar cortex was also confirmed by several studies that used anterograde (6), but mostly retrograde (3,13,17,20–22), tracers in cat, rat (5), opossum (28), and monkey (14). The raphe nuclei found to be involved in the cortical projection were (following the nomenclature of Taber et al. [26]): the nucleus raphe pallidus, obscurus, magnus, pontis, dorsalis, and centralis superior. There was no clear evidence of a localized topographical relationship between the raphe nuclei and cerebellar areas, although some differences were reported in the number of nuclei and the density of neurons involved in the projection. Nevertheless the possibility of a topographical relationship remained open since only the vermis and the flocculus were explored in the cerebellar cortex using retrograde tracers. Less attention was given to the connections to the three pairs of cerebellar nuclei, medialis, interpositus, and lateralis, which receive innervation from the raphe nuclei (9,10,13). No evidence for localization was described. The nucleus lateralis of both rat and monkey was shown to receive fibers from all the raphe nuclei innervating the cerebellar cortex (10), thus suggesting a collateral innervation from the same neurons or pool of neurons. In addition, the raphe cerebellar projection is reported to be bilateral, going either to the cerebellar cortex (17,21) or the cerebellar nuclei (10).

An important discovery came from the work of Bobillier et al. (6), who showed that the same raphe nuclei projecting to the cerebellar cortex also project to many other structures in the brain stem, diencephalon, and telencephalon. Whether these multiple efferents originate in separate neurons of the raphe or whether they are the result of repeated branching of the same neuron is not known.

As pointed out by several authors (5), not all the neurons of the raphe nuclei contain 5-HT. Therefore, in order to demonstrate that raphe neurons projecting to the cerebellar cortex contain 5-HT, the double-labeling method was applied. This consisted of identifying the raphe cerebellar neurons with a retrogradely transported tracer and revealing the presence of 5-HT in the same neurons. This experiment was done in the opossum (28), the rat (5), and the cat (20). The present results were obtained using a complex of colloidal gold/apo horseradish peroxidase (HRP) as the retrogradely transported tracer.

In our experiments the tracer was injected in two selected regions of the cerebellar cortex of the cat: the posterior vermis (around the midline) bilaterally and the hemispheres unilaterally. The cortex was only impregnated by the tracer, with no diffusion to the underlying cerebellar nuclei. The two injected areas were far enough apart to allow the detection of local differences in the raphe nuclei involved in the cerebellar projection. Retrograde labeling was detected using a silver intensification method (1) in free floating 50-μm sections cut with a vibratome. The presence of 5-HT was revealed in the same sections by immunohistochemistry, following the method described elsewhere (11) and using highly specific (7) antibodies raised in the rabbit against 5-HT (courtesy of J. Puizillout). Many neurons of the raphe nuclei were found to be only 5-HT immunoreactive (5-HT-IR). Others were found to be only retrogradely labeled; they are the neurons identified as projecting to the cerebellar cortex. A few were double labeled (the 5-HT-IR neurons projecting to the cerebellar cortex). Figure 1 shows an example of the three types of labeled perikarya.

The distribution in the raphe nuclei of the neurons projecting to the injection site of the cerebellar cortex and those containing 5-HT as well were examined in horizontal sections of the brain stem. Retrogradely labeled neurons were found in several structures of the brain stem. Only those traced in the raphe nuclei and the IO were reported (Figs. 2 and 3). The IO has an exclusive point-to-point topographical relation with the cerebellar cortex (see ref. 8 for the cat) and served as a control of the localization of the injection site. Figure 2 shows a general view of the results obtained in an animal in which the tracer was injected in the posterior vermis. In this

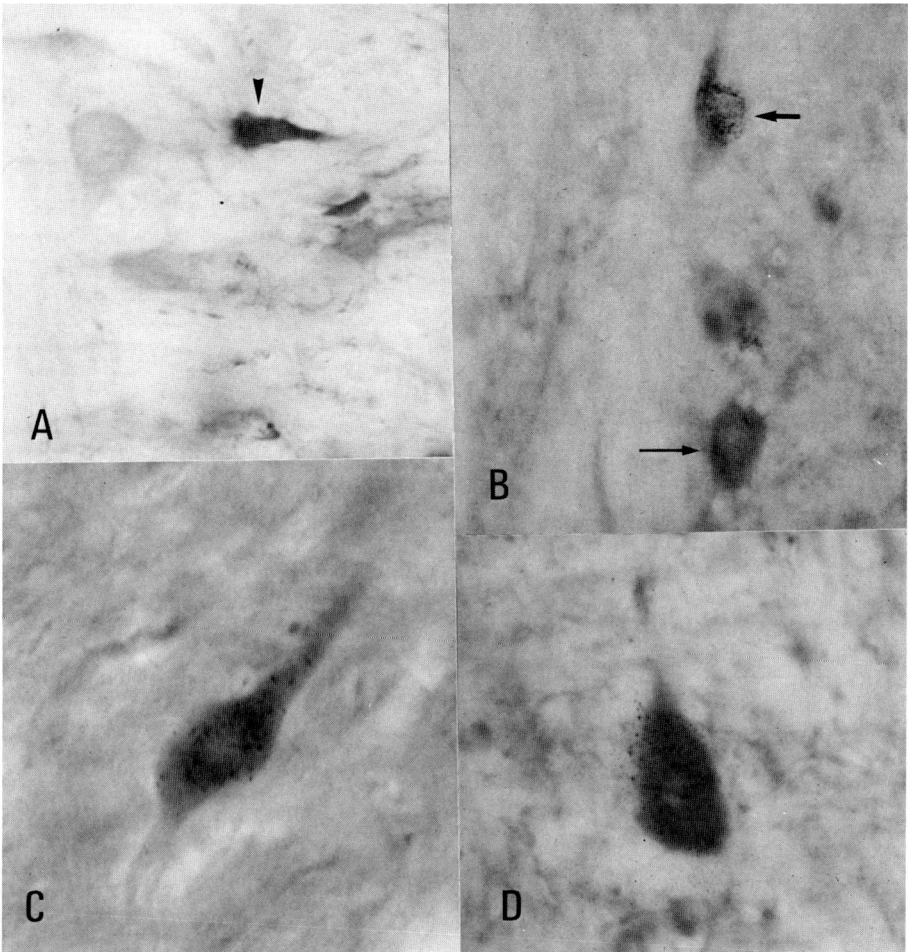

FIG. 1. Photomicrographs showing the retrogradely labeled, the 5-HT-IR, and the double-labeled neurons. **A**: Immunoreactivity in the raphe magnus of a cat; *arrowhead* shows a 5-HT-IR neuron; the other neurons with light staining are considered immunonegative. **B**: Raphe pontis of a cat following an injection of the gold/apo-HRP complex in the cerebellar cortex, and showing a retrogradely labeled neuron (*short arrow*) and a 5-HT-IR retrogradely labeled neuron (*long arrow*). **C** and **D**: Double-labeled neurons at higher magnification found, respectively, in the nucleus lateralis of the cerebellar cortex and the nucleus centralis superior.

case the caudal part of the medial accessory olive was marked bilaterally, and in fact zone A of the posterior vermis had been injected bilaterally. With regard to the raphe cerebellar projection, this experiment illustrates two major points:

a. As in previous studies, the raphe nuclei involved in the projection were the raphe pallidus, obscurus, magnus, pontis, and centralis superior. However, the projection appeared to originate from two distinct main zones of the raphe, one

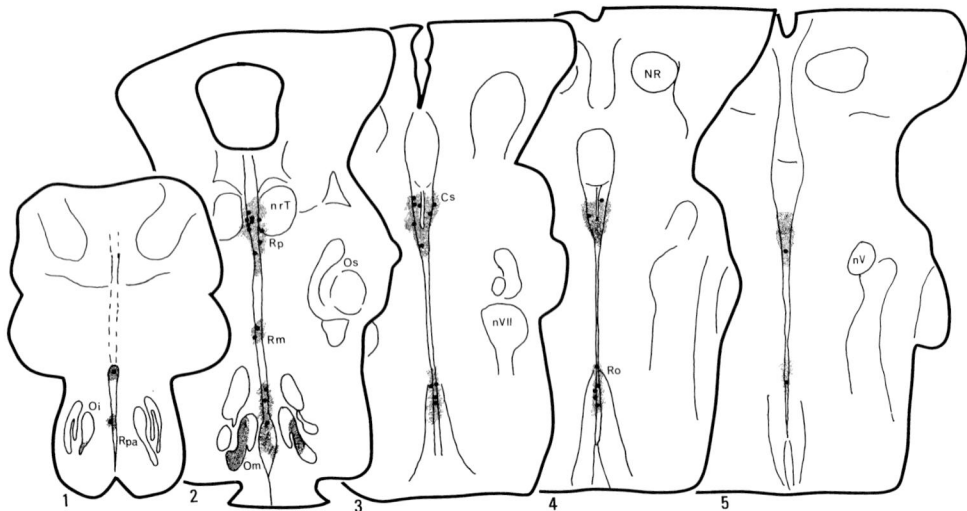

FIG. 2. General view of the brain stem of a cat showing the labeled areas in the raphe nuclei and in the IO, following a bilateral injection of gold/apo-HRP in zone A of the cerebellar cortex. Five sections at equal distance in the brain stem cut horizontally (1 to 5 from ventral to dorsal) are shown. The shaded areas represent the regions of the raphe and the IO where retrogradely labeled neurons were observed. The black spots represent the 5-HT-IR retrogradely labeled neurons identified in the serial sections. Abbreviations in this and the following figures: CE, nucleus cuneatus externus; CS, nucleus centralis superior; NR, nucleus ruber; nrT, nucleus reticularis tegmenti pontis; NspV, nucleus spinalis trigemini; Nst, nucleus subtrigeminalis; nV, nucleus motorius trigemini; nVII, nucleus facialis; Oi, inferior oliva; Om, medial accessory oliva; Op, principal oliva; Os, superior oliva; Ph, nucleus praepositus hypoglossi; Pm, paramedianus; RL, nucleus reticularis lateralis; Rm, nucleus raphe magnus; Ro, nucleus raphe obscurus; Rp, nucleus raphe pontis; Rpa, nucleus raphe pallidus; Vest, vestibular nuclei.

anterior, including the nucleus raphe pontis and centralis superior, and the other posterior, including the nucleus raphe pallidus, obscurus, and magnus. The nucleus raphe dorsalis could not be explored in our study; however, if involved in the projection it will belong to the anterior zone. A larger number of labeled neurons were observed in the anterior zone of the raphe, as compared to the posterior. Labeled neurons were traced bilaterally in the raphe, a result expected, however, from the bilateral injection of the tracer performed in this particular experiment.

b. Some of the retrogradely labeled neurons were 5-HT-IR (double labeled); their proportion, however, appeared to be less than expected.

Figure 3 shows a general view of the brain stem in an experiment in which zone D of the cerebellar hemispheres was injected in one side. The retrogradely labeled neurons were traced in the contralateral principal olive only. In this, as in the previous case, in spite of the different localization of the injection site with no overlapping (with the injection site of the preceding example), similar zones of the raphe nuclei were retrogradely labeled: one anterior, including the nucleus raphe pontis

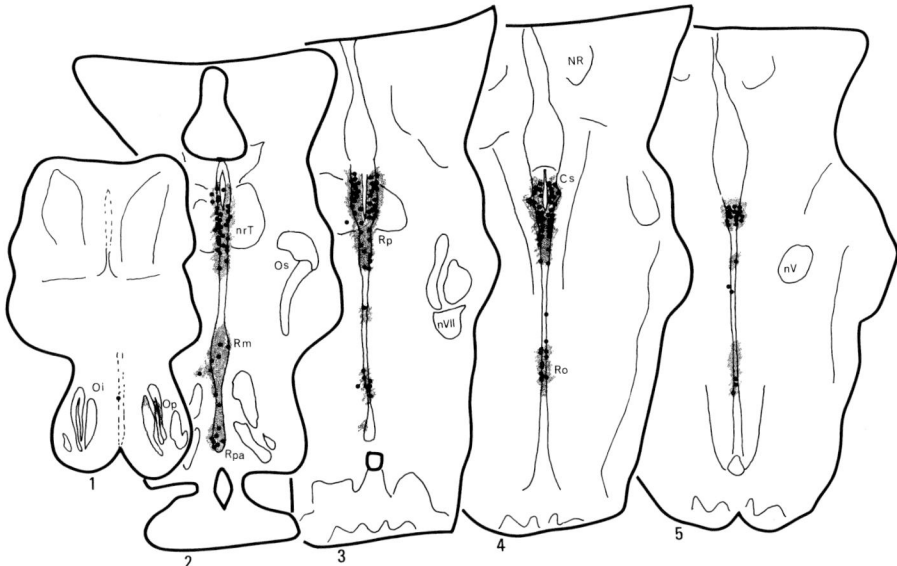

FIG. 3. General view of the brain stem of a cat showing the labeled areas in the raphe nuclei and the IO, following the unilateral injection of gold/apo-HRP in zone D of the cerebellar cortex. Same representation as in Fig. 2.

and centralis superior, and one posterior, including the nucleus raphe pallidus, obscurus, and magnus. The total extent of the two labeled areas was larger than in the previous case (compare Figs. 2 and 3); the total number of retrogradely labeled neurons in each area is larger also. In addition, the labeled neurons were distributed about equally in both sides of the raphe, while the tracer was, in this case, only injected on one side. These results support the previous data (see above), which indicate an absence of localization in the raphe cerebellar projections.

The double-labeled neurons identified in the raphe appeared to be more numerous in the case shown in Fig. 3 than in that in Fig. 2. Their number, however, was still lower than expected. To quantify the proportion of the double-labeled neurons in thick immunostained sections is a difficult problem for several reasons: (i) The antibodies usually do not penetrate completely to the central core of the section, and the impregnation of both surfaces of the free-floating section varies from one experiment to another. The histochemical reaction, however, reveals the retrograde tracer in the entire section thickness (2). Thus, the number of double-labeled elements could be variable and is probably underestimated. (ii) Numerous immunostained fibers and terminal boutons may mimick light immunoreactivity, and therefore only intensely immunostained perikarya can be considered 5-HT-IR. (iii) The silver grains of the retrograde tracer filling the neurons make it difficult to estimate the degree of immunostaining. (iv) The retrogradely labeled neurons were also observed in the raphe and the border structures as a continuum, making it difficult and subjective to count the labeled neurons in the raphe only; this was particularly true in the anterior zone of the raphe where the retrogradely labeled neurons were densely packed. Therefore, we prefer not to quantify the double-labeled neurons, but, to provide an estimate, we counted them in the posterior zone of the raphe where the neurons projecting to the cerebellar cortex were less numerous but easier to distinguish from the neighboring structures. In two experiments in which the tracer was injected in zone A of the cerebellar cortex, the proportion of 5-HT-IR neurons was 12% and 14%, respectively, of the number of retrogradely labeled cells. In two other experiments in which the tracer was injected in zone D of the cortex, the proportion of 5-HT-IR neurons was, respectively, 16% and 23%. In spite of the large variability, these data indicate that the proportion of double-labeled neurons is not negligible and that the proportion of 5-HT neurons projecting to zone D is larger than that projecting to zone A.

In the cat, Rosina and Steinbusch (20) reported 5-HT-IR neurons projecting to the cerebellar cortex from the raphe nuclei, namely, from the nucleus raphe dorsalis, pontis, and centralis superior. Bishop and Ho (5) found in rat very few 5-HT-IR neurons projecting to the cerebellar cortex from the nucleus raphe magnus and centralis superior. Walker et al. (28), in the opossum, and Kerr and Bishop (18), in the cat, were unable to trace 5-HT-IR neurons projecting to the cerebellar cortex from the raphe nuclei. Perhaps the differences in our results depend on the tracer used: the gold/apo-HRP complex is, for us (*unpublished results*), a more sensitive tracer.

These experiments allow us to conclude that, indeed, the raphe nuclei provide 5-HT innervation of the cerebellar cortex, as postulated previously. In addition, they show that the 5-HT-IR neurons, presumed serotoninergic, are only a small part of the raphe cerebellar projection. Thus, the main part of the projection must have another, as yet unknown, function.

They also raise an important question: can the 5-HT-IR neurons of the raphe projecting to the cerebellar cortex account for the extensive serotoninergic cerebellar innervation (see Chapter 6, this volume)? Diffuse branching of the raphe nuclei axons have been described (see Chapter 1, this volume), and this was also suggested by the absence of topographical localization found in our experiments. It could explain the paucity of 5-HT-IR raphe cerebellar neurons. However, serotoninergic neurons have been described in brain stem structures other than the raphe nuclei (5,12,18,19,24,27,28). Of particular interest for the cerebellar functions are the 5-HT-IR periolivary neurons, which send terminals to the IO (11; for the 5-HT innervation of the IO, see Chapter 7, this volume). Recently, 5-HT-IR neurons projecting to the cerebellar cortex from various brain stem structures, including the periolivary neurons, have been described in the rat (5), the opossum (28), and the cat (18,20). Our experiments confirm this.

Figures 4 and 5 show the results obtained from two cats in which the double-labeling method was applied following injection of the gold/apo-HRP complex in the cerebellar cortex. The brain stem was, in these cases, serially cut in the frontal plane. All the retrogradely labeled neurons and the retrogradely labeled 5-HT-IR (double-labeled) neurons found in the lower brain stem were reported in the figures.

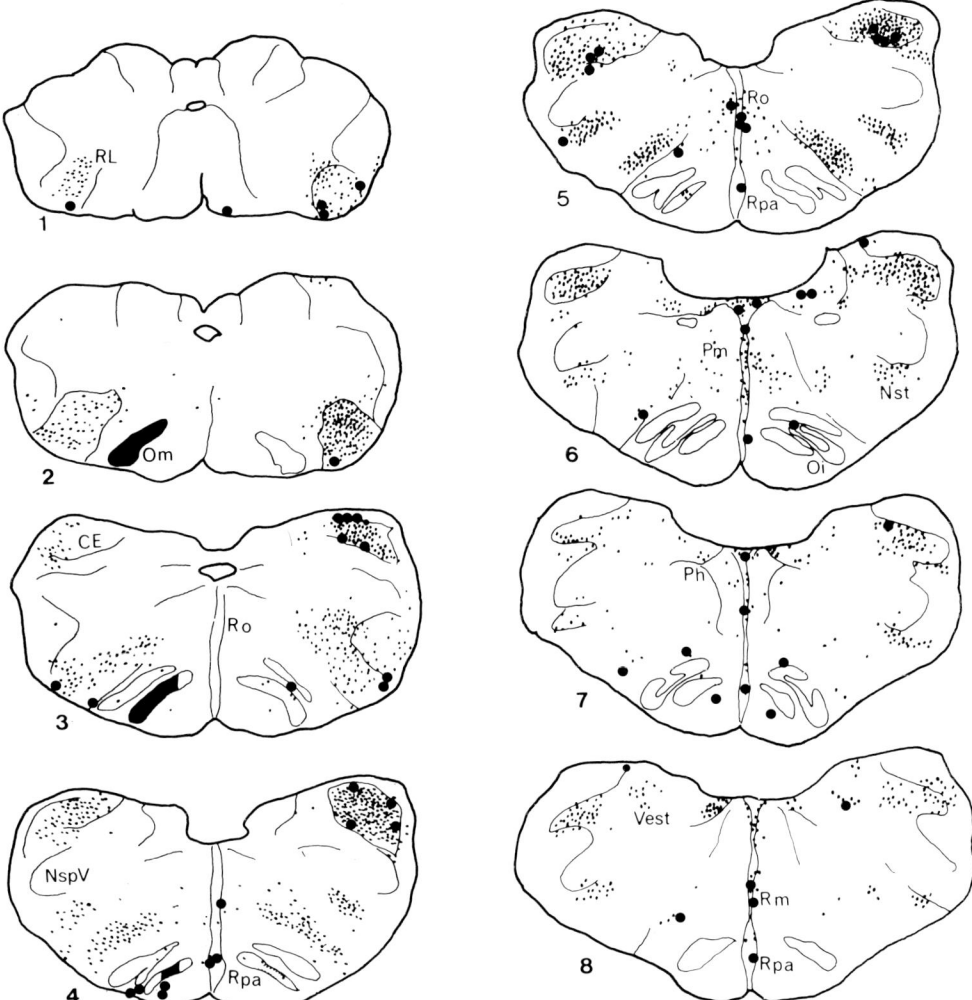

FIG. 4. General view of the lower brain stem of a cat showing the labeled neurons observed following a bilateral injection of gold/apo-HRP in zone A of the cerebellar cortex. Eight sections at equal distance of the brain stem, cut in the frontal plane (1 to 8, from caudal to rostral) are shown. The *small black dots* represent individual neurons retrogradely labeled, and the *large black dots*, 5-HT-IR retrogradely labeled neurons, identified in all the serial sections observed.

In one experiment, zone A of the posterior vermis was injected bilaterally and the caudal part of the medial accessory olive was marked bilaterally (Fig. 4). In the other experiment, zone D of the cerebellar hemisphere was injected unilaterally, and the contralateral principal olive only was marked (Fig. 5). As described above, retrogradely labeled and double-labeled neurons were found in the raphe nuclei in both cases, with no evident differences in the localization.

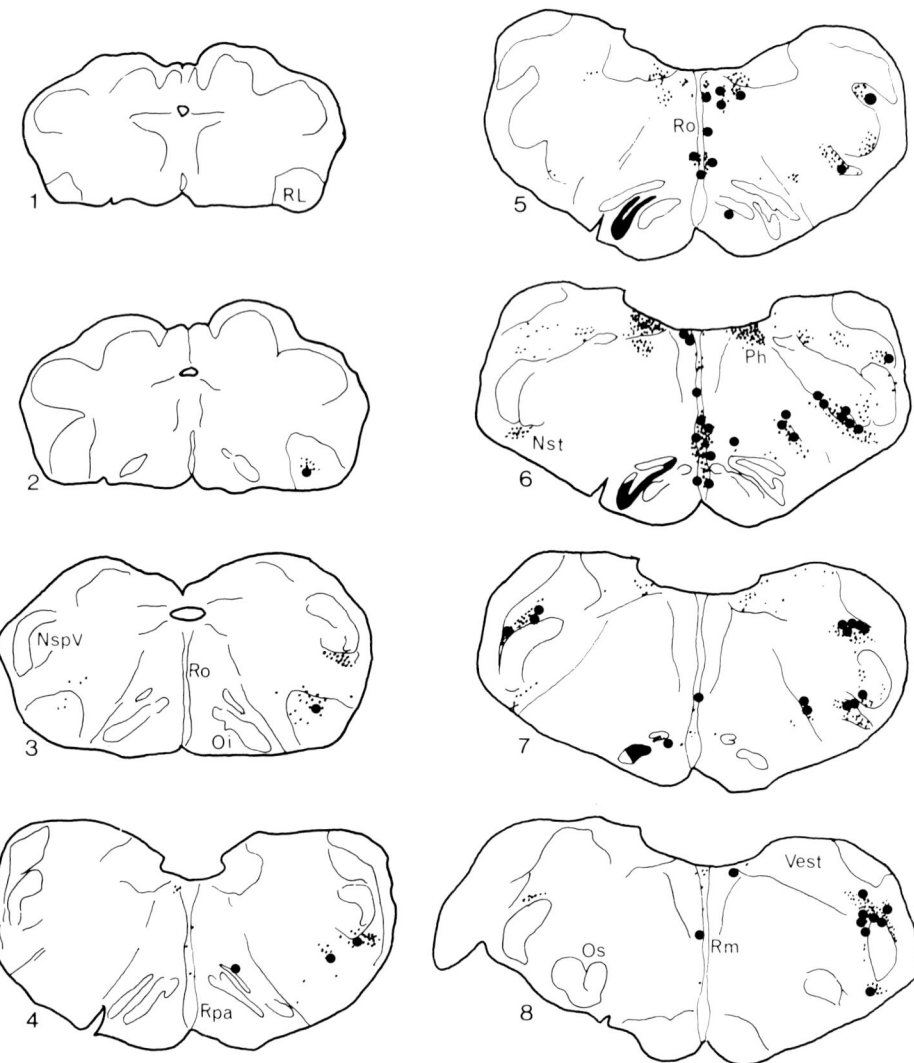

FIG. 5. General view of the lower brain stem of a cat showing the labeled neurons observed following a bilateral injection of gold/apo-HRP in zone D of the cerebellar cortex. Same representation as in Fig. 4.

Several other brain stem structures contained retrogradely labeled neurons: the lateral reticular nucleus, the subtrigeminal nucleus, the paramedian nucleus, the external cuneatus nucleus, the vestibular and perihypoglossal complexes, and the periolivary neurons, as illustrated in Figs. 4 and 5, and also the cerebellar nuclei (not illustrated). All these neurons are described to project to the cerebellar cortex as mossy fibers (16). The projections show clear differences of localization in the two experiments (cf. Figs. 4 and 5), due to the different zone of the cerebellar cortex injected with the tracer (16).

In addition, 5-HT-IR neurons projecting to the cerebellar cortex (double-labeled neurons) were observed in most of these nonraphe structures found marked with the tracer, including the cerebellar nuclei (Fig. 1C). It can be seen that they were found in the nuclei giving mossy fibers to the cerebellar cortex and were always intermingled with the retrogradely labeled neurons only. They therefore follow the localizations obtained in individual experiments according to the different injection sites (cf. Figs. 4 and 5).

The IO, whose axons terminate in the cerebellar cortex as climbing fibers, did not display double-labeled neurons. A few double-labeled elements, however, were located nearby; they are the periolivary neurons, which terminate in the IO. This result suggests that the periolivary neurons innervate both the IO and the cerebellar cortex, but it does not predict whether they are separate neurons or branching of the same neurons.

The number of double-labeled neurons appears to be relatively higher in the experiment in which zone D of the cerebellar cortex was injected, although the injection site was not larger (see also the raphe nuclei illustrated in Figs. 2 and 3). This last observation raises the question of whether the 5-HT innervation of the lateral areas of the cerebellar cortex is more densely represented in the brain stem. Nonetheless, the number of double-labeled neurons, with respect to the retrogradely labeled neurons in a given nucleus, is very low. In both of the cases illustrated in Figs. 4 and 5, the number is less than that described for the raphe nuclei. Kerr and Bishop (18) have also found a low proportion of double-labeled neurons, from 2.1% to 14.5% in different nuclei.

In summary, our results show that the serotoninergic innervation of the cerebellar cortex does not originate solely in the raphe nuclei, but comes from multiple sources. They are the nuclei known to project to the cerebellar cortex as mossy fibers and the periolivary neurons. The raphe cerebellar projection must be considered one of these sources. It appears that a few 5-HT fibers accompany the mossy afferents to the cerebellar cortex and terminate in the same areas. Most of the 5-HT terminals are in the granule cells layer (Chapter 6, this volume), as are the mossy fibers. The IO, which sends climbing afferents to the cerebellar cortex, does not contain 5-HT neurons, but a parallel innervation could be provided by the 5-HT periolivary neurons. Some of the serotoninergic fibers terminate in the molecular layer and in the Purkinje cell layer, as do the climbing fibers, although the proportion varies between different species (5,18,28; Chapter 6, this volume). In the cerebellar cortex 5-HT was shown to control glutamate release from the glutamatergic terminals, which are present in both the molecular and the granular cell layers (see Chapter 11, this volume). It appears that the 5-HT fibers, accompanying each group of afferents to the cerebellar cortex, could provide a specific control of glutamate release in the cortical area reached by a given group of afferents.

Another clear finding was the relative scarcity of serotoninergic neurons projecting to the cerebellar cortex, all sources considered. This might be compensated for by the extensive branching of the 5-HT fibers suggested by our present results. On the other hand, most of the cerebellar 5-HT fibers have nonjunctional terminals (4; Chapter 1, this volume) presumably communicating at a distance by volume transmission (see Chapter 1, this volume). Such a system does not need to rely on the density of neurons. We propose, as a working hypothesis, that the serotoninergic neurons may have a dual role, innervating nonserotoninergic neurons in the same nucleus of origin and in their target areas, the cerebellar cortex and the cerebellar nuclei (the effects of exogenous 5-HT on the cerebellar cortex and the cerebellar nuclei have been described using an electrophysiological method; see Chapters 16 and 17, this volume). The periolivary neurons sending fibers to both the IO and the cerebellar cortex and nuclei, are one example of this type of organization.

ACKNOWLEDGMENTS

The author is grateful to M. Guegan for her excellent technical assistance in histology. The drawings in this chapter were done by M. M. Kado. Thanks are due to P. Turner for revising the English.

REFERENCES

1. Basbaum AI, Menetrey D. Wheat germ agglutinin-apoHRP gold: a new retrograde tracer for light and electron-microscopic single- and double-label studies. *J Comp Neurol* 1987;261:306–318.
2. Batini C, Buisseret-Delmas C, Compoint C, Daniel H. The GABAergic neurones of the cerebellar nuclei in the rat: projections to the cerebellar cortex. *Neurosci Lett* 1989;99:251–256.
3. Batini C, Buisseret-Delmas C, Corvisier C, Hardy O, Jassik-Gerschenfeld D. Brain stem nuclei giving fibers to lobules VI and VII of the cerebellar vermis. *Brain Res* 1978;153:241–261.
4. Beaudet A, Sotelo C. Synaptic remodeling of serotonin axon terminals in rat agranular cerebellum. *Brain Res* 1981;206:305–329.
5. Bishop GA, Ho RH. The distribution and origin of serotonin immunoreactivity in the rat cerebellum. *Brain Res* 1985;331:195–207.
6. Bobillier P, Seguin S, Petitjean F, Salvert D, Touret M, Jouvet M. The raphe nuclei of the cat brain stem: a topographical atlas of their efferent projections as revealed by autoradiography. *Brain Res* 1976;113:449–486.
7. Bras H, Chazal G, Destombes J, Puizillout JJ. Anti-5-hydroxytryptamine antibodies: studies on their cross-reactivity in vitro and their immunohistochemical specificity. *Exp Brain Res* 1986;63:627–638.
8. Brodal A, Kawamura K. Olivocerebellar projections: a review. *Adv Anat Embryol Cell Biol* 1980;64:1–140.
9. Brodal A, Taber E, Walberg S. The raphe nuclei of the brain stem in the cat. II. Efferent connections. *J Comp Neurol* 1960;114:239–259.
10. Chan-Palay V. *Cerebellar dentate nucleus. Organization, cytology and transmitters*. Berlin/Heidelberg/New York: Springer-Verlag, 1977.
11. Compoint C, Buisseret-Delmas C. Origin, distribution and organization of the serotoninergic innervation in the inferior olivary complex of the rat. *Arch Ital Biol* 1988;126:99–110.
12. Dahlström A, Fuxe K. Evidence for the existence of monoamine-containing neurons in the central nervous system. I. Demonstration of monoamines in the cell bodies of brain stem neurons. *Acta Physiol Scand* 1964;62(suppl 232):3–56.
13. Eller TW, Chan-Palay V. Afferents to the cerebellar lateral nucleus. Evidence for retrograde transport of horseradish peroxidase after pressure injections through micropipettes. *J Comp Neurol* 1976;166:285–301.

14. Frankfurter A, Weber JT, Harting JK. Brain stem projections to lobule VII of the posterior vermis in the squirrel monkey: as demonstrated by the retrograde axonal transport of tritiated horseradish peroxidase. *Brain Res* 1977;124:135–139.
15. Hökfelt T, Fuxe K. Cerebellar monoamine nerve terminals, a new type of afferent fibers to the cortex cerebelli. *Exp Brain Res* 1969;9:63–72.
16. Ito M. *The cerebellum and neural control.* New York: Raven Press, 1984.
17. Kawasaki T, Sato Y. Afferent projection from the dorsal nucleus of the raphe to the flocculus in cats. *Brain Res* 1980;197:496–502.
18. Kerr CVH, Bishop GA. Topographical organization in the origin of serotoninergic projections to different regions of the cat cerebellar cortex. *J Comp Neurol* 1991;304:502–515.
19. Kimoto Y, Satoh K, Sakumoto T, Tohyama M, Shimizu N. Afferent fiber connections from the lower brain stem to the rat cerebellum by the horseradish peroxidase method combined with MAO staining, with special reference to noradrenergic neurons. *J Hinforsch* 1978;19:85–100.
20. Rosina A, Steinbusch H. Origin of serotonergic afferents to cat cerebellum. A combined immunohistochemical and retrograde tracing study. *Neurosci Lett* 1983(suppl 14):S315.
21. Sato Y, Kawasaki T, Ikarashi K. Afferent projections from the brainstem to the three floccular zones in cats. II. Mossy fiber projections. *Brain Res* 1983;272:37–48.
22. Shinnar S, Maciewicz RJ, Shofer RJ. A raphe projection to cat cerebellar cortex. *Brain Res* 1975;97:139–143.
23. Simon H, Moal ML, Calas A. Efferents and afferents of the ventral tegmental-A10 region studied after local injection of (^{3}H)leucine and horseradish peroxidase. *Brain Res* 1979;175:1–23.
24. Steinbusch HWM. Distribution of serotonin-immunoreactivity in the central nervous system of the rat cell bodies and terminals. *Neuroscience* 1981;6:557–618.
25. Steinbusch HWM, Nieuwenhuys R. The raphe nuclei of the rat brainstem: a cytoarchitectonic and immunohistochemical study. In: Emson PC, ed. *Chemical neuroanatomy.* New York: Raven Press, 1983:131–207.
26. Taber E, Brodal A, Walberg F. The raphe nuclei of the brain stem in the cat. I. Normal topography and cytoarchitecture and general discussion. *J Comp Neurol* 1960;114:161–187.
27. Takeuchi Y, Kimura H, Sano Y. Immunohistochemical demonstration of serotonin-containing nerve fibers in the cerebellum. *Cell Tissue Res* 1982;226:1–12.
28. Walker JJ, Bishop GA, Ho RH, King JS. Brainstem origin of serotonin and enkephalin immunoreactive afferents to the opossum's cerebellum. *J Comp Neurol* 1988;276:481–497.

*Serotonin, the Cerebellum,
and Ataxia*, edited by
P. Trouillas and K. Fuxe.
Raven Press, Ltd., New York © 1993.

4

Distribution of Tryptophan Hydroxylase Immunoreactive Neurons in the Human Brain Stem

Nicolas Kopp, Michèle Aguerra, Dominique Martin,
*Michel Maitre, and Marie-Françoise Belin

*Laboratoire d'Anatomie Pathologique, Faculté de Médecine Alexis Carrel,
69372 Lyon, France; *INSERM U44, 67085 Strasbourg, France*

Brain serotonergic systems are thought to be involved in many physiological functions (sleep, pain, respiration, memory, aggressive behavior) and in maturation and trophicity of nervous cells. These systems have been implicated in the genesis of many diseases and pathological states, such as depression and suicide, dementia of the Alzheimer type, Parkinson's disease, degeneration altering the cerebellum, Down's syndrome, and the cerebral consequences of chronic undernutrition.

Their anatomical distribution has been widely investigated in different species by histofluorescence (9,17,25), autoradiographic (2,5,8,11,18,22), and immunohistochemical methods (7,28,30,33).

Data are available in nonhuman primates (1,12,15,30) and humans (19) as well as from Olson et al. (20), (using 3- to 4-month-old fetuses), Takahashi et al. (29), (using 3- to 7-month-old fetuses), and Baker et al. (3), and Törk and Hornung (31) (adults, mean age, 65 years).

The work of Nobin and Björklund (19) and Olson et al. (20) was based on the Falck-Hillarp histofluorescence technique. Takahashi et al. (29) used an antibody directed against serotonin; in all these instances, the applicability of the cytochemical method used was limited by post-mortem degradation and diffusion of the neurotransmitter. Thus, the method could be fruitfully performed only in brains for which fixation could be rapid enough, i.e., in brains that had a small volume and were collected shortly after death. For these reasons, only fetal brains could be studied.

Enzyme immunocytochemistry appeared to be less hindered by these pitfalls. Therefore, Törk and Hornung (31) and Baker et al. (3) developed and used a protocol based on the identification and localization of an enzyme implied in the synthesis of serotonin; the enzyme, called PH8, was a monoclonal antibody raised to monkey liver phenylalanine hydroxylase, recognizing all three amino acid decarboxylases: phenylalanine hydroxylase, tyrosine hydroxylase, and tryptophan hydroxylase (13). PH8 was rendered specific to tryptophan hydroxylase-containing neurons by the authors with the use of special fixation and embedding procedures.

To investigate the anatomical distribution of serotonergic neurons in the human post-mortem brain, we chose to use a specific polyclonal antibody against tryptophan hydroxylase (TPOH) (33). TPOH, the rate-limiting enzyme in the biosynthesis of serotonin, is only confined in serotonin neurons; it is, therefore, considered the only marker allowing specification of the serotonergic nature of a neuron. The TPOH polyclonal antibody was used successfully in the rat (33). Experimental conditions were established for its utilization on post-mortem brains obtained at autopsy from neonates, infants, and adults. Another aim of the study was to apply a routine fixation procedure.

MATERIAL AND METHODS

Six brains were obtained at autopsy (Laboratoire d'Anatomie Pathologique, Hôpital Edouard Herriot, Lyon, France) from two neonates, one infant, and three adults considered as devoid of neurologic, psychiatric, and endocrine disorders (see Table 1).

The brain stem was isolated from the brain, and leptomeninges and vessels were stripped out. The brain stem was, after 3 hr of fixation by immersion into eight blocks (mesencephalon, 2; pons, 3; medulla oblongata, 3), perpendicular to its main axis, as indicated by the atlas of Olszewski and Baxter (21). The fixation medium was paraformaldehyde 0.1 M, 4% at pH 7.4 with 0.2 picric acid. The eight blocks remained in the fixation medium at 4°C for 48 to 72 hr (according to the size). The

TABLE 1.

Case	Age	Sex	Post-mortem delay (hr)	Cause of death
D.O.	14 hr (27-week gestation)	F	8	Hyaline membranes
G.I.	2.5 hr (38-week gestation)	M	29	Failure of ligation of umbilical cord
G.I.	50 days (38-week gestation)	M	11.75	Sudden infant death syndrome explained by myocarditis, diffuse hepatic steatosis, moderate pulmonary-intestinal inflammatory infiltrate
C.O.	60 years	M	14.5	Pulmonary lymphoblastic lymphoma
B.A.	68 years	M	7	Myocardial infarction
T.A.	68 years	M	11	Angor pectoris, paroxysmal tachyarrhythmia, myocardial infarctions

blocks were then rinsed for 18 hr in 15% sucrose dissolved in 0.1 M sodium phosphate-buffered saline (PBS), pH 7.4. The blocks were frozen in methylbutane at −60°C. They were stored at −20°C for less than 10 days.

The blocks were cut at 20 μm with a cryostat. Sections were collected on albumin-coated slides. Every fourth consecutive section was used for the study. Four sections were used for immunohistochemistry and the fifth was stained with cresyl violet for location of anatomical landmarks. The immunohistochemical experiment was based on the peroxidase-antiperoxidase (PAP) technique following a procedure already described (33). The immunohistochemical sections and cresyl violet sections were drawn with a photographic enlarger. Schematic graphs were made in 11 planes of each section. Each plane was represented with a slight modification of the cresyl violet-based atlas of Olszewski and Baxter (21) and TPOH immunoreactive (IR) cell bodies were positioned in the anatomical landmarks by dots, one dot corresponding to approximately four cell bodies. The 11 planes (Figs. 3–13) were numbered in a caudorostral direction.

RESULTS

IR dots were found in the ependymal wall of the fourth ventricle (Fig. 1). These could be supraependymal fibers. Subependymal fibers were also seen.

IR cell bodies were observed in six cases, including the one with a post-mortem delay of 29 hr. Cell bodies were usually much more IR than neurites, except for the area of the nucleus raphe pallidus and periaqueductal gray (Fig. 2) where neurites were also very distinctly seen. The intensity of immunoreactivity was greater in neonates and infants than in adults; this discrepancy has already been mentioned for tyrosine hydroxylase IR neurons (23) and neurotensin IR neurons (26). The distribution was mainly confined to the limits of raphe nuclei, as defined by Olszewski and Baxter (21), Braak (6), and Baker et al. (4) but also overlapped with other structures of brain stem.

Medulla at the level of the midolive and area postrema (Fig. 3). TPOH IR cell bodies (TICB) were on both sides of the midline, separated by approximately 200 to 400 μm. They were disposed in a dorsal part (nucleus raphe obscurus) separated from a ventral part (nucleus raphe pallidus). Laterally, TICB were in a dense pack in the nucleus medulla oblongata lateralis, ventral part and, more scattered, in the nucleus medulla oblongata centralis, subnucleus dorsalis. A few TICB were seen in stratum gliosum subependymale.

Upper part of olive at the emergence of the acoustic nerve (Fig. 4). On both sides of midline, TICB were in a continuous straight line (nucleus raphe obscurus dorsally and nucleus raphe pallidus ventrally). Laterally, TICB were in nucleus paragigantocellularis, lateral and ventral parts.

Lower pons at the level of the nucleus of the seventh nerve and crossing by the sixth nerve (Fig. 5). A first group of TICB was on the midline with a dorsal expansion laterally toward the dorsal part of the nucleus pontis centralis caudalis and with

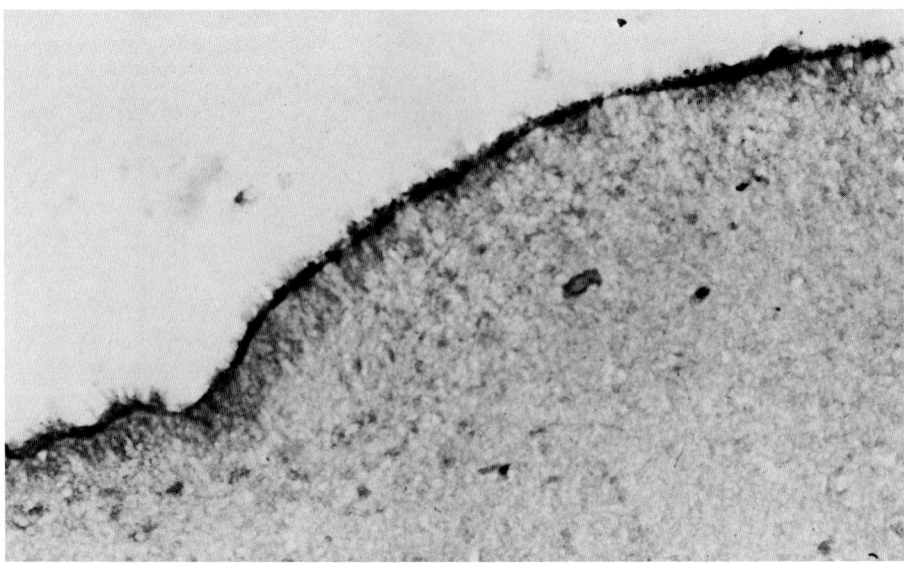

FIG. 1. Wall of the fourth ventricle. Dense TPOH immunoreactivity of the ependymal cells. On the apical area of cells, in the ventricle, small dots are seen (supraependymal fibers?).

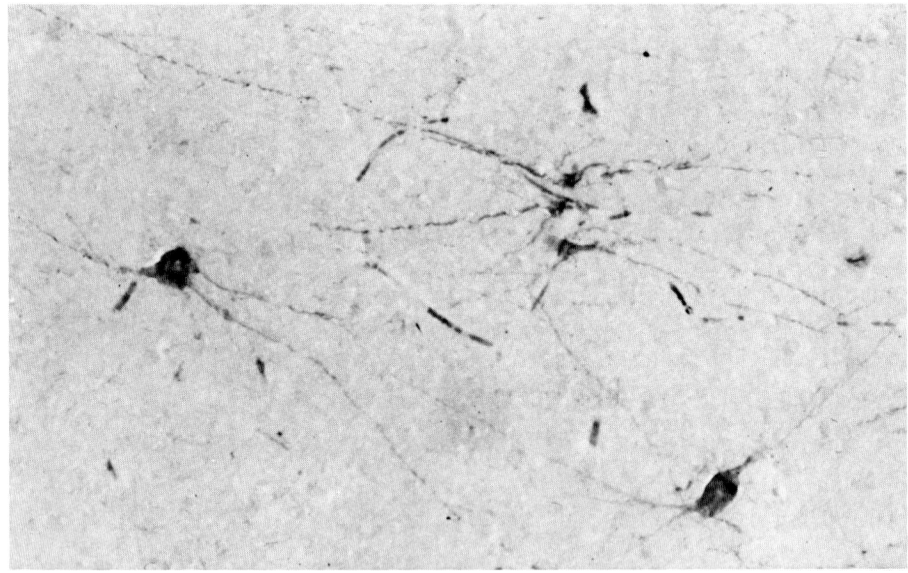

FIG. 2. TICB and fibers in periaqueductal gray.

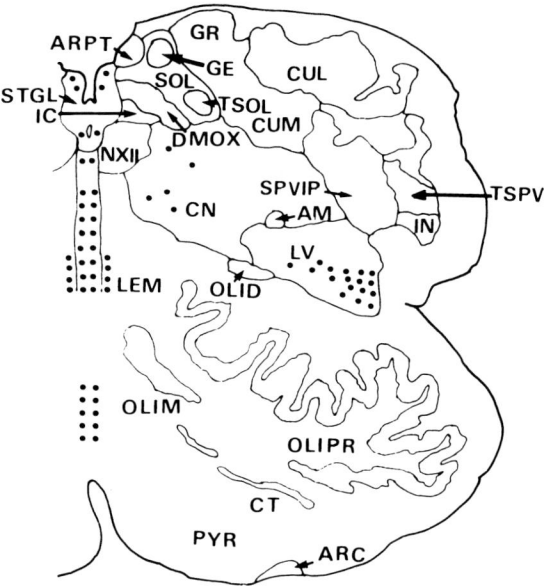

FIG. 3. Rostral medulla. Nucleus raphe obscurus and nucleus raphe pallidus.

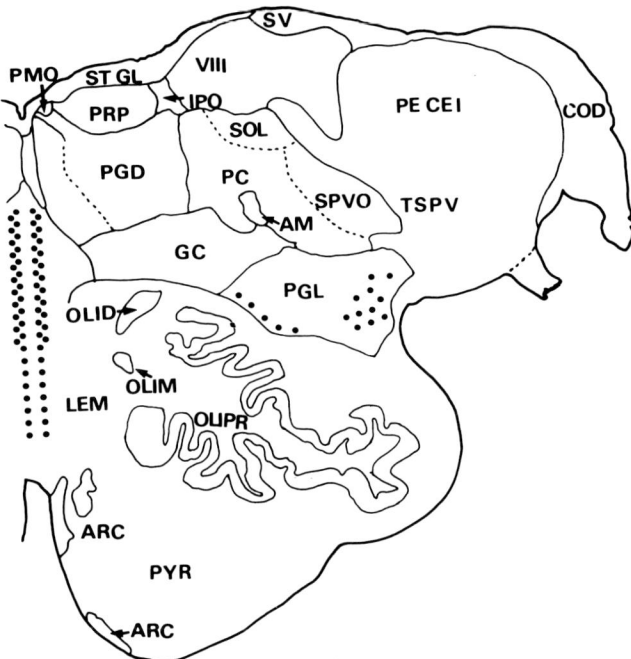

FIG. 4. Rostral medulla. Nucleus raphe obscurus and nucleus raphe pallidus at a more rostral level.

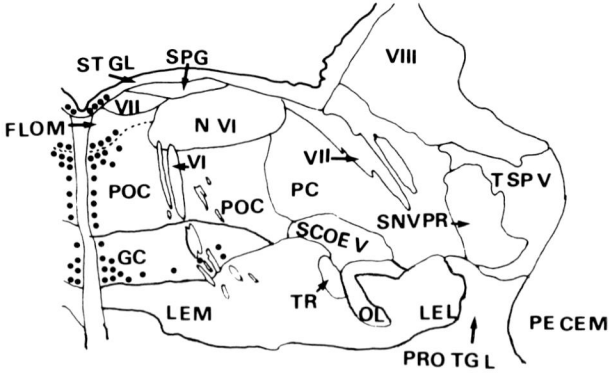

GR PONTIS

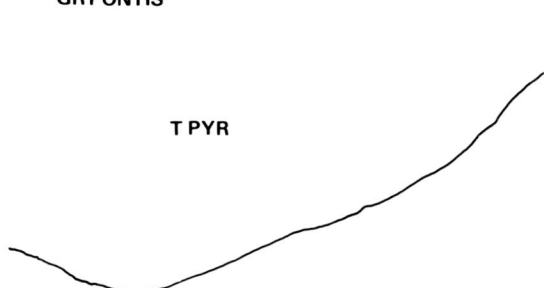

T PYR

FIG. 5. Caudal pons. Nucleus raphe magnus and nucleus raphe obscurus.

a ventral expansion in the ventral part of nucleus gigantocellularis in the part where the sixth nerve crosses it. A second group of TICB was found in stratum gliosum subependymale.

More rostral part of the pons (Fig. 6). This plane of section contained the smallest number of pontine TICB. They were located on both sides of the raphe and, to a lesser extent, in the raphe itself between the two fasciculi longitudinales mediales. These TICB represent the nucleus raphe magnus. Another small group of TICB was seen in the stratum gliosum subependymale.

Pons at the level of the caudal part of the nucleus locus coeruleus (Fig. 7). The nucleus raphe medialis was in griseum centralis pontis, nucleus centralis superior subnucleus dorsalis, nucleus papillioformis, and nucleus centralis superior subnucleus medialis. A ventrolateral extension was seen in the process of griseum pontis supralemniscalis. TICB of the nucleus centralis superior subnucleus dorsalis and griseum centralis pontis were separated from more ventral TICB of the nucleus

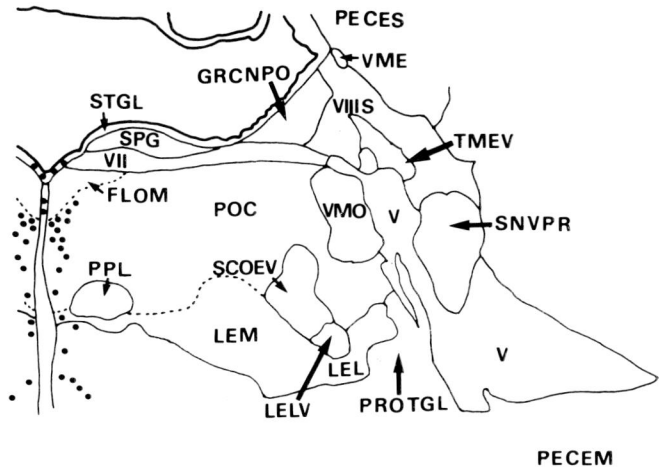

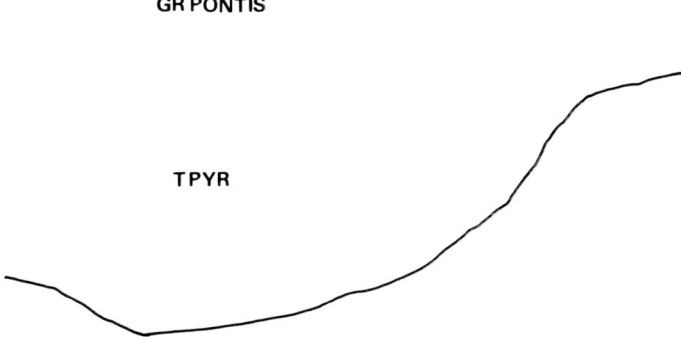

FIG. 6. Pons. Nucleus raphe magnus.

papillioformis and the nucleus centralis superior subnucleus medialis by the fasciculus longitudinalis medialis. More laterally, TICB were found in nucleus pontis oralis.

Pons at the level of the superior cerebellar peduncles (Fig. 8). The nucleus raphe medialis had a dorsal wing around the nucleus compactus suprafascicularis. A few TICB were also found in the fasciculus longitudinalis medialis. The ventral extension of TICB, the nucleus paramedialis, was not very rich and sketched a ring-like profile. More laterally, patches of TICB were found in the ventral part of pedunculus cerebellaris superior and in the nucleus pontalis orallis.

Pons at the level of the decussatio of the pedunculus cerebellaris superior (Fig. 9). The TICB were found in two narrow columns on both sides of midline with a slight thickening dorsally in the supracochlear nucleus where it was probably in

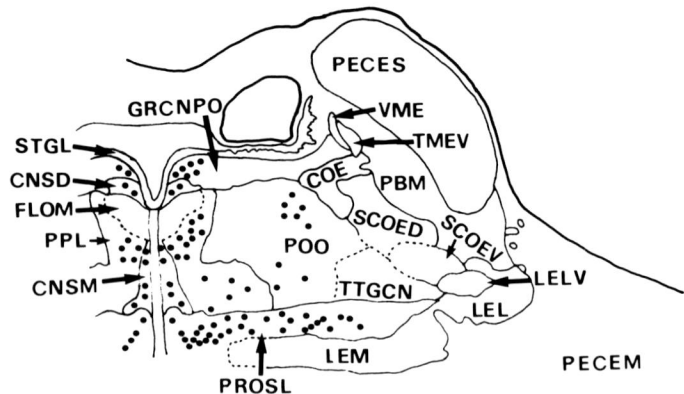
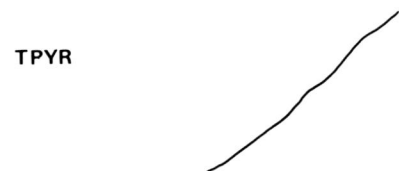

FIG. 7. Pons. Nucleus raphe medialis.

continuity with the caudal part of the nucleus raphe dorsalis. A lateroventral group of TICB was found in the interpeduncularis subnucleus medialis, along the midline and more laterally. A few TICB were present in the dorsal part of the decussatio of the superior cerebellar peduncle as well as in the griseum centralis medialis.

Mesencephalon at the level of the nucleus of the fourth nerve (Fig. 10). Here, the nucleus raphe dorsally was outlined by TICB, at its densest and widest extent. One could distinguish four parts: the dorsal part in the nucleus raphe dorsalis and a small adjacent area of griseum centralis medialis, medial and lateral parts; the lateral part in the nucleus supratrochlearis; the ventrolateral part in the tractus tegmentalis centralis, and the median part in the nucleus subcuneiformis. Scattered TICB were found in the decussatio of the pedunculus cerebellaris superior.

Mesencephalon at a level caudal to the red nucleus (Fig. 11). TICB were less densely packed than in Fig. 10. One could distinguish three groups: a dorsal group

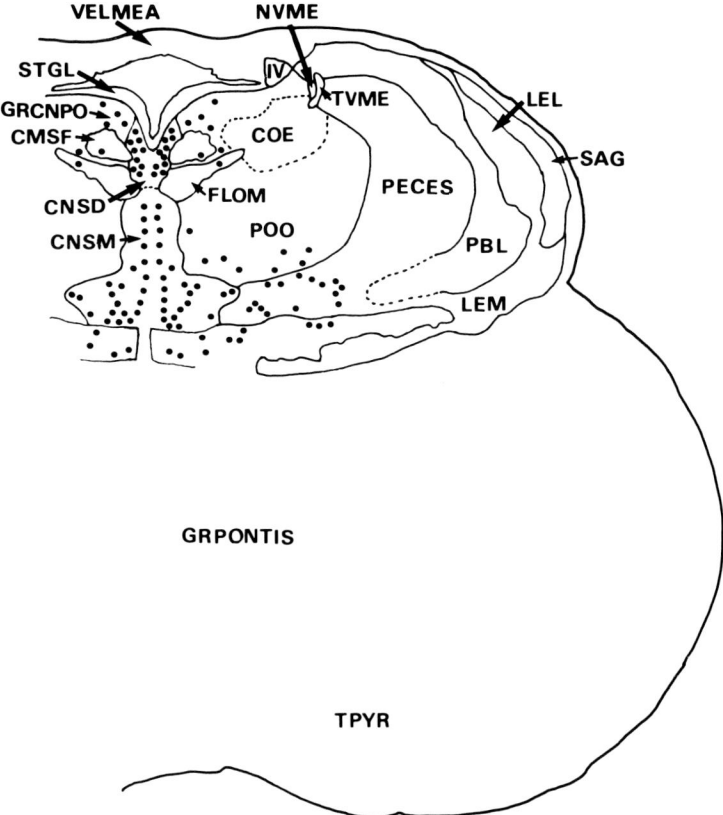

FIG. 8. Rostral pons. Nucleus raphe medialis.

in the dorsal part of the nucleus supratrochlearis, the third nerve oculomotorius caudalis centralis and third nerve nucleus oculomotorius principalis; a ventral group in the ventral part of the nucleus supratrochlearis; and a lateral group in the nucleus subcuneiformis.

Mesencephalon at the level of the junction of the red nucleus and pedunculus cerebellaris superior (Fig. 12). Two groups of TICB could be separated. One group was seen in the griseum centralis medialis (ventral part around the Edinger-Westphall nucleus), the lateral part, and on the midline (third nucleus of Perlia). A second group was found in the fasciculus longitudinalis medialis, intermingled with branches of the third nerve, extending more laterally to the tractus tegmentalis centralis and the lemniscus medialis.

Mesencephalon at the level of the maximal extend of the red nucleus (Fig. 13). TICB were found in a single group on the midline between the two nuclei oculomotori principales and the two Edinger-Westphall nuclei. Dorsally, the group

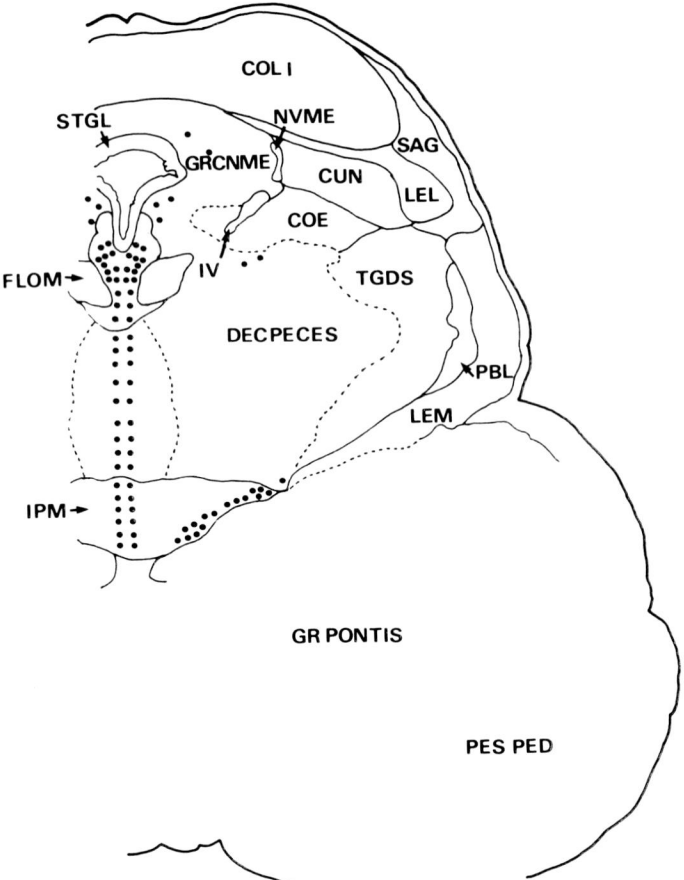

FIG. 9. Rostral pons. Nucleus raphe medialis.

sketched a wing-like profile in the griseum centralis medialis, medial part. This was the most rostral group, known as the caudal linear nucleus.

DISCUSSION

The preparation and specificity of TPOH have been documented in the rat (33).

TPOH is a highly unstable enzyme and thus was difficult to purify; this was an obstacle to the production of antisera. The lability of TPOH during post-mortem degradation made it necessary to restrict the present study to cases with short post-mortem delay (less than 15 hr). However, in a case with a 29-hr delay, no major difference in distribution was found compared with other cases.

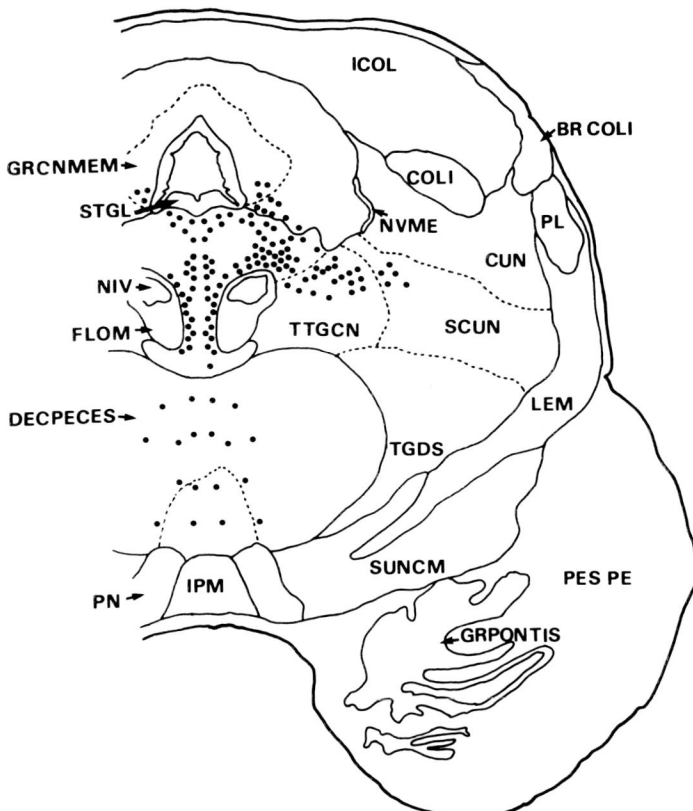

FIG. 10. Caudal mesencephalon. Nucleus raphe dorsalis.

No clear-cut difference in distribution was found in our study among neonates, infants, and adults. This suggests that serotoninergic systems are in place before birth.

We found only minor differences with the distribution reported by Takahashi et al. (29), Baker et al. (4) and Törk and Hornung (3). The lateral extension in the lateral tegmentum was not as wide. The paramedian nucleus was less thick. TICB were found in the interpeduncular nucleus but only in its more caudal part. The rostral extent of TICB, the caudal linear nucleus, extended more rostrally than described by Törk and Hornung. These minor differences could be explained by a better specificity of our antibody.

Dense grouping in the histologically defined raphe nuclei is in agreement with other mammals. The nucleus raphe dorsalis, as marked by TPOH immunoreactivity, has four subdivisions, as described by Baker et al. (ref. 4, Fig. 8). No TICB were found in the nucleus locus coeruleus as in other human studies, in opposition to certain mammals (16,27,28).

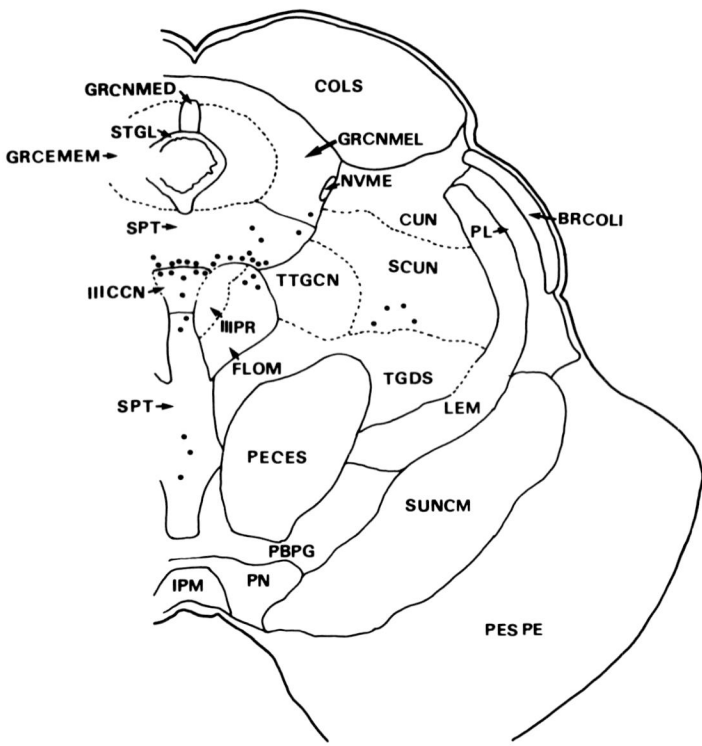

FIG. 11. Mesencephalon. Nucleus raphe dorsalis.

This study could contribute to future studies of diseases supposed to involve serotonergic systems and/or raphe nuclei: Alzheimer's disease (24), Parkinson's disease (14), depression and suicide (10), and disturbances of brain development.

ACKNOWLEDGMENTS

We thank V. Thivolle for typing the manuscript and INSERM (grant no. 87-6013), Département de Biologie Humaine de Lyon and Université Claude Bernard (contrat Jeune Equipe) and Fédération "Naître et Vivre."

ABBREVIATIONS

AM	Nucleus ambiguus	BRCOLS	Brachium colliculi superioris
ARC	Nucleus arcuatus		
ARPT	Area postrema	CAPSRU	Capsule of the nucleus ruber
BRCOLI	Brachium colliculi inferioris		

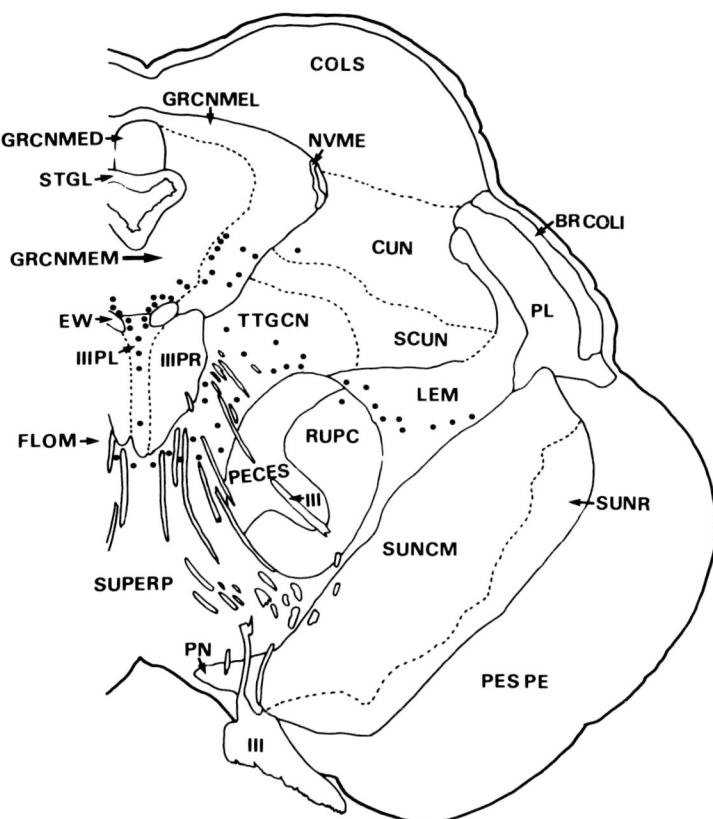

FIG. 12. Mesencephalon. Nucleus raphe dorsalis.

CMSF	Nucleus compactus suprafascicularis	DECPECES	Decussatio pedunculorum cerebellorum superiorum
CN	Nucleus medullae oblongatae centralis	DMOX	Nucleus dorsalis motorius nervi vagi
CNSD	Nucleus centralis superior, subnucleus dorsalis	EW	Nucleus Edinger-Westphall
CNSM	Nucleus centralis superior, subnucleus medialis	FLOM	Fasciculus longitudinalis medialis
		GC	Nucleus gigantocellularis
COD	Nucleus cochlearis dorsalis	GE	Nucleus tractus solitarii, subnucleus gelatinosus
COE	Nucleus locus coeruleus	GR	Griseum
COLI	Nucleus colliculi inferioris	GRCNME	Griseum centrale mesencephali
COLS	Colliculus superior		
CT	Nucleus conterminalis	GRCNMED	Griseum centrale mesencephali, subnucleus dorsalis
CUL	Nucleus cuneatus lateralis		
CUM	Nucleus cuneatus medialis		
CUN	Nucleus cuneiformis	GRCNMEL	Griseum centrale

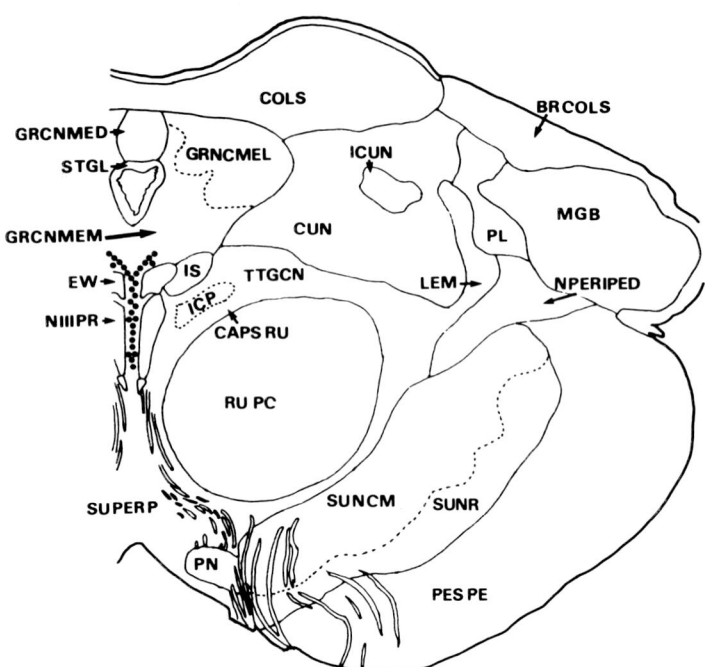

FIG. 13. Rostral mesencephalon. Nucleus caudal linear.

	mesencephali, subnucleus lateralis	IV	Nucleus nervi trochlearis
GRCNMEM	Griseum centrale mesencephali, subnucleus medialis	LEL	Lemniscus lateralis
		LELV	Nucleus lemniscus lateralis ventralis
GRCNPO	Griseum centralis pontis	LEM	Lemniscus medialis
GR PONTIS	Griseum pontis	LV	Nucleus medullae oblongatae lateralis, subnucleus ventralis
IC	Nucleus intercalatus		
ICOL	Nucleus intercollicularis		
ICP	Nucleus intracapsularis		
ICUN	Nucleus intercuneiformis	MGB	Corpus geniculatum mediale
III CCN	Nucleus oculomotorius caudalis centralis	NIII PR	Nucleus oculomotorius principalis
III PL	Nucleus Perlia	NIV	Nucleus nervi trochlearis
III PR	Nucleus oculomotorius principalis	NPERIPED	Nucleus peripeduncularis
		NVJ	Nucleus nervi abducentis
IN	Insulae nuclei cuneati laterales	NVME	Nucleus nervi trigemini mesencephalicus
IPM	Nucleus interpeduncularis, subnucleus medialis	NXII	Nucleus nervi hypoglossi
		OL	Nucleus olivaris
		OLID	Nucleus olivaris inferior accessorius dorsalis
IPO	Nucleus interpositus		
IS	Nucleus interstitialis (Cajal)	OLIM	Nucleus olivaris inferior accessorius medialis

OLIPR	Nucleus olivaris inferior principalis	SCUN	Nucleus subcuneiformis
		SNVPR	Nucleus nervi trigemini sensibilis principalis
PBL	Nucleus parabrachialis lateralis	SOL	Nucleus tractus solitarius
PBM	Nucleus parabrachialis medialis	SPG	Nucleus suprageniculatus
		SPT	Nucleus supratrochlearis
PBPG	Nucleus parabrachialis pigmentosus	SPVIP	Nucleus tractus spinalis trigemini interpolaris
PC	Nucleus parvocellularis	SPVO	Nucleus tractus spinalis trigemini ovalis
PECEI	Nucleus pedonculus cerebelli inferior		
		STGL	Stratum gliosum subependymale
PECEM	Pedunculus cerebelli medialis	SUNCM	Nucleus substantia nigrae, subnucleus compactus
PECES	Pedunculus cerebelli superior	SUNR	Nucleus substantia nigrae, subnucleus reticulata
PESPED	Pes pedunculi		
PGD	Nucleus paragigantocellularis dorsalis	SUPERP	Substantia perforata posterior
		SV	Nucleus supravestibularis
PGL	Nucleus paragigantocellularis lateralis	TGDS	Nucleus tegmenti pedunculopontinus, subnucleus dissipatis
PL	Nucleus paralemniscalis	TMEV	Tractus nervi trigemini mesencephalicus
PMO	Nucleus paramedianus dorsalis oralis		
		TPYR	Tractus pyramidalis
PN	Nucleus paranigralis	TR	Nucleus trapezoidalis
POC	Nucleus pontis centralis	TSOL	Tractus solitarius
POO	Nucleus pontis centralis oralis	TSPV	Tractus nervi trigemini spinalis
PPL	Nucleus papillioformis	TTGCN	Tractus tegmentalis centralis
PROSL	Processus griseum pontis supralemniscalis		
		TVME	Tractus nervi trigemini mesencephalicus
PROTGL	Processus griseum pontis tegmentosus lateralis	V	Nucleus trigeminalis
PRP	Nucleus praepositus hypoglossi	VELMEA	Velum medullare anterior
		VI	Nervus abducentis
PYR	Pyramis	VII	Nervus fascialis
RUPC	Nucleus ruber, subnucleus parvocellularis	VIII	Nucleus vestibularis
		VIIIS	Nucleus vestibularis superior
SAG	Nucleus sagulum		
SCOED	Nucleus subcoeruleus, subnucleus dorsalis	VME	Nucleus nervi trigemini mesencephalicus
SCOEV	Nucleus subcoeruleus, subnucleus ventralis	VMO	Nucleus nervi trigemini motorius

REFERENCES

1. Azmitia EC, Gannon PJ. The primate serotonergic system: a review of human and animal studies and a report on Macacca fascicularis. *Adv Neurol* 1986;43:407–468.
2. Azmitia E, Segal M. An autoradiographic analysis of the differential ascending projections of the dorsal and median raphe nuclei in the rat. *J Comp Neurol* 1978;179:649–668.
3. Baker KG, Halliday GM, Halasz P, et al. Cytoarchitecture of serotonin-synthesizing neurons in the pontine tegmentum of the human brain. *Synapse* 1991;7:301–320.

4. Baker KG, Halliday GM, Török I. Cytoarchitecture of the human dorsal raphe nucleus. *J Comp Neurol* 1990;301:141–161.
5. Beaudet A, Descarries L. Radioautographic characterization of a serotonin-accumulating nerve cell group in adult rat hypothalamus. *Brain Res* 1979;160:231–243.
6. Braak H. Uber die Kerngebiete des menschlichen Hirnstammes. II. Die raphe Kerne. *Z Zellforsch* 1970;107:123–141.
7. Brusco A, Peressini S, Pecci-Saavedra J. Serotonin-like immunoreactivity and anti-5-hydroxytryptamine (5HT) antibodies. *J Histochem Cytochem* 1983;31:524–530.
8. Chan-Palay V. Serotonin axons in the supra and subependymal plexuses and in the leptomeninges; their roles in local alteration of cerebrospinal fluid and vasomotor activity. *Brain Res* 1976;102:103–130.
9. Dahlström A, Fuxe K. Evidence for the existence of monoamine-containing neurons in the central nervous system. I. Demonstration of monoamines in the cell bodies of brainstem neurons. *Acta Physiol Scand* 1964;62(suppl 232):1–55.
10. Dalery J, Kopp N. Depression. In: Riederer P, Kopp N, Pearson J, eds. *An introduction to neurotransmission in health and disease*. New York: Oxford University Press, 1990:278–288.
11. Descarries L, Beaudet A, Watkins KC. Serotonin nerve terminals in adult rat neocortex. *Brain Res* 1975;100:563–588.
12. Felten DL, Sladek JR. Monoamine distribution in primate brain. V. Monoaminergic nuclei: anatomy, pathways and local organization. *Brain Res Bull* 1983;10:171–284.
13. Haan EA, Jennings IG, Cuello AC, et al. Identification of serotonergic neurons in human brain by a monoclonal antibody binding in all three aromatic amino-acid hydrolases. *Brain Res* 1987;426:19–27.
14. Halliday GM, Blumberg PC, Hoh TH, et al. Neuropathology of immunohistochemistry identified brainstem neurons in Parkinson's disease. *Ann Neurol* 1990;27:373–385.
15. Hornung JP, Fritschy JM. Serotonergic system in the brainstem of the marmoset: a combined immunocytochemical and three dimensional reconstruction study. *J Comp Neurol* 1988;270:471–487.
16. Leger L, Wiklund L. Distribution and numbers of indole amine cell bodies in the cat brainstem determined by FALCK HILLARP fluorescence histochemistry. *Brain Res Bull* 1982;9:245–252.
17. Leger L, Wiklund L, Descarries L, Pearson M. Description of an indole aminergic cell component in the cat locus coeruleus; a fluorescence histochemical and radioautographic study. *Brain Res* 1979;168:43–56.
18. Moore RY, Halaris AE, Jones BE. Serotonin neurons of the midbrain raphe: ascending projections. *J Comp Neurol* 1978;80:417–438.
19. Nobin A, Björklund A. Topography of the monoamine neuron systems in the human brain as revealed in fetuses. *Acta Physiol Scand (Suppl)* 1973;388:S1–S40.
20. Olson L, Boreus LO, Seiger A. Histochemical demonstration and mapping of 5-hydroxytryptamine and catecholamine containing neuron systems in the human fetal brain. *Z Anat Entwicklungsgesch* 1973;139:259–282.
21. Olszewski J, Baxter D. *Cytoarchitecture of the human brain stem*. Basel: S. Karger, 1954.
22. Parent A, Descarries L, Beaudet A. Organization of ascending serotonin systems in the adult rat brain. A radioautographic study after intraventricular administration of ^{3}H 5 hydroxytryptamine. *Neuroscience* 1981;5:115–138.
23. Pearson J, Goldstein M, Kitahama K, Sakamoto N, Michel JP. Catecholamine neurons of the human central nervous system. In: Riederer P, Kopp N, Pearson J, eds. *An introduction to neurotransmission in health and disease*. New York: Oxford University Press, 1990:22–36.
24. Price DL, Whitehouse PJ, Strubble RG, Hedreen JC, Uhl GR. Transmitter systems in selected types of dementia. In: Riederer P, Kopp N, Pearson J, eds. *An introduction to neurotransmission in health and disease*. New York: Oxford University Press, 1990:349–357.
25. Richards JG, Long HP, Tranzen JP. Indolalkylamine nerve terminals in cerebral ventricles: identification by electron microscopy and fluorescence histochemistry. *Brain Res* 1973;57:177–288.
26. Sakamoto N, Michel JP, Kopp N, Kiyama H, Tohyama M, Pearson J. Neurotensin immunoreactivity in the human cingulate gyrus, hippocampal subiculum and mammillary bodies. Its potential role in memory processes. *Brain Res* 1986;375:351–356.
27. Sladek JR Jr, Garver DL, Cummings JP. Monoamine distribution in primate brains. IV. Indole amine-containing perikarya in the brain stem of Macacca arctoïdes. *Neuroscience* 1982;7:477–493.
28. Steinbusch HWM. Distribution of serotonin-immunoreactivity in the central nervous system of the rat cell bodies and terminals. *Neuroscience* 1981;6:557–618.

29. Takahashi H, Nakashima S, Ohama E, Takeda S, Ikuta F. Distribution of serotonin-containing cell bodies in the brain stem of the human fetus determined with immunohistochemistry using anti-serotonin serum. *Brain Dev* 1986;8:355–365.
30. Takeuchi Y, Kimura H, Matssuura T, Sano Y. Immunohistochemical demonstration of the organization of serotonergic neurons in the brain of the monkey (Macacca Fuscata). *Acta Anat* 1982;114:106–124.
31. Törk I, Hornung JP. Raphe nuclei and the serotonergic system. In: Paxinos G, ed. *The human nervous system*. New York: Academic Press, 1990:1001–1022.
32. Vogt M. Some functional aspects of central serotonergic neurons. In: Osborne NN, ed. *Biology of serotonergic transmission*. New York: John Wiley, 1982:299–315.
33. Weissmann D, Belin MF, Aguerra M, et al. Immunohistochemistry of tryptophan hydroxylase in the rat brain. *Neuroscience* 1987;23:291–304.

5

Selective Organization of Tryptophan Hydroxylase Expression in the Raphe Dorsalis

D. Weissmann, F. Richard, C. Rousset, and J. F. Pujol

CNRS UMR 105, CERMEP, 69003 Lyon, France

The nucleus raphe dorsalis (NRD) represents the main serotoninergic group of the rat brain stem. Numerous studies have already analyzed the qualitative organization of serotonin (5-HT)-containing perikarya (3,6,14,18) and tryptophan hydroxylase (TpOH)-positive cell bodies (19). Information has also been reported concerning the characterization of cellular elements (8), especially these cells, which accumulate exogenous tritiated 5-HT (7). However, little is known about the quantitative distribution of the TpOH protein and TpOH-expressing cells in this nucleus.

To specifically approach this problem, we have used an improved methodology to measure brain-specific proteins with a high degree of anatomical resolution (20) and a new pharmacological model (16) that allows, after a parachlorophenylalanine (PCPA) single administration, the estimation of the turnover rate of TpOH protein in brain tissue.

In this chapter we present and discuss the main results that were obtained with this strategy. They were an invitation to descend into this important serotoninergic group to try to understand how specifically TpOH protein synthesis can be regulated in these 5-HT neurons in steady-state conditions.

METHODOLOGICAL CONSIDERATIONS

The details of the methods used to obtain the results presented here have been already extensively described (20). The major original purpose was to demonstrate that the direct transfer of unfixed frozen brain section (20 μm) onto nitrocellulose was a sensitive method for quantitative evaluation of specific soluble proteins such as TpOH with a high degree of resolution.

TpOH was selectively detected among the transferred proteins (75% of the total brain tissue proteins) after incubation with TpOH antiserum in saturating conditions. Antigen-antibody complexes were revealed by subsequent incubation with 125-iodinated G protein.

It was thus possible to map the presence of TpOH protein in the whole serotoninergic system, and we focused our first study on the nucleus raphe dorsalis after having considered that (i) the wide projections of this nucleus could involve differential organization of the 5-HT-containing cells and subsequently different expression of TpOH synthesis and (ii) the inhibition of synthesis of TpOH protein by PCPA already demonstrated in the total NRD (16) could provide a dynamic tool for the quantitative estimation of the turnover rate of the protein in each subdivision of the nucleus.

A modified immunohistochemical procedure on the adjacent postfixed sections allowed the staining of TpOH-positive cells with a high sensitivity. This immunohistochemistry enabled the characterization and counting of those cells in the sections adjacent to each transferred slice.

QUANTITATIVE ANALYSIS OF NEURONAL POPULATION THAT SYNTHESIZES TpOH IN THE NRD

The number of TpOH-positive cells and density of such a population were measured at each 200-μm interval along the posteroanterior axis of the NRD (see Fig. 1 and Table 1). This mapping of TpOH-containing neurons in the rat NRD complemented our less quantitative previous observations made at different levels across the midbrain (19) and is quite consistent with the anterior studies on the mapping of 5-HT neurons in that region of the rat brain (1,2,5–7,9,11,13,14,17). The NRD was subdivided into three main subgroups of TpOH-containing cells: they corresponded to the NRD ventromedialis (NRD VM), which extended all along the posteroanterior axis of the structure; the NRD lateralis (NRD LAT), and the NRD dorsomedialis (NRD DM). The subdivisions defined here were initially described by Fuxe and Jonson (9), then by Steinbusch et al. (17,18). In our study, the number of cells was counted at each anatomical level. The posteroanterior distribution of the absolute number of cells was marked in the whole structure and corresponded to the posteroanterior extension of the nucleus. The NRD VM contained the majority of TpOH-positive cells (72% of the total number of cells). It was of interest to note that the density of cells was homogeneous in most of the nucleus. Nevertheless, in the NRD LAT, which contained 18% of the total population of TpOH-positive cells, they were less densely distributed. Our overall estimation of the total population of TpOH-positive cells ($4,089 \pm 620$) of the NRD exhibited a number of cells expressing the TpOH significantly lower than the number of cells accumulating tritiated 5-HT ($11,500 \pm 207$) after ventricular administration of the exogenous amine (7). This difference could result from a lesser degree of sensitivity of the immunocytochemical detection of TpOH as compared to autoradiographic detection of cells that accumulate exogenous [^{3}H]5-HT (7), or of immunocytochemical detection of endogenous 5-HT-containing cells (17,18). However, it cannot be excluded

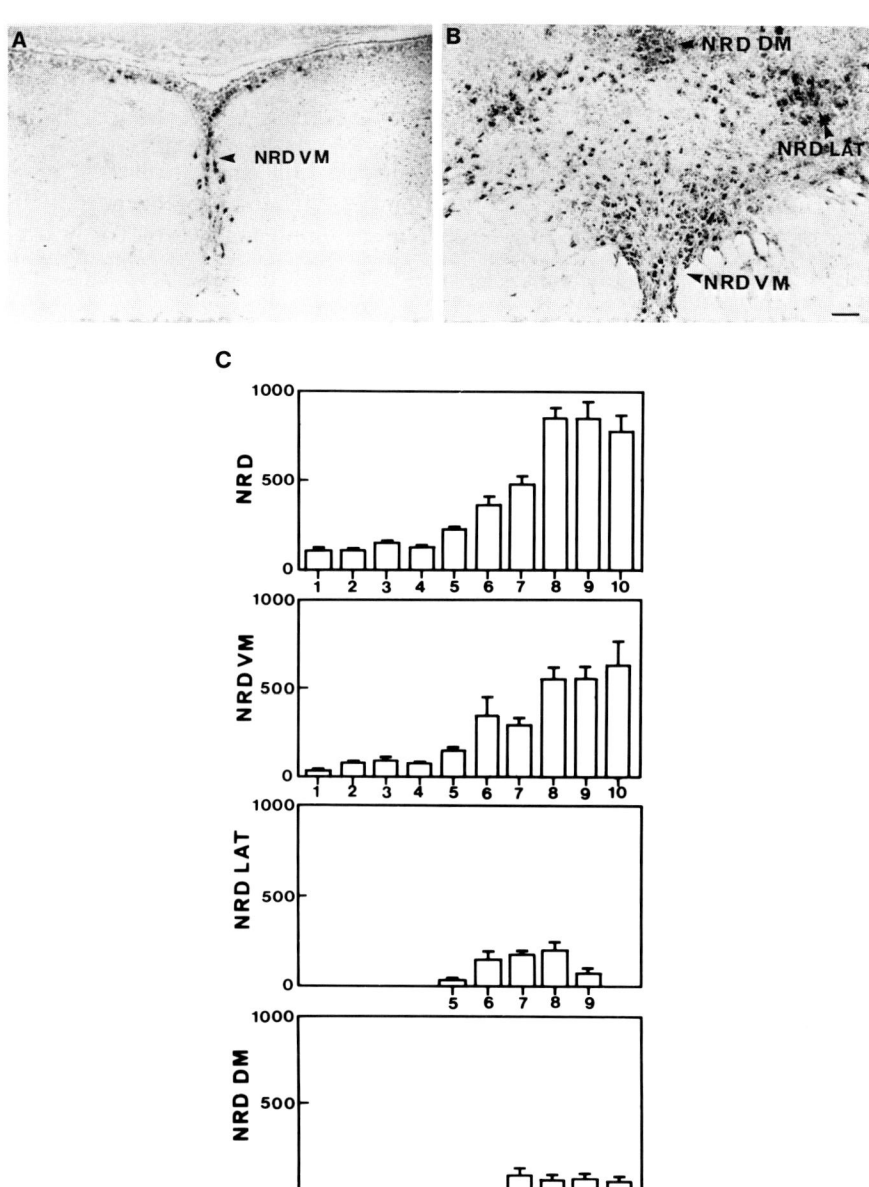

FIG. 1. The NRD as revealed by immunocytochemistry of TpOH protein. **A,B**: TpOH-positive cells in the caudal part of the NRD (A: interaural −0.30 mm in the Paxinos and Watson atlas [15]) and in the rostral part (B: interaural 1.20 mm in the same atlas) where the different subdivisions of this nucleus can be individualized. Calibration bar: 18 μm. **C**: Posteroanterior distribution of the number of cells in the NRD and its subdivisions. Each bar represents the mean ± SEM (n = 5) of this parameter in each anatomical interval (200 μm). The total NRD extends from interaural −0.30 mm in the Paxinos and Watson atlas (15).

TABLE 1. *Distribution of the TpOH-positive cells in the NRD and its subdivisions*

	Number of cells	Volume (mm^3)	Cellular density (cell/mm^3)
NRD	4,089 ± 620	1.17 ± 0.083	3,719 ± 260
NRD VM	2,950 ± 274	0.646 ± 0.02	4,652 ± 284
NRD LAT	757 ± 168[a]	0.385 ± 0.075	2,032 ± 308[a]
NRD DM	392 ± 48[b]	0.1 ± 0.016[b]	5,082 ± 502

The mean ± SEM ($n=5$) of the total number of cells, the volume in which those cells were localized (mm^3), and the cellular density (number of cells/mm^3) are expressed for the total NRD and each of its subdivisions.
[a]$p \leq 0.01$; [b]$p \leq 0.001$ as compared to NRD VM.

that part of the difference reported here would indicate that a significant population of TpOH-containing and/or accumulating cells would express TpOH to a lesser degree. This interpretation has to be evaluated in view of previously reported results that demonstrated that a significant population of 5-HT-containing cells in the NRD were able to express detectable amounts of glutamate decarboxylase (GAD) (4,12). Finally, 5-HT-positive and TpOH-negative cells could belong to a population of serotoninoceptive cells in which the TpOH encoding gene could be inactive enough to make TpOH cell concentration undetectable. Further studies are necessary to explore this hypothesis. Nevertheless, the reproducibility of the results obtained at each anatomical level of each subdivision of the nucleus seems to justify the cell number determined in our experimental conditions as a valid relative index, which allowed the evaluation of the cellular density of the TpOH-expressing cell population, and subsequent relative comparisons performed here between different subgroups of the same nucleus.

STEADY-STATE QUANTITY AND CONCENTRATION OF TpOH PROTEIN IN THE RAT NRD

The absolute amount of TpOH protein (see Fig. 2 and Table 2) closely followed the number of TpOH cells in each interval of each anatomical subdivision. In the

FIG. 2. A,B: TpOH detection obtained after direct transfer of TpOH protein from frontal sections in the posterior (A: interaural −0.30 mm) and the anterior NRD (B: interaural 1.20 mm). **C,D**: Expressed respectively are the posteroanterior distribution of the total amount of TpOH (U·TpOH/interval) and the cellular concentration of TpOH (U·TpOH/cell) in the total NRD, the NRD VM, the NRD LAT, and the NRD DM. Results are expressed as in Fig. 1. **E**: Correlation between transferred TpOH amount and number of TpOH-positive cells. Absolute value of TpOH protein amount was calculated at each 200 μm interval along the posteroanterior axis. The corresponding number of TpOH-positive cells was estimated from postfixed consecutive sections after immunohistochemical detection.

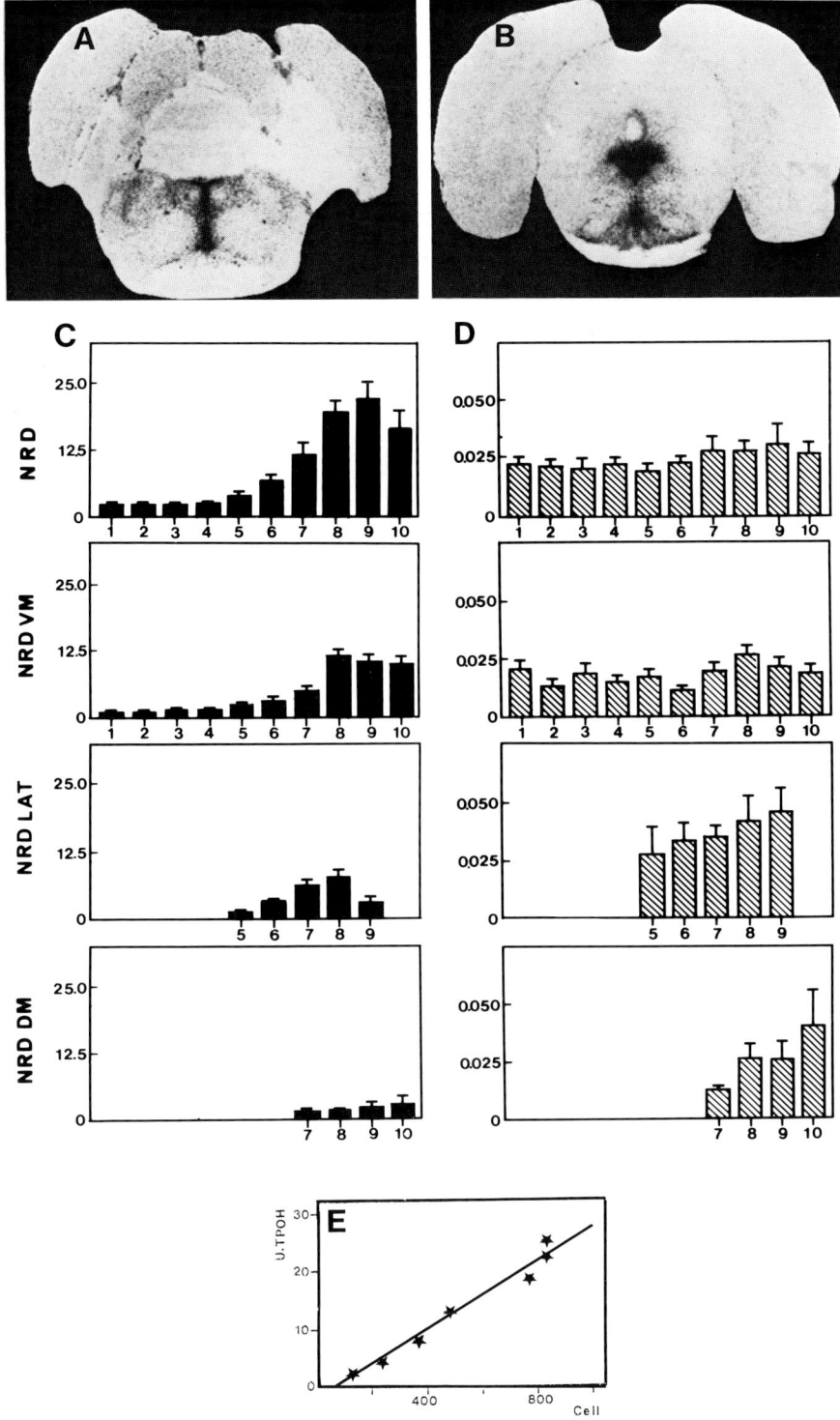

TABLE 2. *Mean tissue and cellular concentration and total amount of TpOH protein in the total NRD and each of its subdivisions*

	Tissue concentration (U·TpOH/mg)	Cellular concentration (U·TpOH/cell)	Total amount of TPOH (U·TpOH)
NRD	78.35 ± 6.15	$(28.98 \pm 3\ 10)^{-3}$	95.5 ± 9.8
NRD VM	78.35 ± 5.41	$(18.08 \pm 1.6\ 10)^{-3}$	54.5 ± 4
NRD LAT	67.40 ± 3.56^a	$(36.04 \pm 3.5\ 10)^{-3a}$	22.5 ± 5.5^b
NRD DM	85.24 ± 4.9	$(23.37 \pm 3\ 10)^{-3}$	8.56 ± 0.96^c

Results are expressed as in Table 1.
$^a p \leq 0.05\%$; $^b p \leq 0.01$; $^c p \leq 0.001$ as compared to NRD VM.

total NRD, a linear relationship between these two parameters was demonstrated. The slope of this relationship was $28.8\ 10^{-3} \pm 1.4\ 10^{-3}$ U·TpOH/cell. As expected, it was very close to the mean cellular concentration calculated for the global structure (see Table 2). These observations hardly suggested that the transferred TpOH protein in the NRD came from TpOH perikarya and dendrites. A similar interpretation had already been suggested for tyrosine hydroxylase (TH) distribution in the catecholaminergic groups of perikarya in which, after subcellular fractionation, TH protein was found mainly located in the cellular fraction (10).

In each raphe subdivision, when analyzed along the posteroanterior axis, the TpOH tissue concentration was quite homogeneous. This reflected the homogeneity of cell density in each subdivision of the structure. In the NRD LAT, however, the TpOH tissue concentration was less even along the posteroanterior axis, and the distribution was significantly correlated to the cell density found at each anatomical interval ($p \leq 0.05\%$). This observation also likely reflects the fact that the majority of transferred TpOH protein was located in cell bodies and dendrites. When divided by cell density, the tissue concentration can thus be reasonably considered as a good approximation of the mean cellular concentration of TpOH protein. Such a calculation showed that the cellular concentration of TpOH was greatest in the NRD LAT. This occurred because, although the tissue concentration of TpOH protein was similar to that measured in the other portions of the nucleus, the cell number per unit of volume was less than half of the population of TpOH-containing cells present in other portions of the nucleus.

ESTIMATION OF THE RATE OF DISAPPEARANCE OF TpOH PROTEIN IN THE RAT NRD

Recently, we (16) demonstrated that PCPA administration (300 mg/kg i.p.) was followed by a first kinetic order decay of TpOH protein quantity measured by Western blotting in the rat NRD. It was also demonstrated that this apparent total inhibition of TpOH protein synthesis was not related to the inhibition of 5-HT synthesis since the injection of similar doses of 6-fluorotryptophan, another inhibitor of

TpOH activity, failed to produce the same effect. We decided to use this property to estimate the rate constant of TpOH protein turnover in steady-state conditions in the rat NRD. This estimation was performed by measuring TpOH protein quantity and concentration 2 days after saline or PCPA administration. This time was chosen because it corresponded to the maximum of the TpOH decrease after PCPA treatment (16). An apparent rate constant of disappearance was thus determined in each subdivision of the NRD (see Fig. 3 and Table 3). For the total NRD an overall -58% decrease of TpOH concentration was found, which was quite similar to the relative decrease measured in similar experiments by the biochemical method (16). A mean k value of 0.434 ± 0.014 on day 1 was estimated corresponding to a half-life of 1.6 days. The constant rate of disappearance was similar in the ventromedial part of the nucleus with an estimated half-life of 1.52 days, but slower in the dorsomedial area ($t_{1/2} = 2.06$ days), and slower again in the lateral portion in which the

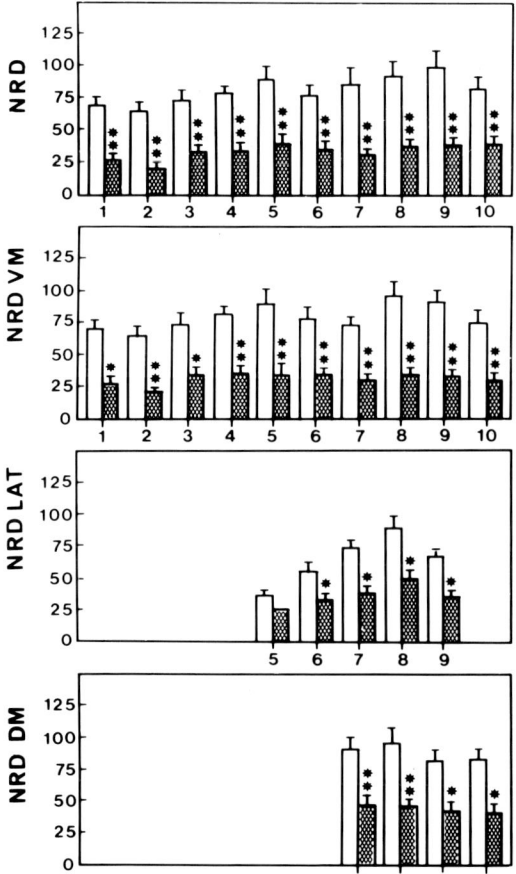

FIG. 3. Distribution of the tissue concentration of TpOH in control (*open bars*) and PCPA-treated animals (*hatched bars*) (U·TpOH/mg of tissue) in the total NRD, the NRD VM, the NRD LAT, and the NRD DM. Results are expressed as in Fig. 1.

TABLE 3. *Effect of PCPA treatment on TpOH tissue concentrations and determination of the rate constant of disappearance (k) of TpOH*

	Tissue concentration (U·TpOH/mg)	k (day^{-1})	TpOH rate of synthesis (U·TpOH/cell/day)
NRD			
Sham	78.35 ± 6.15	0.434 ± 0.014	10.40 ± 0.03 10^{-3}
PCPA	33.17 ± 1.72^a		
NRD VM			
Sham	78.35 ± 5.41	0.456 ± 0.024	8.24 ± 0.4 10^{-3}
PCPA	30.86 ± 2.67^a		
NRD LAT			
Sham	67.40 ± 3.56	0.287 ± 0.03^b	10.34 ± 1.08 $^{-3}$
PCPA	37.89 ± 3.7^a		
NRD DM			
Sham	85.24 ± 4.9	0.336 ± 0.03	7.85 ± 0.7 $^{-3}$
PCPA	42.76 ± 4.9^a		

The mean ± SEM of the tissue concentrations of TpOH in control and PCPA-treated animals (U·TpOH/mg tissue) in the total NRD and each of its subdivisions are given. The rate constant of disappearance (k) and the cellular rate of synthesis of TpOH are calculated for each subgroup of the nucleus.
$^a p \leq 0.001$ as compared to sham animals.
$^b p \leq 0.05$ as compared to NRD VM.

renewing of the TpOH pool took 1.6 times the time required in the VM portion. Thus, the rate of renewing of TpOH protein differs in the anatomical subdivisions of the NRD. At steady state, this implies a differential degree of expression of the gene encoding for TpOH protein. It was interesting to note (i) the lowest values for the constant rate of renewal were found in the NRD LAT in which the cellular concentration was the highest and (ii) the global cellular rate of synthesis at steady state, expressed as the product of k with the corresponding cellular concentration, exhibited only nonsignificant variations (<20%) between the different subdivisions. The expression of TpOH thus seems regulated to keep the number of TpOH molecules synthesized by each cell at a given level. In this context, it will be of great interest to compare these dynamic variations of protein concentration to those of the specific mRNA encoding for it. Further studies are still necessary to determine if TpOH gene expression is in fact regulated by TpOH cellular concentrations and what process modulates the increase of k in the NRD LAT along the posteroanterior axis. It will, of course, be of great interest to compare, in the same context, the dynamic changes occurring in the different groups of the raphe nuclei.

Finally, when precisely analyzed in each subpopulation of the NRD, the TpOH protein expression appeared to be regulated differently in steady-state conditions. Such differences imply a selective process of regulation related to the somatotopic organization of each cell subgroup. The mechanisms of such cellular adaptation to brain organization remain to be elucidated.

REFERENCES

1. Aghajanian GK, Asher IM. Histochemical fluorescence of raphe neurons: selective enhancement by tryptophan. *Science* 1971;172:1159–1161.
2. Aghajanian GK, Kuhar MJ, Roth RH. Serotonin-containing neuronal perikarya and terminals: differential effects of p-chlorophenyl-alanine. *Brain Res* 1973;54:85–101.
3. Azmitia E. The serotonin-producing neurons of the midbrain median and dorsal raphe nuclei. In: Iversen LL, Iversen SD, Snyder SH, eds. *Handbook of psychopharmacology*, vol 9. New York: Plenum, 1978:233–314.
4. Belin MF, Nanopoulos D, Didier M, et al. Immunohistochemical evidence for the presence of gamma-aminobutyric acid and serotonin in one nerve cell. A study on the raphe nuclei of the rat using antibodies to glutamate decarboxylase and serotonin. *Brain Res* 1983;275:329–339.
5. Chan-Palay V. Indoleamine neurons and their processes in the normal rat brain and in chronic diet-induced thiamine deficiency demonstrated by uptake of 3H-serotonin. *J Comp Neurol* 1977;176:467–494.
6. Dahlström A, Fuxe K. Evidence for the existence of monoamine-containing neurons in the central nervous system. I. Demonstration of monoamines in the cell bodies of brainstem neurons. *Acta Physiol Scand* 1964;62(suppl 232):1–55.
7. Descarries L, Watkins CK, Garcia S, Beaudet A. The serotonin neurons in nucleus raphe dorsalis: a light and electron microscope radioautographic study. *J Comp Neurol* 1982;207:239–254.
8. Diaz-Cintra S, Cintra L, Kemper T, Resnick O, Morgane PJ. Nucleus raphe dorsalis: a morphometric Golgi study in rats of three age groups. *Brain Res* 1981;207:1–16.
9. Fuxe K, Jonson G. Further mapping of central 5-hydroxytryptamine neurons: studies with neurotoxic dihydroxytryptamines. *Adv Biochem Pharmacol* 1974;10:1–12.
10. Gillon JY, Labatut R, Renaud B, Pujol JF. Subcellular distribution of tyrosine hydroxylase in some catecholaminergic rat brain areas determined by a quantitative immunoblot assay. *J Neurochem* 1989;52:677–683.
11. Levitt P, Moore RY. Developmental organization of raphe serotonin neuron groups in the rat. *Anat Embryol* 1978;154:241–251.
12. Nanopoulos D, Belin MF, Maitre M, Vincendon G, Pujol JF. Immunohistochemical evidence for the existence of GABA-ergic neurons in the nucleus raphe dorsalis. Possible existence of neurons containing serotonin and GABA. *Brain Res* 1982;232:375–389.
13. Palay SL, Chan-Palay V. A guide to the synaptic analysis of the neuropil. In: *The synapse (Cold Spring Harbor symposia on quantitative biology, vol XL)*. Cold Spring Harbor, NY: Cold Spring Harbor Laboratory, 1976:1–16.
14. Parent A, Descarries L, Beaudet A. Organization of ascending serotonin systems in the adult rat brain. A radioautographic study after intraventricular administration of (3H)5-HT. *Neuroscience* 1981;115–138.
15. Paxinos G, Watson C. *The rat brain in stereotaxic coordinates*. 2nd ed. New York: Academic Press,1986.
16. Richard F, Sanne JL, Bourde O, et al. Variation of tryptophan-5-hydroxylase concentration in the rat raphe dorsalis nucleus after parachlorophenylalanine administration: I. A model to study turnover of the enzymatic protein. *Brain Res (submitted)*.
17. Steinbusch HWM, Nieuwenhuys R, Verhofstad AAJ, Van Der Kooy D. The nucleus raphe dorsalis of the rat and its projections upon the caudatoputamen. A combined cytoarchitectonic, immunohistochemical and retrograde transport study. *J Physiol (Paris)* 1981;77:157–174.
18. Steinbusch HWM. Serotonin-immunoreactive neurons and their projections in the CNS. In: Björklund A, Hökfelt T, Kuhar MJ, eds. *Handbook of Chemical Neuroanatomy*, vol 3. Amsterdam: Elsevier, 1984:68–125.
19. Weissmann D, Belin MF, Aguera M, et al. Immunohistochemistry of tryptophan hydroxylase in the rat brain. *Neuroscience* 1987;23:291–304.
20. Weissmann D, Labatut R, Richard F, Rousset C, Pujol JF. Direct transfer into nitrocellulose and quantitative radioautographic anatomical determination of brain tyrosine hydroxylase protein concentration. *J Neurochem* 1989;53:793–799.

Serotonin, the Cerebellum, and Ataxia, edited by
P. Trouillas and K. Fuxe.
Raven Press, Ltd., New York © 1993.

6

The Serotoninergic System in the Cerebellum: Origin, Ultrastructural Relationships, and Physiological Effects

Georgia A. Bishop, Christopher W. Kerr, Yi Fei Chen, and James S. King

Department of Cell Biology, Neurobiology, and Anatomy, The Ohio State University, Columbus, Ohio 43210-1239

Data from a number of anatomical, pharmacological, and physiological studies have established that serotonin (5-HT) is present in a system of cerebellar afferents and that it appears to function in modulating Purkinje cell activity (16,21,28,34, 47). Immunohistochemical studies (7,8,27,50) have shown that 5-HT is present in a beaded plexus of fine varicose fibers in all species studied, including the rat, opossum, and cat. Although the morphological characteristics of 5-HT immunoreactive (IR) fibers is homogeneous across species, the laminar and lobular distribution of immunoreactivity is species specific and thus may reflect functional heterogeneity for this monoamine. The anatomical and physiological data described in this chapter were derived from the cat, as this species, when compared to the rat or opossum, has the greatest and most uniform distribution of 5-HT in the cerebellar cortex (27). Further, the vast majority of physiological and behavioral studies have been carried out in this species (see ref. 24 for review). However, to date, few studies have attempted to incorporate this chemically defined afferent system into current theories of cerebellar function and dysfunction. In the present account the distribution of 5-HT IR fibers, the identification of the cells of origin of these serotoninergic afferents, the ultrastructural relationships, as well as the physiological actions of this indoleamine in the cat will be reviewed. (Portions of this work have been published previously [27,29,30].)

METHODS

Immunohistochemical Analysis of 5-HT IR Fibers and Cell Bodies

The immunohistochemical techniques used to label 5-HT afferents and cell bodies are identical to those published previously (7,8,27). The 5-HT antibody was obtained from Dr. Robert Elde at the University of Minnesota. Briefly, animals were deeply anesthetized with sodium pentobarbital (40 mg/kg) and perfused through the aorta with saline and either 4% paraformaldehyde in phosphate buffer or a 2% paraformaldehyde-picric acid fixative (45). Some animals were given intraperitoneal injections of pargyline (50 mg/kg body weight) and L-tryptophan (50 mg/kg) prior to perfusion to enhance the level of 5-HT in neuronal cell bodies. The brains were removed, sectioned at 60 μm on a freezing microtome and processed for 5-HT immunohistochemistry by the peroxidase-antiperoxidase (PAP) technique (46). Every section was examined for the presence of 5-HT immunoreactivity. The distribution of 5-HT afferents and cell bodies was photographed and plotted on representative sections through the cerebellum and brain stem, respectively.

Analysis of the Cells of Origin of 5-HT Afferents in the Cerebellum

A double-label paradigm, as described previously (7,8,27,52), that combines retrograde transport of horseradish peroxidase (HRP) and PAP immunohistochemistry was used to positively identify the population of neurons in the brain stem that gives rise to the beaded plexus of serotoninergic fibers found within the cerebellum. Briefly, adult cats were anesthetized with sodium pentobarbital (40 mg/kg) and secured in a Kopf stereotaxic frame. Injections of 30% HRP in saline were made into either the anterior lobe vermis, posterior lobe vermis, paramedian lobule, or hemispheres (Crus I, II, lobus simplex). Following survivals of 24 to 36 hr the animals were reanesthetized and perfused through the aorta as previously described. Some animals were pretreated with pargyline and L-tryptophan, as described earlier, to enhance the level of 5-HT in cell bodies. The tissue was processed first for HRP histochemistry using a cobalt chloride-enhanced DAB procedure (1,7), which produces black granules in retrogradely labeled cells. This procedure was followed by PAP immunohistochemistry to identify serotoninergic cells that project to the cerebellum. All sections were examined. Three types of labeled neurons were observed: (i) cells with a diffuse brown immunostaining of their cytoplasm indicating they were serotoninergic neurons, (ii) cells with uniform black granules in their cytoplasm that delineated retrogradely labeled cells, and (iii) cells with both staining characteristics indicating they were serotoninergic neurons that projected to the cerebellum. The distribution of each type of neuron was plotted on a standardized set of drawings through the brain stem. The source of 5-HT to different regions of the cerebellum were then compared.

Electron Microscopic Analysis of 5-HT IR Fibers

Adult cats were anesthetized with sodium pentobarbital (40 mg/kg i.p.) and perfused through the aorta with saline followed by 4% paraformaldehyde-0.2% glutaraldehyde in phosphate buffer. The brain was removed and sectioned on a vibratome at 60 to 80 μm in the sagittal plane. The sections were then incubated for 30 min in phosphate buffered saline (PBS) to which 0.3% Triton X-100 had been added and then in a primary antibody to 5-HT diluted 1:5,000 in PBS for 24 hr. They were then processed for PAP immunohistochemistry (46) with sheep antirabbit IgG (1:300 in PBS), rabbit PAP (1:500 in PBS), and DAB. Sections that contained IR profiles were blocked and postfixed in 1% osmium tetroxide for 1 hr, rinsed in phosphate buffer, dehydrated through a graded series of acetones, and infiltrated with and flat-embedded in Spurr's resin. When properly hardened selected sections were photographed, mounted on a Beem capsule and sectioned at 80 to 100 nM on a Reichert Ultramicrotome. Sections were viewed and photographed on a Philips 300 electron microscope. Analysis was carried out to determine: (i) the number of approximations formed between immunolabeled profiles and somata and/or dendrites of cerebellar neurons, (ii) the identity, where possible, of the postsynaptic element, and (iii) the number of synaptic specializations formed between 5-HT fibers and their targets.

ANALYSIS OF THE PHYSIOLOGICAL EFFECTS OF 5-HT IN THE CEREBELLUM

Adult cats were anesthetized intraperitoneally with a combination of sodium thialymal (40 mg/kg) and α-chloralose (70 mg/kg) and secured in a Kopf stereotaxic frame. The bone overlying the cerebellum was removed for placement of multibarrel recording electrodes, as well as for placement of stimulating electrodes into the inferior cerebellar peduncle. These were used to activate climbing fibers, which allowed positive identification of the neuron from which data were obtained as a Purkinje cell. The center barrel of the recording electrode was filled with 4 M NaCl as was one of the drug barrels. This latter channel functions in an automatic balancing circuit that insures that observed effects are due to the drug applied and not a current effect. The remaining barrels were filled with combinations of 0.1 M 5-HT; 0.2 M glutamate; 0.2 M aspartate, 0.5 M GABA; 20 mM ($\pm$)-8-hydroxy-2-(di-n-propylamino)tetralin hydrobromide, a 5-HT_{1A} receptor agonist (8-OH-DPAT); 0.2 M ipsapirone (IPS), another 5-HT_{1A} agonist; 10 mM ($\pm$)-1-(2,5-dimethoxy-4-iodophenyl)-2-aminopropane hydrochloride (DOI), a $5\text{-HT}_{1C/2}$ receptor agonist; 10 mM spiperone hydrochloride, a 5-HT_{1A} receptor antagonist; 10 mM ritanserin, a $5\text{-HT}_{1C/2}$ receptor antagonist; and 0.2 M ($\pm$)-2-methyl-5-hydroxytryptamine maleate (2-methyl 5-HT), a 5-HT_3 receptor agonist. Solutions were adjusted for pH and an appropriate retaining current was applied to all barrels during advancement of the electrode to prevent leakage of all substances. This current was reversed to iontophoretically apply specific compounds to neurons isolated extracellularly. Records were stored on film as well as on a computer disc for later off-line analysis. The amplified signal was also monitored on an oscilloscope and converted to a uniform voltage pulse by passage through a window discriminator. These pulses were counted on a ratemeter over 1-sec intervals and displayed on a strip chart recorder.

The results presented here on the anatomical distribution and origin of 5-HT are a summary of previously published material (27). Some of the results have been presented in abstract form (28).

RESULTS

Anatomical Studies

Distribution and Ultrastructure of Serotoninergic Afferents

In the cat, as well as other mammals, 5-HT IR is localized within a fine beaded plexus of fibers (Fig. 1). This plexus forms an extensive network that is confined almost entirely to the granule cell and lower Purkinje cell layers (Figs. 2 and 3); a few beaded fibers extend into the molecular layer (Fig. 1A). This 5-HT plexus has a uniform distribution throughout the cerebellum (Figs. 2A and 3A,B), with the exception of vermal lobule X (Figs. 1C,D and 2C) and the flocculus (Fig. 3B), where only sparse labeling is observed as compared to other regions of the cerebellum. In addition to the cortex, an extensive plexus of 5-HT IR fibers and varicosities is also present throughout all of the deep cerebellar nuclei (Fig. 3A,B).

An ultrastructural analysis of 5-HT IR terminals was carried out to determine the cytological characteristics and synaptic relationships of this chemically defined afferent system. 5-HT IR profiles are observed throughout the granule cell layer. Thin (0.2–0.5 μm) fibers connect 5-HT-positive swellings that measure 0.95 to 1.8 μm in diameter. Both the thin fibers and swellings contain vesicles that range in size from 30 to 60 nm (Fig. 4E). 5-HT IR profiles are in direct apposition to granule cell bodies (Fig. 4A,B) as well as dendritic profiles in the granule cell layer. Further, 5-HT IR profiles are present within the mossy fiber glomerulus, where they approximate dendritic profiles (Fig. 4C,D). A few 5-HT IR swellings are juxtaposed to Purkinje cell bodies. To date, over 1,200 profiles have been examined in serial sections. Of these, only 140 form "classic" junctional complexes with either granule cell bodies ($n = 40$) or dendritic profiles ($n = 100$) in the granule cell layer.

Origin of Serotoninergic Afferents

Injections of HRP were made into the (i) anterior lobe vermis, (ii) posterior lobe vermis, (iii) paramedian lobule, and (iv) laterally in lobus simplex, crus I, and crus II to determine if there was a topographical organization in the serotoninergic pro-

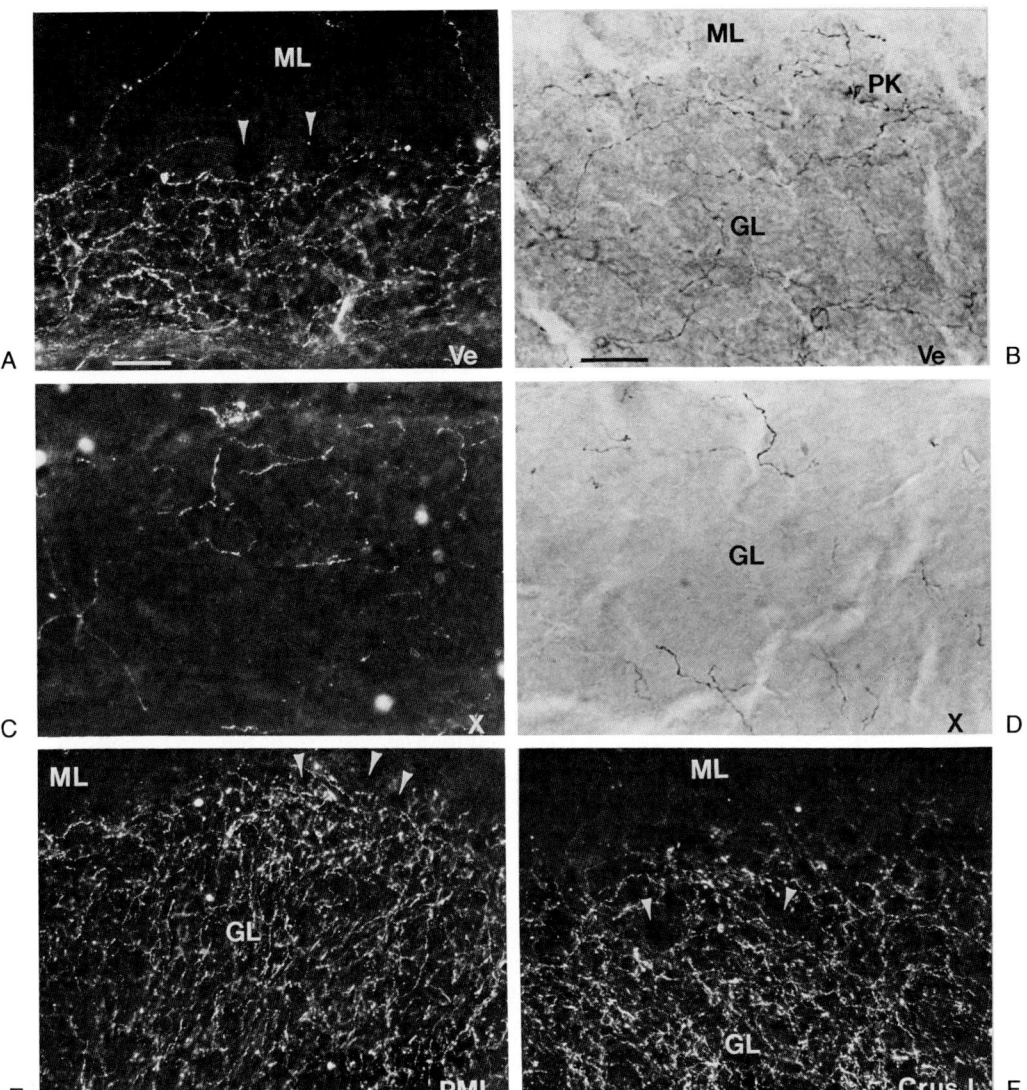

FIG. 1. Dark- and bright-field photomicrographs illustrating the distribution of 5-HT IR fibers and varicosities in vermal lobules Ve (**A,B**) and X (**C,D**) as well as the paramedian lobule (PML) (**E**) and Crus I (**F**). Regardless of the area the vast majority of 5-HT IR is located within the granule cell layer (GL). A few fibers (A) enter the molecular layer (ML) or approximate Purkinje cells (PK) (A,E,F, *arrowheads*). Note the relative paucity of 5-HT IR in lobule X (C,D) as compared to other areas. Calibration bar in A = 50 μm and also applies to C; in B, 25 μm; in D, 25 μm; and in E, 50 μm and also applies to F.

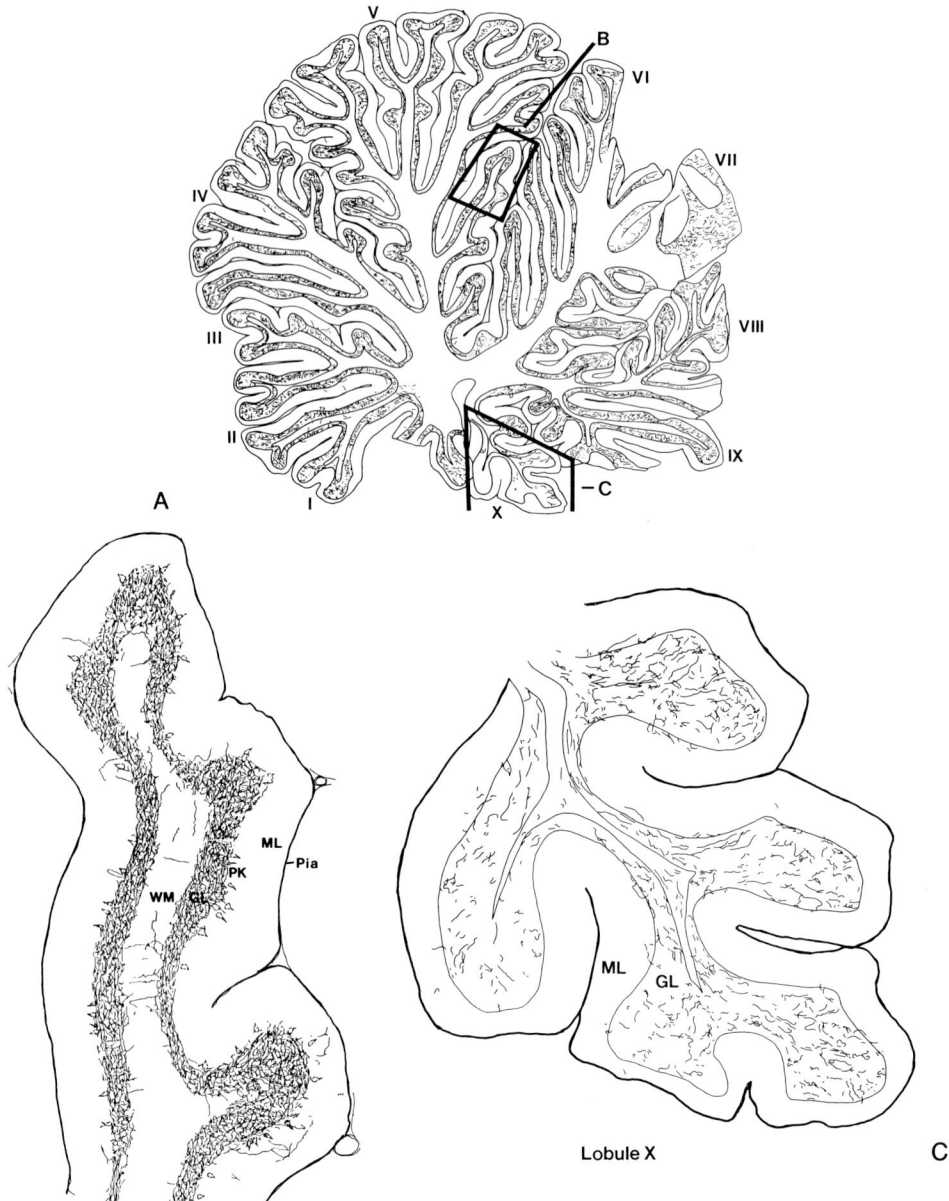

FIG. 2. A: Low-power camera lucida drawing of a midsagittal section of the cat's cerebellum illustrating the near uniform lobular distribution of 5-HT IR fibers. **B,C**: High-power drawings of lobule Ve (B) and lobule X (C), as indicated by the boxes in A. Note the sparse 5-HT IR in lobule X as compared to lobule Ve. Labeling is confined to the granule cell layer (GL) in all lobules. WM, white matter; other abbreviations as in Fig.1.

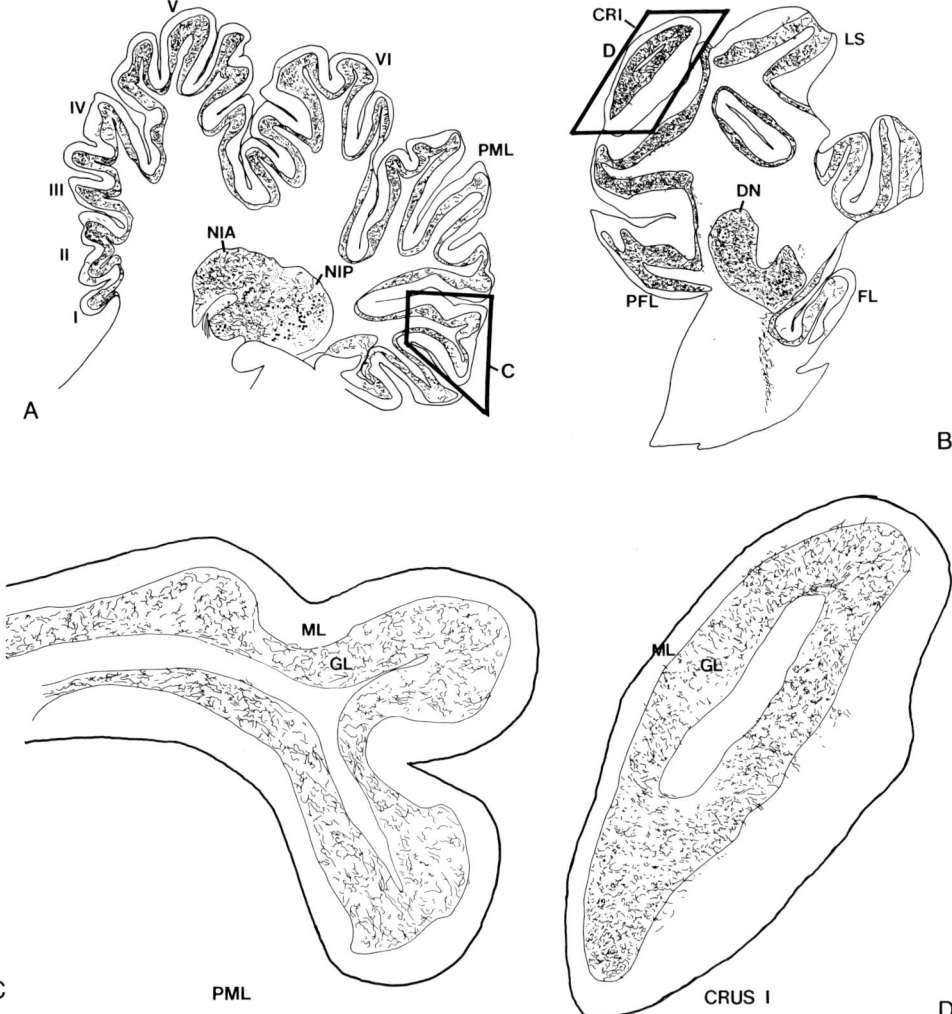

FIG. 3. A,B: Low-power camera lucida drawings through the intermediate (A) and lateral (B) aspect of the cerebellum illustrating the uniform lobular and laminar distribution of 5-HT IR fibers and varicosities. The enclosed areas in A and B are shown at higher magnification in **C** and **D**, respectively. CRI, crus I; DN, dentate nucleus; FL, flocculus; GL, granule cell layer; LS, lobus simplex; ML, molecular layer; NIA, nucleus interpositus anterior; NIP, nucleus interpositus posterior; PFL, paraflocculus; PML, paramedian lobule.

jection to the cat's cerebellum. Following tissue processing for the double-label technique, three types of labeled cells, including those (i) immunoreactive for 5-HT alone (Fig. 5A,B), (ii) retrogradely labeled alone (Fig. 5C, open block arrow), or (iii) both immunohistochemically and retrogradely labeled (Fig. 5C–F), were plotted on a series of standardized sections through the brain stem. These studies reveal similarities and some differences with respect to the populations of serotoninergic

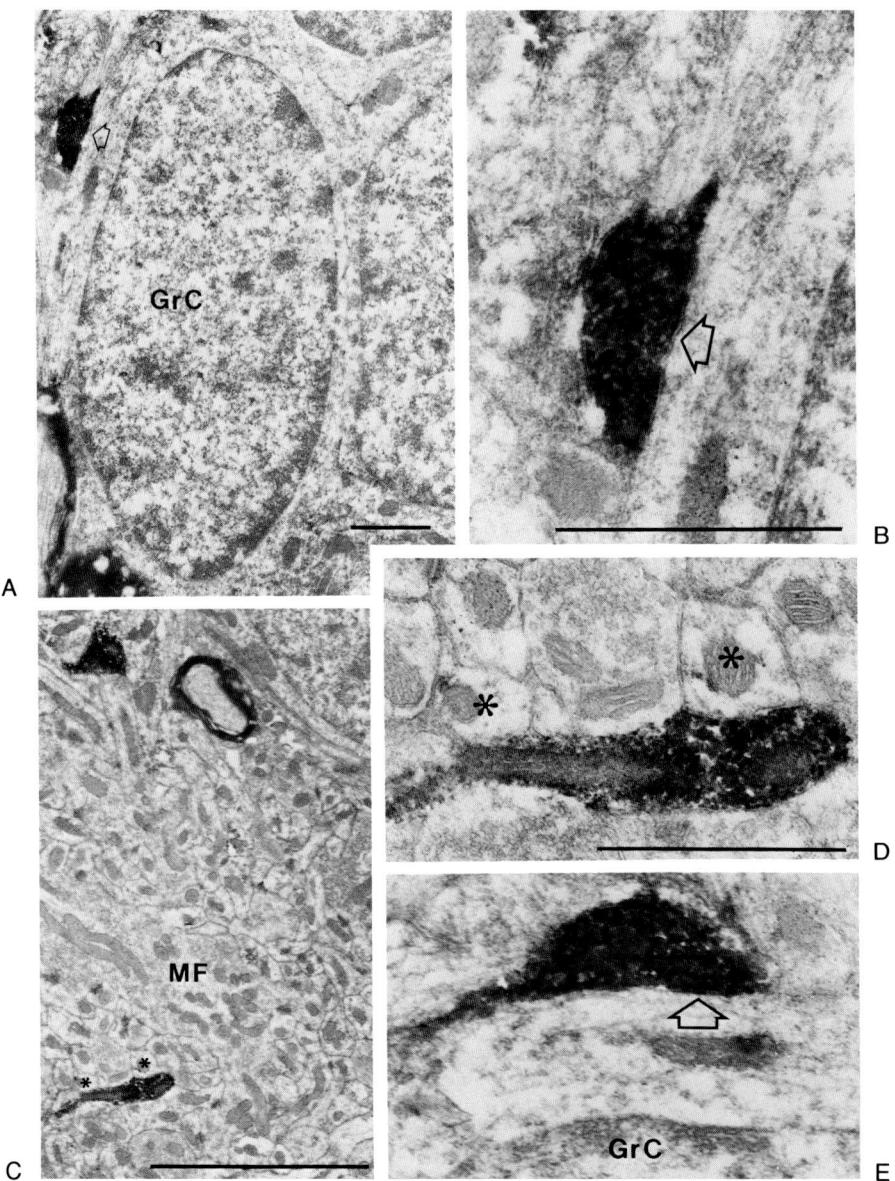

FIG. 4. A–E: Low- and high-power electron micrographs illustrating 5-HT IR profiles in apposition to granule cell (GrC) bodies (A,B,E) and dendritic profiles (*asterisks*) within a mossy fiber glomerulus (C,D). A junctional complex is illustrated in Fig. 5A (block arrow). Calibration bars in A,B,D, 1 μm and in C, 5 μm. Bar in D also applies to E.

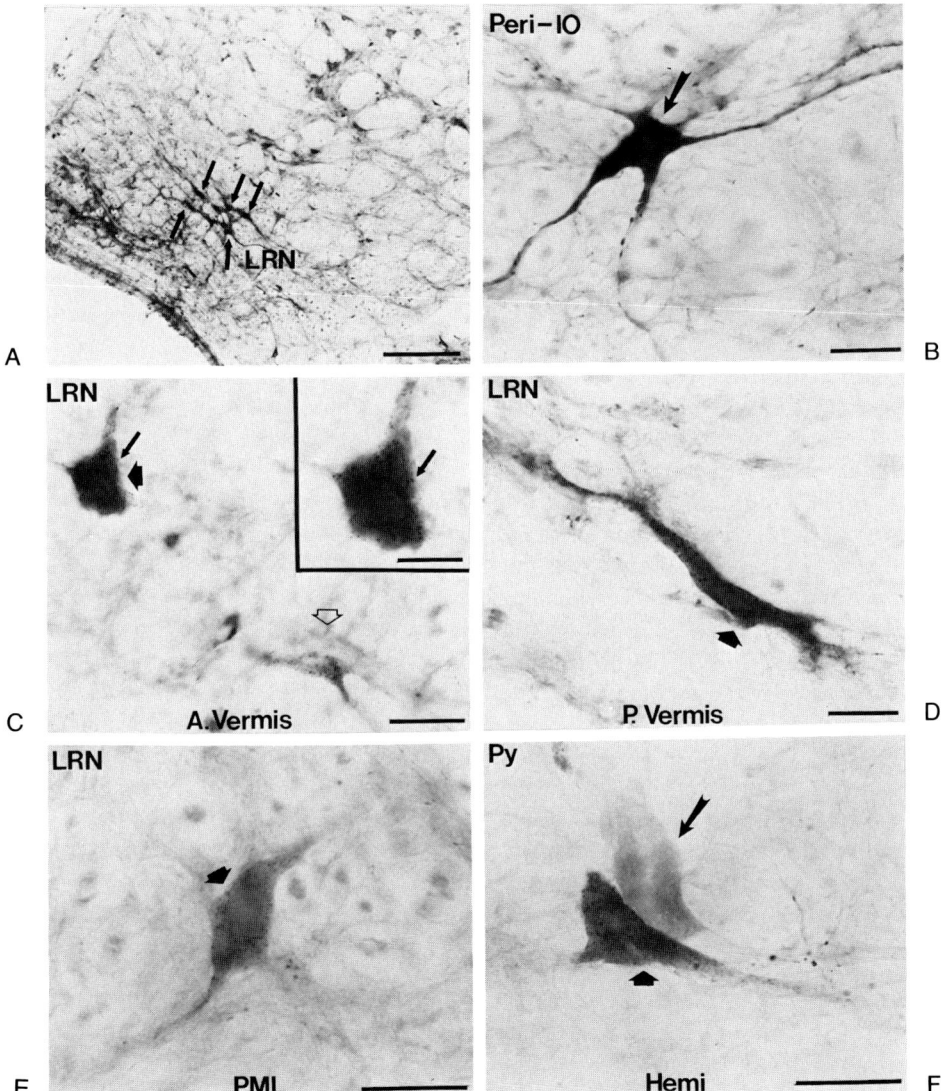

FIG. 5. Photomicrographs illustrating the results of double-label studies. **A,B**: Examples of 5-HT IR neurons in the lateral reticular nucleus (LRN) (A) and the periolivary reticular formation (Peri-IO) (B). **C–F**: Representative examples of double-labeled cells following HRP injections into the anterior lobe vermis (A. Vermis) (C), the posterior lobe vermis (P. Vermis) (D), the paramedian lobule (PML) (E), or the hemisphere (Hemi) (F). Calibration bar in A, 100 μm; in B, C, 25 μm; in D, 10 μm; in E, F, 15 μm; and in the inset of C, 10 μm.

neurons that project to disparate regions of the cerebellar cortex. The data are summarized in Fig. 6. 5-HT IR cells are present in nuclei of the raphe and the reticular formation of the medulla and pons. These cells are represented by the triangles on the right side of Fig. 6. The nomenclature for the nuclei was taken from the atlas of Berman (6). In the caudal medulla, 5-HT-containing somata are located principally within the raphe (Fig. 6B–H) and lateral reticular nuclei (Fig. 6B–E). At more rostral levels (Fig. 6E–H), serotoninergic neurons extend into the lateral tegmental field as well as the nuclei reticularis gigantocellularis and magnocellularis. Additional 5-HT-positive cell bodies are found within the medullary pyramids (Fig. 6D–G) and the periolivary reticular formation (Fig. 6E–H). The brain stem distribution of serotoninergic neurons is in agreement with that previously reported in the cat (25,49). The locations of neurons that give rise to the serotoninergic projection to different regions of the cat's cerebellum are represented on the left side of Fig. 6. The neuronal source to each injected area of the cerebellum is represented by a different symbol that is keyed on the drawing of the unfolded cerebellum shown in Fig. 6A. The serotoninergic projection to the anterior lobe vermis is derived from three different brain stem nuclei including the lateral reticular nucleus, paramedian reticular nucleus, and lateral tegmental fields (Figs. 5C and 6, open stars). The hemispheric portion of the cerebellum also receives a projection from serotoninergic neurons in the lateral and paramedian reticular nuclei, as well as from neurons located within the reticular formation immediately adjacent to the rostral aspect of the inferior olive (Figs. 5F and 6, closed circles). The lateral tegmental fields do not appear to project to lateral lobes of the cerebellum. In contrast to a convergent 5-HT input to the anterior lobe vermis and hemispheres, the projections to the posterior lobe vermis (Figs. 5D and 6, closed stars) and paramedian lobule (Figs. 5E and 6, open circles) arise solely from the lateral reticular nucleus. Although a few retrogradely labeled and many 5-HT IR neurons were observed within various raphe nuclei, no double-labeled cells were identified. Thus, it does not appear that the raphe nuclei contribute to the serotoninergic plexus of afferents that distribute within the four areas of the cerebellar cortex of the cat covered by our HRP injec-

FIG. 6. A: Camera lucida drawing of the unfolded cerebellum illustrating the extent of representative HRP injections in the anterior lobe vermis (*open stars*), posterior lobe vermis (*closed stars*), paramedian lobule (*open circles*), and hemispheres (*closed circles*). **B–H**: Camera lucida drawings of representative sections through the brain stem that illustrate the distribution of 5-HT IR neurons on the right side (*closed triangles*) and double-labeled cells following the injections shown in A on the left side. The symbols on the brain stem sections correspond to those illustrating the injection site. CUN, nucleus cuneatus; DAO, dorsal accessory olivary nucleus; DMN, dorsal motor vagal nucleus; ECN, external cuneate nucleus; FTL, lateral tegmental fields; GRA, nucleus gracilis; ICP, inferior cerebellar peduncle; LRN, lateral reticular nucleus; MAO, medial accessory olivary nucleus; NRG, nucleus reticularis gigantocellularis; PERI IO, periolivary reticular formation; PH, perihypoglossal nucleus; PO, principal olivary nucleus; PRN, paramedian reticular nucleus; SOL, nucleus solitarius; VIN, inferior vestibular nucleus; VMN, medial vestibular nucleus; XIIN, hypoglossal nerve.

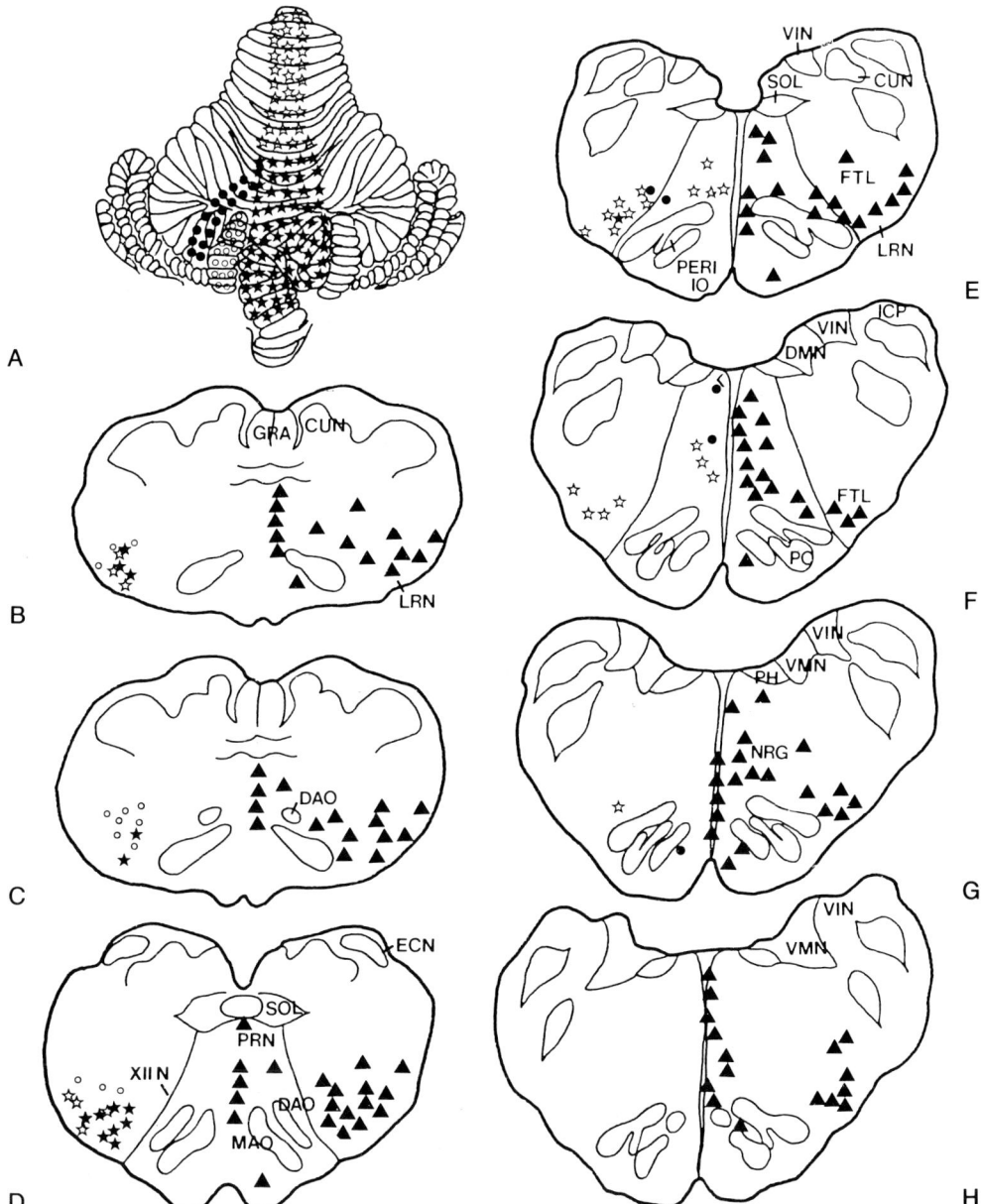

tions. As illustrated in Fig. 5C, both double-labeled and retrogradely labeled alone cells were intermingled in all precerebellar nuclei that contributed to the 5-HT projection to the cerebellum. The proportion of neurons within a given nucleus that gave rise to the 5-HT projection to the cerebellum was compared to that derived from non-5-HT neurons (retrogradely labeled alone). As summarized in Fig. 7, the double-labeled cells comprised only a small percentage of the projection to the cerebellar cortex derived from a particular brain stem nucleus.

Physiological Studies

Effects on Spontaneous Activity

In these experiments, 5-HT was iontophoretically applied to neurons that were identified as Purkinje cells on the basis of their spontaneous or amino acid-induced activity (Fig. 8A) or their response to stimulation of the inferior cerebellar peduncle (Fig. 8B,C). Stimulation of this fiber tract activates climbing fibers, which elicit a characteristic response in Purkinje cells (Fig. 8B,C, arrow). The extracellular response of spontaneously active Purkinje cells is characterized by simple, unitary action potentials (Fig. 8A, asterisks). Occasionally, a high-frequency burst interrupts the simple spike activity (Fig. 8A, arrow). This high-frequency burst has been shown to be caused by activation of the climbing fiber system of afferents (19), whereas the simple spikes have been correlated with activation of the mossy fiber-parallel fiber afferent system. Physiological data were taken directly from the oscilloscope (Figs. 8A–C and 9A–H) as well as from chart recordings (Figs. 8D–F, 9I,J, and 10A–F) to illustrate the effects of 5-HT and other compounds on the extended firing rate of a unit. Application of 5-HT to spontaneously active units (Fig. 8D,E) suppresses the simple spike firing in 100% of cells tested ($n=12$). In the chart recordings shown in Fig. 9I it can be seen that this effect is repeatable and dose dependent. Neural activity is reduced within 2 to 3 sec after iontophoresis of 5-HT is initiated, with maximal suppression occurring within 10 sec. For most cells, there is a minimal delay between the cessation of 5-HT application and the return to the control firing rate. In some cases, a prolonged application of 5-HT induces a rhythmic firing pattern in cells that is characterized by regular periods of activity interspersed with quiescent intervals (Fig. 8F). When 5-HT iontophoresis is terminated, the unit returns to a continuous firing pattern until 5-HT is reapplied (Fig. 8F).

Interactions with Amino Acids

Interactions between 5-HT and various amino acids were also analyzed in this study. As with spontaneous activity, 5-HT suppresses activity in 100% of cells activated by glutamate ($n=62$) and 90% of those driven by aspartate ($n=19$) in a

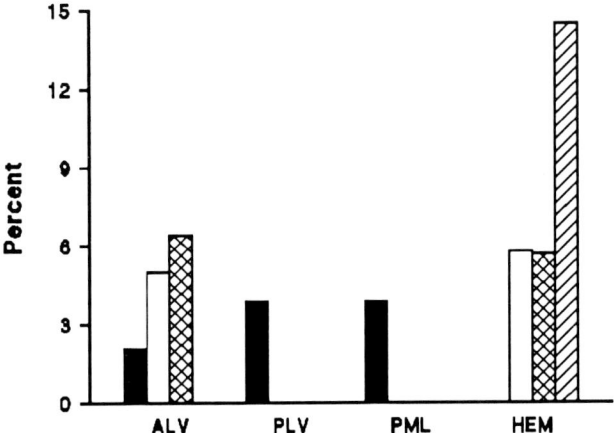

FIG. 7. Histogram illustrating the percentage of double-labeled cells as compared to cells retrogradely labeled alone, found in four brain stem nuclei following injections into different regions of the cerebellar cortex. ALV, anterior lobe vermis; PLV, posterior lobe vermis; PML, paramedian lobule; Hem, hemisphere; LRN, lateral reticular nucleus (■); FTL, lateral tegmental fields (□); PRN, paramedian reticular nucleus (▨); PERI IO, periolivary reticular formation (▧).

dose-dependent manner (Fig. 9A–I). In addition, 5-HT potentiates the suppressive effects of GABA (Fig. 9J), even in the presence of the excitatory amino acids glutamate and aspartate. This potentiation of GABA is seen even if both substances are applied at subthreshold levels, as shown in Fig. 9J (open block arrow). Application of 5-HT at +15 nA or GABA at +10 nA partially suppresses unit activity, whereas currents of 5 nA for either substance is subthreshold for the response. If both are simultaneously applied, there is a partial suppression of the units glutamate-induced activity initially. The unit's activity is completely suppressed with continued application of the two chemical messengers. If the cell is "preconditioned" with subthreshold doses of either 5-HT or GABA, prior to simultaneous application of both substances the delay to complete suppression is eliminated.

Receptor Identification

Several agonists and antagonists to various 5-HT receptor subtypes were applied to identify which receptor(s) are responsible for mediating the observed effects. It should be noted that the effects of these substances were tested on glutamate-activated cells. 8-OH-DPAT (8-OH) and IPS, two 5-HT$_{1A}$ receptor agonists, completely mimicked the effects of 5-HT (Fig. 10A–C). Further, simultaneous application of 5-HT and 8-OH led to a potentiation that exceeds the suppressive effects elicited by each substance applied separately (Fig. 10A). In the unit shown in Fig. 10A, 5-HT or 8-OH applied at +30 nA each led to a 23% reduction in glutamate-induced activity. Upon reversal of the current to either barrel the cell immediately

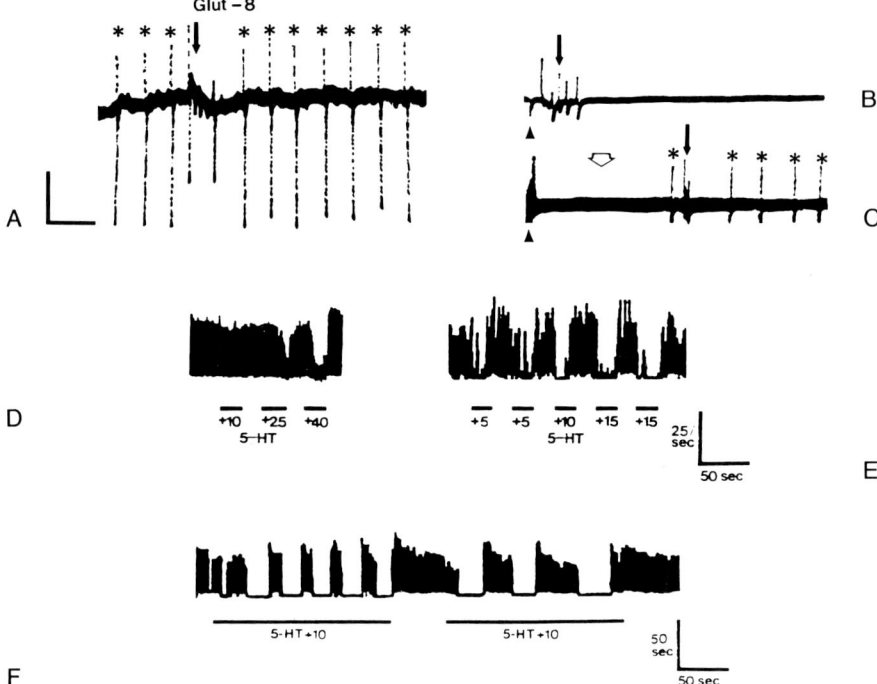

FIG. 8. A–C: Oscillographic traces illustrating glutamate-(Glut 8) (A) and stimulus-induced (B,C) activity recorded extracellularly from Purkinje cells. Purkinje cell activity is characterized by action potentials with two different configurations. *Asterisks* in A and C indicate a simple action potential and the *arrows* in A–C, indicate a complex action potential characterized by a high-frequency burst consisting of an initial positive going spike followed by several low-amplitude action potentials. Also note that following the complex spike there is a period of suppression of the simple spike activity for a variable period of time. The second complex spike in C is spontaneous. Calibration bar = 30mV, 20 msec for the traces in A; 20 mV, 10 msec for those in B; and 20 mV, 70 msec for those in C. **D–F**: Chart recordings illustrating the suppressive effects of 5-HT on spontaneous activity. Note the suppression is dose dependent. In some cases prolonged application of 5-HT induces a rhythmic pattern of firing in the Purkinje cell (F).

returns to control levels of firing. When both 5-HT and 8-OH are applied simultaneously, however, there is complete suppression of unit activity. Even when 5-HT is removed, the suppressive effect of 8-OH alone is enhanced such that there is still a 60% reduction in unit activity. After the current to the 8-OH barrel is reversed, the unit activity remains decreased by 23% as compared to control for an additional 25 sec before recovering completely.

To confirm the presence of a 5-HT$_{1A}$ receptor, the antagonist spiperone was applied (Fig. 10C). Iontophoresis of 5-HT or 8-OH suppresses glutamate-induced activity. However, when spiperone, a 5-HT$_{1A}$ receptor antagonist, is applied simultaneously, the suppressive effects of both ligands are blocked. When spiperone is removed, 5-HT and 8-OH again suppress unit activity. As spiperone also acts on

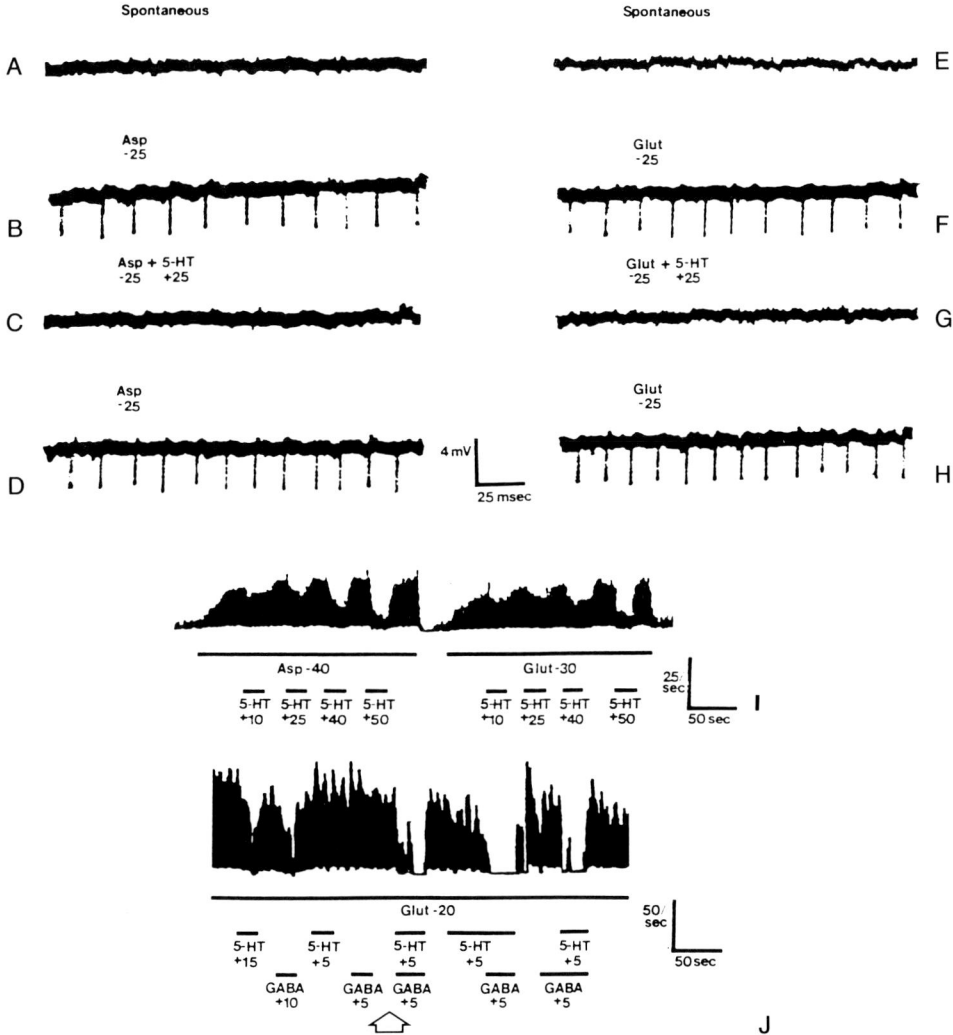

FIG. 9. Oscillographic traces (**A–H**) and a chart recording (**I**) illustrate the suppressive effect of 5-HT on aspartate- (Asp) (A–D,I) and glutamate- (Glut) (E–H,I) induced activity. Note in I that the suppressive effect of 5-HT is dose dependent. **J**: Chart recording illustrating interactions between 5-HT and GABA in a glutamate-activated unit. Note potentiation of effects of 5-HT and GABA even when both are applied at subthreshold levels (*block arrow*).

$5\text{-HT}_{1C/2}$ receptors, DOI, which has a high affinity for the 5-HT_2 receptor and low affinity for the 5-HT_{1A} receptor, was applied (Fig. 10D). DOI has no effect on the activity of a unit that was suppressed by application of 5-HT or 8-OH. To further confirm the absence of a 5-HT_2 or 5-HT_{1C} receptor, the effect of ritanserin, a $5\text{-HT}_{2/1C}$ receptor antagonist, was tested. Simultaneous application of ritanserin is

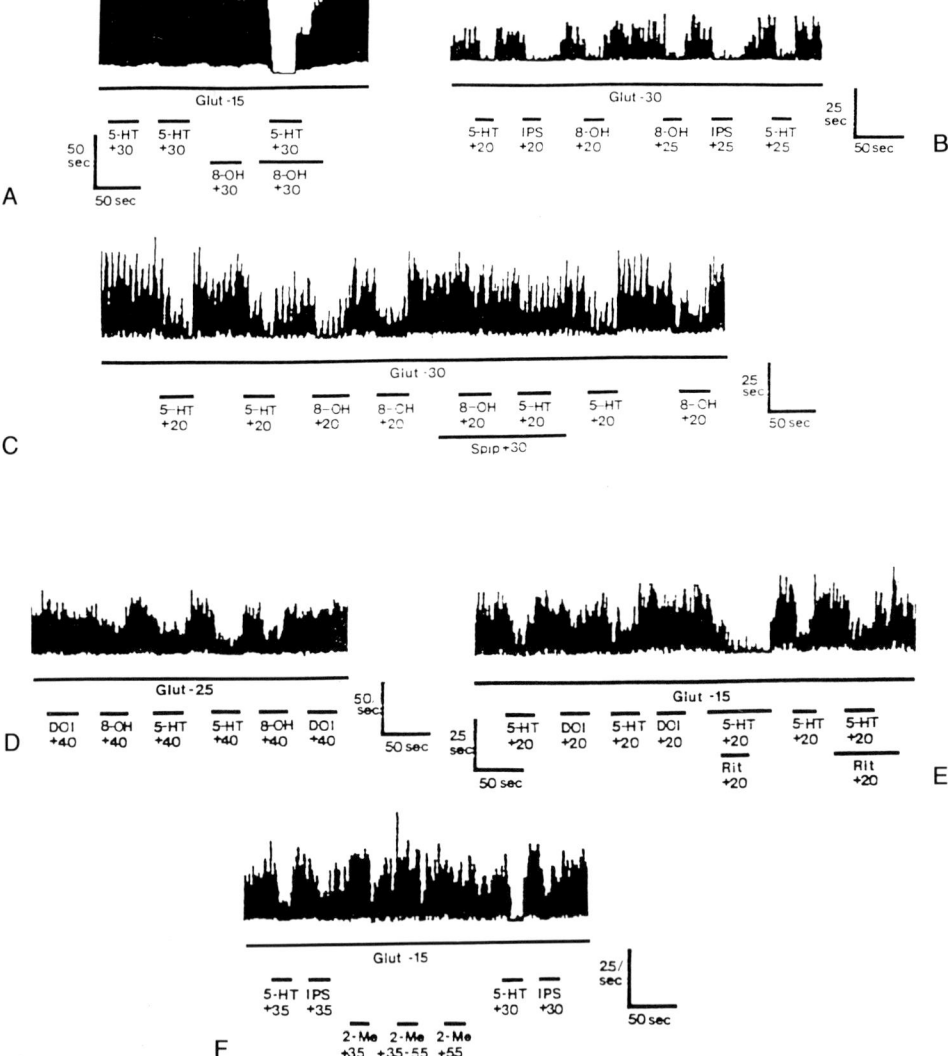

FIG. 10. A–F: Chart recordings illustrating interactions between 5-HT and various 5-HT receptor agonists and antagonists. 8-OH and IPS, both 5-HT$_{1A}$ receptor agonists, mimic the action of 5-HT (A–C). The 5-HT$_{1A}$ receptor antagonist spiperone (Spip) blocks the suppressive effects of both 5-HT and 8-OH (C). The 5-HT$_2$ receptor agonist DOI, as well as the 5-HT$_3$ receptor agonist 2-ME, has little to no effect on Purkinje cell activity (D–F). Ritanserin (Rit), a 5-HT$_2$ receptor antagonist, is ineffective in blocking 5-HT-induced suppression of Purkinje cell activity (E).

ineffective in blocking the suppressive effects of 5-HT (Fig. 10E). These data suggest the presence of a 5-HT_{1A}, but not a 5-HT_2 or 5-HT_{1C}, receptor in the cat's cerebellar cortex.

The presence of a 5-HT_3 receptor was tested by applying methyl-5-HT (2-ME). This 5-HT_3 receptor agonist has no effect on Purkinje cells, which are suppressed by either 5-HT, 8-OH (not shown), or IPS (Fig. 10F).

DISCUSSION

5-HT is a chemical messenger that is present throughout the mammalian central nervous system (CNS), including the cerebellum. Based on immunohistochemical preparations of the cerebellum from several species, serotoninergic afferents give rise to a network of fine fibers and small varicosities (7,8,32,50). In the cat cerebellum, this beaded plexus of fibers has a relatively uniform lobular distribution as it is present throughout all areas of the cortex with the exception of lobule X and the flocculus. With respect to laminar distribution, 5-HT IR profiles arc confined almost exclusively to the granule cell layer.

Brain Stem Origin of 5-HT

It has been suggested that neurons in the raphe nuclei are the source of serotoninergic afferents to the cerebellum (14). It is well established that 5-HT-positive cells are present in medullary and pontine raphe nuclei (17,25,39,40,49). Different studies, including the present one, have found retrogradely labeled cells within these nuclei following injections of tracers into the cerebellum or degenerating neurons following lesions of the cortex (5,9,12,22,43,48). Therefore, it was assumed that these nuclei were the source of 5-HT afferents to the cerebellum. To positively identify the cells of origin of 5-HT in the cerebellum, a double-labeling technique has been used in the rat, opossum, and cat (7,27,52). The results are consistent across species. The primary source of 5-HT to the cerebellar cortex appears to arise from neurons located in the medullary reticular formation. However, a recent study by King et al. (32) has shown that a few double-labeled cells can be detected in the locus coeruleus, pars alpha when fluorescent microspheres are injected into the posterior lobe vermis of the opossum. Further, a few raphe dorsalis neurons are double labeled when injections of fluorescent microspheres are made into the cerebellar nuclei of the cat (*unpublished observations*). However, to date no double-labeled cells have been found in any medullary raphe nuclei following injections of HRP or fluorescent microspheres into disparate regions of the cerebellar cortex or the deep cerebellar nuclei. Thus, it appears that the 5-HT neurons within these caudal raphe nuclei project to other targets such as the spinal cord (10,11,15,36,44). Taken together these data suggest that the medullary raphe projection to the cerebellum is likely derived from a population of neurons that is chemically distinct from those that contain 5-HT. The conclusion is based on negative findings with respect to the raphe; however, the positive findings in three different species, using two different retrograde tracers, establishes nuclei within the reticular formation as a primary source of 5-HT to the cerebellar cortex.

Physiological Effects of 5-HT

It is of interest that the cells of origin of 5-HT to the cat, rat, and opossum cerebellum are interspersed with neurons that give rise to mossy fibers, an accepted excitatory input (19,24). When applied iontophoretically, 5-HT appears to uniformly suppress both spontaneous as well as glutamate- and/or aspartate-induced activation of Purkinje cells. The data derived from these studies indicate that the reported effects are mediated primarily, if not exclusively, by 5-HT$_{1A}$ receptors. Most biochemical studies show few to no 5-HT receptors in the cerebellum (31,38, 42,51). However, physiological studies using the same ligands, have positively established a functional role for this indoleamine in regulating Purkinje cell activity. It is not clear why there are differences in the two approaches to receptor identification. The present findings regarding the suppressive effects of 5-HT on spontaneous activity are not consistent with those described by others. In slices of the rat cerebellum, 5-HT was found to enhance the spontaneous activity of deep cerebellar nuclear neurons (21) and to have no effect on the spontaneous activity of Purkinje cells (23). Lee et al. (34) found a similar lack of effect of 5-HT on spontaneously active Purkinje cells in the rat recorded *in vivo*. There are several reasons why differences are seen in these studies. First is the preparation used. Both Gardette et al. (21) and Hicks et al. (23) used cerebellar slices from neonatal rats (postnatal day [PD] 16–25). Morphologically, the rat's cerebellum is not mature until PD 30 (4, 13) when the EGL is no longer evident and parallel fiber synaptogenesis is complete. Thus, cerebellar circuitry is not mature at the ages used in these studies and neurons may not respond as those in the adult to application of 5-HT. Several studies have suggested that 5-HT may have a different role during brain development (for review, see refs. 32 and 33). Whereas 5-HT may play a trophic role in establishing normal neural circuitry, at later stages it appears to function as a chemical messenger that modulates neuronal activity. A second factor that may account for the differences in the effect of 5-HT on spontaneous activity in different species is the fact that the data in the rat were obtained in slice preparations. Thus the Purkinje cells were removed from their normal extrinsic synaptic inputs and may have been under the tonic influence of local circuitry, which is predominantly inhibitory in nature. It is more difficult to reconcile the differences between the study by Lee et al. (34) and the present one as they used adult animals (rat) and recorded *in vivo*. As noted above, the distribution of serotoninergic afferents is not uniform in the rat and thus different neuronal circuits may be involved, depending on the area from which the data were obtained. Further, different anesthesia was used (α-chloralose in the cat versus urethane in the rat). Finally, there may be different receptors or receptor sensitivity in the two species that mediate different effects.

All studies to date appear to be in agreement with respect to interactions between 5-HT and excitatory amino acids. Uniformly, 5-HT suppresses glutamate- and aspartate-induced activity in all species and cell preparations. The mechanism by which this suppression occurs is currently unknown. It has been suggested that 5-HT blocks the release of glutamate (41). These data would not be confirmed in the present study as unit activity is blocked following exogenous application of the amino acid. Hicks et al. (23) found that the suppression of glutamate-induced responses occurred with virtually no changes in the intrinsic membrane properties of Purkinje cells, which suggested a true pharmacological interaction between the two chemical messengers rather than an effect of 5-HT on membrane properties of the neuron. This interaction could occur at the level of the receptor or the transduction mechanism. With respect to the latter, it has been shown in several areas of the brain that most 5-HT receptors are linked to either the adenylate cyclase-cAMP or the inositol trisphosphate second messenger system (20). Involvement of these second messenger pathways may lead to changes in the cellular environment or metabolism that directly alter its ability to respond to excitatory amino acids.

5-HT may also alter neuronal responsiveness through its interactions with the GABAergic system. In the present study, 5-HT potentiated the effects of GABA even when one or both were applied at subthreshold levels. In our paradigm 5-HT is iontophoresed into the extracellular space, thus any neuron in the vicinity may be affected. 5-HT could enhance GABA release from adjacent terminals; however, this mechanism is unlikely as Lee et al. (35) used specific GABA reuptake and release blockers to show that the action of 5-HT did not involve alterations in release or reuptake of GABA. The mechanism of interaction of GABA and 5-HT may occur at the level of signal transduction. 5-HT acting through the 5-HT$_{1A}$ receptor appears to activate potassium channels (2,3,20,37). Nicoll (37) has suggested that different ligands and their receptors may exert their effects on the same ionic channels; thus, there may be a potentiation of effects following application of relatively small quantities of one or more chemical messenger. For example, it is known that the activation of a GABA$_B$ receptor results in selective opening of K$^+$ channels. Further, data (37) suggest that 5-HT acts on the same channels as GABA leading to a potentiation of effects that results in neuronal hyperpolarization. In addition, chemical messengers may also have effects on different ionic channels that may result in the same net effect on membrane polarization. For example, activation of GABA$_A$ receptor leads to the opening of a Cl$^-$ channel, whereas, as noted previously, application of 5-HT results in opening of K$^+$ channels. The net effect is a potentiation of hyperpolarization of the cell with a resulting decrease in both spontaneous and amino acid-induced excitation.

Functional Considerations

Functionally, 5-HT can be analyzed at the cellular level by relating known mechanisms of action to specific cerebellar phenomena described in previous studies. In addition, we can speculate on its overall impact on cerebellar activity. The findings of the present and previous studies indicate that 5-HT is involved in decreasing Purkinje cell activity through complex mechanisms that involve primarily the 5-HT_{1A} receptor. This receptor appears to be linked to the adenylate cyclase-cAMP second messenger system (18,20), thus suggesting a metabotropic action for 5-HT; this type of action is generally associated with chemical messengers referred to as neuromodulators (26).

To date we can only speculate on the role of 5-HT in regulating motor activity mediated through the cerebellum. There are several theories of cerebellar function (24). There are significant physiological, neurochemical, and biochemical differences between the classically defined extrinsic afferents to the cerebellar cortex, namely, climbing fibers and mossy fibers, and the serotoninergic system. Climbing fibers and mossy fibers appear to act as ionotropic neurotransmitters that depolarize and thus excite Purkinje cells. This in turn leads to suppression of neurons in the deep cerebellar nuclei and a resultant decrease in cerebellar outflow (24). In contrast serotoninergic afferents acting through metabotropic mechanisms may be involved in decreasing the firing rate of a Purkinje cell, perhaps through opening of K^+ channels and/or decreasing Purkinje cell responsiveness to glutamate. Regardless, the net effect is a decrease of Purkinje cell input to the cerebellar nuclei, which in turn results in a subsequent increase in cerebellar output. A major question that remains to be addressed in defining the role of 5-HT in cerebellar circuitry is related to mechanisms that regulate the physiological release of 5-HT and the location of the 5-HT receptors. Further, the possible direct physiological effects of 5-HT on neurons in the cerebellar nuclei must be determined to understand more completely the role of 5-HT in the regulation of motor activity.

ACKNOWLEDGMENTS

This work was supported by grant NS 18028. The authors gratefully acknowledge the technical expertise of Katharine Dillingham. The photographic assistance of Karl Rubin is also appreciated.

REFERENCES

1. Adams JC. Technical considerations on the use of HRP as a neuronal marker. *Neuroscience* 2 1977; 2:141–146.
2. Aghajanian GK, Lakoski JM. Hyperpolarization of serotonergic neurons by serotonin and LSD: studies in brain slices showing increased K+ conductance. *Brain Res* 1984;305:181–185.
3. Aghajanian GK, Sprouse JS, Sheldon P, Rasmussen K. Electrophysiology of the central serotonin system: receptor subtypes and transducer mechanisms. *Ann NY Acad Sci* 1990;600:93–103.
4. Altman J. Postnatal development of the cerebellar cortex in the rat. II. Phases in the maturation of Purkinje cells and of the molecular layer. *J Comp Neurol* 1972;145:399–464.
5. Batini C, Buisseret-Delmas C, Corvisier J, Hardy O, Jassik-Gerschenfeld D. Brain stem nuclei giving fibers to lobules VI and VII of the cerebellar vermis. *Brain Res* 1978;153:241–261.
6. Berman AL. *The brainstem of the cat*. Madison: University of Wisconsin Press, 1969.

7. Bishop GA, Ho RH. The distribution and origin of serotonin immunoreactivity in the rat cerebellum. *Brain Res* 1985;331:195–207.
8. Bishop GA, Ho RH, King JS. Localization of serotonin immunoreactivity in the opossum cerebellum. *J Comp Neurol* 1985;235:301–321.
9. Bobillier P, Seguin S, Petitjean F, Salvert D, Touret M, Jouvet M. The raphe nuclei of the cat brain stem: a topographical atlas of their efferent projections as revealed by autoradiography. *Brain Res* 1976;113:449–486.
10. Bowker RM, Steinbusch HWM, Coulter JD. Serotonergic and peptidergic projections to the spinal cord demonstrated by a combined retrograde HRP histochemical and immunocytochemical staining method. *Brain Res* 1981;211:412–417.
11. Bowker RM, Westlund KN, Sullivan MC, Wilber JF, Coulter JD. Descending serotonergic, peptidergic and cholinergic pathways from the raphe nuclei: a multiple transmitter complex. *Brain Res* 1983;288:33–48.
12. Brodal A, Taber E, Walberg F. The raphe nuclei of the brain stem in the cat. II. Efferent connections. *J Comp Neurol* 1960;114:239–260.
13. Calvet M-C, Calvet J. Computer-assisted analysis of the developing Purkinje neuron. I. Effects of the age of the animal at the moment of explantation on the subsequent dendritic development in organotypic cultures. *Brain Res* 1988;462:322–333.
14. Chan-Palay V. Fine structure of labelled axons in the cerebellar cortex and nuclei of rodents and primates after intraventricular infusions with tritiated serotonin. *Anat Embryol* 1975;148:235–265.
15. Chiba T, Masuko S. Coexistence of varying combinations of neuropeptides with 5-hydroxytryptamine in neurons of the raphe pallidus et obscurus projecting to the spinal cord. *Neurosci Res* 1989; 7:13–23.
16. Crepel F, Krupa M. Modulation of the responsiveness of cerebellar Purkinje cells to excitatory amino acids. In: Ben-Ari Y, ed. *Excitatory amino acids and neuronal plasticity*. New York: Plenum 1990:323–329.
17. Dahlström A, Fuxe K. Evidence for the existence of monoamine-containing neurons in the central nervous system. I. Demonstration of monoamines in the cell bodies of brain stem neurons. *Acta Physiol Scand [Suppl]* 1964;232:1–80.
18. DeVivo M, Maayani S. 5-HT receptors coupled to adenylate cyclase. In: Sanders-Bush E, ed. *The serotonin receptors*. Clifton, NJ: Humana Press, 1988:141–179.
19. Eccles JC, Ito M, Szentagothai J. *The cerebellum as a neuronal machine*. Berlin/Heidelberg/New York: Springer-Verlag, 1967.
20. Frazer A, Maayani S, Wolf BB. Subtypes of receptors for serotonin. *Annu Rev Pharmacol Toxicol* 1990;30:307–348.
21. Gardette R, Krupa M, Crepel F. Differential effects of serotonin on the spontaneous discharge and on the excitatory amino acid-induced responses of deep cerebellar nuclei neurons in rat cerebellar slices. *Neuroscience* 1987;23:491–500.
22. Gould BB. Organization of afferents from the brain stem nuclei to the cerebellar cortex in the cat. *Adv Anat Embryol Cell Biol* 1980;62:1–90.
23. Hicks TP, Krupa M, Crépel F. Selective effects of serotonin upon excitatory amino acid-induced depolarizations of Purkinje cells in cerebellar slices from young rats. *Brain Res* 1989;492:371–376.
24. Ito M. *The cerebellum and neural control*. New York: Raven Press, 1984.
25. Jacobs BL, Gannon PJ, Azmitia EC. Atlas of serotonergic cell bodies in the cat brainstem: an immunocytochemical analysis. *Brain Res Bull* 1984;13:1–31.
26. Kaczmarek LK, Levitan IB. *Neuromodulators*. New York: Oxford University Press, 1987.
27. Kerr CHW, Bishop GA. Topographical organization in the origin of serotoninergic projections to different regions of the cat's cerebellar cortex. *J Comp Neurol* 1991;304:502–515.
28. Kerr CW, Bishop GA. Suppression of Purkinje cell activity by chemically coded extrinsic afferents. *Soc Neurosci Abstr* 1989;15:466.
29. Kerr CW, Bishop GA. Serotonin suppression of Purkinje cell activity through selective activation of the 5-HT1A receptor. *Brain Res(in press)*.
30. Kerr CW, Chen YF, King JS, Bishop GA. 5-HT in the cat's cerebellar cortex: ultrastructural analysis and identification of receptors. *Soc Neurosci Abstr* 1991;17(*in press*).
31. Kilpatrick GJ, Jones BJ, Tyers MB. Identification and distribution of 5-HT3 receptors in rat brain using radioligand binding. *Nature* 1987;330:746–748.
32. King JS, Walker JJ, Bishop GA. The brainstem origin and development of serotonin in the opossum cerebellum. In: Trouillas P, Fuxe K, eds. *Serotonin, the cerebellum, and ataxia*. New York: Raven Press, 1993:137–154.

33. Lauder JM. Ontogeny of the serotonergic system in the rat: serotonin as a developmental signal. *Ann NY Acad Sci* 1990;600:297–314.
34. Lee M, Strahlendorf JC, Strahlendorf HK. Modulatory action of serotonin on glutamate-induced excitation of cerebellar Purkinje cells. *Brain Res* 1986;361:107–113.
35. Lee M, Strahlendorf JC, Strahlendorf HK. Picrotoxin but not bicuculline antagonizes 5-hydroxytryptamine-induced inhibition of cerebellar Purkinje neurons. *Exp Neurol* 1987;97:577–591.
36. Millhorn DE, Hökfelt T, Verhofstad AAJ, Terenius L. Individual cells in the raphe nuclei of the medulla oblongata in rat that contain immunoreactivities for both serotonin and enkephalin project to the spinal cord. *Exp Brain Res* 1989;75:536–542.
37. Nicoll RA. The coupling of neurotransmitter receptors to ion channels in the brain. *Science* 1988;241:545–551.
38. Peroutka SJ, Snyder SH. Two distinct serotonin receptors: regional variations in receptor binding in mammalian brain. *Brain Res* 1981;208:339–347.
39. Pin C, Jones B, Jouvet M. Topographie des neurones monoaminergiques du tronc cérébral du chat: étude par histofluorescence. *C R Soc Biol (Paris)* 1968;162:2136–2141.
40. Poitras D, Parent A. Atlas of the distribution of monoamine-containing nerve cell bodies in the brain stem of the cat. *J Comp Neurol* 1978;179:699–718.
41. Raiteri M, Maura G, Bonanno G, Pittaluga A. Differential pharmacology and function of two 5-HT1 receptors modulating transmitter release in rat cerebellum. *J Pharmacol Exp Ther* 1986;237:644–648.
42. Sanders-Bush E. *The serotonin receptors*. Clifton, NJ: Humana Press, 1988.
43. Shinnar S, Maciewicz RJ, Shofer RJ. A raphe projection to cat cerebellar cortex. *Brain Res* 1973;97:139–143.
44. Skagerberg G, Björklund A. Topographic principles in the spinal projections of serotonergic and non-serotonergic brainstem neurons in the rat. *Neuroscience* 1985;15:445–480.
45. Stephanini M, DeMartino C, Zamboni L. Fixation of ejaculated spermatozoa for electron microscopy. *Nature* 1967;216:173–174.
46. Sternberger LA. *Immunocytochemistry*, 2nd ed. New York: John Wiley, 1979.
47. Strahlendorf JC, Lee M, Strahlendorf HK. Modulatory role of serotonin on GABA-elicited inhibition of cerebellar Purkinje cells. *Neuroscience* 1989;30:117–125.
48. Taber PE, Hoddevik GH, Walberg F. The cerebellar projection from the raphe nuclei in the cat as studied with the method of retrograde transport of horseradish peroxidase. *Anat Embryol (Berl)* 1977; 152:73–87.
49. Takeuchi Y, Kimura H, Sano Y. Immunohistochemical demonstration of the distribution of serotonin neurons in the brainstem of the rat and cat. *Cell Tissue Res* 1982;224:247–267.
50. Takeuchi Y, Kimura H, Sano Y. Immunohistochemical demonstration of serotonin-containing nerve fibers in the cerebellum. *Cell Tissue Res* 1982;226:1–12.
51. Waeber C, Dietl MM, Hayer D, Palacios JM. 5-HT1 receptors in the vertebrate brain: regional distribution examined by autoradiography. *Naunyn Schmiedebergs Arch Pharmacol* 1989;340:486–494.
52. Walker JJ, Bishop GA, Ho RH, King JS. Brainstem origin of serotonin- and enkephalin immunoreactive afferents to the opossum's cerebellum. *J Comp Neurol* 1988;276:481–497.

*Serotonin, the Cerebellum,
and Ataxia*, edited by
P. Trouillas and K. Fuxe.
Raven Press, Ltd., New York © 1993.

7

Serotonergic Innervation of the Inferior Olive and Tremor Generated in the Olivocerebellar Climbing Fiber System

Leif Wiklund

Laboratoire de Physiologie Nerveuse, CNRS, 91190 Gif-sur-Yvette, France

The inferior olive is the origin of climbing fibers to the cerebellum, and these afferents synapse directly on the Purkinje cells of the cerebellar cortex (11,20). Each Purkinje cell receives a single climbing fiber, but this forms several synaptic junctions with the soma and primary dendrites of the Purkinje cell. The powerful climbing fiber excitation evokes a complex spike in the Purkinje cells (14).

The olivocerebellar projection demonstrates a strict topographical organization. Different compartments of the olivary subnuclei project to different sagittal zones of the cerebellar cortex and cerebellar nuclei (2,17,18,35). The caudal part of the medial accessory olivary nucleus (MAO) projects to the medial A zone of vermis, the caudal dorsal accessory nucleus (DAO) to the B zone of vermis, the rostromedial DAO to the C1 and C3 zones of pars intermedia, the rostral MAO to the C2 zone, and the principal nucleus (PO) to the hemisperal D zones (17,18).

Olivary neurons normally fire at a relatively low frequency of up to a few impulses per second and cannot be driven at frequencies above 10 to 12 per second (1). It has been noted that groups of olivary neurons have a tendency to synchronize their activity (14,22), which may be explained by their electrotonic coupling through dendritic gap junctions (23,33).

Systemic administration of harmaline elicits whole-body tremor in different experimental animals. Careful electrophysiological experiments by De Montigny and Lamarre (10) and Llinás and Volkind (24) have demonstrated that this tremor is generated in the olivocerebellar climbing fiber system. Harmaline administration provokes in caudal parts of the accessory olivary nuclei rhythmic, synchronous activity of 8 to 12 Hz in large groups of neurons. The rhythmic activity is transmitted to the cerebellum through the olivocerebellar system, and via cerebellofugal systems to the brain stem and spinal cord motoneurons, where it results in tremor.

This chapter reviews a series of studies that indicate that harmaline exerts its tremogenic action on olivary neurons by interaction with serotonergic regulatory control of certain olivary compartments.

SEROTONERGIC INNERVATION OF THE INFERIOR OLIVE

Serotonergic innervation of olivary nuclei has been studied with several techniques. Using Falk-Hillarp fluorescence histochemistry, Wiklund et al. (36) studied the distribution of serotonergic innervation in cat inferior olive. A distinct topographical organization was demonstrated and found to correspond to the topographical organization of the olivocerebellar projection. The densest serotonergic innervation was found in caudal DAO, which projects to the B zone. Dense serotonergic innervation was also found in caudal MAO projecting to the A zone. Sparse innervation was found in the regions of DAO projecting to the C1 and C3 zones, while rostral MAO projecting to the C2 zone was devoid of serotonergic innervation. Later investigations using the immunocytochemical technique (6,28) have indicated that the distribution of serotonergic innervation of rat inferior olive has a relatively similar organization, although some species differences exist.

Serotonergic innervation of the rat DAO has been investigated with autoradiographic technique at the light and electron microscopic levels (39). The density of innervation was estimated to be around 4 million boutons per cubic millimeter of tissue. Ultrastructurally, the serotonergic boutons formed few synaptic junctions, but were regularly apposed to small dendrites and dendritic spines. Aggregation of presumed transmitter storing organelles toward the membrane facing dendritic profiles and glial investment of the serotonergic boutons suggested a directed action of serotonergic innervation onto such distal dendritic profiles. Interestingly, the distal dendritic compartment seems to contain most gap junctions coupling olivary neurons (33).

The origin of serotonergic innervation to the different olivary subnuclei is probably incompletely known, but interesting information is provided by Bishop and Ho (7) in the rat. These authors used horseradish peroxidase retrograde tracing combined with immunocytochemical detection of neurons containing serotonin. Retrogradely labeled serotonergic neurons were detected in the bulbar tegmentum immediately overlying the DAO, suggesting that very short projections may represent the major origin of serotonergic innervation to the olive. The study of Vergé et al. (this volume) reports 5-HT$_{1A}$ receptors on olivary neurons in the rat.

RELATION OF HARMALINE-INDUCED AND SEROTONERGIC INNERVATION

The study of De Montigny and Lamarre (10) demonstrated that harmaline-induced activity did not appear in all parts of the inferior olive, but that it was most prevalent in the caudal MAO and DAO. Sjölund et al. (31) used the known topography of the cat olivocerebellar projection to quantify harmaline-induced activity in different olivocerebellar compartments. Surface electrodes were placed in identified zones of the anterior lobe of the cerebellar cortex, harmaline was administered systematically, and mass Purkinje cell activity evoked by rhythmic, synchronous climbing fiber activity was recorded. Periods with climbing fiber activity of 10 to 12-Hz frequency were separated by silent periods. Such waxing and waning of harmaline-induced activity are also seen in recordings from the inferior olive itself (10), and probably reflect variations in olivary neuron excitability. Sjölund and co-workers quantified the harmaline-induced activity in different cortical zones: the average frequency indicating the prevalence of rhythmic firing, the average amplitude indicating the number of Purkinje cells and corresponding olivary neurons that fired in synchrony. Both these parameters indicated that harmaline induced most rhythmic and synchronous activity in the B zone receiving climbing fibers from the caudal DAO, which received the densest serotonergic innervation. Strong activity was also recorded in the A zone connected to caudal MAO, which receives a rather rich serotonergic innervation. Weaker activity was recorded in the C1 and C3 zones, which receive climbing fibers from the rostral DAO, which is sparsely innervated by serotonergic fibers. No harmaline-induced activity was recorded in the C2 zone receiving climbing fibers from the rostral MAO, which was devoid of serotonergic innervation. Thus, the harmaline-induced activity appeared in olivary regions receiving serotonergic innervation, and the amount of recorded activity seemed proportional to the density of serotonergic innervation.

In another series of experiments, Sjölund and co-workers (31) studied the effect of lesioning the serotonergic system on harmaline-induced activity. In rats, the serotonergic system was lesioned by intraventricular injection of 5,6- or 5,7-dihydroxytryptamine (4). With fluorescence histochemistry, it was shown that such treatment induced an efficient lesion of serotonergic innervation of the olive. Functionally, it was found that both harmaline-induced tremor and electrophysiologically recorded rhythmic, synchronous activity in the olivocerebellar system were markedly decreased in rats with lesions of the serotonergic system. These experiments, therefore, suggest that harmaline needs intact serotonergic innervation to exert its action on olivary neurons. Indeed, harmaline has pharmacological properties that are compatible with such a mode of action, being an inhibitor of monoamine oxidase (15,34), as well as having less well-studied effects such as serotonin uptake inhibition (8,29).

TREMOR COMPONENT OF SEROTONERGIC MOTOR SYNDROME

A "serotonergic motor syndrome" in the rat has frequently been used in psychopharmacological research (16,21). The syndrome can be induced by several pharmacological regimens resulting in increased stimulation of serotonergic receptors, e.g., systemic administration of serotonin receptor agonists, serotonin-releasing drugs, or monoamine oxidase inhibition combined with L-tryptophan loading, which causes an "overflow" of transmitter from serotonergic nerve terminals. The syndrome consists of stereotypic motor behavior including hyperactivity, tremor, lateral head weaving, forepaw treading, and Straub's tail. The appearance of the syndrome varies somewhat depending on which drugs are used, but tremor is a constant component. The suggestion that harmaline-induced tremor depends on interaction with serotonergic innervation of the inferior olive raised the question whether the tremor component of the serotonergic motor syndrome depends on a similar mechanism.

Electrophysiologically, it was demonstrated that systemic administration of serotonin receptor agonists, such as 5-methoxy-N, N-dimethyltryptamine (32,37,38) or quipazine (3), resulted in rhythmic, synchronous olivocerebellar activity. Similarly, monoamine oxidase inhibition combined with L-tryptophan loading resulted in rhythmic climbing fiber activity (32,37,38). That the induced rhythmic climbing fiber activity results in tremor was demonstrated in experiments in which tremor was recorded with the method of Dill et al. (13). Pronounced tremor was recorded in normal rats after administration of monoamine oxidase inhibitor and L-tryptophan, but in rats in which the inferior olive had been destroyed by the method of Desclin and Escubi (12), the tremor component of the serotonergic motor syndrome was efficiently suppressed.

Taken together, these observations show that the tremor component in the serotonergic motor syndrome is generated in the inferior olive by a mechanism similar to that of harmaline-induced tremor.

CONCLUSIONS

Specific parts of the olivary complex receive rich serotonergic innervation, which presumably originates from serotonergic cell groups in the bulbar tegmentum. The olivary compartments projecting to the vermal B and A zones, which are related to spinal motor functions, receive especially dense serotonergic innervation. The serotonergic terminals act on distal dendrites of olivary neurons.

The evidence presented indicates that harmaline acts through serotonergic innervation of the olivary neurons. Moreover, the tremor component of the serotonergic motor syndrome is generated in the inferior olive and olivocerebellospinal systems. In addition to the evidence reviewed above, Barragan et al. (3) showed that harmaline-induced rhythmic activity in the olive could be partially antagonized with serotonin receptor antagonists. Taken together, these findings indicate that serotonergic innervation is critically involved in eliciting rhythmic, synchronous firing in olivary neurons.

Olivary neurons demonstrate a complex action potential consisting of a fast initial spike, followed by a large delayed depolarization and a long hyperpolarization, which is terminated by a rebound potential (9,25). Llinás and Yarom (25) showed that the initial spike is classical sodium conductance and the delayed depolarization dendritic calcium conductance. Since an increase in cytoplasmic calcium is known to block the conductivity over gap junctions (5,27,30), it has been suggested that one effect of dendritic calcium conductance is a transient decrease in electrotonic coupling of olivary neurons (39). Further, Llinás and Yarom (25) reported that hyperpolarization of the olivary neuron markedly augments the rebound potential, which facilitates elicitation of a new action potential and oscillatory activity of the neuron. With extracellular recordings, Headley et al. (19) investigated some properties of iontophoretically applied serotonin on olivary cells. Interestingly, they found two effects. First, serotonin selectively suppressed the delayed depolarization, i.e., the dendritic calcium conductance. According to our hypothesis (39), this would mean that the gap junctions would be kept open and that the olivary neurons tend to synchronize their activity. Second, serotonin had a hyperpolarizing effect on the olivary neurons that, according to Llinás and Yarom (25), would bring about rhythmic, oscillatory activity. By the suggested modulatory action of olivary neurons, serotonin may account for both the synchrony and rhythmicity of the olivary neuronal activity, which have been shown to result in tremor. This hypothesis was partly supported by recent findings by Llinás and Yarom (26) in guinea pig inferior olivary neurons.

It is not known whether harmaline- and serotonin-induced tremor generated in the inferior olive corresponds to any clinical condition of pathological tremor. Nevertheless, it is of considerable interest that malfunction of serotonergic regulation of a single brain stem nucleus can result in drastic motor symptoms, such as whole body tremor.

REFERENCES

1. Armstrong DM, Harvey RJ. Responses of a spino-olivo cerebellar pathway in the cat. *J Physiol (Lond)* 1968;194:147–168.
2. Azizi SA, Woodward DJ. Inferior olivary nuclear complex of the rat: morphology and comments on the principle of organization within the olivocerebellar system. *J Comp Neurol* 1987;263:467–484.
3. Barragan LA, Dehaye-Bouchaud N, Laget P. Drug-induced activation of the inferior olivary nucleus in young rabbits. Differential effects of harmaline and quipazine. *Neuropharmacology* 1985;24:645–654.
4. Baumgarten HG, Lachenmayer L, Björklund A. Chemical lesioning of indolamine pathways. In: Myers RD, ed. *Methods in psychobiology*, vol 3. New York: Academic Press, 1977:47–98.
5. Baux G, Simmonneu M, Tauc L, Segundo JP. Uncoupling of electrotonic synapses by calcium. *Proc Nat Acad Sci USA* 1978;75:4577–4581.
6. Bishop GA, Ho RH. Substance P and serotonin immunoreactivity in the rat inferior olive. *Brain Res Bull* 1984;12:105–113.
7. Bishop GA, Ho RH. Cell bodies of origin of serotonin-immunoreactive afferents to the inferior olivary complex of the rat. *Brain Res* 1986;399:369–373.
8. Buckholz NS, Boggan WO. Effects of tetrahydro-beta-carbolines on monoamine oxidase and serotonin uptake in mouse brain. *Biochem Pharmacol* 1977;25:2319–2321.
9. Crill WE. Unitary multi-spiked responses in cat inferior olive nucleus. *J Neurophysiol* 1970;33:199–209.
10. De Montigny C, Lamarre Y. Rhythmic activity induced by harmaline in the olivocerebellobulbar system of the cat. *Brain Res* 1973;53:81–95.
11. Desclin JC. Histological evidence supporting the inferior oliva as the major source of cerebellar climbing fibres in the rat. *Brain Res* 1974;77:365–384.

12. Desclin JC, Escubi J. Effects of 3-acetylpyridine on the central nervous system of the rat, as demonstrated by silver methods. *Brain Res* 1974;77:349–364.
13. Dill RE, Dorman HL, Nickey WM. A simple method for recording tremors in small animals. *J Appl Physiol* 1968;24:598–599.
14. Eccles JC, Ito M, Szentágothai J. *The cerebellum as a neuronal machine*. New York: Springer, 1967.
15. Fuller RW, Wong CJ, Hemrick-Luecke SK. MD 240928 and harmaline: opposite selectivity in antagonism of the inactivation of types A and B monoamine oxidase by pargyline in mice. *Life Sci* 1986;38:409–412.
16. Green AR, Grahame-Smith DG. Effects of drugs on the processes regulating the functional activity of brain 5-hydroxytryptamine. *Nature* 1976;260:487–491.
17. Groenewegen HJ, Voogd J. The parasagittal zonation within the olivo-cerebellar projection. I. Climbing fiber distribution in the vermis of cat cerebellum. *J Comp Neurol* 1977;174:417–488.
18. Groenewegen HJ, Voogd J, Freedman SL. The parasagittal zonation within the olivo-cerebellar projection. II. Climbing fiber distribution in the intermediate and hemispheric parts of cat cerebellum. *J Comp Neurol* 1979;183:551–602.
19. Headley PM, Lodge D, Duggan AW. Drug-induced rhythmical activity in the inferior olivary complex of the rat. *Brain Res* 1976;101:461–478.
20. Ito M. *The cerebellum and neural control*. New York: Raven Press, 1984.
21. Jacobs BL. An animal behavior model for studying central serotoninergic synapses. *Life Sci* 1976;19:777–786.
22. Llinás R. Electrophysiological properties of the olivocerebellar system. In: Strata P, ed. *The olivocerebellar system in motor control* (*Exp Brain Res*, series 17). Berlin: Springer-Verlag, 1988:201–208.
23. Llinás R, Baker R, Sotelo C. Electrotonic coupling between neurons in the cat inferior olive. *J Neurophysiol* 1974;37:560–571.
24. Llinás R, Vollkind RA. The olivocerebellar system: functional properties as revealed by harmaline-induced tremor. *Exp Brain Res* 1973;18:69–87.
25. Llinás R, Yarom Y. Electrophysiological properties of mammalian inferior olivary cells in vitro. In: Courville J, De Montigny C, Lamarre Y, eds. *The inferior olivary nucleus*. New York: Raven Press, 1980:379–388.
26. Llinás R, Yarom Y. Oscillatory properties of guinea-pig inferior olivary neurones and their pharmacological modulation: an in vitro study. *J Physiol (Lond)* 1986;376:163–182.
27. Loewenstein WR. Cell-to-cell membrane channels: permeability, formation, genetics and functions. In: Andreoli et al., eds. *The physiological basis for disorders in biomembranes*. Plenum Press, New York: Plenum Press, 1977.
28. Paré M, Descarries L, Wiklund L. Innervation and reinnervation of rat inferior olive by neurons containing serotonin and substance P: an immunohistochemical study after 5,6-dihydroxytryptamine lesioning. *J Neurocytol* 1987;16:155–167.
29. Rommelspacher H, Strauss SM, Rehse K. Beta-carbolines: a tool for investigating structure-activity relationships of the high affinity uptake of serotonin, noradrenaline, GABA and choline into a synaptosome-rich fraction of various regions from rat brain. *J Neurochem* 1978;30:1573–1578.
30. Rose B, Loewenstein WR. Permeability of cell junction depends on local cytoplasmic calcium activity. *Nature* 1975;254:250–252.
31. Sjölund B, Björklund A, Wiklund L. The indolaminergic innervation of the inferior olive. II. Relation to harmaline induced tremor. *Brain Res* 1977;131:23–37.
32. Sjölund B, Wiklund L, Björklund A. Functional role of serotoninergic innervation of inferior olivary cells. In: Courville J, De Montigny C, Lamarre Y, eds. *The inferior olivary nucleus*. New York: Raven Press, 1980:163–168.
33. Sotelo C, Llinás R, Baker R. Structural study of inferior olivary nucleus of the cat: morphological correlates of electrotonic coupling. *J Neurophysiol* 1974;37:541–559.
34. Udenfriend S, Witkop B, Redfield BG, Weissbach H. Studies with reversible inhibitors of monoamine oxidase: harmaline and related compounds. *Biochem Pharmacol* 1958;1:160–165.
35. Van der Want JJL, Wiklund L, Guegan M, Ruigrok T, Voogd J. Anterograde tracing of the rat olivocerebellar system with Phaseolus vulgaris leucoagglutinin (PHA-L). Demonstration of climbing fiber collateral innervation of the cerebellar nuclei. *J Comp Neurol* 1989;288:1–18.
36. Wiklund L, Björklund A, Sjölund B. The indolaminergic innervation of the inferior olive. I. Convergence with the direct spinal afferents in the areas projecting to the cerebellar anterior lobe. *Brain Res* 1977;131:1–21.

37. Wiklund L, Descarries L, Mollgård K. Serontoninergic axon terminals in the rat dorsal accessory olive: normal ultrastructure and light microscopic demonstration of regeneration after 5,6-dihydroxytryptamine lesioning. *J Neurocytol* 1981;10:1009–1027.
38. Wiklund L, Sjölund B, Björklund A. Inferior olivary nucleus: serotonergic basis for a tremor phenomenon. In: Schott B, et al., eds. *Les neuromédiateurs du tronc cérébrale*. Paris: Laboratoires Sandoz, 1980:177–186.
39. Wiklund L, Sjölund B, Björklund A. Morphological and functional studies on the serotoninergic innervation of the inferior olive. *J Physiol (Paris)* 1981;77:183–186.

*Serotonin, the Cerebellum,
and Ataxia*, edited by
P. Trouillas and K. Fuxe.
Raven Press, Ltd., New York © 1993.

8

A Small Population of Purkinje Cells in the Posterior Vermis Is Specifically Labeled by a Tyrosine Hydroxylase Antibody

B. Berthie, H. Axelrad, *C. Verney, and M. E. Marc

*Laboratoire de Neurophysiologie, Faculté de Médecine Pitié-Salpêtrière,
75013 Paris, France; *INSERM U106, Neuromorphologie, Hôpital Salpêtrière,
75013 Paris, France*

The vertebrate and particularly the mammalian cerebellar cortex Purkinje cells (PCs) are categorized as a unique morphological and physiological type of neuron. Arguments in favor of this classification come from (i) their highly recognizable appearance in the classical silver impregnations (26,27), (ii) recent immunocytological labeling with calbindin, which specifically labels the sole PCs in the cerebellar cortex (21,30), and (iii) the extensive electrophysiological recordings of this cell type obtained, during the past 30 years, from different species (11,17,18,20,22–24). Their common morphological features, particular position in respect to the cerebellar cortical circuit, and identical physiological properties seem to specify PCs throughout the phylogenetic spectrum.

Albeit the abundance of data confirming the uniqueness of this cell type, it is now a well-demonstrated fact that PCs also have a diversity of biochemical and immunocytological properties (1,6,7,10,31). Factors common to this molecular differentiation seem to be the important number of each particularly labeled subset of PC and their anatomical organization in parasagittal bands (8,13,14). The exact numerical importance of each differently labeled population and whether there exists overlap between the different markers have not been clearly ascertained. Moreover, no clear functional implications have been convincingly proposed to correlate with such a molecular heterogeneity.

In the course of a more general study of the functional dynamics of the cerebellar cortex we have undertaken a complete three-dimensional (3D) and quantitative morphometric analysis of the different neuronal elements of this structure. During the reconstruction of the spatial organization of the tyrosine hydroxylase (TH)-positive fibers that span the whole depth of the cortex, we encountered, to our surprise, a small number of completely and well-stained PCs.

We, therefore, report here the finding of a very restricted group of PCs that were selectively stained by a monoclonal TH antibody (TH+). In contrast to the other descriptions of cerebellar cortex molecular markers, these TH+ PCs number very few and are all found in a well-delineated zone of the posterior vermis.

MATERIAL AND METHODS

All experiments were carried out on young adult male Wistar rats (180–220 g).

After fixation of the tissue (4% paraformaldehyde), the immunocytochemistry labeling was done on serial 40 μm thick parasagittal sections of the vermis, according to the method described in Febvret et al. (12). We used a monoclonal TH antiserum (Instar 1:2,000) and a polyclonal anti-TH antibody (Boy 1:2,000) revealed by the streptavidin-biotin-peroxydase method (Amersham). The chromogen was diaminobenzidine and, if needed, the reaction product was intensified with nickel. Nomarsky optics was used throughout. The 3D computer reconstruction programs were developed in our laboratory.

RESULTS

The existence of noradrenergic fibers in the cerebellar cortex is now a well-documented fact (9). The advent of immunocytochemical techniques using a monoclonal antibody against TH, the rate-limiting enzyme in the synthesis of catecholamine, has allowed precise and reproducible labeling of such fibers in the central nervous system (CNS). An example of cerebellar cortical TH+ fibers, labeled in such conditions, is illustrated in Fig. 1A. In this photomicrograph of a parasagittal section, illuminated with Nomarsky optics, the fibers are clearly viewed against a clear background. These fibers are thin, with a beaded appearance, and course throughout the cortical layers in oblique, horizontal, and vertical directions. In some instances, as the one illustrated here, these fibers seem to have a greater density in the vicinity of the PC layer, while in other areas the density seems higher in portions of the molecular or granular layers.

While systematically scanning the parasagittal serial sections to get insight into the TH+ fiber density, we were quite astonished to find a few well-stained neurons. These were unmistakably PCs, as judged from the characteristic appearance of the dendritic arbor and the dimensions and localization of the soma. One of these neurons is illustrated in Fig. 1B. As can be seen, its soma is located in the PC layer and the dendritic trunks rise through the molecular layer. These primary and secondary dendrites form the proximal compartment of the arbor (28) and are clearly visible due to their important dimensions. The distal compartment of the dendritic tree, made up by the numerous and very small spiny branchlets, can only be grossly

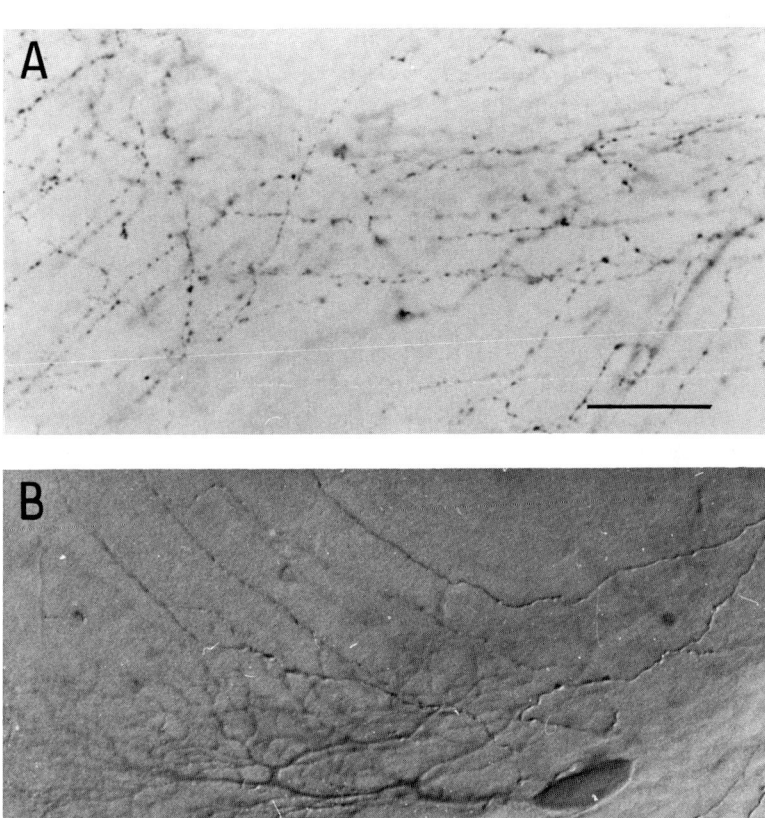

FIG. 1. A: Cerebellar cortical TH+ fibers. Parasagittal section. The fibers are thin, with a beaded appearance, and course throughout the cerebellar layers in oblique, vertical, or horizontal directions. Note the higher density of fibers at the level of the PC layer. **B**: PC completely visualized using the TH antibody. Note the characteristic morphological features of this cell type, particularly the proximal compartment of the dendritic tree. Nomarsky optics. Calibration bars are 50 μm.

delineated by the uniform stain of the neuropil around the proximal compartment, in contrast with the rest of the background.

The labeling of PCs by the TH antibody is numerically restricted to a very small number of neurons in each studied vermis. The specificity of the labeling is validated by the fact that, as could be predicted, if a PC is labeled in a given section and part of its dendritic tree is cut, the rest of the missing dendrite(s) is easily found in the immediately adjacent section due to the contrast between its darker stain against the unlabeled background neuropil.

Apart from the few number of stained cells, another characteristic that differentiates this TH+ labeling of PCs from the other markers known to stain these neurons is the circumscribed localization of the TH+ PCs. All the neurons found up to now (61 in 13 cerebella) are located in the posterior vermis. Figure 2 illustrates four such neurons chosen to show the entire span of positions found. All the neurons are symmetrically located in the posterior vermis, caudal to the secondary fissure, in the different folds of folia IX and X. A kind of clustering of these neurons is observed, distributed mainly in two groups, one in the superficial part of folium IX a+b, the other along the deep part of the lateroposterior fissure.

To see if the 3D spatial spread of the dendritic arbors of these TH+ PCs were comparable to that found for PCs stained with the Golgi technique (3,4), some of the labeled cells were drawn with a camera lucida at high magnification, the x, y, and z coordinates calculated, and a 3D computer reconstruction performed. Such a reconstructed PC is illustrated in Fig. 3 and is the same neuron as the one represented in Fig. 1B. The computer reconstruction allows a rotation of the neuron in space and, thus, a view from different angles. The comparison of these different views with the usual parasagittal view, due to the plane of section, is important to

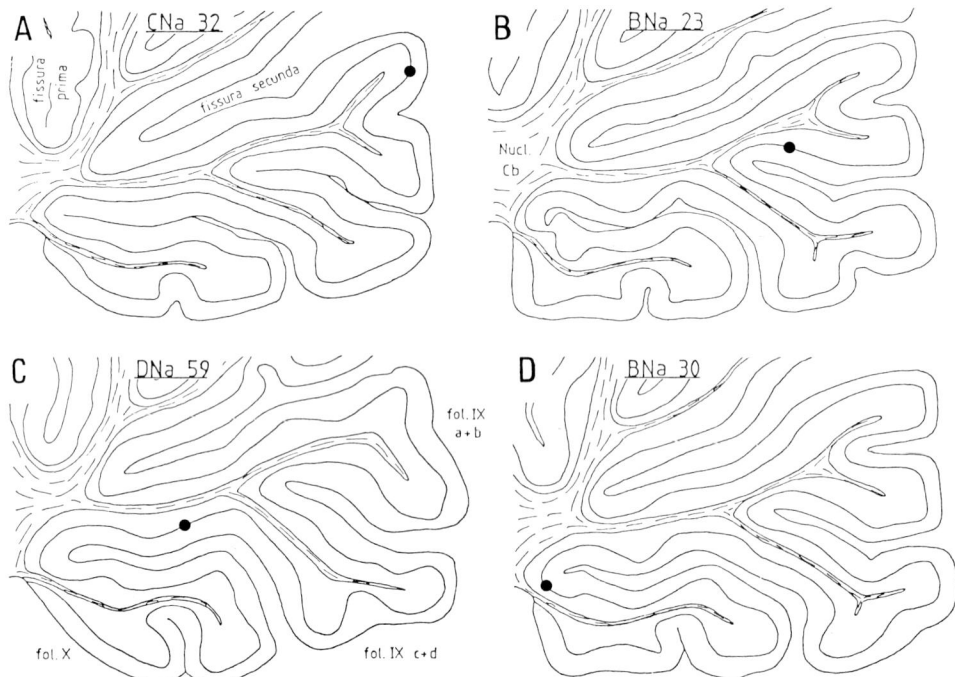

FIG. 2. Localization of Th+ PCs in the posterior vermis. Four different cells illustrate the entire span of different positions found. Note that all PCs lie in folia IX a+b, IX c+d, and X.

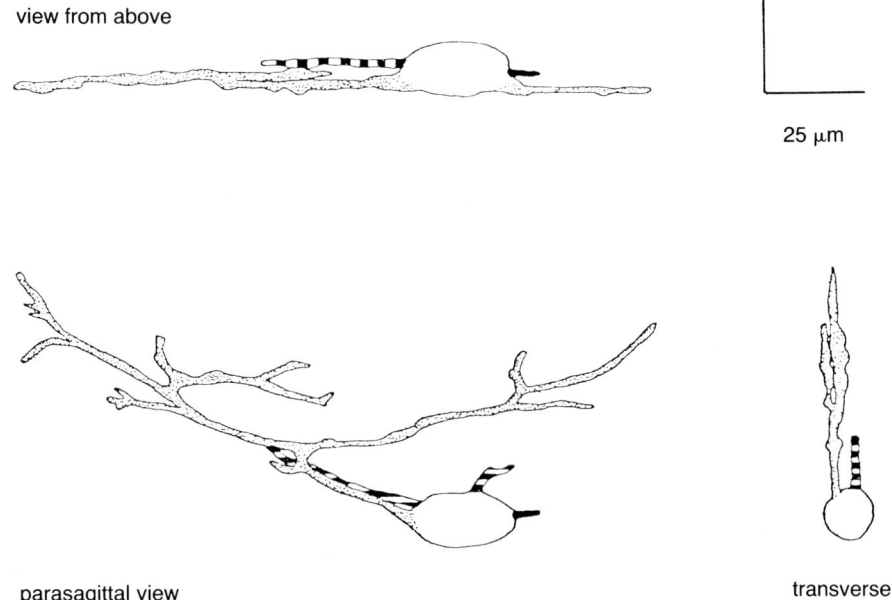

FIG. 3. 3D reconstruction of a TH+ PC illustrating that it is composed of a biplanar dendritic tree. Same cell as in Fig. 1B. Note that only a computer 3D reconstruction allows rotatation of the cell in space, thus determining the number of planes of its dendritic tree.

understand the spatial spread of the dendritic tree. In the present case it allows us to see that the flat dendritic tree is not monoplanar but that the different dendrites form two parallel planes with respect to the axis of the folium (i.e., the direction of the parallel fibers). From a reconstruction of six such stained neurons it appears that they are in all aspects comparable to the silver-stained PCs, from which the main morphological descriptions characterizing this cell type are derived.

DISCUSSION AND CONCLUSION

We present here preliminary results indicating that there is, in the rat posterior cerebellum, a small population of neurons selectively labeled by a specific monoclonal TH antibody. The specificity was ascertained by similar results obtained using polyclonal anti-TH antibodies. These TH+ neurons can be classified as PCs on the basis of their location in the cortex and the typical spatial spread of their dendritic tree. They are symmetrically clustered in the vermis in two distinct groups centered in the superficial part of folium IX a+b and along the deep part of the lateroposterior fissure.

From our knowledge, this is the first time that PCs denoting a catecholaminergic property are demonstrated in the adult mammalian cerebellum. Some PCs, visualized by catecholamine histofluorescence, had been shown in the cat cerebellar cortex (9), but these authors attributed this property to autofluorescence. On the other hand, it seems that the immature mouse PCs are labeled by TH antibodies (16). These authors claimed that this last feature disappeared when the animals were 3 to 4 weeks old. Such developmentally correlated transient expression of TH+ neurons was described in different areas of the CNS, especially the neocortex (2). On the other hand, TH mRNA has been detected in the adult rat cerebellum (25), a fact that positively correlated with our own finding.

The exact functional significance of PCs with such specialized molecular properties is open to speculation. One possible hypothesis would be that these different molecular markers could act as cues during development (29,31) to help the orientation of incoming fibers. Another hypothesis takes in account the fact that the cerebellar cortex is made up of an array of hundreds of structurally distinct modules (15), a suggestion that had been made, in functional arguments, nearly a decade ago (20).

An interesting feature is that all of these TH+ PCs cells are located in the posterior vermis. This region is known to present a great number of minor morphological abnormalities. It has recently been shown that the dopamine D3 receptor is present on PCs in this zone (15) and that a quite dense net of cholinergic fibers is also present in this part of the cerebellum (19). This region could, therefore, be a strongly differentiated part of the cerebellar cortex.

Further extensions of our work on these neurons include *in situ* hybridization, dopamine β-hydroxylase immunocytochemistry labeling specifically the noradrenergic neurons, double GABA-TH staining, and an ontogenetic approach.

ACKNOWLEDGMENT

This research was supported by grant INSERM CRE 899001.

REFERENCES

1. Batini C. Cerebellar localization and colocalization of GABA and calcium binding protein—D28k. *Arch Ital Biol* 1990;128:127–149.
2. Berger B, Verney C, Gaspar P, Febvret A. Transient expression of tyrosine hydroxylase immunoreactivity in some neurons of the rat neocortex during postnatal development. *Dev Brain Res* 1985;23:141–144.
3. Berthie B, Axelrad H. Variations in the shape of the dendritic tree of Purkinje cells stained by silver impregnation in the rat cerebellar cortex. *Eur J Neurosci* 1988(suppl 1):136.
4. Berthie B, Axelrad H. Morphometric analysis of fully impregnated Purkinje cells in the rat cerebellar cortex shows that the flat dendritic tree is not monoplanar in all cases. In: Llinas R, Sotelo C, eds. *Neurobiology of the cerebellar system: a centenary of Ramon y Cajal's description of the cerebellar circuits*. Barcelona, 1988.
5. Bouthenet ML, Souil E, Martres MP, Sokoloff P, Giros B, Schwartz JC. Localization of dopamine D3 receptor mRNA in the rat brain using in situ hybridization histochemistry: comparison with dopamine D2 receptor mRNA. *Brain Res* 1991;564:203–219.
6. Chan-Palay V. Purkinje cells of the cerebellum: localization and function of multiple neuroactive substances. *Exp Brain Res* 1984(suppl 9):129–144.

7. Chan-Palay V, Nilaver G, Palay S, et al. Chemical heterogeneity in Purkinje cells: existence and coexistence of glutamic acid decarboxylase-like and motilin-like immunoreactivities. *Proc Natl Acad Sci USA* 1981;78:7787–7791.
 8. Chan-Palay V, Palay S, Wu JY. Sagittal cerebellar microbands of taurine neurons: immunocytochemical demonstration by using antibodies against the synthesizing enzyme cysteine sulfinic acid decarboxylase. *Proc Natl Acad Sci USA* 1982;79:4221–4225.
 9. Chu NS, Bloom FE. The catecholamine-containing neurons in the cat dorso-lateral pontine tegmentum: distribution of the cell bodies and some axonal projections. *Brain Res* 1974;66:1–21.
10. De Camilli P, Miller PE, Levitt P, Walter U, Greengard P. Anatomy of cerebellar Purkinje cells in the rat determined by a specific immunohistochemical marker. *Neuroscience* 1984;11:761–817.
11. Eccles JC, Ito M, Szentagothai J. *The cerebellum as a neuronal machine.* New York: Springer-Verlag, 1974.
12. Febvret A, Berger B, Gaspar P, Verney C. Further indication that distinct dopaminergic subsets project to the rat cerebral cortex: lack of colocalization with neurotensin in the superficial dopaminergic fields of the anterior cingulate, motor, retrosplenial and visual cortices. *Brain Res* 1991;547:37–52.
13. Hawkes R, Colonnier M, LeClerc N. Monoclonal antibodies reveal sagittal banding in the rodent cerebellar cortex. *Brain Res* 1985;333:359–365.
14. Hawkes R, LeClerc N. Antigenic map of the rat cerebellar cortex: the distribution of parasagittal bands as revealed by monoclonal anti-Purkinje cell antibody mabQ113. *J Comp Neurol* 1987;256:29–41.
15. Hawkes R, Gravel C. The modular cerebellum. *Prog Neurobiol* 1991;36:309–327.
16. Hess EJ, Wilson MC. Tottering and leaner mutations perturb transient developmental expression of tyrosine hydroxylase in embryologically distinct Purkinje cells. *Neuron* 1991;6:123–132.
17. Hounsgaard J, Midtgaard J. Intrinsic determinants of firing pattern in Purkinje cells of the turtle cerebellum in vitro. *J Physiol (Lond)* 1988;319:143–152.
18. Hounsgaard J, Midtgaard J. Synaptic control of excitability in turtle cerebellar Purkinje cells. *J Physiol (Lond)* 1989;409:157–170.
19. Illing R-B. A subtype of cerebellar Golgi cells may be cholinergic. *Brain Res* 1990;522:267–274.
20. Ito M. *The cerebellum and neuronal control.* New York: Raven Press, 1984.
21. Jande SS, Maler L, Lawson DEM. Immunocytochemical mapping of vitamine D-dependent calcium-binding protein in brain. *Nature* 1981;294:765–767.
22. Llano I, Marty A, Armstrong CM, Konnerth A. Synaptic and agonist-induced excitatory currents of Purkinje cells in rat cerebellar slices. *J Physiol (Lond)* 1991;434:183–213.
23. Llinas R, Sugimori M. Electrophysiological properties of in vitro Purkinje cell somata in mammalian cerebellar slices. *J Physiol (Lond)* 1980;305:171–195.
24. Llinas R, Sugimori M. Electrophysiological properties of in vitro Purkinje cell dendrites in mammalian cerebellar slices. *J Physiol (Lond)* 1980;305:197–213.
25. Mallet J, Faucon Biguet N, Buda M, Lamouroux A, Samolyk D. Detection and regulation of the tyrosine hydroxylase mRNA levels in rat adrenal medulla and brain tissues. *Cold Spring Harb Symp Quant Biol* 1983;48:305–308.
26. Palay S, Chan-Palay V. *Cerebellar cortex.* New York: Springer-Verlag, 1974.
27. Ramon y Cajal S. Histologie du système nerveux, vol 2. Paris: Maloine, 1911.
28. Sotelo C. Purkinje cell ontogeny: formation and maintenance of spines. *Prog Brain Res* 1978;48:149–170.
29. Sotelo C, Wassef M. Cerebellar development: afferent organization and Purkinje cell heterogeneity. *Philos Trans R Soc Lond [Biol]* 1991;331:307–313.
30. Thomasset M, Parkes CO, Cuisinier-Gleizes P. Rat calcium-binding proteins: distribution, development, and vitamin D dependence. *Am Physiol Soc* 1982;E483–E488.
31. Wassef M, Angaut P, Arsenio-Nunes L, Bourrat F, Sotelo C. Purkinje cell heterogeneity: its role in organizing the topography of the cerebellar cortex connections. In: Llinas R, Sotelo C, eds. *The cerebellum revisited.* New York: Springer-Verlag, 1992.

*Serotonin, the Cerebellum,
and Ataxia,* edited by
P. Trouillas and K. Fuxe.
Raven Press, Ltd., New York © 1993.

9

GABA Neurons and Innervation by Tryptophan Hydroxylase (PH8) and Monoamine Oxidase B Immunoreactive Axons in the Human Cerebellum

T. Zetzsche and V. Chan-Palay

Neurology Clinic, University Hospital, CH-8091 Zurich, Switzerland

In 1950 the detection of high amounts of gamma-aminobutyric acid (GABA) in the central nervous system was reported (1,2). In the meantime considerable evidence has been accumulated that indicates that GABA is a major inhibitory neurotransmitter in the central nervous system (3–5). It was demonstrated that subpopulations of neurons have the capacity to synthesize GABA by the enzyme glutamate decarboxylase (GAD) via a shunt of the citrate cycle. GABA was released from nerve terminals after stimulation, and uptake and degradation mechanisms for GABA were studied in neurons and glial cells (for review, see refs. 3–5). The effects of GABA were shown to be mediated by $GABA_A$ and $GABA_B$ receptors, located in the pre- and postsynaptic membranes of GABA elements. GABA receptor complexes contain binding sites for GABA and ion channels in close association (6,7).

Substantial knowledge about the neuronal circuitry in the cerebellum resulted from morphological studies that used Golgi staining, tracing techniques, and electron microscopy (8–10). By means of electrophysiology (11,12) it was demonstrated in animals that subpopulations of cerebellar neurons may use GABA as an inhibitory neurotransmitter. Activation of basket cells, whose axons form a so-called basket plexus around Purkinje cell somata, were shown to inhibit the spontaneous activity of Purkinje cells (13,14). Purkinje cells themselves, whose axons make synaptic contacts with neurons of the deep cerebellar nuclei and the nucleus of Deiters' were shown to depress the activity of these cells (15–18). Similar results were obtained when GABA was applied by iontophoresis and both effects could be blocked by bicuculline, an antagonist of the $GABA_A$ receptor (19–21). Other candidates of cerebellar neurons that might use GABA as a neurotransmitter are Golgi and stellate cells (11,22,23). Both cell types have axons that terminate locally on the Purkinje or granule cell dendrites, respectively (9). The hypothesis that several cerebellar neurons are GABAergic was supported by histochemical, immunohistochemical, and autoradiographic studies, which have demonstrated that subpopulations of these neurons accumulate GABA or contain enzymes of the GABA metabolism (12,24–29).

In animals it has been demonstrated that the cerebellum is innervated by fibers that contain serotonin (30–33). These fibers pass through the dentate nucleus and constitute a fiber plexus in the granular layer, the Purkinje cell layer, and the molecular layer of the cerebellar cortex. In addition, serotonin receptors could be detected, although in low concentration in the cerebellum (Palacios et al., this volume). Finally electrophysiological studies have demonstrated that serotonin influenced various electrophysiological properties of cerebellar cortex neurons (see Chapter 16).

To study GABA neurons in the human cerebellum, immunohistochemical techniques were used to detect several GABA markers (34): GAD is the rate-limiting enzyme of GABA synthesis (3). It was detected in presynaptic elements of GABA neurons (26,35). An antiplasma against rat GAD was used (28,36). Parvalbumin and calbindin D-28k are cytoplasmic calcium-binding proteins that were shown in animals to coexist with GABA in some subpopulations of neurons (37–40). The function of these calcium-binding proteins is as yet unknown; they may serve to buffer intracellular calcium (40,41). We used polyclonal antibodies (42) against rat muscle parvalbumin and bovine cerebellar calbindin D-28k to localize these antigens. Monoclonal antibodies against the α_1 subunit of the $GABA_A$ benzodiazepine receptor complex (bd 24) (43,44) were applied to detect postsynaptic GABA elements.

Two different antibodies were used to label serotonin-monoamine related structures. The first monoclonal antibody, PH8, immunoreactive for tryptophan hydroxylase (45), was demonstrated to stain specifically serotoninergic raphe neurons (46; Chapter 2, this volume). In the human brain stem immunoreactivity for the second monoclonal antibody against human platelet monoamine oxidase (MAO) B (47) was also detected in nonneuronal structures such as glial cells. Regarding the staining of neurons, MAO B was found in serotoninergic nuclei and other monoaminergic brain stem nuclei such as the locus coeruleus or the substantia nigra were typically non-immunoreactive (48; Chapter 2, this volume). This indicates that MAO B may be used as a marker for serotonin-containing neurons and their processes, although one has to be aware that the staining is not specifically neuronal, but, in addition, nonneuronal elements may be labeled.

Only postmortem brains of control patients in the Zürich study on dementia (Chapter 2, this volume), who had no history of neurological or psychiatric disease, were used. A total of four patients was included (age: 74–91 years; postmortem delay: 4–10 hr). In every case the diagnosis was confirmed by neuropathological examination. The brains were perfused with 4% paraformaldehyde for 2 hr at autopsy. Afterward approximately 8 mm thick tissue blocks were cut out and immersion fixed overnight. Vibratome sections, 70 μm thick of the cerebellar cortex and the dentate nucleus were cut in the sagittal, transverse, and horizontal planes. These sections were freeze-thawed and subjected to free-floating immunocytochemistry and/or counterstained with cresyl violet (Nissl) to detect cytoarchitectural boundaries. After preincubation with 5% normal goat serum (NGS) for 1 hr, sections were incubated in primary antibodies for 4 days (or 5 days with the GAD antibody) at 4°C. The primary antibodies were diluted in 1% NGS in following concentrations: GAD, 1:4,000; calbindin D-28k, 1:100,000; parvalbumin, 1:5,000; $GABA_A$ receptor, 1:2,500; PH8, 1:6,000; MAO-B, 1:500,000. Visualization was performed with gold-labeled secondary antibodies and the IGSS method (49) or with the avidin-biotin-peroxidase-diaminobenzidine method with cobalt-nickel enhancement (50) in case of the GAD antibody.

GAD. In the cerebellar cortex we found GAD immunoreactivity predominantly in axons and axonal varicosities; the staining of somata was mostly very faint and dendritic staining was restricted to the proximal segments. Some but not all Purkinje cells showed GAD immunoreactivity in their somata, axons, and proximal dendrites. In sagittal sections GAD-immunoreactive (GAD-i) basket cell axons were seen in the lower molecular layer, running parallel to the Purkinje cell layer. They gave rise to collaterals that formed dense basket plexus around Purkinje cell somata. In the molecular and the granular layers numerous GAD-i axonal varicosities were detected. In the molecular layer these varicosities were sometimes seen on the surface of Purkinje cell dendrites. The somata of basket, stellate, and Golgi cells were only faintly stained. Granule cells were never GAD-i. In the dentate nucleus we found a dense accumulation of GAD-i axons and axonal varicosities. Large dentate neurons were not immunoreactive by themselves, but the surface of their somata and dendrites was covered by GAD-i varicosities. In the white matter small bipolar and multipolar neurons were found to be GAD-i in the cytoplasm of somata and dendrites.

Calbindin D-28k. In the cerebellar cortex all Purkinje cells were specifically immunoreactive for calbindin D-28k. Dendrites including terminal arborizations and dendritic spines, somata, and axons were readily immunoreactive. In the dentate nucleus nonimmunoreactive cells were surrounded by a dense accumulation of immunoreactive axons and axonal varicosities.

Parvalbumin. In the cerebellar cortex stellate, basket, and Purkinje cells were immunoreactive for parvalbumin. Granule cells or Golgi cells were never stained. Only a subpopulation of Purkinje cells was parvalbumin immunoreactive (parv-i), and the staining of distal dendrites or dendritic spines was mostly very weak. Basket cells, their dendrites, horizontal basket cell axons, and basket fiber plexus around Purkinje cell somata were readily stained. Also numerous stellate cells and their processes were parv-i. In the dentate nucleus neurons were not parv-i, but they were surrounded by a dense accumulation of parv-i axons and varicosities.

$GABA_A$ receptor. In the cerebellar cortex the highest density of immunoreactivity for the $GABA_A$ receptor was found in the granular layer. In the molecular and the Purkinje cell layers we found weaker $GABA_A$ receptor immunoreactivity, which was confined to the surface of the neurons. In the dentate nucleus all types of large

and small neurons (10) were readily immunoreactive and showed an intense staining of the surface membranes of their dendrites including spines, somata, and axon initial segments.

PH8. Immunoreactivity was detected in fine axonal fibers and small varicosities that were scattered in the molecular layer, the Purkinje cell layer around nonimmunoreactive Purkinje cells, and the granular layer of the cerebellar cortex (Fig. 1).

MAO-B. In all three layers of the human cerebellar cortex fine axonal fibers and numerous varicosities immunoreactive for MAO B were detected (Fig. 1). The majority of varicosities of the cerebellar cortex was clearly located in the granular layer where the density of immunoreactive structures was consistently higher compared to the molecular layer. Local accumulations of varicosities were encountered around nonimmunoreactive somata in the Purkinje cell layer, especially at their lower border. The white matter of the folia contained numerous astrocytes and immunoreactive processes that were stained for MAO B. No immunoreactive astrocytes were detected in the molecular layer. The dentate nucleus was clearly immunoreactive due to accumulations of small fibers and varicosities that surrounded the nonimmunoreactive large dentate neurons. Astrocytes were stained inside the dentate gray matter and in the surrounding white matter.

Conclusively we found in the human cerebellar cortex only stellate, basket, Purkinje, and Golgi cells and in the dentate nucleus only small neurons to be immunoreactive for GAD, which is in accordance with previous studies in animals (26,35). The staining was mostly axonal, which might represent the actual distribution of GAD in human nervous tissue. The specific immunoreactivity of Purkinje cells for calbindin D-28k is in accordance with studies in animals (40,51). We found no Golgi cells (52) to be immunoreactive for calbindin D-28k. The intense immunoreactivity even in fine dendrites and dendritic spines might be correlated to the results of biochemical studies that have found, that the concentration of calbindin D-28k is 10 times higher in the cerebellum than in other brain regions (41,53). The immunoreactivity of parvalbumin might be different from the distribution in rats (40) with respect to the fact that not all Purkinje cells were readily stained in the human cerebellum. $GABA_A$ receptor immunoreactivity in the human cerebellar cortex was quite similar to that previously observed in the cerebellum of rodents and monkeys (54,55). The intense immunoreactivity of granule cell somata is somewhat astonishing because their surfaces have no synapses (9). The high concentration of GAD-i axons and axonal varicosities in the dentate nucleus and the intense staining of the cell surface membrane of dentate neurons for the $GABA_A$ receptor are in accordance with the view that the dentate nucleus might be under inhibitory control through GABA (12) in humans as well.

We found fine axonal fibers and varicosities in the cerebellar cortex to be immunoreactive for the MAO-B and PH8 antibody. The existence of PH8 immunoreactive fibers in the cerebellar cortex might be due to a serotoninergic innervation, which was described for animals (30–33). The sources of this innervation of the human cerebellar cortex have to be elucidated. In animals several brain stem neu-

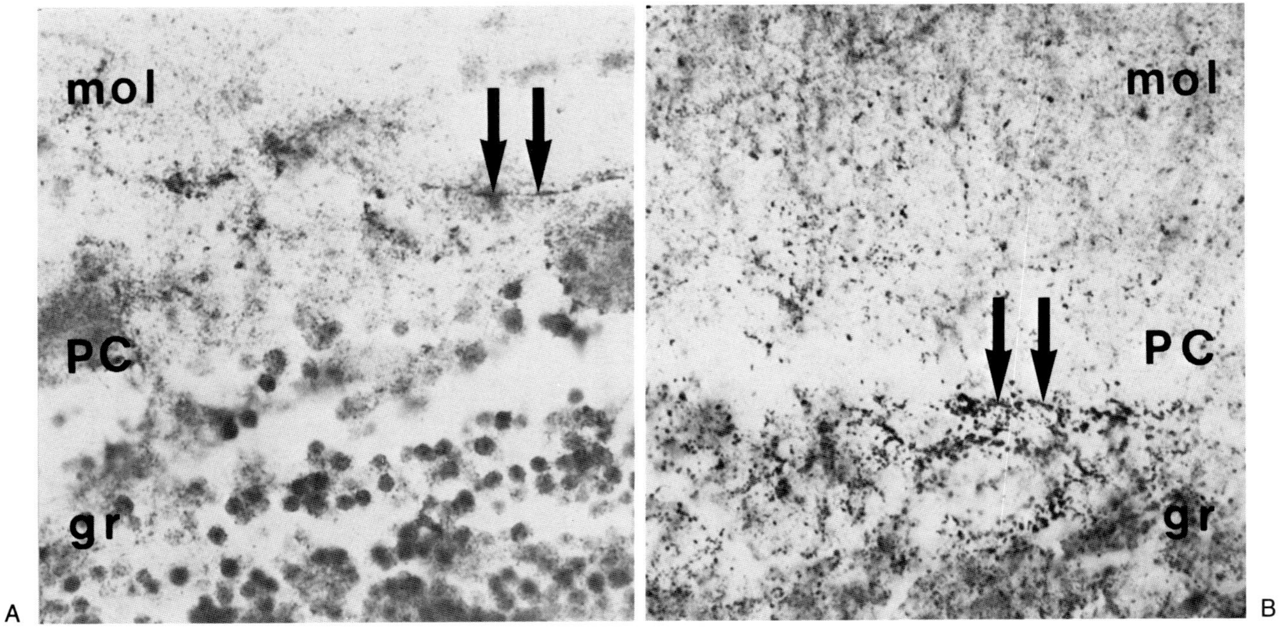

FIG. 1. PH8 (**A**) and MAO B (**B**) immunoreactivity in the human cerebellar cortex. A: PH8 immunoreactive axonal fibers (*arrows*) and varicosities in the three layers of the cerebellar cortex. Granule cell nuclei are stained by cresyl violet. B: MAO B immunoreactive varicosities (*arrows*), which are accumulated at the lower border of the PC and in the granular layer (gr). IGSS (A,B); with cresyl violet counterstain (A). Magnification: ×560 (A,B). mol, molecular layer; PC, Purkinje cell layer.

rons outside the raphe nuclei, which were immunoreactive for serotonin antibodies, were also retrogradely labeled by tracers injected into the cerebellum (Chapter 6, this volume). In humans raphe nuclei might also be possible candidates for the origin of cerebellar serotonin (46,56). Human raphe neurons were demonstrated to be immunoreactive for MAO B and PH8 (48,56; Chapter 2, this volume). Correspondingly cerebellar fibers may contain serotonin and MAO B in coexistence. We found more processes and varicosities in the cerebellar cortex to be immunoreactive for MAO-B than for PH8. It cannot be excluded that this staining pattern is caused by postmortem alterations due to a higher susceptibility of tryptophan hydroxylase compared to MAO B. Another explanation could be that MAO B occurs not only in serotonin-synthesizing fibers but also in structures that contain monoamines other than serotonin or that accumulate serotonin by an uptake mechanism but do not synthesize it. Further studies are necessary to clarify these points.

ACKNOWLEDGMENTS

This work was supported in part by Swiss National Foundation grant 31-26396-89. We are grateful to Dr. C. W. Abell (University of Texas at Austin) (MAO B), Dr. K. G. Baimbridge (University of Vancouver, British Columbia, Canada) (calbindin D-28k, parvalbumin), Dr. R. G. H. Cotton (Murdoch Institute, Melbourne, Australia) (PH8), Dr. I. J. Kopin (National Institute of Mental Health, Rockville, Maryland) (GAD), and Dr. H. Möhler (University of Zürich, Switzerland) (bd 24) for kindly providing the antibodies for this study. T.Z. was supported by a German Research Foundation postdoctoral grant for part of these studies.

REFERENCES

1. Awapara J, Landau AJ, Fuerst R, Seale B. Free gamma-aminobutyric acid in brain. *J Biol Chem* 1950;187:35–39.
2. Roberts E, Frankel S. Gamma-aminobutyric acid in brain. Its formation from glutamic acid. *J Biol Chem* 1950;187:55–63.
3. Baxter CF. The nature of gamma-aminobutyric acid. In: Lajtha A, ed. *Handbook of neurochemistry*, vol 3. New York: Plenum, 1970:289–353.
4. Roberts E, Chase TN, Tower DB. *GABA in nervous system function*. New York: Raven Press, 1976.
5. McIlwain H, Bachelard HS. *Biochemistry and the central nervous system*. New York: Churchill Livingstone, 1985.
6. Costa E. The supramolecular organization of receptors for gamma-aminobutyric acid (GABA). In: Biggio G, Costa E, Gessa GL, Spano PF, eds. *Receptors as supramolecular entities* (*Advances in the biosciences*, vol 44). New York: Pergamon, 1983: 213–235.
7. Bowery NG. GABA receptors. In: Webster RA, Jordan CC, eds. *Neurotransmitters, drugs and disease*. London: Blackwell, 1989:182–197.
8. Ramon Y Cajal S. *Histologie du système nerveux de l'homme et des vertébrés* (Azoulay L, trans. vols 1 and 2). Madrid: Consejo Superior de Investigaciones Cientificas, 1911 (reprinted Paris: Maloine, 1955).
9. Palay SL, Chan-Palay V. *Cerebellar cortex*. New York: Springer, 1974.
10. Chan-Palay V. *Cerebellar dentate nucleus*. New York: Springer, 1977.
11. Eccles JC, Ito M, Szentagothai J. *The cerebellum as a neuronal machine*. New York: Springer, 1967.

12. Ito M. *The cerebellum and neural control*. New York: Raven Press, 1984.
13. Eccles JC, Llinas R, Sasaki K. The inhibitory interneurons within the cerebellar cortex. *Exp Brain Res* 1966;1:1–16.
14. Eccles JC, Llinas R, Sasaki K. Intracellularly recorded responses of the cerebellar Purkinje cells. *Exp Brain Res* 1966;1:161–183.
15. Ito M, Yoshida M. The cerebellar-evoked monosynaptic inhibition of Deiters' neurons. *Experientia* 1964;20:515–516.
16. Ito M, Yoshida M. The origin of cerebellar-induced inhibition of Deiters' neurones. I. Monosynaptic initiation of the inhibitory postsynaptic potentials. *Exp Brain Res* 1966;2:330–349.
17. Ito M, Yoshida M, Obata K. Monosynaptic inhibition of the intracerebellar nuclei induced from the cerebellar cortex. *Experientia* 1964;20:575–576.
18. Ito M, Yoshida M, Obata K, Kawai N, Udo M. Inhibitory control of intracerebellar nuclei by the Purkinje cell axons. *Exp Brain Res* 1970;10:64–80.
19. Curtis DR, Felix D. The effect of bicuculline upon synaptic inhibition in the cerebral and cerebellar cortices of the cat. *Brain Res* 1971;34:301–321.
20. Curtis DR, Duggan AW, Felix D. GABA and inhibition of Deiters' neurones. *Brain Res* 1970;23:117–120.
21. Curtis DR, Duggan AW, Felix D, Johnston GA, McLennan H. Antagonism between bicuculline and GABA in the cat brain. *Brain Res* 1971;33:57–73.
22. Eccles JC, Llinas R, Sasaki K. The action of antidromic impulses on the cerebellar Purkinje cells. *J Physiol (Lond)* 1966;182:316–345.
23. Krnjevic K. GABA and other transmitters in the cerebellum. In: Palay SL, Chan-Palay V, eds. *The cerebellum—new vistas*. New York: Springer, 1982:533–549.
24. Hökfelt T, Ljungdahl A. Autoradiographic identification of cerebral and cerebellar cortical neurons accumulating labeled gamma-aminobutyric acid (3H-GABA). *Exp Brain Res* 1972;14:354–362.
25. Hyde JC, Robinson N. Gamma-aminobutyrate transaminase activity in rat cerebellar cortex: a histochemical study. *Brain Res* 1974;82:109–116.
26. Saito K, Barber R, Wu JY, Matsuda T, Roberts E, Vaughn JE. Immunohistochemical localization of glutamic acid decarboxylase in rat cerebellum. *Proc Natl Acad Sci USA* 1974; 71:269–273.
27. Chan-Palay V, Palay SL, Wu J-Y. Gamma-aminobutyric acid pathways in the cerebellum studied by retrograde and anterograde transport of glutamic acid decarboxylase antibody after in vivo injections. *Anat Embryol* 1979;157:1–14.
28. Oertel WH, Schmechel DE, Mugnaini E, Tappaz ML, Kopin IJ. Immunocytochemical localization of glutamate decarboxylase in rat cerebellum with a new antiserum. *Neuroscience* 1981;6:2715–2735.
29. Chan-Palay V. Neurotransmitters and receptors in the cerebellum: immunocytochemical localization of glutamic acid decarboxylase, GABA-transaminase, and cyclic GMP and autoradiography with 3H-muscimol. In: Palay SL, Chan-Palay V, eds. *The cerebellum—new vistas*. New York: Springer, 1982:552–584.
30. Chan-Palay V. Fine structure of labelled axons in the cerebellar cortex and nuclei of rodents and primates after intraventricular infusions with tritiated serotonin. *Anat Embryol* 1975;148:235–265.
31. Yamamoto M, Chan-Palay V, Palay SL. Autoradiographic experiments to examine uptake, anterograde and retrograde transport of tritiated serotonin in the mammalian brain. *Anat Embryol* 1980;159:137–149.
32. Takeuchi Y, Kimura H, Sano Y. Immunohistochemical demonstration of serotonin-containing nerve fibers in the cerebellum. *Cell Tissue Res* 1982;226:1–12.
33. Bishop GA, Ho RH, King JS. Localization of serotonin immunoreactivity in the opossum cerebellum. *J Comp Neurol* 1985;235:301–321.
34. Zetzsche T, Baimbridge KG, Möhler H, Chan-Palay V. Subsets of GABA neurons in the human cerebellum in normal controls and senile dementia of the Alzheimer type patients detected by glutamate decarboxylase, $GABA_A$/benzodiazepine receptor protein, calbindin D-28k and parvalbumin immunocytochemistry. *Dementia* 1990;1:237–252.
35. Mugnaini E, Oertel WH. An atlas of the distribution of GABAergic neurons and terminals in the rat CNS as revealed by GAD immunohistochemistry. In: Björklund A, Hökfelt A, Kuhar MJ eds. *Handbook of chemical neuroanatomy*, vol 4. Amsterdam: Elsevier, 1985:436–608.
36. Oertel WH, Schmechel DE, Tappaz ML, Kopin IJ. Production of a specific antiserum to rat brain glutamic acid decarboxylase by injection of an antigen-antibody complex. *Neuroscience* 1981;6:2689–2700.

37. Celio MR. Parvalbumin in most gamma-aminobutyric acid-containing neurons of the rat cerebral cortex. *Science* 1986;231:995–997.
38. Katsumaru H, Kosaka T, Heizmann CW, Hama K. Immunocytochemical study of GABAergic neurons containing the calcium-binding protein parvalbumin in the rat hippocampus. *Exp Brain Res* 1988;72:347–362.
39. Hendry SHC, Jones EG, Emson PC, Lawson DEM, Heizmann CW, Streit P. Two classes of cortical GABA neurons defined by differential calcium binding protein immunoreactivities. *Exp Brain Res* 1989;76:467–472.
40. Celio MR. Calbindin D-28k and parvalbumin in the rat nervous system. *Neuroscience* 1990;35:375–475.
41. Baimbridge KG, Miller JJ, Parkes CO. Calcium-binding protein distribution in the rat brain. *Brain Res* 1982;239:519–525.
42. Sloviter RS. Calcium binding protein (calbindin-D28k) and parvalbumin immunocytochemistry: localization in the rat hippocampus with specific reference to the selective vulnerability of hippocampal neurons to seizure activity. *J Comp Neurol* 1989;280:183–196.
43. Schoch P, Richards JG, Häring P, et al. Co-localization of GABA$_A$-receptors and benzodiazepine receptors in the brain shown by monoclonal antibodies. *Nature* 1985;314:168–171.
44. Ewert M, Shivers BD, Lüddens H, Möhler H, Seeburg PH. Subunit selectivity and epitope characterization of mAbs directed against the GABA$_A$/benzodiazepine receptor. *J Cell Biol* 1990;110:2043–2048.
45. Haan EA, Jennings IG, Cuello AC, et al. A monoclonal antibody recognizing all three aromatic amino acid hydroxylases allows identification of serotonergic neurons in human brain. *Brain Res* 1987;426:19–27.
46. Baker KG, Halliday GM, Halasz J-P, et al. Cytoarchitecture of serotonin-synthesizing neurons in the pontine tegmentum of the human brain. *Synapse* 1991;7:301–320.
47. Denney RM, Patel NT, Fritz NT, Abell CW. A monoclonal antibody elicited to human platelet monoamine oxidase. Isolation and specificity for human monoamine oxidase B but not A. *Mol Pharmacol* 1982;22:500–508.
48. Westlund KN, Denney RM, Rose RM, Abell CW. Localization of distinct monoamine oxidase A and monoamine oxidase B cell populations in human brainstem. *Neuroscience* 1988;25:439–456.
49. Chan-Palay V. Somatostatin immunoreactive neurons in the human hippocampus and cortex shown by immunogold/silver intensification on vibratome sections: coexistence with neuropeptide Y neurons, and effects in Alzheimer-type dementia. *J Comp Neurol* 1987;260:201–223.
50. Adams JC. Heavy metal intensification of DAB-based HRP reaction product. *J Histochem Cytochem* 1981;29:775.
51. Baimbridge KG, Miller JJ. Immunohistochemical localization of calcium-binding protein in the cerebellum, hippocampal formation and olfactory bulb of the rat. *Brain Res* 1982;245:223–229.
52. Garcia-Segura LM, Baetens D, Roth J, Norman AW, Orci L. Immunohistochemical mapping of calcium-binding protein immunoreactivity in the rat central nervous system. *Brain Res* 1984;296:75–86.
53. Christakos S, Rhoten WB, Feldman SC. Rat calbindin D28k: purification, quantitation, immunocytochemical localization and comparative aspects. *Meth Enzymol* 1987;139:534–551.
54. Richards JG, Schoch P, Häring P, Takacs B, Möhler H. Resolving GABA$_A$/benzodiazepine receptors: cellular and subcellular localization in the CNS with monoclonal antibodies. *J Neurosci* 1987;7:1866–1886.
55. Somogyi P, Takagi H, Richards JG, Möhler H. Subcellular localization of benzodiazepine/GABA$_A$ receptors in the cerebellum of rat, cat, and monkey using monoclonal antibodies. *J Neurosci* 1989;9:2197–2209.
56. Törk I, Hornung JP. Raphe nuclei and the serotonergic system. In: Paxinos G, ed. *The human nervous system*. New York: Academic Press, 1990:1001–1022.

*Serotonin, the Cerebellum,
and Ataxia,* edited by
P. Trouillas and K. Fuxe.
Raven Press, Ltd., New York © 1993.

10

The Brain Stem Origin and Development of Serotonin in the Opossum Cerebellum

James S. King, James J. Walker, and Georgia A. Bishop

Department of Cell Biology, Neurobiology, and Anatomy, The Ohio State University, Columbus, Ohio 43210-1239

It is well established that serotonin (5-HT) is expressed in the rat brain stem very early during embryonic stages of central nervous system (CNS) development (21). Lauder and colleagues (22–24) have provided evidence that 5-HT acts as a developmental signal to alter the morphological and biochemical differentiation of raphe neurons. In addition, the number of high-affinity 5-HT receptors in the brain stem reach their highest levels at birth, decline, and then increase to adult levels, further suggesting a role for 5-HT in development that may be distinct from its adult function (38). At postnatal day (PD) 10, binding sites for 5-HT$_{1A}$ receptors are relatively abundant, but become greatly reduced in the adult, and it has been suggested that this transient expression of receptors may be correlated with cell migration (12).

We have previously described the distribution of 5-HT in the cerebellum of the adult opossum (7) and have used this species to study the maturation of chemically identified afferents because of its unique embryology. At birth the opossum brain is embryonic when compared to other species (36). The immaturity of the opossum cerebellum at birth and its relatively slow development make it possible to analyze events that occur rapidly and *in utero* in most other mammals. On PD 1, the day of birth, specific brain stem nuclei are difficult to identify because of the relative immaturity of the brain (31). However, 5-HT is present within neurons located in the raphe and adjacent reticular formation as well as in a fiber bundle located within the rostral cerebellum. Because of the possible role of 5-HT in regulating brain development we have described its distribution in the cerebellum and correlated its developmental time course with that of other developmental events (i.e., neuronal migration, synaptogenesis, and morphogenesis) (5,8).

In this chapter we will review our previous results documenting the adult distribution of 5-HT, the early arrival of 5-HT axons, and the transient expression of 5-HT during cerebellar development and provide evidence that this system of afferents is derived from the medullary reticular formation. More recent experiments indicate that other brain stem sources include the dorsal raphe nucleus and the locus coeruleus, pars alpha (see ref. 30 for localization of this cell group in the opossum).

MATERIALS AND METHODS

Imunohistochemistry

The trajectory of serotoninergic axons, as well as the distribution of serotoninergic fibers in the cerebellum and cell bodies in the brain stem, was analyzed using the peroxidase-antiperoxidase (PAP) technique (35). The primary antibody (194D) was obtained from Dr. R. Elde (University of Minnesota). Adult opossums were anesthetized with sodium pentobarbital (40 mg/kg, i.p.) and perfused through the aorta with saline followed by a 2% paraformaldehyde-picric acid fixative (34) at room temperature. Pouch young animals between PD 1 and 80 were anesthetized with metofane and perfused transcardially with a 2% paraformaldehyde-picric acid fixative (34). Briefly, the brain was removed and postfixed in the same fixative for 4 to 6 hr at 4°C and then transferred to a 30% sucrose-0.2 M phosphate buffer (pH 7.2) solution at 4°C and left overnight. The tissue was sectioned at 60 to 80 μm on a freezing microtome in either the transverse or sagittal plane. Unmounted sections were incubated consecutively in a primary antibody to 5-HT (194D, diluted 1:10,000, 24–48 hr at 4°C), sheep antirabbit IgG serum (diluted 1:300, 1–1.5 hr at room temperature), and finally rabbit PAP serum (diluted 1:1,000, 1.5 hr at room temperature). All sections were rinsed with borate-buffered saline after each incubation. The tissue was then incubated in 0.05% 3,3-diaminobenzidine tetrahydrochloride (DAB) and 0.006% H_2O_2 for 5 to 10 min at room temperature. After a final wash in borate-buffered saline, the sections were mounted on gelatin-coated slides, dehydrated through alcohols, cleared with xylene, and coverslipped.

Double-Labeling Techniques

Horseradish Peroxidase–Peroxidase-Antiperoxidase Method

Adult animals ($n = 11$) were anesthetized by intraperitoneal injections of sodium pentobarbital (Nembutal, 40 mg/kg) and secured in a stereotaxic headholder. The cerebellum was exposed via a dorsal craniotomy and the dura was cut. Multiple pressure injections (0.2 μl/injection) of HRP (30% in saline) were centered in the posterior lobe vermis (lobules VI–IX) or the cerebellar nuclei. Following survival times of 20 to 24 hr, the animals were anesthetized and perfused with 4% paraformaldehyde in phosphate buffer (0.2 M). To enhance the level of 5-HT in brain stem somata, the animals received the monoamine oxidase inhibitor pargyline (50 mg/kg i.p.) followed by L-tryptophan (50 mg/kg i.p.). Brains were blocked and cut serially on a freezing microtome at 60 μm in the transverse plane. Serial sections were collected in phosphate-buffered saline (PBS) and processed for HRP histochemistry using cobalt chloride-intensified DAB as the chromogen. The same tissue sections were then processed for 5-HT immunohistochemistry. The specific details of this double-labeling paradigm have been published previously (6) and follow the procedure described by Bowker et al. (10,11). A series of pouch young opossums ranging in age from PD 9 to 77 were processed using the HRP-PAP double-label paradigm, described above for adult animals. The only difference was that pargyline and L-tryptophan were not used.

Fluorescent Microspheres

Green or red fluorescent microspheres were injected into the cerebellar cortex and/or the cerebellar nuclei of six adult opossums to confirm or extend the results of the HRP-PAP double-label technique. In this procedure, the animals were anesthetized with sodium pentobarbital (40 mg/kg i.p.) and secured in a stereotaxic frame. The bone and dura over the posterior lobe vermis were removed. Multiple injections 0.1–0.3 μl each) of fluorescein- or rhodamine-labeled microspheres (Luma Fluor, Inc.) were made in lobules VII–IX of the vermis or in the cerebellar nuclei through a Hamilton syringe (17). The wound was sutured and the animals allowed to survive 24 to 30 hr. Prior to perfusion the animals were given an intraperitoneal injection of pargyline (50 mg/kg). They were given an intraperitoneal injection (50 mg/kg) of L-tryptophan, a precursor of 5-HT, 30 to 45 min later. These injections were given to increase 5-HT labeling of neuronal cell bodies. After an additional 30 to 45 min, the animals were deeply anesthetized with sodium pentobarbital and perfused through the aorta with saline followed by 4% paraformaldehyde in phosphate buffer. The brains were removed, stored in fixative for 4 to 6 hr, and then transferred to Sorenson's phosphate buffer with 15% sucrose until they sunk. Serial sections of the brain stems were cut in the transverse plane at 60 μm on a freezing microtome and the cerebellum at 90 μm in the sagittal plane. The brain stem sections were rinsed in PBS and placed in 194D (diluted 1:5,000) for 48 hr at 4°C with constant agitation. They were then placed into either a rhodamine- or fluorescein-tagged rabbit IgG (1:300) for 2 hr at room temperature with constant agitation. The sections were rinsed in PBS, mounted on clean slides, cleared in xylene for 1 min, and coverslipped with Krystalon (EM Diagnostic Systems). The sections were examined with a Zeiss fluorescent microscope equipped with rhodamine and fluorescein filters. Each section was examined for the presence of double-labeled cells. Photomicrographs of the same area or neuron were taken with each filter to demonstrate double- or single-labeled neurons.

RESULTS

Adult Distribution

Cerebellar Cortex

The majority of 5-HT immunoreactive (IR) fibers are located in the internal granule layer (IGL), particularly at the granule cell-Purkinje cell (PK) interface (Fig. 1). Here they arborize, forming a plexus within the IGL and around the PK bodies (Fig. 1D–F). A few axons extend into the molecular layer and course either vertically or tangentially toward the pial surface (Fig. 1E). 5-HT axons are varicose and do not terminate as either mossy fibers or climbing fibers (Fig. 1D–F). The majority of the axonal swellings measure 1.5 μm or less and have an average intervaricosity distance of 5.3 μm (7). Within the cerebellar lobules there is a differential distribution of 5-HT. Folia within the vermis and hemispheres of the anterior lobe contain few IR fibers (Fig. 1A–C). The posterior lobules generally display more 5-HT fibers, with the densest labeling found in lobule VIII and the dorsal folia of IX (Fig. 1E).

Cerebellar Nuclei

5-HT fibers enter the cerebellum via the superior cerebellar peduncle and form a bundle that courses immediately dorsal to the ependymal lining of the fourth ventricle (Fig. 2). Individual varicose axons enter the ventral aspect of all four cerebellar nuclei. Upon reaching the caudal aspect of the deep nuclei, fibers within this bundle turn dorsally and course toward lobules VIII and IX (Fig. 2D). In contrast to the generally sparse and differential lobular distribution of 5-HT in the cerebellar cortex, all the cerebellar nuclei contain numerous beaded 5-HT axons (Fig. 3). The density of the 5-HT immunoreactivity appears to increase in more caudal levels of the cerebellar nuclei (compare Fig. 3A and C). Varicosities within the cerebellar nuclei measure 1.5 μm or less and the mean distance between these swellings is 3.85 μm (7).

Ontogeny of 5-HT in the Cerebellum

Early Arrival

At birth, (PD 1) 5-HT axons are present within the cerebellar anlage. At this age the cerebellum, when viewed from the dorsum of the brain, is shaped like the letter U. Transverse sections through the most rostral regions of the cerebellum reveal that it is continuous with the tectum through the isthmus region (Fig. 4A) and more caudally the body of the U overlies the medulla (Fig. 4B). Histologically the cerebellum consists of a densely packed ventricular (germinal) layer, an intermediate cellular layer, and more superficial acellular areas (Fig. 4C). Individual 5-HT fibers

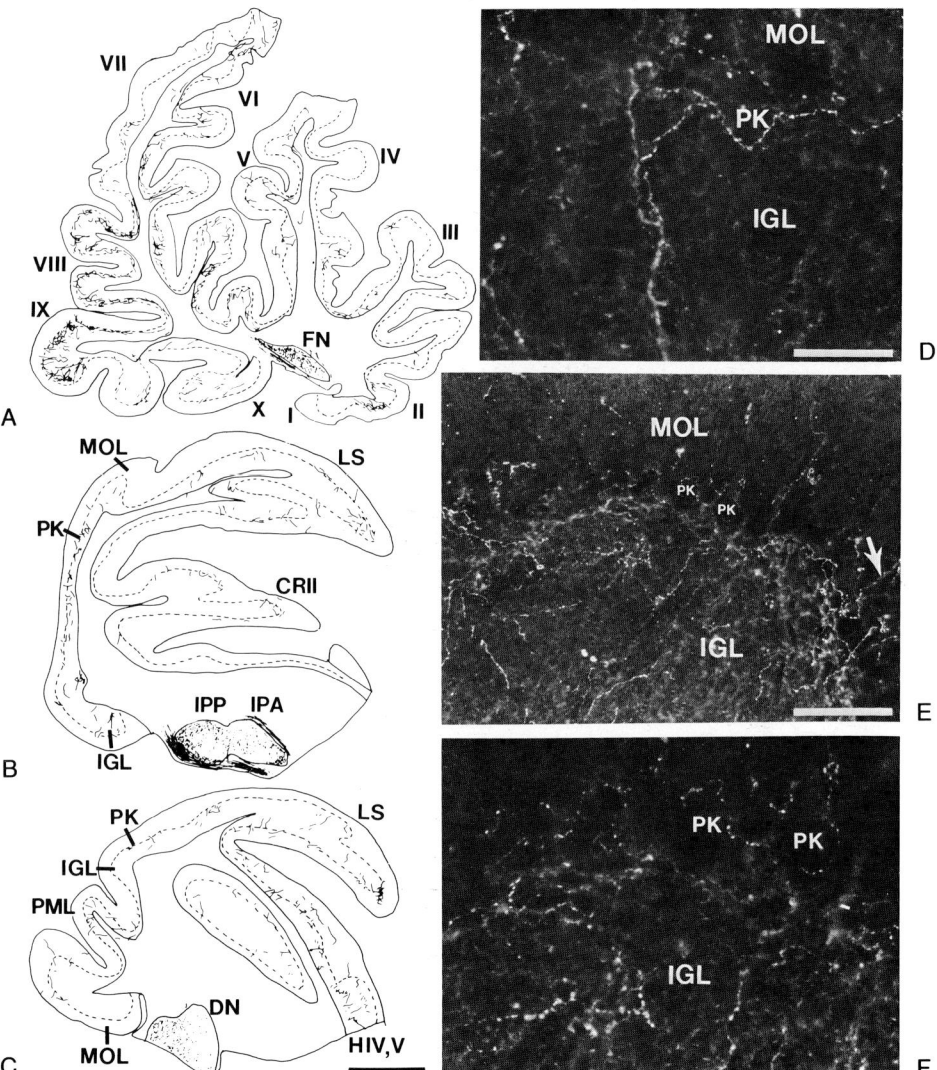

FIG. 1. A–C: Camera lucida drawings of three representative sagittal sections from the adult cerebellum illustrating the distribution of 5-HT fibers (*irregular lines* and *dots*). Section in A is most medial and C is most lateral. The vermal lobules are labeled I–X, and some of the intermediate and lateral lobules are identified, as are the cerebellar nuclei (CRII, crus two; HIV,V, lateral hemispheres of the anterior lobe; LS, lobus simplex; PML, paramedian lobule; DN, dentate nucleus; FN, fastigial nucleus; IPA, interpositus anterior; IPP, interpositus posterior). The PK layer is indicated by the *broken line* and the IGL and the molecular layer (MOL) are labeled. **D–F:** Dark-field photomicrographs taken from lobules II (D) and IX (E,F). The varicose axons course through the IGL and many course along the PK layer. Fibers occasionally continue into the molecular layer (E, *arrow*). Calibration bar in C = 2 mm; in D, 50 μm and also applies to F; in E, the bar = 100 μm.

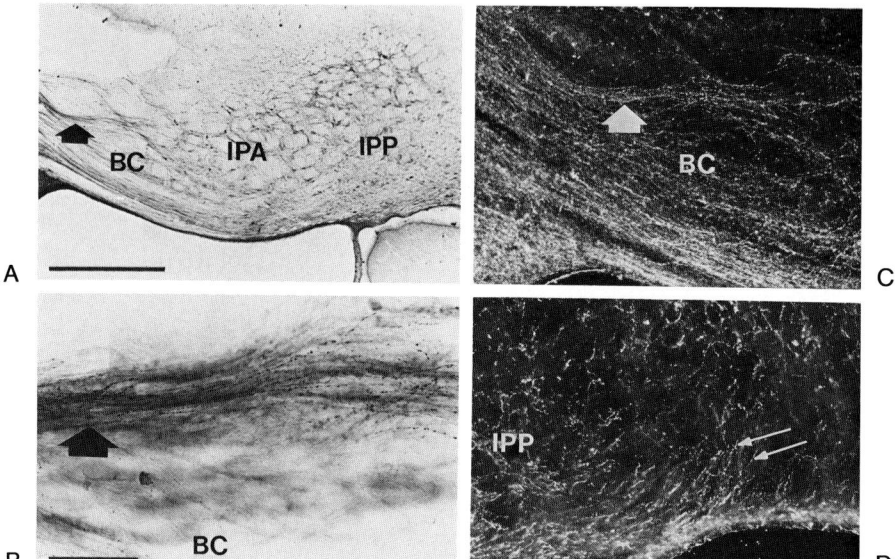

FIG. 2. 5-HT fibers enter the cerebellum via the brachium conjunctivum (BC) and are illustrated in bright- and dark-field photomicrographs (**A–C**, *block arrows*). They course through the cerebellar nuclei, and as they reach the caudal pole of the interpositus posterior (IPP), they continue into the cerebellar cortex (**D**, *arrows*). IPA, interpositus anterior. Calibration bar in A = 500 μm; in B, 200 μm and also applies to C and D.

enter the cerebellum from a distinct bundle of axons that is present within the isthmus region (Fig. 4F, arrows). Within the cerebellar anlage they aggregate adjacent to the pia mater in an acellular region as revealed in histological sections (compare Fig. 4C and F, block arrows). Individual beaded fibers also are present in the intermediate layer (Fig. 4E) and some terminate in growth cone-like expansions within the ventricular layer (Fig. 4D, arrow).

By PD 12 the external granule layer (EGL) covers the cerebellar surface, the ventricular layer is reduced in depth, a multitiered PK layer is present, and an acellular zone is evident between the EGL and the PK layer. 5-HT IR fibers enter the cerebellum through the isthmus region and course within the cerebellum in the bundles just deep to the pia mater described at PD 1. At this age, 5-HT fibers also enter via the incipient inferior cerebellar peduncle. Varicose 5-HT axons, many ending in growth cones, are present throughout the cellular zone that extends between the ventricular layer and the nascent PK layer.

By PD 21 the primary fissure divides the cerebellum into anterior and posterior lobes; in addition, individual cerebellar nuclei can be differentiated in Nissl preparations (Fig. 5A). 5-HT IR fibers reach the cerebellum via the two routes described at PD 12 (Fig. 5A–C, arrows) and form a dense plexus along the ventricular layer (Fig. 5B, block arrow) and within the cerebellar nuclei. Varicose axons are present

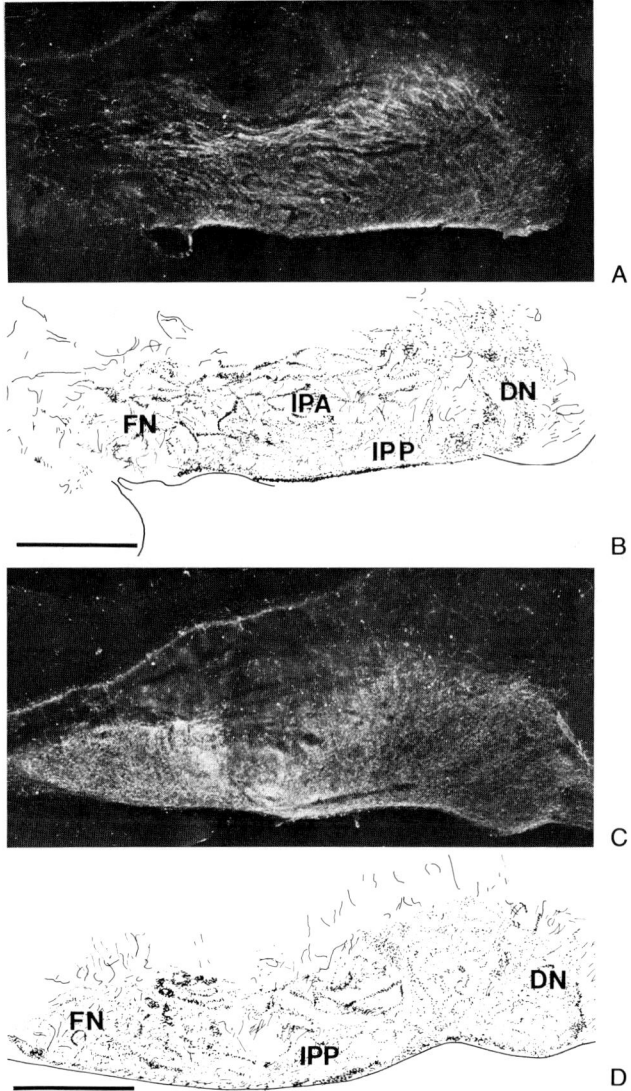

FIG. 3. A,C: Dark-field photomicrographs of transverse sections through the cerebellar nuclei to illustrate 5-HT fibers in the fastigial nucleus (FN), interpositus anterior and posterior (IPA, IPP), and dentate nucleus (DN). The drawings (**B,D**) were made from the same sections shown in the photomicrographs (A,C) to illustrate the relative density of the 5-HT fibers. Calibration bars in B and D = 1 mm and also apply to A and C.

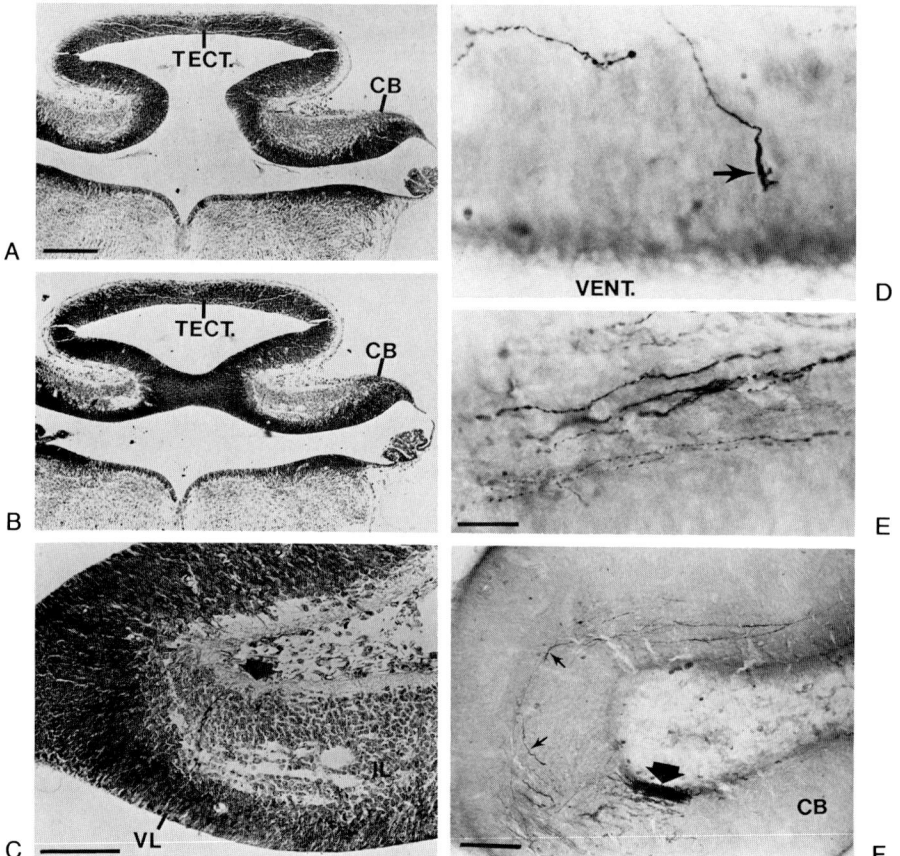

FIG. 4. A–C: Transverse sections of a PD 1 brain stem stained for Nissl substance. The cerebellum (CB) is U shaped and is comprised of three layers: a ventricular layer (VL), an intermediate layer, and a superficial acellular zone (C, *block arrow*). At this age 5-HT fibers terminate in growth cones (**D**, *arrow*), are beaded (**E**), and enter the cerebellum through the isthmus region between the tectum (TECT.) and the cerebellum (**F**, *arrows*). 5-HT axons form a bundle within the cerebellum rostrally just beneath the pia mater (F, *block arrow*). Calibration bar in A = 250 μm and applies to B, the bar in C = 100 μm and applies to D, the bar in E = 25 μm and the bar in F = 100 μm.

within the medullary core of the cerebellum but do not penetrate into the PK layer or the EGL (Fig. 5C–E). At this age, they are distributed throughout both the anterior and posterior lobes (Fig. 5C–E).

Transient Expression

By PD 30, cerebellar foliation is evident in the incipient vermis and the hemispheres (Fig. 6A–D). The PK layer is still multitiered and small basophilic migrat-

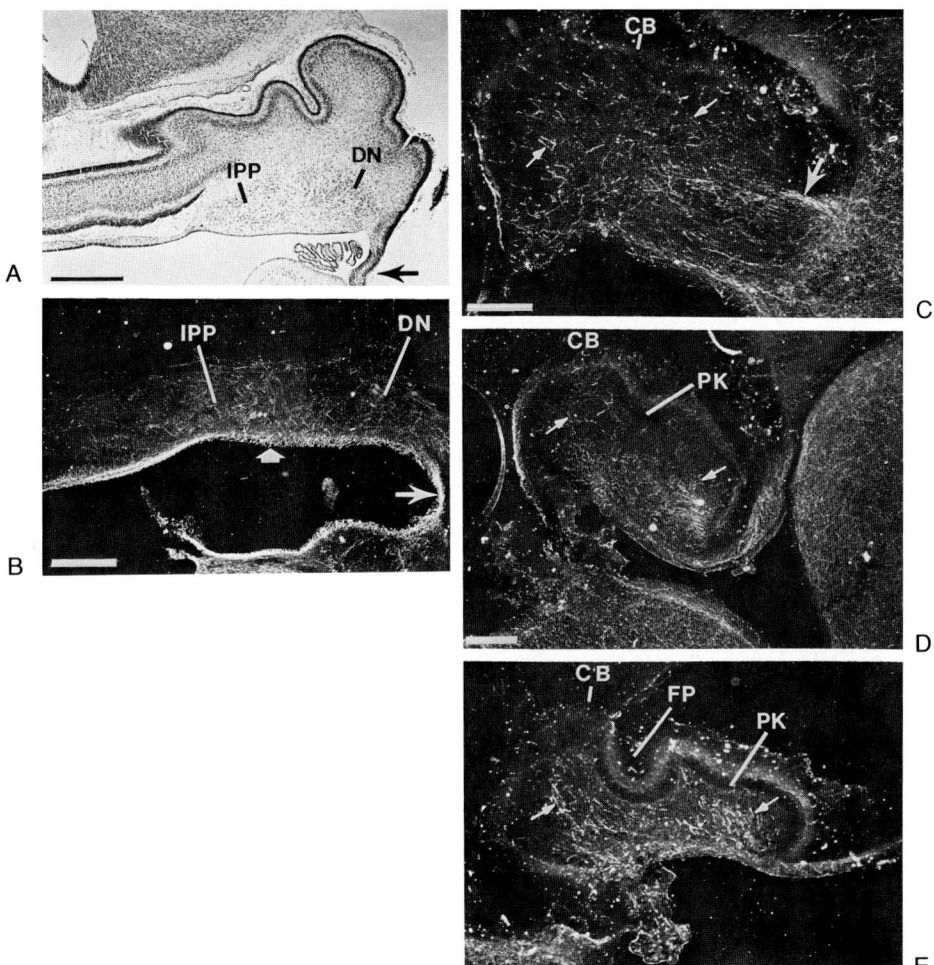

FIG. 5. A: Photomicrograph of a transverse section of the cerebellum from a PD 33 opossum stained for Nissl substance. The interpositus posterior (IPP) and the dentate nucleus (DN) are labeled. The inferior cerebellar peduncle is indicated by the *arrow*. Serotoninergic fibers enter the cerebellum via the incipient inferior cerebellar peduncle (**B**, *arrow*) and distribute throughout the cerebellar nuclei, as well as along the ventricular layer (B, *block arrow*). Interpositus posterior and dentate nucleus are present at this level. **C–E**: Dark-field photomicrographs of representative sagittal sections from a PD 25 opossum cerebellum (CB); C is lateral and E is medial. The primary fissure (FP) demarcates the anterior and posterior lobes; both contain 5-HT IR fibers C–E, *small arrows*) that enter the cerebellum via the peduncular stalk (C, *large arrow*). The 5-HT axons arborize within the medullary core of the cerebellum but do not penetrate the PK layer (D,E). Calibration bar in A = 500 μm; in B, 500 μm; in C, 250 μm; in D, 250 μm and also applies to E.

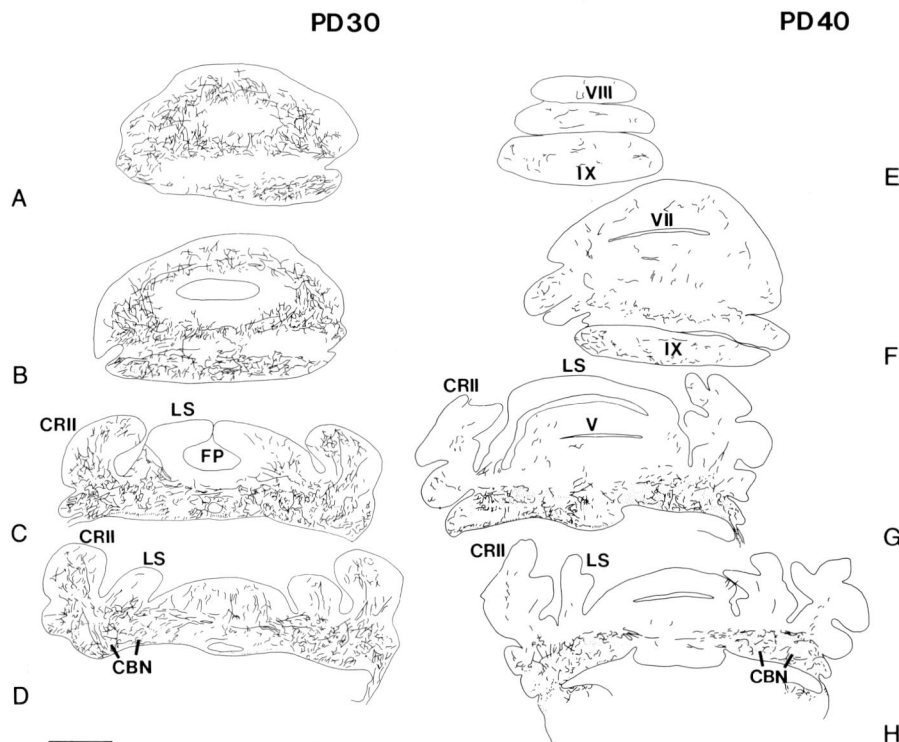

FIG. 6. Camera lucida drawings of 5-HT fibers seen in representative transverse sections through caudal (**A,E**) to rostral (**D,H**) levels of the developing cerebellum (**A–D**, PD 30 animal; **E–H**, PD 40 animal). The cerebellar nuclei (CBN), vermal lobules V, VII, VIII, IX and crus II (CRII), lobus simplex (LS), and paramedian lobule (PML) are labeled for reference. The primary (FP) is labeled in C. Calibration bar in D = 1 mm and applies to A–C, E–H.

ing cells are evident between the EGL and the PK layer. 5-HT axons reach the cerebellum via the superior cerebellar peduncle and the inferior cerebellar peduncle. At this age 5-HT axons, many with growth cones, are present throughout the rostral to caudal extent of the cerebellum. They do not distribute within the PK layer or the EGL but are confined to the incipient IGL, which can be differentiated histologically for the first time between PD 30 and 33. The density of 5-HT fibers is greater in the posterior lobe of the cerebellar cortex than in the anterior lobe (compare Fig. 6A and D). Numerous 5-HT axons are present in the cerebellar nuclei (Fig. 6D). By PD 40 (Fig. 6E–H) there is a decrease in the density of 5-HT IR fibers throughout the cerebellar cortex (compare Fig. 6A–D and E–H). In contrast, the cerebellar nuclei (Fig. 6H, CBN) still display a plexus of immunolabeled fibers comparable to that seen at PD 30. Within the cerebellar cortex the laminar distribution has not changed, but the number of growth cones has greatly diminished. Between PD 40 and 70 the number of 5-HT fibers in the inferior cerebellar peduncle decreases, but they are still present within the superior cerebellar peduncle, which in the adult is the primary route of entry. By PD 70 the adult pattern of distribution is achieved within the cerebellar cortex.

Brain Stem Origin

Adult Animals

In the opossum brain stem, serotoninergic cell bodies span the rostro-caudal extent of the pons and medulla and are located, as described in several species (6,14, 16,19,30) throughout the raphe nuclei and the adjacent reticular formation (Fig. 7A). Subsequent to injections of retrograde tracers into the posterior lobe vermis and processing the brain stem for 5-HT immunohistochemistry, double-labeled neurons are present in the medulla (Fig. 7C) and pons. They are located primarily in the nucleus reticularis gigantocellularis (Fig. 7C); the nucleus reticularis gigantocellularis, pars ventralis; as well as around the inferior olive and within the medullary pyramids. These observations also were confirmed using fluorescent-labeled microspheres and 5-HT immunohistochemistry. The latter method also revealed double-labeled neurons in the locus coeruleus, pars alpha (Fig. 8A–C) and the dorsal raphe nucleus (Fig. 8D,E). Double-labeled neurons are present in the same brain stem nuclei labeled after cortical injections when the injection sites included the cerebellar nuclei or were centered in the cerebellar nuclei.

Developing Animals

By PD 9, double-labeled neurons are present within many of the same brain stem regions as seen in adult animals, including the medullary reticular formation and the region of the locus coeruleus (Fig. 7B,D,E). The incidence of double-labeled neurons in the medulla and pons increases as the animals mature. By PD 60, a few double-labeled neurons also are present in the dorsal raphe nucleus.

DISCUSSION

Species Differences

Distribution of 5-HT in the Cerebellar Cortex

Analysis of tissue sections processed for immunohistochemistry in the cat, rat, and opossum reveals significant differences in the quantity as well as the laminar and lobular distribution of 5-HT afferents. Of the three species, the cat has the most extensive distribution of 5-HT IR fibers and varicosities, followed by the rat, and then the opossum. In the cat, 5-HT IR afferents have a dense, uniform distribution

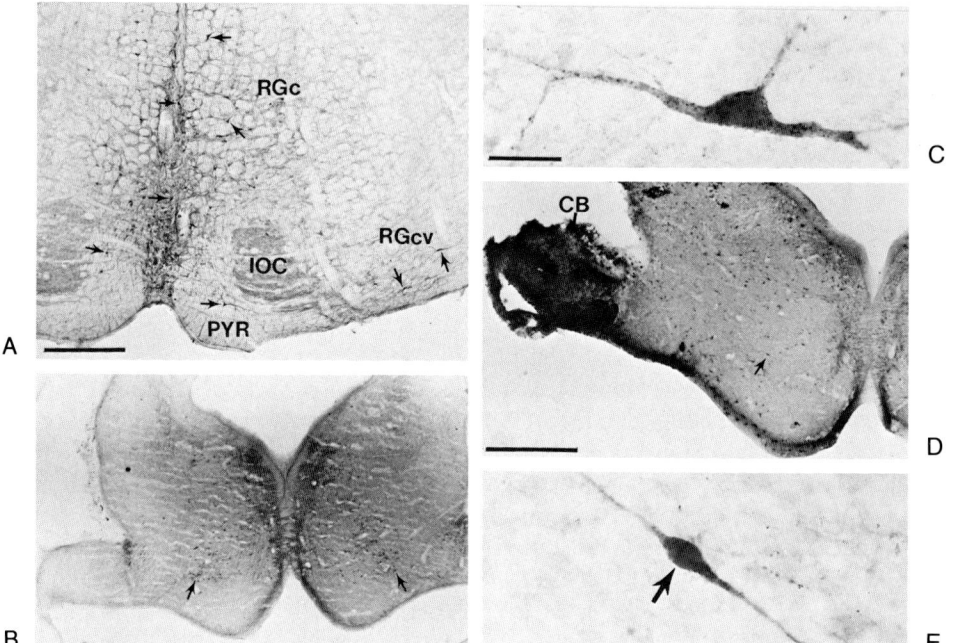

FIG. 7. A: Photomicrograph through the medulla illustrating the location of 5-HT neurons (*arrows*). Neurons in the nucleus reticularis gigantocellularis (RGc), nucleus reticularis gigantocellularis pars ventralis (RGcv) as well as 5-HT neurons in the pyramidal bundle (PYR) and around the inferior olive complex (IOC) give rise to the 5-HT projection to the cerebellum. **C**: High-power magnification of a double-labeled cell in RGc. **B**: Distribution of 5-HT neurons in the pons in a PD 9 animal. Following injections of HRP in the cerebellum (CB) (**D**, CB), double-labeled cells are found in an area that corresponds to the locus coeruleus (D, *arrow*). The double-labeled neuron indicated by the *arrow* in D is shown at higher magnification in **E**. Calibration bar in A = 500 μm and also applies to B; the bar in C = 20 μm and also applies to E; the bar in D = 500 μm.

throughout the medial to lateral extent of the cerebellum including the vermis, intermediate cortex, and hemispheres (9,19). The rat has a similar lobular distribution, although the density of the 5-HT plexus is not as great, particularly in the anterior lobe vermis (6). In contrast, 5-HT in the opossum is most prominent in the posterior lobe vermis, in particular lobules VIII and IX; some IR fibers and varicosities are present in the anterior lobe vermis. Scattered 5-HT axons also are present in the paramedian lobule, hemispheres, and flocculus of this marsupial.

Laminar differences in the distribution of 5-HT IR axons also are apparent in these three species. In the cat, 5-HT IR fibers and varicosities distribute throughout the granule cell layer, regardless of the area of the cerebellum examined. In contrast, 5-HT has a nearly equal distribution between the granule cell and molecular layers in the rat (6). However, there are some regional variations with respect to this general pattern of laminar distribution. For example, in lobule VI, only scattered

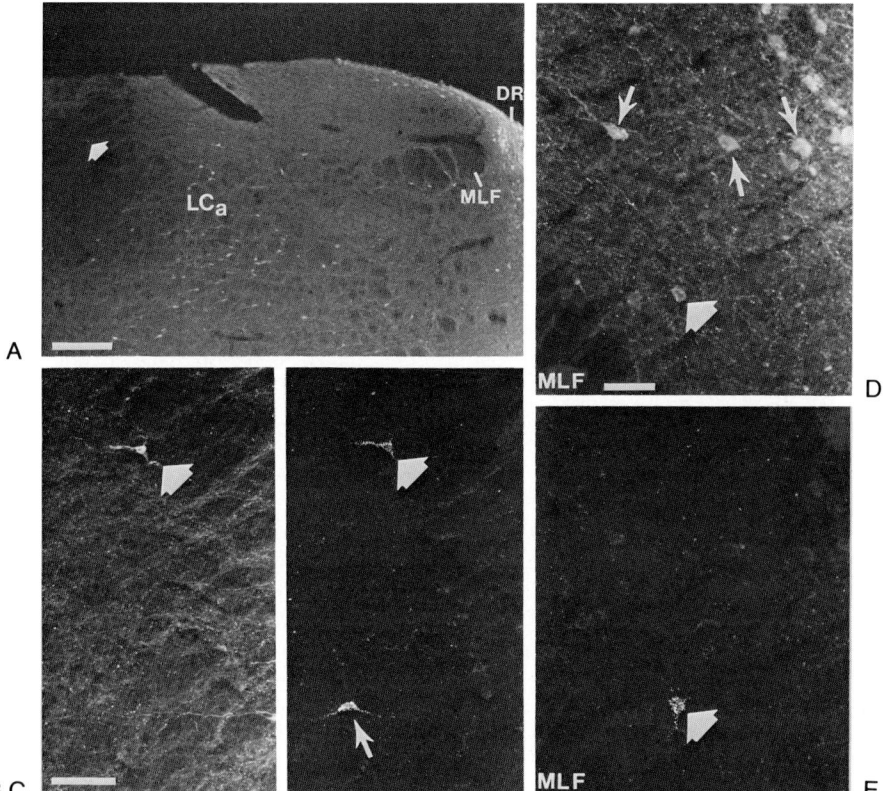

FIG. 8. Photomicrographs illustrating the location of double-labeled neurons in the locus coeruleus, pars alpha (LC$_a$) (**A–C**) and dorsal raphe nucleus (**D,E,**) following injections of fluorescent microspheres into the posterior vermis of an adult opossum. The dorsal raphe (DR) and medial longitudinal fasciculus (MLF) are labeled for reference. The cell in B (*block arrow*) is 5-HT positive and in C (*block arrow*) also is retrogradely labeled by the microspheres. A cell that projects to the cerebellum, but is not 5-HT positive is shown in C (arrow). D illustrates four 5-HT neurons (*arrows, block arrow*) in the dorsal raphe nucleus. Only one is retrogradely labeled (E, *block arrow*) after an injection of microspheres in the cerebellum. The 5-HT cells were visualized with a rhodamine filter and the retrogradely labeled cells with a FITC filter. Calibration bar in A = 200 μm; in B,C, 100 μm and also applies to C; in D, 50 μm and also applies to E.

5-HT labeling is present within the granule cell layer. As with the lobular distribution, the opossum also has the most restricted laminar distribution of 5-HT in the three species. In the areas where 5-HT is most prevalent, immunolabeling is most extensive in the upper part of the granule cell layer, that is, the portion located immediately subjacent to the PK layer. In addition, numerous 5-HT IR fibers appear to surround PK bodies, especially in lobules VIII and IX of the posterior lobe vermis.

The significance of the differential laminar and lobular distribution of 5-HT in various species is not clear. In one respect, the laminar differences may prove inconsequential as the targets of 5-HT afferents may not necessarily be within the lamina in which 5-HT varicosities are located. 5-HT-positive axon terminals and varicosities have been examined in electron micrographs in several areas of the CNS including the cerebral cortex (13) and inferior olive (20). These studies indicate a paucity of classically defined synaptic junctions (33) between serotoninergic terminals and an apposed neuronal membrane even when examined in serial sections. This paucity of synaptic contacts also appears to be true in the cat cerebellum (9). In the latter study, two findings are of particular interest, first vesicles are present in both the axonal shafts and varicosities. Second, as in other areas of the nervous system, few synaptic junctions have been identified. This suggests that 5-HT may interact with its postsynaptic targets at nonjunctional sites via the mechanism recently defined as "volume transmission" (15). An analysis of the distribution of 5-HT receptors in tissue sections taken from the cerebella of various species needs to be carried out in order to address possible mechanisms of action. Once these data are known, differences in laminar distribution may be more easily addressed and their significance, if any, better understood.

Differences in lobular distribution have implications as to a differential role for 5-HT in cerebellar function. In the opossum, 5-HT innervation is focused primarily, although not exclusively, in the posterior lobe vermis as compared to the near uniform distribution to both anterior and posterior lobes seen in the cat and to some extent in the rat. This suggests that 5-HT is involved in modulating the activity of more restricted populations of neurons in the former species. In the opossum, the posterior lobe vermis receives a primary input from the spinal trigeminal nucleus as well as from the caudal medial accessory olive and the dorsal cap of Kooy, as revealed by analyzing the distribution of retrogradely labeled cells following HRP (37) or fluorescent microsphere injections (*unpublished observations*) into the caudal vermis. This area of the inferior olive receives input from the reticular formation, the inferior vestibular nucleus, the dorsal column nuclei, the superior colliculus, the pretectal nuclei, and the subparafascicular nucleus (29). In part, these olivary neurons appear to be involved in relaying visual and/or vestibular information to the caudal cerebellum (1,3,27,28). Thus, 5-HT in the opossum could be related to cerebellar processing of specific sensory information. However, in the rat and cat, 5-HT has the potential to interact with all afferent systems to the cerebellum, including spinal, to more anterior vermal regions and corticopontine to lateral aspects of the cortex.

5-HT in the Cerebellar Nuclei

In sharp contrast to the cerebellar cortex, the cerebellar nuclei of the opossum (7), rat (6), and cat (19) display a relatively uniform distribution of 5-HT axons. Figure 9 summarizes this distribution in three representative sagittal sections from the fastigial, interpositus, and dentate nuclei of each of these three species. These data suggest that this system of afferents directly influences the output neurons of the

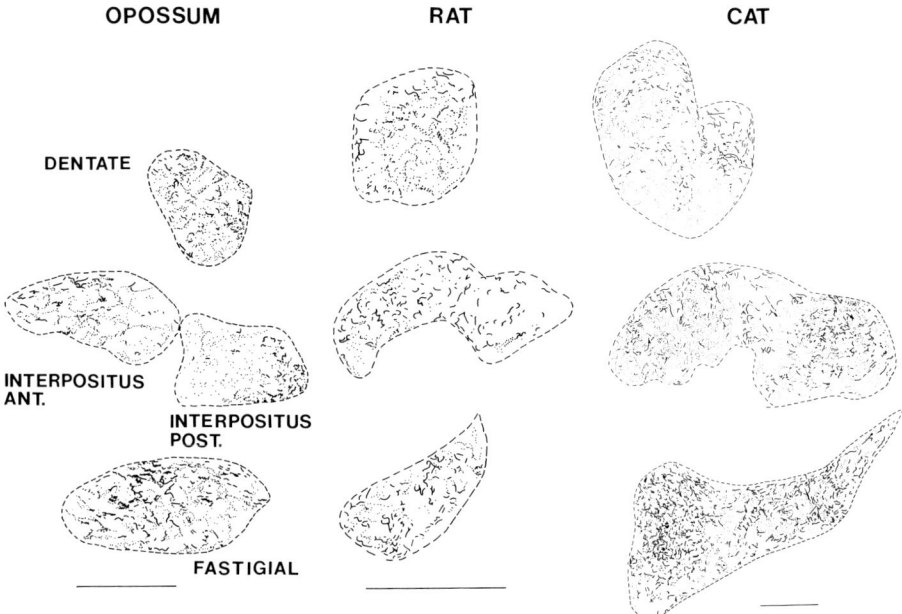

FIG. 9. Camera lucida drawings of 5-HT axons (*dots* and *irregular lines*) from representative sagittal sections through the cerebellar nuclei, dentate, interpositus posterior, interpositus anterior, and fastigial nuclei of three species, opossum, rat, and cat. Calibration bar for each species = 1 mm.

cerebellum. Based on these findings, the physiological effects of 5-HT on the cerebellar nuclei should be investigated to determine if 5-HT has the same suppressive effect on these neurons as it does on PK in the cat (18).

Brain Stem Source of Cerebellar 5-HT

The data from our double-labeling experiments in developing and adult animals suggest that 5-HT in the cerebellar cortex is derived primarily from the medullary reticular formation including neurons scattered around the inferior olivary complex and in the medullary pyramids, as well as a few neurons in the locus coeruleus, pars alpha. The only raphe neurons containing 5-HT that project to the cerebellum were found in the dorsal raphe nucleus. When the injection sites included the cerebellar nuclei, neurons in the same brain stem locations were double labeled. These data could be interpreted to suggest that the source of cerebellar 5-HT is the same as that for the cerebellar nuclei and cortex; however, this will have to be documented by additional experiments.

Developmental Expression

A detailed analysis of 5-HT ontogeny in the rat brain by Lidov and Molliver (26) described the initial 5-HT axons in the developing cerebellum on gestational day 21. At this age the cerebellum has a well-defined EGL, a thin molecular layer, and a poorly organized PK layer. A primary feature of the 5-HT afferent system in the rodent during postnatal development is the temporal sequence of the formation of terminal fields. In the cerebellum at PD 1 to 3, 5-HT axons ramify beneath the cerebellar cortex and do not penetrate the molecular layer or the EGL. At PD 6, 5-HT axons extend into the IGL with occasional axons in the PK layer. By PD 10, the PK are nearly in a uniform monolayer and 5-HT axons ramify in the IGL, the PK cell layer, and the molecular layer. Between PD 10 and 21, the 5-HT axons are thinner and increase in density (26) when compared to younger animals.

In contrast to the developing rat (26), the opossum cerebellum has 5-HT fibers present when the histological layers have not begun to differentiate, on PD 1. 5-HT axons are present in the intermediate zone located between the ventricular layer and the pial surface. This area is characterized by migrating neurons that, in the rat, will give rise to PK, Golgi neurons, and cerebellar nuclear neurons (2). Between PD 1 and 30, 5-HT axons with growth cones remain ("wait") in the intermediate zone and extend throughout the rostral to caudal extent of the cerebellum. In the opossum, a distinct IGL is not apparent in histological sections until PD 30 to 33, although granule cells probably begin to migrate prior to this time (25,32). This time frame (PD 30–33), is coincident with the time (PD 30) that 5-HT IR fibers have their greatest distribution throughout the cerebellum. After PD 40, 5-HT decreases throughout the developing cerebellar cortex, particularly the anterior lobe, until the adult pattern of distribution is reached by PD 40 to 47 (7). The reduction of 5-HT fibers in the inferior cerebellar peduncle after PD 40 provides further evidence for a transient expression of 5-HT during cerebellar development. A transient expression of 5-HT during development of the cerebral cortex also has been described by Bennett-Clarke et al. (4). Thus, this finding is not unique to the cerebellum, yet the precise role of 5-HT in the developing nervous system has not been determined. The early arrival, the waiting period in the medullary core of the cerebellum, and the coincident transient distribution of 5-HT axons with the formation of the IGL support a role for 5-HT in cerebellar development. Based on this temporal sequence, 5-HT may be involved in the maturation of neurons in the cerebellar nuclei, the migration of granule cells, and/or mossy fiber synaptogenesis.

ACKNOWLEDGMENTS

The authors would like to thank Mrs. Barbara Diener-Phelan for her technical and photographic assistance and Mrs. Kate Dillingham for typing the manuscript. We thank Dr. George Martin for reading the manuscript and his assistance in data analysis. This work was supported by grant NS 08789.

REFERENCES

1. Alley K, Baker R, Simpson JI. Afferents to the vestibulo-cerebellum and the origin of the visual climbing fibers in the rabbit. *Brain Res* 1975;98:582–589.
2. Altman J, Bayer SA. Prenatal development of the cerebellar system in the rat. 1. Cytogenesis and histogenesis of the deep nuclei and the cortex of the cerebellum. *J Comp Neurol* 1978;179:23–48.
3. Barmack NH, Young WS. Optokinetic stimulation increases corticotropin-releasing factor mRNA in inferior olivary neurons of rabbits. *J Neurosci* 1990;10:631–640.
4. Bennett-Clarke CA, Chiaia NL, Crissman RS, Rhoades RW. The source of the transient serotoninergic input to the developing visual and somatosensory cortices in rat. *Neuroscience* 1991;43:163–183.
5. Bishop G, Ho R, King JS. A temporal analysis of the origin and distribution of serotoninergic afferents in the cerebellum of pouch young opossums. *Anat Embryol* 1988;179:33–48.
6. Bishop GA, Ho RH. The distribution and origin of serotonin immunoreactivity in the rat cerebellum. *Brain Res* 1985;331:195–207.
7. Bishop GA, Ho RH, King JS. Localization of serotonin immunoreactivity in the opossum cerebellum. *J Comp Neurol* 1985;235:301–321.
8. Bishop GA, Ho RH, King JS. An immunohistochemical study of serotonin development in the opossum cerebellum. *Anat Embryol* 1985;17:325–338.
9. Bishop GA, Kerr CW, King JS, Chen YF. The serotoninergic system in the cat's cerebellum: origin, ultrastructural relationships and physiological effects. In: Trouillas P, Fuxe K, ed. *Serotonin, the cerebellum, and ataxia*. New York: Raven Press, 1993:91–112.
10. Bowker RM, Steinbusch HWM, Coulter JD. Serotonergic and peptidergic projections to the spinal cord demonstrated by a combined retrograde HRP histochemical and immunocytochemical staining method. *Brain Res* 1981;211:412–417.
11. Bowker RM, Westlund KN, Sullivan MD, Coulter JD. A combined retrograde transport and immunocytochemical staining method for demonstrating the origins of serotonergic projections. *J Histochem Cytochem* 1982;30:805–810.
12. Daval G, Verge D, Becerril A, Gozlan H, Spampinato U, Hamon M. Transient expression of 5-HT 1A receptor binding sites in some areas of the rat CNS during postnatal development. *Int J Dev Neurosci* 1987;5:171–180.
13. Descarries L, Beaudet A, Watkins KC. Serotonin nerve terminals in adult rat neocortex. *Brain Res* 1974;100:563–588.
14. Felten DL, Sladek JR. Monoamine distribution in primate brain. V. Monoaminergic nuclei: anatomy, pathways and local organization. *Brain Res Bull* 1983;10:171–284.
15. Fuxe K, Agnati LF. Two principal modes of electrochemical communication in the brain: volume versus wiring transmission. In: Fuxe K, Agnati LF, eds. *Volume transmission in the brain: novel mechanisms for neural transmission*. New York: Raven Press, 1991:1–9.
16. Jacobs BL, Gannon PJ, Azmitia EC. Atlas of serotonergic cell bodies in the cat brainstem: an immunocytochemical analysis. *Brain Res Bull* 1984;13:1–31.
17. Katz LC. Specificity in the development of vertical connections in cat striate cortex. *Eur J Neurosci* 1991;3:1–9.
18. Kerr CW, Bishop GA. Serotonin suppression of Purkinje cell activity through selective activation of the 5-HT 1A receptor. *Brain Res(in press)*.
19. Kerr CWH, Bishop GA. Topographical organization in the origin of serotoninergic projections to different regions of the cat cerebellar cortex. *J Comp Neurol* 1991;304:502–515.
20. King JS, Ho RH, Burry RW. The localization of serotonin in the opossum inferior olivary complex. *J Comp Neurol* 1984;227:357–368.
21. Lauder JM. Ontogeny of the serotonergic system in the rat: serotonin as a developmental signal. *Ann NY Acad Sci* 1990;600:297–314.
22. Lauder JM, Krebs H. Serotonin as a differentiation signal in early embryogenesis. *Dev Neurosci* 1978;1:15–30.
23. Lauder JM, Towle AC, Patrick K, Henderson P, Krebs H. Decreased serotonin content of embryonic raphe neurons following maternal administration of p-chlorophenylalanine: a quantitative immunocytochemical study. *Dev Brain Res* 1985;20:107–114.
24. Lauder JM, Wallace JA, Krebs H, Petrusz P, McCarthy K. In vivo and in vitro development of serotonergic neurons. *Brain Res Bull* 1983;9:605–625.
25. Laxson LC, King JS. The formation and growth of the cortical layers in the cerebellum of the opossum. *Anat Embryol* 1983;167:391–409.

26. Lidov HGW, Molliver ME. An immunohistochemical study of serotonin neuron development in the rat: ascending pathways and terminal fields. *Brain Res Bull* 1982;8:389–430.
27. Maekawa K, Simpson JI. Climbing fiber responses evoked in vestibulocerebellum of rabbit from visual system. *J Neurophysiol* 1973;36:649–666.
28. Maekawa K, Takeda T. Electrophysiological identification of the climbing and mossy fiber pathways from the rabbit's retina to the contralateral cerebellar flocculus. *Brain Res* 1976;109:169–174.
29. Martin G, Culberson J, Waxson C, Tinauts M, Panneton M, Tschismadia I. Afferent connections of the inferior olivary nucleus with preliminary notes on their development: studies using the North American opossum. In: Courville J, deMontigny C, Tamarre Y, eds. *The inferior olivary nucleus* 1980:35–72.
30. Martin G, DeLorenzo G, Ho R, Humbertson A, Waltzer R. Serotonergic innervation of the forebrain in the North American opossum. *Brain Behav Evol* 1985;26:196–228.
31. Martin GF, Ghooray G, Ho RH, Pindzola RR, Xu XM. The origin of serotoninergic projections to the lumbosacral spinal cord at different stages of development in the North American opossum. *Dev Brain Res* 1991;58:203–213.
32. O'Donoghue DL, Martin GF, King JS. The timing of granule cell differentiation and mossy fiber morphogenesis in the opossum. *Anat Embryol* 1987;175:341–354.
33. Palay SL. The morphology of synapses in the central nervous system. *Exp Cell Res* 1958;5(suppl):275–293.
34. Stephanini M, DeMartinio C, Zamboni L. Fixation of ejaculated spermatozoa for electron microscopy. *Nature* 1967;216:173–174.
35. Sternberger LA. *Immunocytochemistry*. New York: Wiley, 1979.
36. Ulinski PS. External morphology of pouch young opossum brains: a profile of opossum neurogenesis. *J Comp Neurol* 1971;142:33–58.
37. Walker JJ, Bishop GA, Ho RH, King JS. Brainstem origin of serotonin- and enkephalin immunoreactive afferents to the opossum's cerebellum. *J Comp Neurol* 1988;276:481–497.
38. Whitaker-Azmitia PM, Shemer AV, Caruso J, Molino L, Azmitia EC. Role of high affinity serotonin receptors in neuronal growth. *Ann NY Acad Sci* 1990;600:315–330.

*Serotonin, the Cerebellum,
and Ataxia*, edited by
P. Trouillas and K. Fuxe.
Raven Press, Ltd., New York © 1993.

11

Serotonergic Control of Glutamatergic Systems in the Cerebellum

Maurizio Raiteri, Guido Maura, Pierpaola Lottero, and Licia Gastaldo

*Istituto di Farmacologia e Farmacognosia, Università degli Studi di Genova,
16148 Genova, Italy*

Serotonergic afferents to the cerebellar cortex were identified by Hökfelt and Fuxe (10) by using the fluorescence technique. These 5-hydroxytryptamine (5-HT) projections reach the three layers of the cerebellar cortex (3,5). The 5-HT fibers originate from the raphe nuclei (4,21) as well as from other nuclei including some in the reticular formation (2).

Excitatory amino acids (EAAs), in particular glutamate (GLU) and/or aspartate (ASP), are the cerebellar neurotransmitters released from parallel fibers (20), climbing fibers (25), and mossy fibers (7,15).

5-HT and EAAs interact in rat cerebellum. In particular, 5–HT exerts a potent inhibitory control on the release of both GLU (15,16,19) and ASP (14). The inhibition of EAA release is brought about through activation of 5-HT receptors located on the EAA-releasing terminals. Activation of these presynaptic 5-HT receptors produces profound postsynaptic effects (18) and may have therapeutic relevance in the treatment of some human cerebellar syndromes.

INHIBITION OF EAA RELEASE BY 5-HT

Slices or synaptosomes from rat cerebellum depolarized, respectively, with 35 or 15 mM K^+ released endogenous GLU and ASP in a calcium-dependent manner. The release of both EAAs was inhibited by 5-HT (14–16,19). Figure 1 illustrates the concentration-dependent inhibition of the endogenous GLU release evoked by depolarization of rat cerebellar slices. It is noteworthy that the potency of 5-HT is unusually high ($EC_{50} = 0.4$ nM).

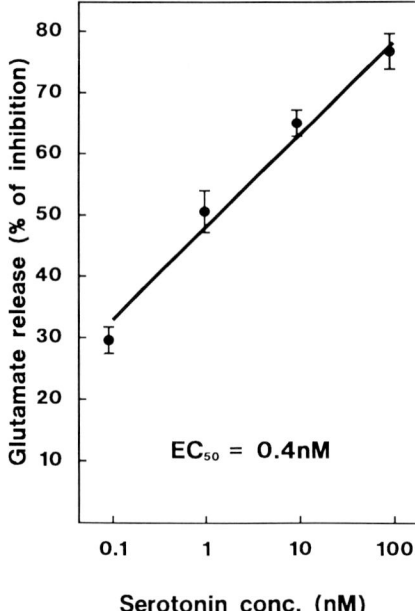

FIG. 1. Inhibition by 5-HT of the K^+-evoked release of endogenous GLU from rat cerebellar slices. Slices were prepared and superfused as described in Maura et al. (16). Depolarization was carried out with high K^+ (35 mM) at min 38 (S_1) and min 66 (S_2) of superfusion. 5-HT was added concomitantly with high K^+ (S_2). GLU was determined by high performance liquid chromatography with fluorescent detection following precolumn derivation with o-phthalaldehyde. Means ± SEM of four to six experiments in duplicate are shown.

HETEROGENEITY OF THE 5-HT RECEPTORS INVOLVED

Mammalian 5-HT receptors are highly heterogeneous and have been classified into four major types termed 5-HT_1-like, 5-HT_2, 5-HT_3, and 5-HT_4. Several subtypes of the 5-HT_1-like type have been proposed to exist: 5-HT_{1A}, 5-HT_{1B}, 5-HT_{1C}, 5-HT_{1D}, and 5-HT_1-like (24).

In cerebellar slices, the K^+-evoked release of GLU (16) and ASP (14) was inhibited by both 8-hydroxy-2-(di-n-propylamino)tetralin (8-OH-DPAT), a 5-HT_{1A} receptor agonist, and by 1-(2,5-dimethoxy-4-iodophenyl)-2-aminopropane (DOI), a 5-HT_2 receptor agonist. The effects of the two drugs on the release of endogenous GLU are illustrated in Fig. 2. Thus, the release of EAAs induced by depolarization of rat cerebellar slices can be inhibited through the activation of 5-HT receptors of both the 5-HT_1-like and 5-HT_2 types. The findings that the effects of 5-HT on GLU and ASP release were prevented in part by ketanserin (a 5-HT_2 receptor antagonist) and totally by methiothepin (a mixed $5\text{-HT}_1/5\text{-HT}_2$ receptor antagonist) confirm this view (14,16).

It is likely that the serotonergic receptors regulating EAA release play a physiological role inasmuch as ketanserin and, particularly, methiothepin increased on their own the K^+-evoked release of GLU (Fig. 3) and ASP (14).

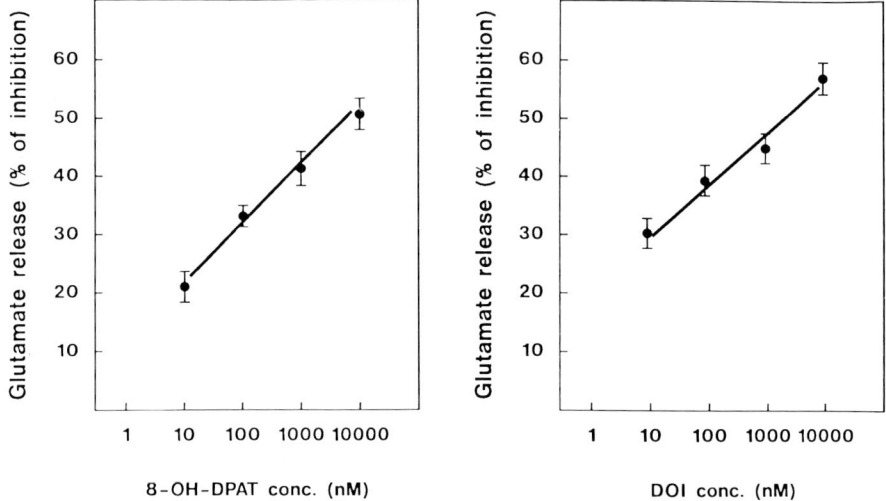

FIG. 2. Inhibition by 8-OH-DPAT or DOI of the K^+-evoked release of endogenous GLU from cerebellar slices. Experimental details as in the legend to Fig. 1. Data are means ± SEM of three to five experiments in duplicate.

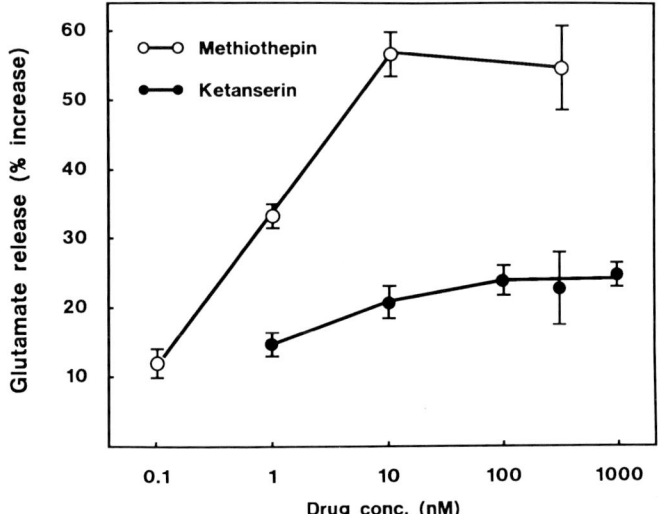

FIG. 3. Effects of methiothepin or ketanserin on the K^+-evoked release of endogenous GLU from cerebellar slices. The antagonists were added 8 min before high K^+ (S_2). Other experimental details as in the legend to Fig. 1. Means ± SEM of three to five experiments in duplicate are shown.

LOCALIZATION OF THE 5-HT RECEPTORS REGULATING GLU RELEASE

Studies with cerebellar synaptosomes showed that the 5-HT_1-like receptors are located on GLU-releasing axon terminals, while the receptors of the 5-HT_2 type are located on structures that do not survive the preparation of "standard" synaptosomes (16,19). The effect of varying concentrations of 5-HT on the K^+ (15 mM)-evoked release of endogenous GLU from cerebellar synaptosomes is shown in Fig. 4.

A detailed pharmacological analysis of the 5-HT_1 receptor located on "standard" glutamatergic synaptosomes (see Table 1) shows that, although the receptor is sensitive to the 5-HT_{1A} receptor agonist 8-OH-DPAT, it does not conform entirely to the criteria defining the 5-HT_{1A} binding site. Thus, it could represent an isoform of the 5-HT_{1A} subtype and be classified as a 5-HT_{1A}-like receptor.

Where are the 5-HT_2 receptors located? It is known that during homogenization of cerebellar tissue, two species of synaptosomes, respectively termed "standard" and "giant," are formed. Giant synaptosomes appear to originate from the endings of mossy fibers. They can be separated from standard synaptosomes due to differences in sedimentation characteristics and can be partly purified from the nuclear fraction of the cerebellar homogenate (9,11). Mossy fibers make excitatory synapses with granule cells (12). Immunochemical (22) and electrophysiological (7) studies suggest that GLU is a major mossy fiber transmitter in the cerebellum.

Depolarization of giant synaptosomes with high K^+ provoked release of endogenous GLU, which was highly calcium dependent (Table 2), in keeping with the idea that GLU is a mossy fiber transmitter.

Interestingly, 5-HT and DOI, but not 8-OH-DPAT, inhibited the K^+-evoked GLU release from giant synaptosomes (Fig. 5), suggesting the presence of 5-HT_2 receptors. This is confirmed by the finding that the 5-HT_2 receptor antagonist ketanserin blocked the 5-HT inhibition of GLU release (Fig. 6). Thus, the 5-HT_2 receptors mediating inhibition of GLU release in rat cerebellum appear to be located at least on some of the mossy fiber terminals synapsing onto the granule cells.

POSTSYNAPTIC CONSEQUENCES OF PRESYNAPTIC 5-HT RECEPTOR ACTIVATION

Changes of postsynaptic events consequent to manipulation of presynaptic receptors have rarely been described in the central nervous system. It is known that activation of postsynaptic EAA receptors in cerebellum can cause increase of cGMP levels (1,6,8,13). It was of interest to establish whether manipulation of the 5-HT receptors located on the EAA-releasing nerve terminals could affect the levels of cGMP produced when the postsynaptic EAA receptors are activated by endogenous EAAs released during depolarization.

In cerebellar slices, depolarization with 35 mM K^+ produced an increase of cGMP levels. This increase, similar to the release of GLU and ASP from the same

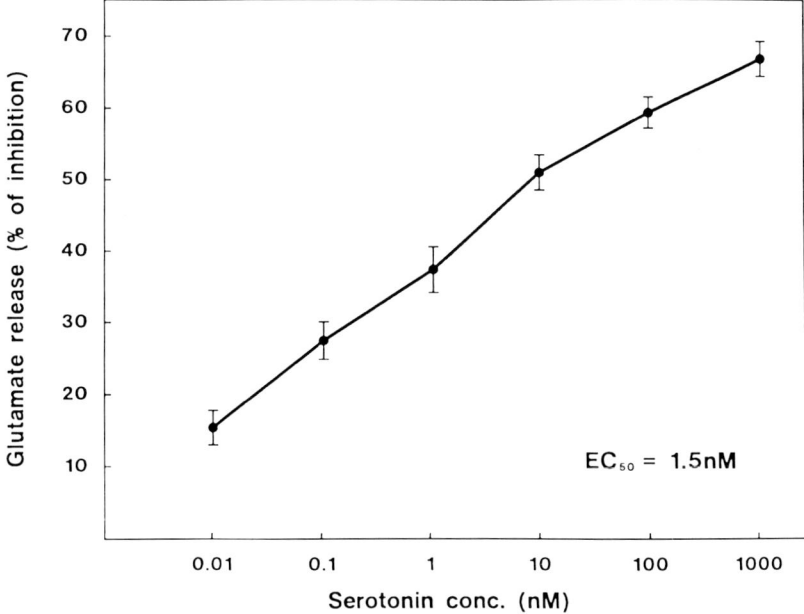

FIG. 4. Inhibition by 5-HT of endogenous GLU release evoked by 15 mM KCl from rat cerebellar standard synaptosomes. Synaptosomes were prepared and superfused as previously described (19). GLU was determined as indicated in the legend to Fig. 1. 5-HT was added concomitantly with high K^+. Means ± SEM of seven experiments in triplicate are presented.

preparation, was calcium dependent (18). The cGMP production due to K^+ depolarization was concentration dependently inhibited by D-(−)-2-amino-5-phosphonopentanoic acid (D-AP5) ($IC_{50} = 0.019$ μM; maximal inhibition 70%) (see Fig. 7), an antagonist at the EAA receptor of the N-methyl-D-aspartate (NMDA) type. The result indicates the involvement of NMDA receptors in the cGMP production by endogenous EAAs released during depolarization.

The cGMP response was potently inhibited by 5-HT, 8-OH-DPAT, and DOI (see

TABLE 1. *Pharmacological profile of the 5-HT receptor mediating inhibition of GLU release from cerebellar standard synaptosomes*

Agonists		
RU 24969	$5\text{-HT}_{1A/B/C}$	Active
8-OH-DPAT	5-HT_{1A}	Active
DOI	5-HT_2	Inactive
Antagonists		
Methiothepin	$5\text{-HT}_1/5\text{-HT}_2$	Active
Ketanserin	5-HT_2	Inactive
Methysergide	$5\text{-HT}_{1C/D}/5\text{-HT}_2$	Inactive
(−)Propranolol	$5\text{-HT}_{1A/B}$	Inactive
Spiperone	$5\text{-HT}_{1A}/5\text{-HT}_2$	Inactive
ICS 205-930	5-HT_3	Inactive

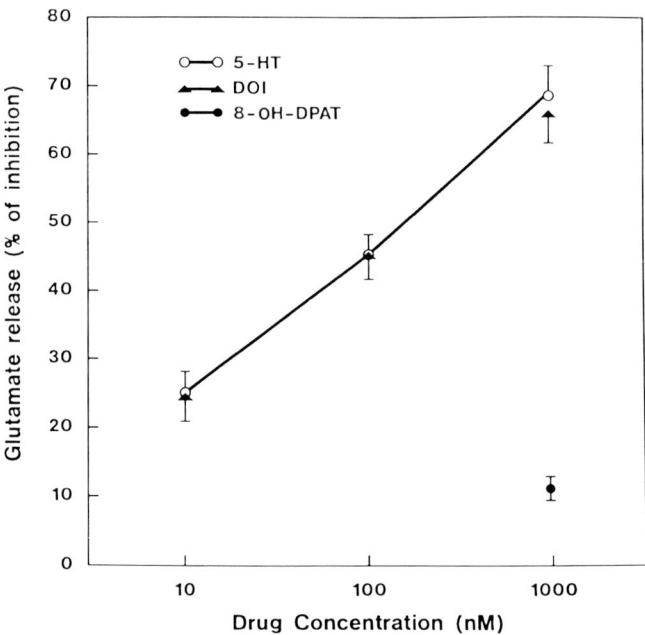

FIG. 5. Effects of 5-HT, DOI, and 8-OH-DPAT on the K^+-evoked release of endogenous GLU from cerebellar giant synaptosomes. Agonists were added concomitantly with high K^+. Other experimental details as in the footnote to Table 2. Means ± SEM of three to five experiments in duplicate are shown.

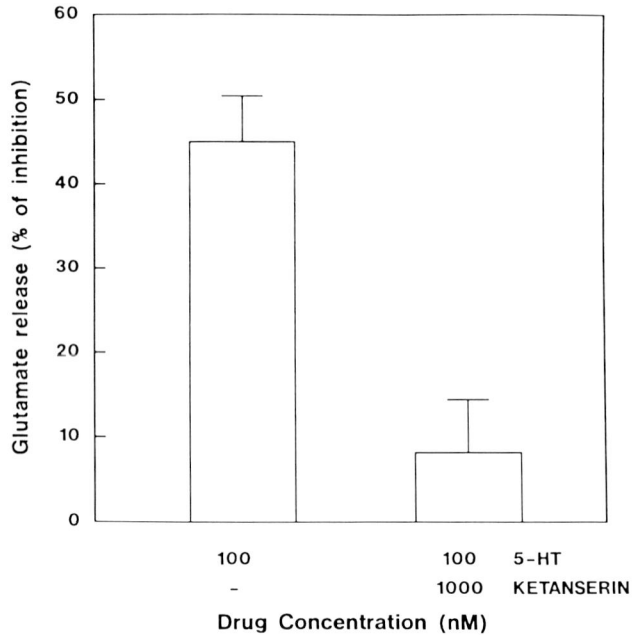

FIG. 6. Effects of ketanserin on the 5-HT inhibition of the K^+-evoked release of endogenous GLU from cerebellar giant synaptosomes. Ketanserin was added 8 min before high K^+ and 5-HT concomitantly with the depolarizing stimulus. Other experimental details as in the footnote to Table 2. Data are means ± SEM of three to five experiments in duplicate.

TABLE 2. *Depolarization-evoked release of endogenous GLU from cerebellar giant synaptosomes and its calcium dependence*

	Endogenous GLU (pmoles/mg protein)	
	Standard medium	Ca^{2+}-free medium
Basal release	216 ± 18.7	200 ± 20.8
K^+-evoked release	658 ± 52.3	301 ± 28.0

Giant synaptosomes were prepared from rat cerebellum as previously described (15) and superfused according to Raiteri et al. (17). Calcium ions were omitted 8 min before depolarization with 15 mM KCl. Basal release represents the total amount in the two 3-min fractions collected before and after the 6-min fraction corresponding to K^+ depolarization. GLU was determined as reported in the legend to Fig. 1. Means ± SEM of six to eight experiments in duplicate are presented.

Fig. 8) (18). The IC_{50} values amounted to about 1 nM. The effect of 8-OH-DPAT was antagonized by methiothepin, but not by ketanserin, whereas the effect of DOI was sensitive to both antagonists (Fig. 9). The data clearly suggest that activation of both presynaptic 5-HT_{1A}-like and 5-HT_2 receptors can potently inhibit the cGMP production stimulated postsynaptically when EAA receptors are activated.

Methiothepin or ketanserin, added alone to the depolarized cerebellar slices, produced a concentration-dependent increase of cGMP (see Fig. 10) (18), suggesting that both 5-HT_{1A}-like and 5-HT_2 receptors may be physiologically activated by the endogenous transmitter released during the depolarizing stimulus.

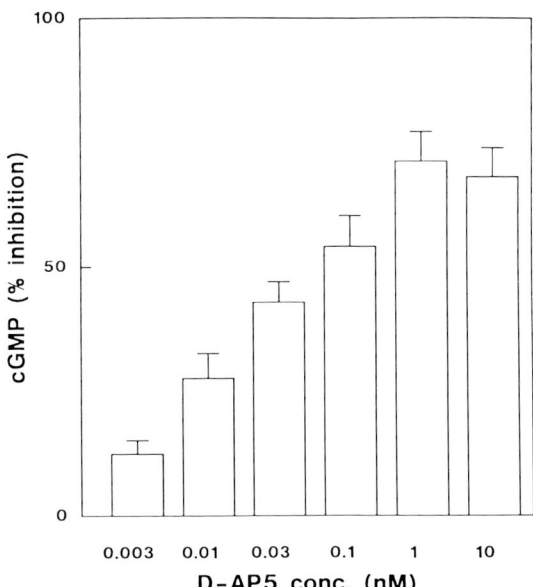

FIG. 7. Effect of D-AP5 on the cGMP response produced by 35 mM KCl in cerebellar slices. Slices were prepared and cGMP was determined by radioimmunoassay as described in Raiteri et al. (18). D-AP5 was added 15 min before depolarization. Means ± SEM of four to six experiments in duplicate are shown.

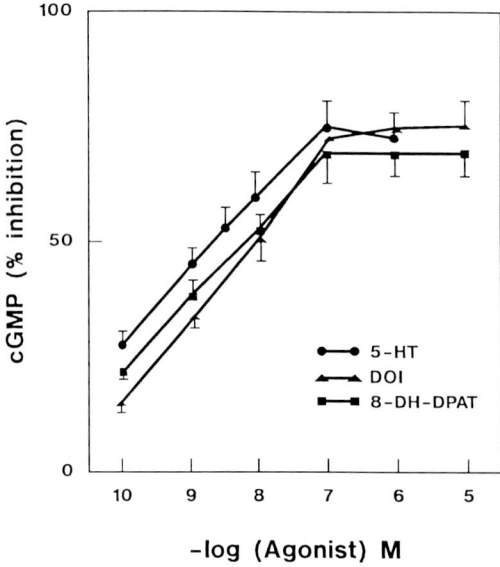

FIG. 8. Inhibition by 5-HT, 8-OH-DPAT, and DOI of the K^+-evoked cGMP response in cerebellar slices. Agonists were added concomitantly with high K^+. Other experimental details as in the legend to Fig. 7. Means + SEM of three to five duplicate experiments are shown.

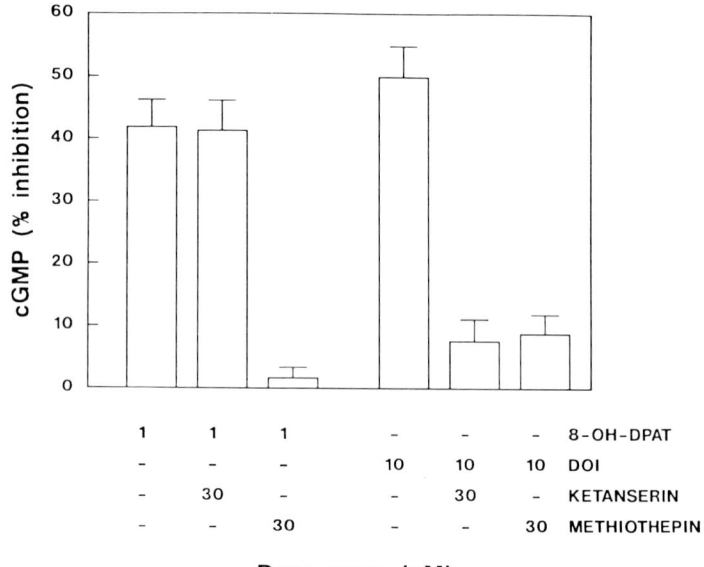

FIG. 9. Antagonism by ketanserin and methiothepin of the inhibition by 8-OH-DPAT and DOI of the cGMP response evoked by 35 mM KCl in cerebellar slices. Antagonists were added 15 min before depolarization; agonists concomitantly with high K^+. Other experimental details as in the legend to Fig. 7. Means ± SEM of three to five duplicate experiments are presented.

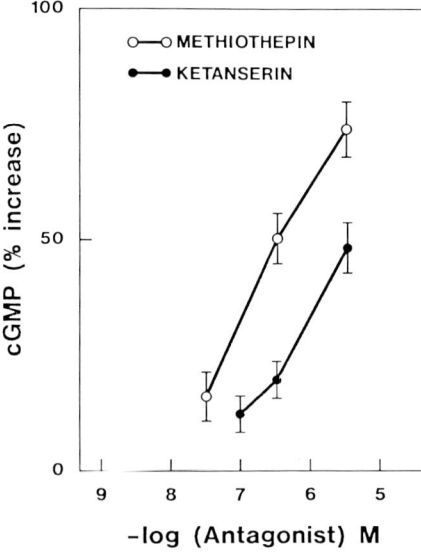

FIG. 10. Effects of methiothepin and ketanserin on the K^+-evoked cGMP response in cerebellar slices. The antagonists were added 15 min before high K^+. Other experimental details as in the legend to Fig. 7. Means ± SEM of three to five experiments in duplicate are presented.

It seemed of interest to ascertain whether the cGMP system linked to EAA receptor activation was sensitive to changes of 5-HT concentration induced in the biophase of the presynaptic 5-HT receptors by drugs that, for instance, release 5-HT or prevent its reuptake. Figure 11 illustrates the inhibition of cGMP levels caused by citalopram (a 5-HT uptake blocker) and the anorectic agent (+)fenfluramine (a 5-HT releaser). Indirect activation of the presynaptic 5-HT receptors can therefore lead to inhibition of EAA release and the consequent cGMP production.

CONCLUDING REMARKS

Our studies of the interaction between 5-HT and EAA transmitters in rat cerebellum allow us to draw the following conclusions (see Fig. 12):

1. *Nanomolar* concentrations of 5-HT can inhibit the depolarization-evoked release of endogenous GLU and ASP.
2. The inhibition of EAA release occurs through activation of presynaptic receptors of the 5-HT_{1A}-like subtype and the 5-HT_2 type located, respectively, on the axon terminals of parallel/climbing fibers and mossy fibers.
3. Both 5-HT_{1A}-like and 5-HT_2 receptors may be activated physiologically by the endogenous indoleamine released during depolarization.
4. Activation of both 5-HT_{1A}-like and 5-HT_2 receptors can inhibit the production of cGMP occurring postsynaptically when EAA receptors (largely of the NMDA type) are activated by EAAs released during depolarization.

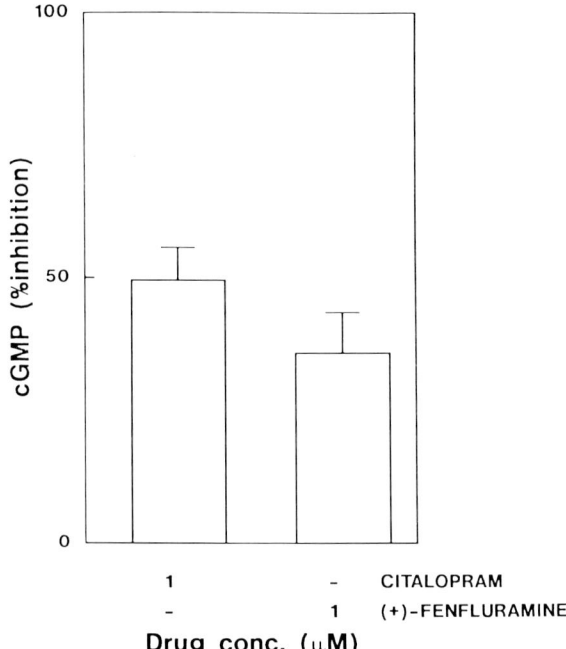

FIG. 11. Effects of citalopram or (+)fenfluramine on the K^+-evoked cGMP response in cerebellar slices. The compounds were added 15 min before depolarization. Other experimental details as in the legend to Fig. 7. Means ± SEM of four to five experiments in duplicate are shown.

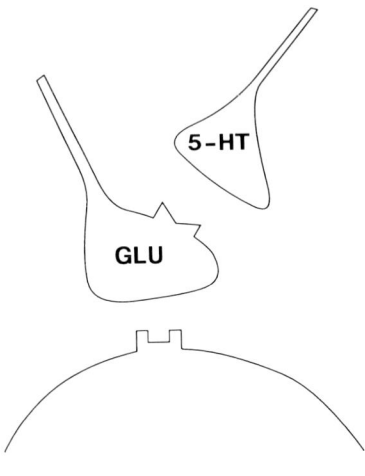

FIG. 12. Hypothetical neuronal connections underlying the serotonergic control of GLU transmission in rat cerebellum. The scheme represents a 5-HT terminal causing presynaptic inhibition (through the activation of $5-HT_{1A}$-like receptors in the case of parallel and/or climbing fibers and of $5-HT_2$ receptors in the case of mossy fibers) of GLU release onto NMDA receptors coupled to cGMP production in a postsynaptic cell.

5. Drugs selective for the 5-HT$_{1A}$-like (8-OH-DPAT or the novel anxiolytics of the 5-HT$_{1A}$ receptor agonist group) or the 5-HT$_2$ (DOI) receptor or that can increase the 5-HT concentration in the receptor biophase (e.g., the antidepressants acting as 5-HT uptake inhibitors such as citalopram, fluoxetine, or (+)fenfluramine) can decrease EAA release and cGMP production.
6. Like 5-OH-tryptophan, the 5-HT precursor that has been reported to be beneficial in some human cerebellar ataxias (23), some of the above drugs may be useful in the treatment of these syndromes.

ACKNOWLEDGMENTS

Supported by grants from the Italian M.U.R.S.T. (40% and 60%) and the Italian C.N.R. (Target Projects "Biotechnology and Bioinstrumentation" and "Chimica Fine II"). The authors wish to thank Mrs. Maura Agate for her assistance in the preparation of the manuscript.

REFERENCES

1. Biggio G, Guidotti A. Climbing fibers activation and 3'-5'-cyclic guanosine monophosphate (cGMP) content in cortex and deep nuclei of cerebellum. *Brain Res* 1976;107:365–373.
2. Bishop GA, Ho RH. The distribution and origin of serotonin immunoreactivity in the rat cerebellum. *Brain Res* 1985;331:195–207.
3. Bobillier P, Seguin S, Petitjean F, Salvert D, Touret M, Jouvet M. The raphe nuclei of the cat brain stem: a topographical atlas of their efferent projections as revealed by autoradiography. *Brain Res* 1976;113:449–486.
4. Chan Palay V. The indoleamine afferent axons to the cerebellum. In: *Cerebellar dentate nucleus: organization, cytology and transmitters.* New York: Springer-Verlag, 1977:390–454.
5. Chan-Palay V. Fine structure of labelled axons in the cerebellar cortex and nuclei of rodents and primates after intraventricular infusions with tritiated serotonin. *Anat Embryol* 1975;148:235–265.
6. Ferrendelli JA, Chang MM, Kinscherf DA. Elevation of cyclic GMP levels in central nervous system by excitatory and inhibitory amino acids. *J Neurochem* 1974;22:535–540.
7. Garthwaite J, Brodbelt AR. Glutamate as the principal mossy fibre transmitter in rat cerebellum: pharmacological evidence. *Eur J Neurosci* 1990;2:177–180.
8. Garthwaite J. Excitatory amino acid receptors and guanosine 3'-5'-cyclic monophosphate in incubated slices of immature and adult rat cerebellum. *Neuroscience* 1982;7:2491–2497.
9. Hajós F, Wilkin G, Wilson J, Balazs R. A rapid procedure for obtaining a preparation of large fragments of the cerebellar glomeruli in high purity. *J Neurochem* 1975;24:1277–1278.
10. Hökfelt T, Fuxe K. Cerebellar monoamine nerve terminals, a new type of afferent fibers to the cortex cerebelli. *Exp Brain Res* 1969;9:63–72.
11. Israel H, Whittaker VP. The isolation of mossy fibre endings from the granular layer of the cerebellar cortex. *Experientia* 1965;21:325–326.
12. Ito M. *The cerebellum and neural control.* New York: Raven Press, 1984.
13. Mao CC, Guidotti A, Costa E. The regulation of cyclic guanosine monophosphate in rat cerebellum: possible involvement of putative amino acid neurotransmitters. *Brain Res* 1974;79:510–514.
14. Maura G, Barzizza A, Folghera S, Raiteri M. Release of endogenous aspartate from rat cerebellum slices and synaptosomes: inhibition mediated by a 5-HT$_2$ receptor and by a 5-HT$_1$ receptors of a possibly novel subtype. *Naunyn Schmiedebergs Arch Pharmacol* 1991;343:229–236.
15. Maura G, Carbone R, Guido M, Pestarino M, Raiteri M. 5-HT$_2$ presynaptic receptors mediate inhibition of glutamate release from cerebellar mossy fibre terminals. *Eur J Pharmacol* 1991;202:185–190.
16. Maura G, Roccatagliata E, Ulivi M, Raiteri M. Serotonin-glutamate interaction in rat cerebellum: involvement of 5-HT$_1$ and 5-HT$_2$ receptors. *Eur J Pharmacol* 1988;145:31–38.

17. Raiteri M, Angelini F, Levi G. A simple apparatus for studying the release of neurotransmitters from synaptosomes. *Eur J Pharmacol* 1974;25:411–414.
18. Raiteri M, Maura G, Barzizza A. Activation of presynaptic 5-hydroxytryptamine$_1$-like receptors on glutamatergic terminals inhibits N-methyl-D-aspartate-induced cyclic GMP production in rat cerebellar slices. *J Pharmacol Exp Ther* 1991;257:1184–1188.
19. Raiteri M, Maura G, Bonanno G, Pittaluga A. Differential pharmacology and function of two 5-HT$_1$ receptors modulating transmitter release in rat cerebellum. *J Pharmacol Exp Ther* 1986;237:644–648.
20. Sandoval ME, Cotman CW. Evaluation of glutamate as a neurotransmitter of cerebellar parallel fibers. *Neuroscience* 1978;3:199–206.
21. Shinnar S, Maciewicz RJ, Shofer RJ. A raphe projection to cat cerebellar cortex. *Brain Res* 1975;97:139–143.
22. Somogyi P, Halasy K, Somogyi J, Storm-Mathisen J, Ottersen OP. Quantification of immunogold labelling reveals enrichment of glutamate in mossy and parallel fibre terminals in cat cerebellum. *Neuroscience* 1986;19:1045–1050.
23. Trouillas P, Brudon F, Adeleine P. Improvement of cerebellar ataxia with levorotatory form of 5-hydroxytryptophan. A double-blind study with quantified data processing. *Arch Neurol* 1988;5:1217–1222.
24. Watson S, Abbott A. Receptor nomenclature supplement. *Trends Pharmacol Sci* 1991(suppl):17.
25. Wiklund L, Toggenburger G, Cuenod M. Aspartate: possible neurotransmitter in cerebellar climbing fibers. *Science* 1982;216:78–80.

*Serotonin, the Cerebellum,
and Ataxia*, edited by
P. Trouillas and K. Fuxe.
Raven Press Ltd., New York © 1993.

12

Visualization of 5-HT Receptors in the Cerebellum and Related Brain Stem Areas

*†J. M. Palacios, ‡M. Pompeiano, §O. Pompeiano, and †G. Mengod

*Research Institute, Laboratorios Almirall, 08024 Barcelona, Spain;
†Department of Neurochemistry, Centro Investigación y Desarrollo, Consejo Superior Investigaciones Científicas, 08034 Barcelona, Spain;
‡Institute of Biological Chemistry, University of Pisa, I-56100 Pisa, Italy;
§Department of Physiology and Biochemistry, University of Pisa, I-56127 Pisa, Italy

The cerebellar cortex receives afferent projections that terminate on the Purkinje (P) cells either directly as climbing fibers (CF) or indirectly (through granular cells) as mossy fibers (MF) (see ref. 8 for references). In addition to these systems that utilize excitatory amino acids as neurotransmitters, there are other afferent projections, which are of different neurochemical specificity. One of these systems is represented by serotoninergic fibers that originate from the raphe complex (and other structures) and project to the different cerebellar lobules and layers, as shown in several animal species, including the rat (4,5,18).

While the presynaptic component of the serotoninergic synapses in the cerebellar cortex is relatively well documented, less is known about the distribution of the corresponding receptors in the mammalian cerebellum.

Serotonin (5-HT) receptors have been pharmacologically divided in four classes: 5-HT_1, 5-HT_2, 5-HT_3, and 5-HT_4 (25). The 5-HT_4 subtype, described originally in the periphery, has been biochemically and electrophysiologically characterized in the brain (12,13), but at present there are no ligands available that permit the visualization of this receptor. The 5-HT_1 receptor class includes three principal subtypes in the rat: the 5-HT_{1A}, 5-HT_{1B}, and 5-HT_{1C}. The 5-HT_{1C} receptor should be more properly classified into the 5-HT_2 class because of structural, biochemical, and pharmacological reasons (27). Recently, a new receptor subtype has been reported in the rat, the 5-HT_{1D}-like (3). With the exception of the 5-HT_3 subtype, they all belong to the G protein-coupled receptor family (11) and are thought to modulate channel activity indirectly through G proteins (see ref. 6 for a review). The 5-HT_3 receptors, on the contrary, directly gate a cation channel (10).

To understand the role that the serotoninergic system plays in cerebellar functions, we decided to study the distribution of various subtypes of 5-HT receptors not only in the different corticonuclear areas of the cerebellum, but also in the main precerebellar nuclei as well as in the most relevant target regions of the efferent cerebellar systems.

METHODOLOGY FOR RECEPTOR VISUALIZATION

To date, three main methodologies have been used to visualize receptors at the microscopic level: receptor autoradiography, receptor immunohistochemistry, and *in situ* hybridization histochemistry (ISHH) of receptor mRNA. In the present study, we have combined receptor autoradiography and ISHH to visualize the distribution of 5-HT receptor subtypes and the cells expressing these receptors in the previously mentioned regions of the rat brain.

The results reported here were obtained in tissues from Wistar rats (male, 200–300 g, BRL). The animals were killed by decapitation, and the brains were quickly removed, frozen in dry ice, and stored at $-70°C$ until sectioned. Sections (20 μm thick) were cut with a microtome cryostat (Leitz 1720), thaw-mounted on gelatinized slides, and kept at $-20°C$ until used.

The existence of selectively labeled ligands has allowed the use of receptor autoradiographic techniques for the visualization of the different 5-HT receptor subtypes in the rat brain (24). The conditions for the selective labeling of 5-HT receptors with these ligands were as previously established (see ref. 23 for references). Briefly, 5-HT_{1A} receptors have been visualized using [^{3}H]8-hydroxy-2-(di-n-propylamino)tetralin (8-OH-DPAT). 5-HT_{1B} receptors have been selectively labeled with [^{125}I]iodocyanopindolol in the presence of 3 μM isoproterenol and 100 nM 8-OH-DPAT to block binding to β-adrenergic and 5-HT_{1A} receptors, respectively. For labeling 5-HT_{1C} and 5-HT_2 receptors, we used [^{125}I]1-(2,5-dimethoxy-4-iodophenyl)-2-aminopropane ([^{125}I]DOI) in the presence of spiperone or 5-HT, respectively. 5-HT_{1C} receptors were also labeled with [^{3}H]mesulergine in the presence of 100 nM spiperone and 5-HT_2 receptors with the more specific ligand [^{3}H]ketanserin. (S)-[^{3}H]zacopride was used to visualize 5-HT_3 receptors. The density of 5-HT terminals was indirectly visualized by using [^{3}H]citalopram, a ligand that binds to 5-HT uptake sites (9).

The recent molecular cloning of many 5-HT receptor subtypes has allowed the application of ISHH to study the expression of these 5-HT receptors in the rat brain. In fact, this technique takes advantage of the possibility of generating molecular probes (such as cDNA, RNA, or oligonucleotides) complementary to selected regions of a mRNA that will hybridize in intact tissue sections to this mRNA. By labeling the probes, for example, radioactively, it is possible to visualize the cells containing the mRNA of interest, in particular the mRNA coding for a receptor protein.

The first 5-HT receptors to be cloned were the rat 5-HT_{1C} (17) and 5-HT_2 (27) subtypes. Later, both human and rat 5-HT_{1A} receptors were cloned (1,14). Recently, the cloning of two new receptors has been reported, the 5-HT_{1B} (20,30) and the 5-HT_{1D}-like (3). A human 5-HT_{1D} receptor was also cloned (7). Finally, the cloning of a 5-HT_3 receptor gene has been reported (19).

In the present study, we visualized cells in the rat brain expressing 5-HT_{1A}, 5-HT_{1C}, or 5-HT_2 receptors. We used synthetic oligodeoxyribonucleotides: they were 48 base long and chosen for their lack of homology with published sequence of other G protein-coupled receptor genes. They were complementary to the base sequences encoding either the amino- or the carboxy-terminal portions or the third cytoplasmic loop of the receptor proteins. The oligonucleotides were synthesized, purified, and finally labeled at their 3'-end by using $[\alpha^{32}P]dATP$, as already described (21). The hybridization conditions were as previously assessed (22,26; Pompeiano et al., *in preparation*).

In preliminary experiments we also used oligonucleotides derived from the rat 5-HT_{1B} (30) and 5-HT_{1D} (Bach et al., *in preparation*) receptor genes to study the distribution of neurons expressing these 5-HT receptor subtypes.

DISTRIBUTION OF 5-HT RECEPTORS IN THE CEREBELLUM AND RELATED AREAS

The cerebellar cortex receives afferent projections from different precerebellar structures that convey information from different brain areas ranging from the cerebral cortex to the spinal cord. While MF originate from several relay stations such as the pontine nuclei, precerebellar reticulotegmental nucleus (nucleus reticularis tegmenti pontis), lateral and paramedian reticular nuclei, vestibular nuclei, and dorsal column (gracile and cuneate) nuclei, CF originate exclusively from the inferior olive (8,15). Concerning the efferent projections from the cerebellum, only some of the P cell axons project directly to the vestibular nuclei, while the majority of them terminates in the cerebellar nuclei. These nuclei are divided into the medial (fastigial), intermediate (interpositus), and lateral (dentate) nuclei. On the other hand, these nuclei convey cerebellar signals to the cerebral cortex, spinal cord, and other structures by utilizing interposed areas such as some thalamic nuclei (ventroanterior, ventrolateral, and ventroposterolateral nuclei), red nucleus, vestibular nuclei, and different nuclei of the main reticular formation.

The distribution of the different subtypes of 5-HT receptors in these structures is summarized in Table 1. While 5-HT_{1A}, 5-HT_{1B}, 5-HT_{1C}, and 5-HT_2 receptors were differently distributed, we could not detect 5-HT_3 receptors in any of the analyzed regions. Because of the lack of very selective ligands, it may be difficult to map in detail 5-HT_{1C} and 5-HT_2 receptors. For this reason data from ISHH study are partic-

TABLE 1. *Distribution of different 5-HT receptor subtypes in the cerebellum and related areas in the rat*

Brain regions	5-HT receptor subtypes			
	$5\text{-}HT_{1A}$	$5\text{-}HT_{1B}$	$5\text{-}HT_{1C}$	$5\text{-}HT_2$
Cerebellum				
CbCx	−	+	−	−
CbN	−	+ + +	+ +	−
Precerebellar nuclei (MF)				
Pn	−	+ +	−	+ + +
RtTg	−	+	−	+ + +
PMn	−	−	−	−
LRt	+	−	−	+ +
DCN	+	−	+	+ +
Precerebellar nuclei (CF)				
IO	−	+ +	−	+ +
Vestibular nuclei	+	+ +	+ +	+
Red nucleus	−	+	−	+ + +
Thalamic nuclei	−	−	−	−
Reticular formation nuclei				
DpMe	+	+	+ +	−
PRF	−	−	+ +	−
Gi	+	+	+ +	+ +
PCRt	−	+	+ +	+
MdRF	−	+	+ +	+
PGi	+	−	−	−

Data are expressed in semiquantitative measures.

CbCx, cerebellar cortex; CbN, cerebellar nuclei; DCN, dorsal column nuclei; DpMe, deep mesencephalic nucleus; Gi, gigantocellular reticular nucleus; IO, inferior olive; LRt, lateral reticular nucleus; MdRF, medullary reticular formation (reticular nucleus of the medulla, dorsal and ventral parts); PGi, paragigantocellular reticular nucleus; PCRt, parvocellular reticular nucleus; PMn, paramedian reticular nucleus; Pn, pontine nuclei; PRF, pontine reticular formation (pontine reticular nucleus, oral and caudal parts); RtTg, reticulotegmental nucleus of the pons.

ularly useful. As to the $5\text{-}HT_{1A}$ receptor subtype, the distribution of the message was in perfect accord with that of the binding sites in the examined regions.

In the cerebellar cortex, the concentration of 5-HT uptake sites was very low (Figs. 1A and 2A) except in lobules VIII–X of the vermis where it was higher (Fig. 1A). These sites were mainly present in the granular and P cell layers. The only receptor observed was the $5\text{-}HT_{1B}$ (Figs. 1B and 2B), which was present at low concentration in the molecular layer. There were no regional differences in the distribution of this receptor subtype, which was thus found to be homogeneously distributed in the medial (vermis), intermediate, and lateral parts of the cerebellar cortex, including the flocculus. $5\text{-}HT_{1B}$ receptor message was also quite abundant in the P cell layer, while $5\text{-}HT_{1D}$ receptor mRNA was not significantly present in the cerebellar cortex. In the cerebellar nuclei, [^{3}H]citalopram binding sites were present at intermediate density, except in the lateral nucleus, where the density was higher (Fig. 2A). These nuclei were rich in $5\text{-}HT_{1B}$ receptors (Fig. 2B), particularly in the lateral nucleus, and they also presented high levels of $5\text{-}HT_{1C}$ receptor transcript (Fig. 2C).

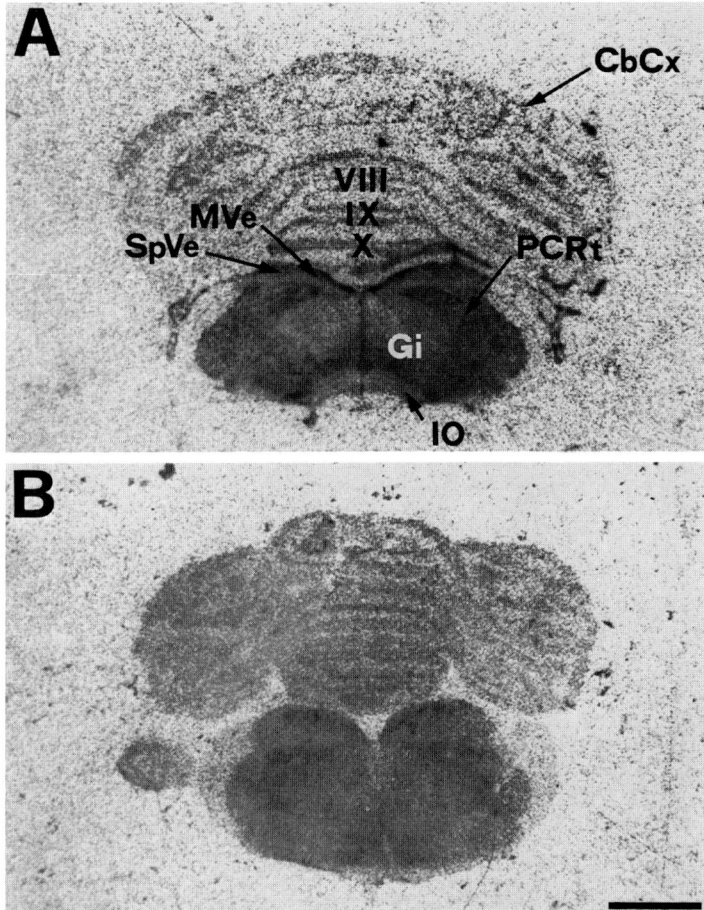

FIG. 1. Autoradiograms generated by incubating rat brain sections with either [^{3}H]citalopram (**A**) or [^{125}I]iodocyanopindolol (**B**) to label 5-HT uptake sites and 5-HT$_{1B}$ receptors, respectively. CbCx, cerebellar cortex; Gi, gigantocellular reticular nucleus; IO, inferior olive; MVe, medial vestibular nucleus; PCRt, parvocellular reticular nucleus; SpVe, spinal vestibular nucleus; VIII–X, lobules VIII–X of the cerebellar vermis. Scale bar is 2 mm.

Among the precerebellar areas, the nuclei sending MF to the cerebellar cortex appeared enriched with 5-HT$_2$ receptors. The pontine nuclei (Fig. 3B) and the reticulotegmental nucleus showed high levels, while the lateral reticular (Fig. 3D) and cuneate nuclei presented intermediate levels of 5-HT$_2$ receptor message. In addition, the pontine nuclei and the reticulotegmental nucleus presented intermediate levels of 5-HT$_{1B}$ receptors and the lateral reticular nucleus showed 5-HT$_{1A}$ receptors, although at low concentration. The dorsal column nuclei presented low levels of 5-HT$_{1A}$ receptors in both nuclei and very low levels of 5-HT$_{1C}$ receptors only in the gracile nucleus. All these structures presented intermediate levels of 5-HT up-

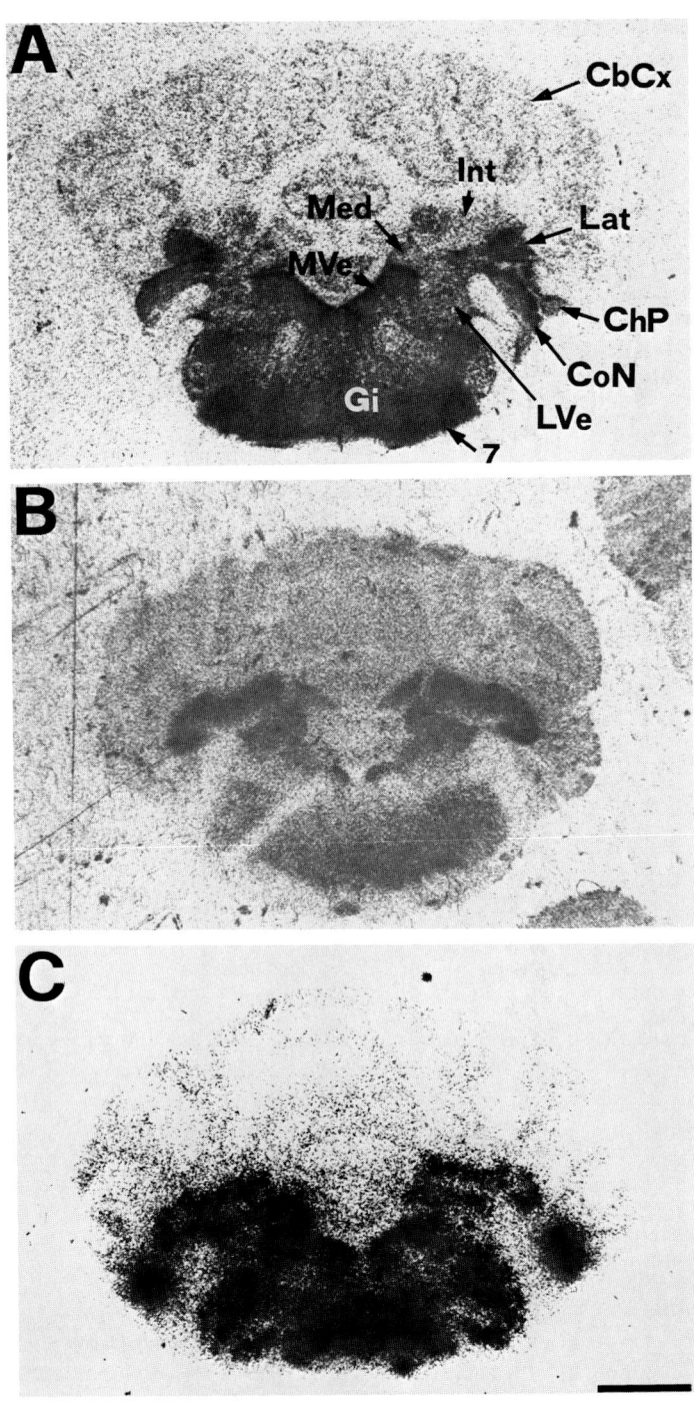

take sites. We could not detect any 5-HT receptor subtype in the paramedian reticular nucleus, which accordingly was not labeled by [^{3}H]citalopram. Another precerebellar region, the inferior olive, sending CF to the cerebellar cortex, showed an intermediate-to-low density of 5-HT uptake sites (Fig. 1A) and intermediate levels of both 5-HT$_{1B}$ receptors (Fig. 1B) and 5-HT$_2$ receptor transcript (Fig. 3D).

Among the structures that receive efferent projections from the cerebellar nuclei, there are some thalamic nuclei (see above), the red nucleus, and the vestibular nuclei. These projections originate from the fastigial, interpositus, and dentate nuclei, respectively (8,15). We could not detect any 5-HT receptor subtype in the thalamic nuclei, which were also devoid of 5-HT uptake sites. The red nucleus presented a high density of 5-HT uptake sites and, in addition, high levels of 5-HT$_2$ receptors and low levels of 5-HT$_{1B}$ receptors. The vestibular nuclei showed intermediate levels of [^{3}H]citalopram binding sites (Figs. 1A and 2A). They presented all four subtypes of 5-HT receptors, but were particularly rich in 5-HT$_{1B}$ (Figs. 1B and 2B) and 5-HT$_{1C}$ (Fig. 2C) subtypes. 5-HT$_{1A}$ receptors were seen only in the superior nucleus.

In addition to the nuclei reported above, which receive specific efferent projections from the cerebellar nuclei, we also investigated the distribution of the different 5-HT receptor subtypes in the main reticular formation, namely, in those reticular areas that do not project to the cerebellar cortex, but rather contribute with their efferent fibers to ascending projections to thalamic nuclei as well as to descending projections to the spinal cord. These reticular structures are mainly under the control of cortical descending and spinal ascending pathways, but they may also receive efferent projections from the cerebellar nuclei. The structures contributing to the main reticular formation include the deep mesencephalic nucleus, pontine and medullary reticular formation, and gigantocellular and parvocellular reticular areas. They showed intermediate levels of 5-HT uptake sites. In all these reticular structures we observed an enrichment of 5-HT$_{1C}$ receptor message, which was present at intermediate density (Figs. 2C and 3A and C). In addition, the deep mesencephalic nucleus showed low levels of 5-HT$_{1A}$ and 5-HT$_{1B}$ sites, and the gigantocellular nucleus showed intermediate levels of 5-HT$_2$ receptor transcript and low levels of 5-HT$_{1A}$ and 5-HT$_{1B}$ (Figs. 1B and 2B) sites. The parvocellular reticular nucleus and the medullary reticular formation also presented low levels of 5-HT$_{1B}$ receptors and 5-HT$_2$ receptor mRNA (Fig. 3D).

←

FIG. 2. Autoradiograms generated by incubating rat brain sections with either radioligands or ^{32}P-labeled oligonucleotide probes. Section in **A** has been incubated with [^{3}H]citalopram to label 5-HT uptake sites. **B:** consecutive section incubated with [^{125}I]iodocyanopindolol to label 5-HT$_{1B}$ receptors. **C:** Section hybridized with an oligonucleotide complementary to 5-HT$_{1C}$ receptor mRNA to visualize the neurons expressing this 5-HT receptor subtype. CbCx, cerebellar cortex; ChP, choroid plexus; CoN, cochlear nuclei; Gi, gigantocellular reticular nucleus; Int, intermediate cerebellar nucleus; Lat, lateral cerebellar nucleus; LVe, lateral vestibular nucleus; Med, medial cerebellar nucleus; MVe, medial vestibular nucleus; 7, facial nucleus. Scale bar is 2 mm.

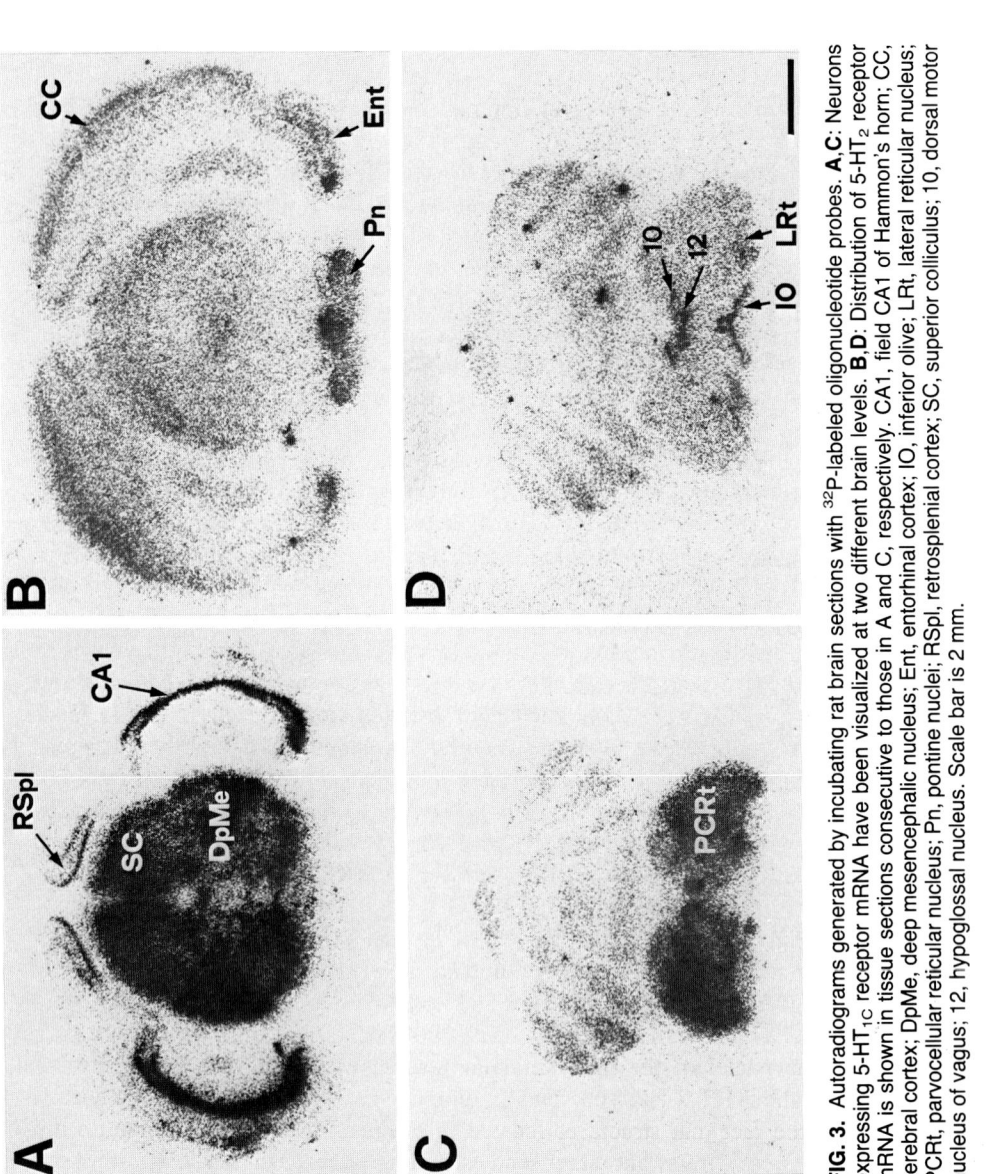

FIG. 3. Autoradiograms generated by incubating rat brain sections with ^{32}P-labeled oligonucleotide probes. **A,C:** Neurons expressing 5-HT$_{1C}$ receptor mRNA have been visualized at two different brain levels. **B,D:** Distribution of 5-HT$_2$ receptor mRNA is shown in tissue sections consecutive to those in A and C, respectively. CA1, field CA1 of Hammon's horn; CC, cerebral cortex; DpMe, deep mesencephalic nucleus; Ent, entorhinal cortex; IO, inferior olive; LRt, lateral reticular nucleus; PCRt, parvocellular reticular nucleus; Pn, pontine nuclei; RSpl, retrosplenial cortex; SC, superior colliculus; 10, dorsal motor nucleus of vagus; 12, hypoglossal nucleus. Scale bar is 2 mm.

In contrast with these findings, the paragigantocellular nucleus presented only a very low density of [^{3}H]citalopram binding sites and 5-HT receptors, which were of the 5-HT$_{1A}$ subtype.

CONCLUSIONS

It is known that the serotoninergic neurons located mainly in the raphe complex send efferent projections to most of the brain regions, although with varying densities (28).

Previous observations made on the cerebellar cortex have shown that the highest density of 5-HT axons is present in the granular cell layer, particularly in the vermal lobules VIII–X. However, only few synaptic contacts were identified in electron microscopic studies (see ref. 29 for a review). In agreement with these findings we observed low levels of 5-HT uptake sites labeled with [^{3}H]citalopram in the cerebellar cortex. Moreover, these sites were more abundant in the posterior vermis and were mainly present in the granular cell layer. The only 5-HT receptor subtype that could be detected in this region was the 5-HT$_{1B}$; the binding sites were observed in the molecular layer, while the corresponding mRNA was seen in the P cell layer. These data then suggest that 5-HT$_{1B}$ receptors are mainly expressed on the dendrites of the P cells. Further experiments are required, however, to identify the 5-HT receptor subtype that should be present in the granular cell layer, where the majority of 5-HT terminals are located.

In the cerebellar nuclei, there was complete agreement between 5-HT uptake sites and receptors, which were both present in all the nuclear regions, although more abundant in the lateral nucleus. At this level 5-HT$_{1B}$ and 5-HT$_{1C}$ reached an intermediate-to-high density. It is worth mentioning that similar distribution was observed in the vestibular nuclei, where in fact the predominant 5-HT receptors were the 5-HT$_{1B}$ and 5-HT$_{1C}$ subtypes. This finding is of interest in view of the close ontogenetic and phylogenetic relations between the cerebellar and the vestibular nuclei (16).

The precerebellar nuclei, sending either MF or CF, represent areas not particularly rich in 5-HT terminals (28) and uptake sites. Interestingly, the predominant 5-HT receptor found in all these areas was of the 5-HT$_2$ subtype, which was absent in the cerebellar cortex. In contrast to the results obtained in the precerebellar reticular areas, the nuclei of the main reticular formation showed a predominance of receptors of the 5-HT$_{1C}$ subtype. This finding can be of some functional relevance in view of the fact that structures located in the main reticular formation do not project to the cerebellum, but rather send ascending fibers to the cerebral cortex and descending fibers to the spinal cord (see ref. 8 for ref.).

A final comment concerns the paragigantocellular nucleus, which in the rat has been found to project direct excitatory afferents to the ipsilateral locus coeruleus complex (LC) (2). The paragigantocellular nucleus showed only very low levels of 5-HT$_{1A}$ receptors. This finding should be compared with the fact that the LC, which contains noradrenergic neurons, receives serotoninergic input (28,29) and expresses 5-HT$_{1C}$, 5-HT$_2$ (Pompeiano et al., *in preparation*), and 5-HT$_{1D}$ receptors (J. M. Palacios, *unpublished observations*). It appears, therefore, that the serotoninergic control of the noradrenergic system does not occur at the level of its main source of excitation, but rather at the level of the LC itself.

REFERENCES

1. Albert P, Zhou QY, Van Tol HHM, Bunzow JR, Civelli O. Cloning, functional expression and mRNA tissue distribution of the rat 5-hydroxytryptamine$_{1A}$ receptor gene. *J Biol Chem* 1990;265: 5825–5832.
2. Aston-Jones G, Shipley MT, Chouvet G, et al. Afferent regulation of locus coeruleus neurons: anatomy, physiology and pharmacology. In: Barnes CD, Pompeiano O, eds. *Neurobiology of the locus coeruleus (Progress in brain research*, vol 88). Amsterdam: Elsevier, 1991:47–75.
3. Bach AWJ, Unger L, Wozny M, Seeburg PH. A new member of the serotonin receptor family: structure and functional expression of a 5-HT$_{1D}$-like receptor. International Conference on 5-Hydroxytryptamine—CNS receptors and brain function, Birmingham, U.K., 1991:28 (abstract).
4. Bishop GA, Ho RH. The distribution and origin of serotonin immunoreactivity in the rat cerebellum. *Brain Res* 1985;331:195–207.
5. Bishop GA, Ho RH, King JS. Localization of serotonin immunoreactivity in the opossum cerebellum. *J Comp Neurol* 1985;235:301–321.
6. Bobker DH, Williams JT. Ion conductances affected by 5-HT receptor subtypes in mammalian neurons. *Trends Neurosci* 1990;13:169–173.
7. Branchek T, Zgombick J, Macchi M, Hartig P, Weinshank R. Cloning and expression of a human 5-HT$_{1D}$ receptor. In: Fozard JR, Saxena PR, eds. *Serotonin: molecular biology, receptors and functional effects*. Basel: Birkhauser, 1991:21–32.
8. Brodal A. *Neurological anatomy*. New York: Oxford University Press, 1981.
9. D'Amato RJ, Largent BL, Snowman AM, Snyder SH. Selective labeling of serotonin uptake sites in rat brain by [^{3}H]citalopram contrasted to labeling of multiple sites by [^{3}H]imipramine. *J Pharmacol Exp Ther* 1987;242:364–371.
10. Derkach V, Surprenant A, North RA. 5-HT$_3$ receptors are membrane ion channels. *Nature* 1989; 339:706–709.
11. Dohlman HG, Caron MG, Lefkowitz RJ. A family of receptors coupled to guanine nucleotide regulatory proteins. *Biochemistry* 1987;26:2657–2664.
12. Dumuis A, Bouhelal R, Sebben M, Cory R, Bockaert J. A nonclassical 5-hydroxytryptamine receptor positively coupled with adenylate cyclase in the central nervous system. *Mol Pharmacol* 1988; 34:880–887.
13. Fagni L, Dumuis A, Sebben M, Bockaert J. The 5-HT$_4$ receptor subtype inhibits K$^+$ current in colliculi neurones via activation of a cyclic AMP-dependent protein kinase. *Br J Pharmacol* 1992;105:973–979.
14. Fargin A, Raymond JR, Lohse MJ, Kobilka BK, Caron MG, Lefkowitz RJ. The genomic clone G-21 which resembles a β-adrenergic receptor sequence encodes the 5-HT$_{1A}$ receptor. *Nature* 1988; 335:358–360.
15. Ito M. *The cerebellum and neural control*. New York: Raven Press, 1984.
16. Jansen J, Brodal A. Das kleinhirn. In: *Möllendorff's Handbuch der mikroskopischen Anatomie der Menschen*, vol IV:8. Berlin: Springer, 1958.
17. Julius D, MacDermott AB, Axel R, Jessel TM. Molecular characterization of a functional cDNA encoding the serotonin lc receptor. *Science* 1988;241:558–564.
18. Kerr CWH, Bishop GA. Topographical organization in the origin of serotoninergic projections to different regions of the cat cerebellar cortex. *J Comp Neurol* 1991;304:502–515.
19. Marick AV, Peterson AS, Brake AJ, Myers RM, Julius D. Primary structure and functional expression of the 5-HT$_3$ receptor, a serotonin-gated ion channel. *Science* 1991;254:432–437.
20. Maroteaux L, Saudou F, Amlaiky N, Boschert U, Plassat JL, Hen R. The mouse 5-HT$_{1B}$ serotonin receptor: cloning, functional expression and localization in motor control centers. *Proc Natl Acad Sci USA* 1992;89:3020–3024.

21. Mengod G, Martinez-Mir MI, Vilaro' MT, Palacios JM. Localization of the mRNA for the dopamine D_2 receptor in the rat brain by in situ hybridization histochemistry. *Proc Natl Acad Sci USA* 1989;86:8560–8564.
22. Mengod G, Pompeiano M, Martinez-Mir MI, Palacios JM. Localization of the mRNA for the 5-HT_2 receptor by in situ hybridization histochemistry. Correlation with the distribution of receptor sites. *Brain Res* 1990;524:139–143.
23. Palacios JM, Waeber C, Hoyer D, Mengod G. Distribution of serotonin receptors. *Ann NY Acad Sci* 1990;600:36–52.
24. Palacios JM, Waeber C, Mengod G, Hoyer D. Autoradiography of 5-HT receptors: a critical appraisal. *Neurochem Int* 1991;18:17–25.
25. Peroutka SJ. 5-Hydroxytryptamine receptor subtypes. *Pharmacol Toxicol* 1990;67:373–383.
26. Pompeiano M, Palacios JM, Mengod G. Distribution and cellular localization of mRNA coding for 5-HT_{1A} receptor in the rat brain: correlation with receptor binding. *J Neurosci* 1992;12:440–453.
27. Pritchett DB, Bach AW, Wozny M, et al. Structure and functional expression of cloned rat serotonin 5-HT_2 receptor. *EMBO J* 1989;7:4135–4140.
28. Steinbush HWM. Serotonin-immunoreactive neurons and their projections in the CNS. In: Björklund A, Hökfelt T, Kuhar MJ, eds. *Handbook of chemical neuroanatomy, vol 3: classical transmitter and transmitter receptors in the CNS, pt. II*. Amsterdam: Elsevier, 1984:68–125.
29. Törk I. Raphe nuclei and serotonin containing systems. In: Paxinos G, ed. *The rat nervous system, vol 2: hindbrain and spinal cord*. Marrickville: Academic Press Australia, 1985:43–78.
30. Voigt MM, Laurie DJ, Seeburg PH, Bach A. Molecular cloning and characterization of a rat brain cDNA encoding a 5-hydroxytryptamine$_{1B}$ receptor. *EMBO J* 1991;10:4017–4023.

Serotonin, the Cerebellum, and Ataxia, edited by
P. Trouillas and K. Fuxe.
Raven Press, Ltd., New York © 1993.

13

5-HT$_{1A}$ Receptors in the Olivocerebellar Complex

*Daniel Vergé, *Line Matthiessen, *Hossein K. Kia,
†Henri Gozlan, †Michel Hamon, ‡Yannick Bailly,
and *Geneviève Daval

Department of Cytology, ‡Developmental Neurobiology Laboratory, Institut des Neurosciences, CNRS UA 1199, Université Pierre et Marie Curie, 75252 Paris, France; †Cellular and Functional Neurobiology Laboratory, INSERM U288, Faculté de Médicine Pitié-Salpêtrière, 75013 Paris, France

The innervation of the cerebellar cortex by serotonin (5-HT) was first demonstrated by fluorescence histochemistry (18) and subsequently confirmed by autoradiography (4,9) and immunocytochemistry (6,32). 5-HT fibers terminating in the cerebellar cortex mainly arise from the nucleus reticularis gigantocellularis, the nucleus reticularis paragigantocellularis, and the nucleus reticularis pontis oralis (6). 5-HT fibers were also found in the inferior olive of the rat by fluorescence histochemistry (40), autoradiography (41), and immunocytochemistry (5,30,33). The origin of this innervation lies in the nucleus reticularis paragigantocellularis (7).

Quantitative autoradiography with selective radioligands has shown that both 5-HT$_1$ and 5-HT$_2$ binding sites exist in the inferior olive (22,23), where they may be located on the neurons at the origin of the climbing fibers within the cerebellum (8). In addition, electrophysiological experiments demonstrated that Purkinje cells are endowed with 5-HT receptors, particularly of the 5-HT$_{1A}$ subtype (10,11,31), and biochemical studies strongly suggested that parallel, climbing, and mossy fibers also have 5-HT receptors in the rat cerebellum (21; Raiteri et al., this volume). Thus, *in vitro* experiments showed that 5-HT controls glutamate release through 5-HT$_{1A}$ receptors located on nerve endings from parallel and/or climbing fibers (Raiteri et al., this volume) and 5-HT$_2$ receptors on mossy fiber terminals (21). However, 5-HT receptors are hardly detectable in the adult rat cerebellum by autoradiographic techniques (12,22,23,26). In contrast, high densities of 5-HT$_{1A}$ binding sites have been found in the cerebellum of young rats (12). This chapter presents recent data concerning the anatomical and cellular localization of 5-HT$_{1A}$ receptors and their quantitative evolution during the postnatal development of the cerebellum.

Some evidence supporting the location of 5-HT_{1A} receptors on olivary neurons in the adult rat is also presented.

Sagittal sections of cerebellar vermis from 8-day-old and adult male Wistar rats were incubated with 50 pM [^{125}I]Bolton-Hunter-8-methoxy-2-(N-propyl-N-propylamino)tetralin ([^{125}I]BH-8-MeO-N-PAT) (15) for the specific labeling of 5-HT_{1A} binding sites (25) and processed for autoradiography with sensitive films. In agreement with previous data (12), 5-HT_{1A} sites were found in a relatively high density during the early postnatal period, whereas no specific binding could be detected in the adulthood (Fig. 1). When adjacent sections from 8-day-old rats were incubated either with the radioligand (Fig. 2A) or anti–5-HT_{1A} receptor antibodies revealed by [^{35}S]-labeled secondary antibodies (14) (Fig. 2B), the distribution of 5-HT_{1A} binding sites appeared similar to that of the receptor protein (34). This result indi-

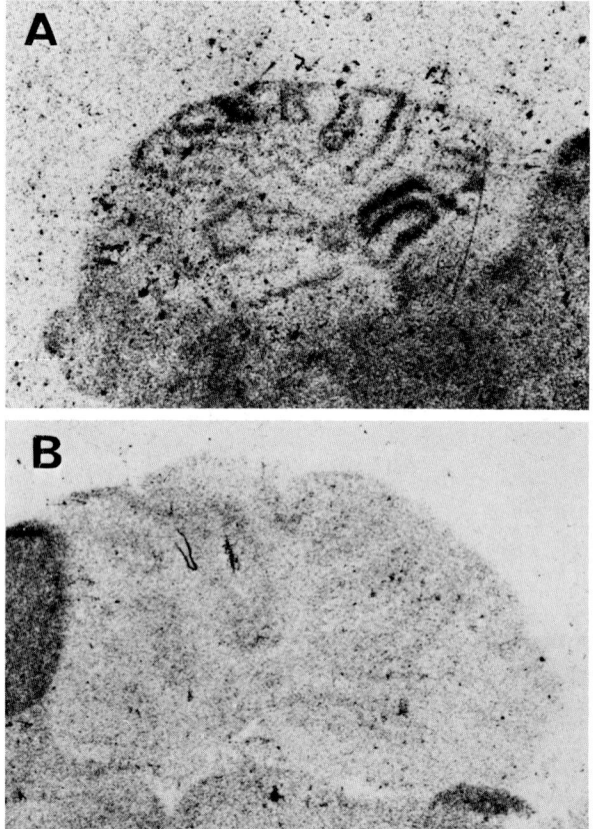

FIG. 1. Autoradiograms of sagittal sections of the cerebellar vermis exposed to [^{125}I]BH-8-MeO-N-PAT. **A**: 8-day-old rat; **B**, 30-day-old rat. Sagittal cryostat sections of cerebellar vermis were incubated with 50 pM [^{125}I]BH-8-MeO-N-PAT and processed for autoradiography (25).

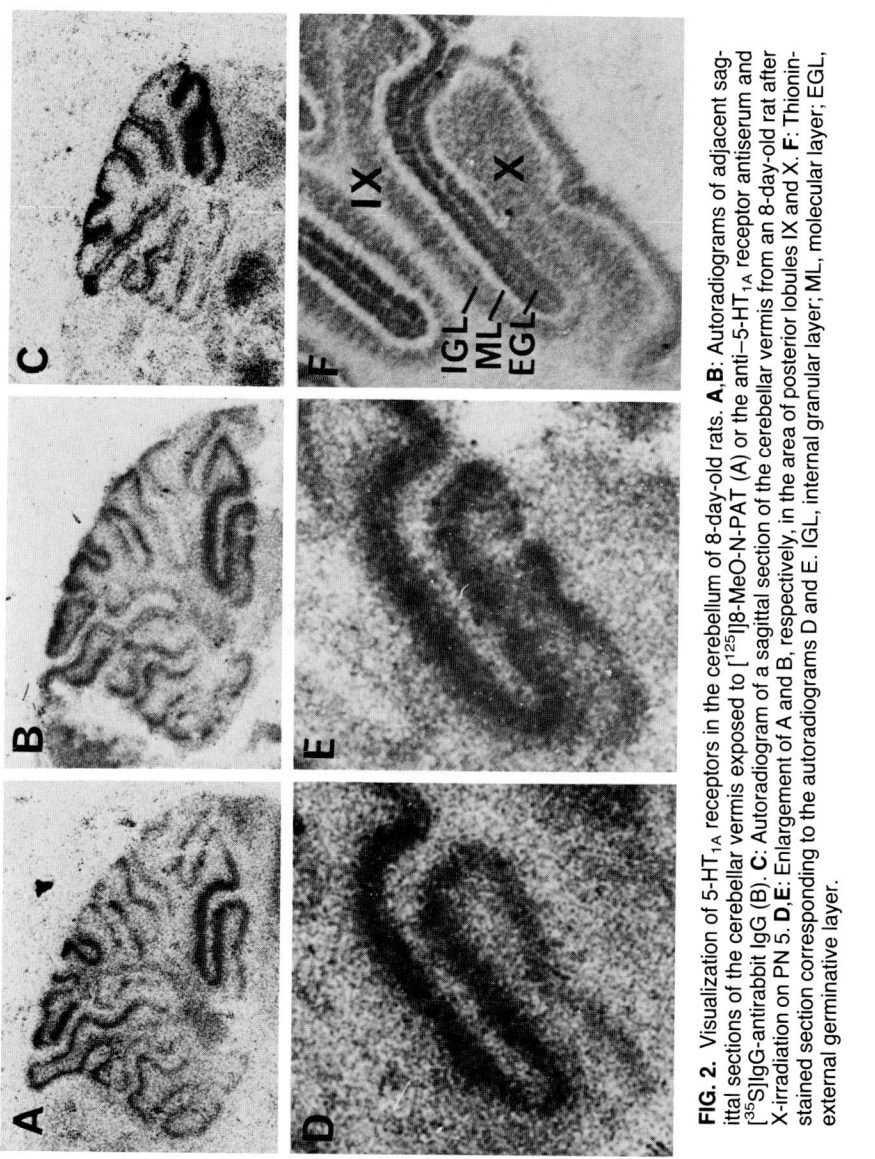

FIG. 2. Visualization of 5-HT$_{1A}$ receptors in the cerebellum of 8-day-old rats. **A,B:** Autoradiograms of adjacent sagittal sections of the cerebellar vermis exposed to [^{125}I]8-MeO-N-PAT (A) or the anti–5-HT$_{1A}$ receptor antiserum and [^{35}S]IgG-antirabbit IgG (B). **C:** Autoradiogram of a sagittal section of the cerebellar vermis from an 8-day-old rat after X-irradiation on PN 5. **D,E:** Enlargement of A and B, respectively, in the area of posterior lobules IX and X. **F:** Thionin-stained section corresponding to the autoradiograms D and E. IGL, internal granular layer; ML, molecular layer; EGL, external germinative layer.

cated that antibodies raised against an intracellular portion of the 5-HT_{1A} receptor (14) recognize the same molecule as the radioligand. Therefore, the observed labeling was actually due to the presence of a high density of 5-HT_{1A} receptors in the cerebellum of young rats. This conclusion is strengthened by the observation that 5-HT_{1A} agonists significantly inhibit forskolin-stimulated adenylate cyclase in the immature rat cerebellum, whereas such an effect cannot be found in the adult animal (16).

As shown in Fig. 2, 5-HT_{1A} receptors are confined to a continuous narrow layer in all the lobules of the vermis. However, this distribution is heterogeneous. Thus, the density of sites is markedly higher in posterior than in anterior lobules, with the posterior part of lobule IXB and the anterior part of lobule X exhibiting the highest level of labeling. The regional heterogeneity of 5-HT_{1A} labeling in sagittal sections is not well correlated with the timing of development of the different lobules, as it was assessed by Altman (1) from [^{3}H]thymidine incorporation experiments. For example, lobules I and X, both of which form early, exhibit a low and high density of binding sites, respectively. On the other hand, a better correlation can be found with the regional distribution of 5-HT innervation in the adult cerebellum. Thus, posterior lobules, where 5-HT_{1A} receptors are particularly abundant, receive a relatively dense innervation when compared to anterior lobules (6).

When autoradiograms were examined at a higher magnification (Fig. 2D,E) at the level of the posterior lobules and compared to the corresponding thionin-stained section (Fig. 2F), it appeared that the external germinative and internal granular layers were devoid of labeling. 5-HT_{1A} receptors seemed to be located in the molecular/Purkinje cell layer. To test this hypothesis, X-irradiated cerebellum was used as a model in which the granule cell population had been drastically reduced.

Five-day-old rats were X-irradiated in the cerebellar area with a single dose of 450 rad for 15 min in order to destroy the external germinative layer. Previous studies have shown that maximal multi-innervation of Purkinje cells by climbing fibers persisted in the resulting agranular cerebellum in adult rats (2). On postnatal day (PN) 8, the distribution of 5-HT_{1A} receptors in sagittal sections of cerebellar vermis visualized either by the specific labeling with [^{125}I]BH-8-MeO-N-PAT (Fig. 2C) or [^{35}S]-labeled antibodies (not shown) remained unchanged in X-irradiated rats (34). However, the density of 5-HT_{1A} binding sites seemed slightly higher than in age-paired normal animals. This result further showed that 5-HT_{1A} receptors in the immature cerebellum are located neither on mature granule cells nor on their precursors in the external germinative layer.

Examination of autoradiograms obtained with sections from the cerebellar vermis of normal rats at various stages of development (PN 5, 8, 12, 21, and 30) after labeling with [^{125}I]BH-8-MeO-N-PAT showed that the overall distribution of 5-HT_{1A} binding sites was roughly conserved throughout the first postnatal month. However, the density of labeling, which was the highest during the first week, then decreased rapidly in all the lobules. The time course of receptor density changes was studied in each lobule by computer-assisted densitometry (20a). An example is given for the anterior part of lobule X (Xa) in Fig. 3. The density of 5-HT_{1A} sites did not change

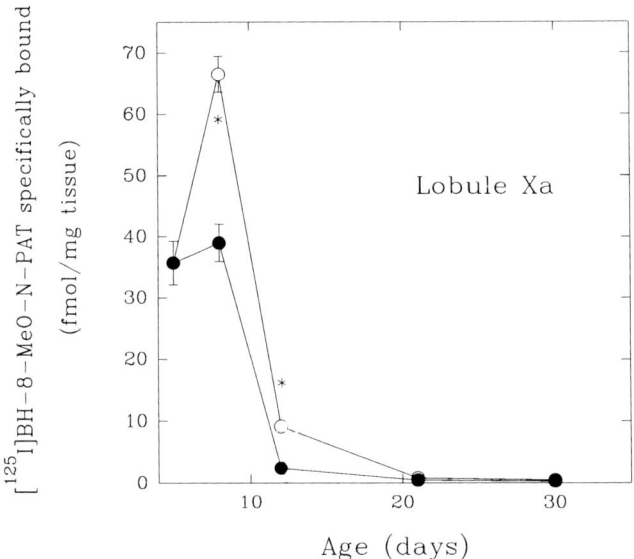

FIG. 3. Evolution of the density of 5-HT$_{1A}$ binding sites labeled with [^{125}I]BH-8-MeO-N-PAT in the anterior part of lobule X of the cerebellar vermis from normal (●) and X-irradiated (○) rats during postnatal development. Sagittal sections of the cerebellar vermis from normal or X-irradiated rats sacrificed at PN 5, 8, 12, 21, or 30 were incubated with 50 pM [^{125}I]BH-8-MeO-N-PAT and processed for quantitative autoradiography. Each value is the means ± SEM of 12 to 18 densitometric measurements from three rats and expressed as fmoles of [^{125}I]BH-8-MeO-N-PAT specifically bound per milligram of tissue. *$p<0.001$ compared to age-paired control rats.

between PN 5 and 8 in this lobule, as in some others (I, II, III, VIB, posterior part of IXB), whereas it decreased significantly in lobules IV, V, VIA, VII, VIII, IXA, and the anterior part of IXB (20a). After PN 8, the specific labeling decreased dramatically in all lobules. By PN 21, it was not significantly different from nonspecific binding. Similar results were obtained with radioimmunohistochemistry using specific anti–5-HT$_{1A}$ receptor antibodies (20a). Densitometric measurements on autoradiograms obtained from cerebella irradiated at PN 5 showed that at PN 8 and 12, the 5-HT$_{1A}$ receptor density was significantly higher than in age-paired animals (Fig. 3). However, the density of labeling then markedly decreased as in normal rats.

Measurements of [^{3}H]8-hydroxy-2-(di-n-propylamino)tetralin ([^{3}H]8-OH-DPAT) specific binding to cerebellar membranes further demonstrated that the density of 5-HT$_{1A}$ binding sites decreased between PN 5 and 30 (Fig. 4A,B). In contrast, the total number of 5-HT$_{1A}$ sites per cerebellum increased during this period (Fig. 4C). This indicated that the decrease in receptor density was not related to a transient expression of 5-HT$_{1A}$ receptors in the cerebellum of newborn rats, but resulted from a dilution phenomenon, the cerebellar volume increasing more rapidly than the number of receptors. Interestingly, the total number of 5-HT$_{1A}$ receptors in the

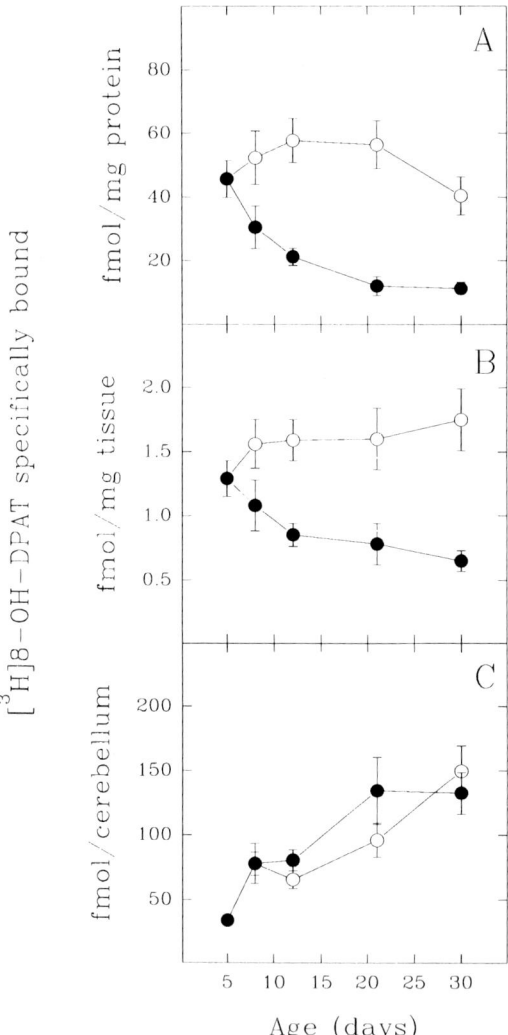

FIG. 4. Evolution of 5-HT$_{1A}$ binding sites in the cerebellum of normal rats (●) and rats X-irradiated at PN5 (○) as determined from measurements of [^{3}H]8-OH-DPAT specific binding to membranes. Membranes from pooled cerebella of rats sacrificed at PN 5, 8, 12, 21, or 30 were incubated with 0.32 to 3.78 nM [^{3}H]8-OH-DPAT. B$_{max}$ values (means ± SEM of three independent determinations) were calculated from saturation studies using nonlinear computer-assisted regression analysis.

cerebellum was not modified by the irradiation at PN 5 (Fig. 4C). This result also indicated that the enhanced density of 5-HT$_{1A}$ sites in the irradiated cerebellum was due to the reduction in volume after irradiation (see Fig. 2). The density of 5-HT$_{1A}$ sites in cerebellar membranes from 30-day-old irradiated animals was relatively high compared with the low level of 5-HT$_{1A}$ receptor labeling in sections from animals in the same group. This discrepancy can probably be explained by methodological differences: first, studies on the whole cerebellum versus the vermis could lead to different results because the postnatal changes in receptor density do not follow similar time courses in the cerebellar vermis and the hemispheres (*un-*

published data); second, membrane binding assays allow the determination of the total number of sites (B_{max}) per milligram of tissue or proteins, whereas autoradiographic studies give only the concentration of bound ligand at a single concentration of free ligand. Thus, densitometric measurements are dependent on the affinity (K_d^{-1}) of the receptor for the radioligand. In particular, a slight but significant increase in K_d was found from PN 5 to 30, leading to an underestimation of the density of 5-HT$_{1A}$ sites in sections of 30-day-old animals. Third, the response of the autoradiographic film is not linear, particularly for low levels of binding, and receptor densities in the adult cerebellum are probably under the threshold of the film response.

The above results showed that 5-HT$_{1A}$ receptor is expressed by cells located in the molecular/Purkinje cell layers, the density of which is increased by irradiation. Parallel fibers can be excluded from the elements expressing 5-HT$_{1A}$ receptors, because irradiation led to a dramatic degeneration of granule cells. Basket and stellate microneurons are also unlikely to bear 5-HT$_{1A}$ receptors, since high densities of labeling were found before PN 5, when the peak of proliferation of these cells had not yet occurred. Therefore, the main candidates for the location of 5-HT$_{1A}$ receptors are Purkinje cells and glial cells. Indeed, electrophysiological studies have revealed the presence of 5-HT$_{1A}$ sites on Purkinje cells (10,11). Binding sites for tritiated 5-HT were found on astrocytes in culture (35). Interestingly, the timing of maturation of Bergmann glial cells is well correlated with changes in 5-HT$_{1A}$ receptor density (28). In line with a possible trophic role for 5-HT, 5-HT$_{1A}$ sites on astroglial cells have been implicated in the regulation of the development of serotoninergic neurons in culture (36).

Autoradiographic studies with [^{125}I]BH-8-MeO-N-PAT using the coverslip technique (42) confirmed the presence of 5-HT$_{1A}$ binding sites in the Purkinje cell/molecular layer, in a manner consistent with their location on both Purkinje and glial cells (Fig. 5). Particularly, in lobules IXB and X, Purkinje cell soma and dendrites seemed to be labeled by the radioligand (arrows, Fig. 5).

Immunocytochemical studies with the anti–5-HT$_{1A}$ receptor antibodies were performed to clarify this point. Eight-day-old rats were anesthetized with diethylether and perfused intracardially with 4% paraformaldehyde in 0.1 M phosphate-buffered saline (PBS), pH 7.4. The cerebellum was postfixed by immersion in the same fixative for 90 min and cryoprotected with 0.1 M phosphate buffer containing 25% sucrose for 48 hr at 4°C. Cryostat sections (20 μm) were preincubated in 50 mM PBS, pH 7.4, containing 3% bovine serum albumin for 30 min, and after washing, they were incubated overnight at 4°C with antirat 5-HT$_{1A}$ receptor antibodies (14) (final dilution 1:1,000 in 50 mM PBS containing 0.1% bovine serum albumin and 0.2% Triton-X 100). The immunoreactivity was revealed by a combination of the peroxidase-antiperoxidase and avidin-biotin-peroxidase techniques (13). A strong immunoreactivity could be observed on sagittal sections of the cerebellar vermis (Fig. 6), particularly at the level of the posterior lobules. Under similar conditions, the main areas of location of 5-HT$_{1A}$ receptors in the adult brain were also labeled (dorsal raphe nucleus, septum, hippocampus, interpeduncular nucleus, entorhinal

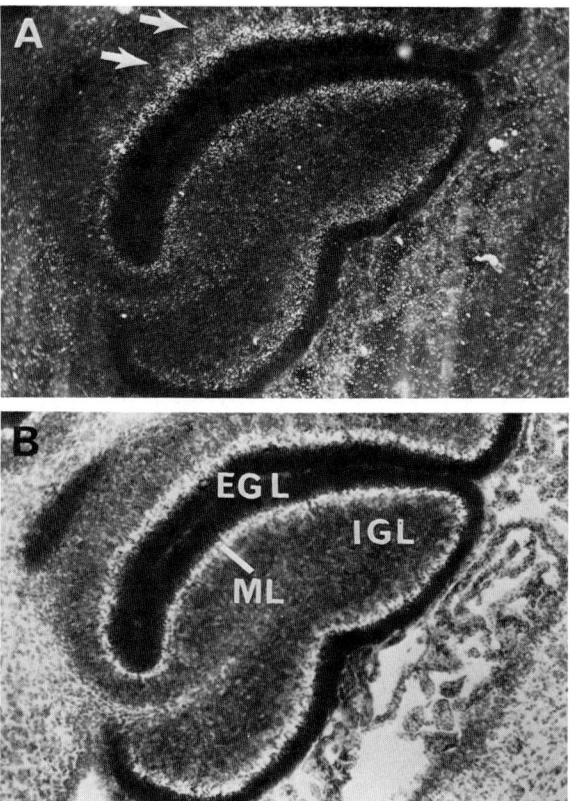

FIG. 5. Autoradiographic visualization of 5-HT$_{1A}$ binding sites in the cerebellar vermis using the emulsion-coated coverslip technique. **A**: Dark-field illumination of an autoradiogram of a sagittal section of the cerebellar vermis (area of the posterior lobules) exposed to [^{125}I]BH-8-MeO-N-PAT. **B**: Thionin-stained corresponding section. Autoradiographic grains are found in the molecular layer (ML) but not in the external germinative layer (EGL) or the internal granular layer (IGL). Purkinje cell somas are also labeled (*arrows*).

cortex). The specificity of the immunostaining was assessed by the following controls: when incubated in preimmune serum, or in the presence of an excess of the synthetic peptide that has been used as antigen to raise anti–5-HT$_{1A}$ receptor antibodies in rabbits (14), no immunoreactive signal could be detected on consecutive sections. Immunocytochemical staining was found in the molecular layer and on Purkinje cell somas (Fig. 6A). At higher magnification (Fig. 6B), Purkinje cells appeared to be labeled on their plasmic membrane and dendritic shafts. Interestingly, the staining was often discontinuous on the membrane. Sometimes staining could also be found on the beginning of the axon. In the molecular layer, the immunoreactivity was probably mainly located on the dendrites of Purkinje cells, but it cannot be excluded that other cell types, for example, glial cells, were also labeled.

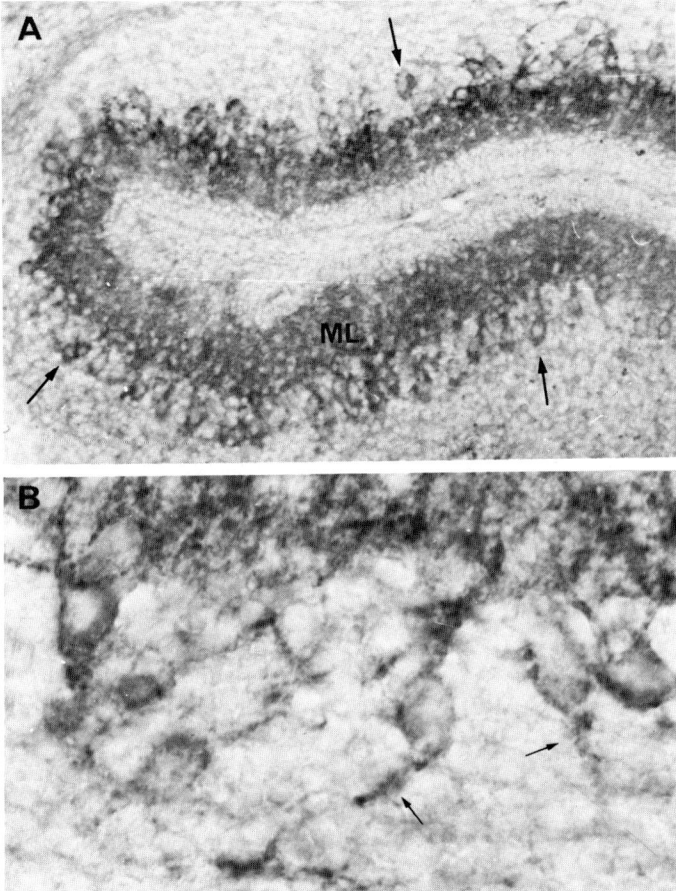

FIG. 6. Immunocytochemical visualization of 5-HT$_{1A}$ receptors in the cerebellum of a normal 8-day-old rat at the level of the posterior lobules. Sagittal cryostat sections were exposed to the anti–5-HT$_{1A}$ receptor antiserum, and immunoreactivity was revealed by the avidin-biotin-peroxidase complex–peroxidase-antiperoxidase technique. **A**: Immunostaining is found in the molecular layer (ML) and at the level of Purkinje cell somas (*arrows*). **B**: At a higher magnification, staining is found on the membrane of Purkinje cell somas and dendrites, and occasionally on the beginning of axons (*small arrows*).

Thus, it has been suggested that 5-HT$_{1A}$ receptors could be located on climbing fiber terminals in the cerebellum (Raiteri et al., this volume). 5-HT$_{1A}$ binding sites have been also detected in the inferior olive containing the cell bodies of these neurons in the rat (22,23). In the mouse, this structure exhibits a high density of labeling with [^{125}I]BH-8-MeO-N-PAT (Kia et al., *unpublished results*). Olivary neurons can be selectively destroyed by the neurotoxic 3-acetylpyridine (3-AP) (3). The 3-AP lesion results in abnormal movements of the trunk and limbs (17,24,27). Behavioral studies have suggested the implication of 5-HT systems in this effect. In particular, Wieland et al. (38) have shown that the 5-HT syndrome due to the selective 5-HT$_{1A}$ agonist 8-OH-DPAT is more pronounced in 3-AP-treated rats than in age-paired controls. Interestingly, the motor abnormalities produced by the injection of 3-AP are similar to the behavioral symptoms reported for the genetically dystonic (dt) rat (19). Furthermore, this mutant also exhibits an increased sensitivity to 8-OH-DPAT for the production of the 5-HT syndrome, with the exception of the tremor component of the syndrome (39). In fact, the dt rat does not show tremor in response to 8-OH-DPAT. Interestingly, the dt rat is also insensitive to the tremorogenic effect of harmaline (20), which is mediated by the inferior olive in normal rats (29). Indeed, a 3-AP-induced lesion of the latter structure suppresses the effect of harmaline (29). These data indicate that 5-HT$_{1A}$ receptors in the olivocerebellar system could be involved in the control of motor behavior. We used 3-AP lesions to examine further with quantitative autoradiography the cellular localization of 5-HT$_{1A}$ sites in the rat inferior olive.

Male Wistar rats (250 g) were injected with 3-AP (65 mg/kg i.p.). After 5 days, they were sacrificed by intracardiac perfusion of 0.15 M phosphate buffer, pH 7.4, and frontal cryostat sections were processed for the labeling of 5-HT$_{1A}$ sites with 2 nM [^{3}H]8-OH-DPAT and quantitative autoradiography as above. The density of 5-HT$_{1A}$ binding sites in the inferior olive was reduced by 39% after 3-AP administration (control: 47.3 ± 2.1 fmol/mg tissue, $n=5$; 3-AP-treated: 28.9 ± 1.7, $n=10$; $p<0.001$). This result indicated that 5-HT$_{1A}$ sites in this structure are at least partly located on the cell bodies of olivary neurons. Further experiments with immunocytochemistry are in progress to define precisely the localization of 5-HT$_{1A}$ receptors and their relationship with the serotoninergic innervation in the inferior olive.

In conclusion, 5-HT$_{1A}$ receptors are not actually expressed in the cerebellum, only for the early postnatal life, and their decrease in density during postnatal development resulted simply from the progressive dilution of these sites in a growing structure. Purkinje cell bodies and dendrites, but not granule cells, are endowed with 5-HT$_{1A}$ receptors in the immature cerebellum. In addition, expression of 5-HT$_{1A}$ receptors in glial cells cannot be excluded. In the adult rat, 5-HT$_{1A}$ receptors are also expressed in olivary neurons. The presence of a high density of 5-HT$_{1A}$ receptors in the cerebellar cortex at an early developmental stage, when the serotoninergic innervation has not yet invaded this region, raises the question of their possible involvement in function(s) unrelated to neurotransmission. 5-HT$_{1A}$ receptors probably do not participate in the regression of the multi-innervation of Purkinje cells by climbing fibers, as these sites are unaffected when the latter process is prevented by X-irradiation. However, it could be possible, as suggested by recent data (37) that 5-HT acts as a neurohormone at 5-HT$_{1A}$ receptors to modulate the development of cerebellar (serotoninergic?) afferents. The presence in the same area (the posterior lobules) of a dense 5-HT innervation in the adult cerebellum and a high density of 5-HT$_{1A}$ receptors in the developing cerebellum suggests that these receptors may serve as a guide for the growth of 5-HT nerve fibers.

ACKNOWLEDGMENTS

We thank Mrs. Touret and Mrs. Cloup for excellent photographic work. We are grateful to the Service des Molécules Marquées of CEA (Gif-sur-Yvette, France) for generous gifts of [^{3}H]8-OH-DPAT and [^{125}I]BH-8-MeO-N-PAT. This research has been supported by grants from CNRS, INSERM, DRED (Ministère de l'Education Nationale), and Bayer-Pharma.

REFERENCES

1. Altman J. Morphological development of the rat cerebellum and some of its mechanisms. In: Palay SL, Chan-Palay V, eds. *The cerebellum: new vistas*. Berlin: Springer-Verlag, 1982:8–49.
2. Bailly Y, Debain C, Delhaye-Bouchaud N, Mariani J. The multiple innervation of cerebellar Purkinje cells by climbing fibers is totally maintained in adult rats which receive a single postnatal irradiation. In: *Proceedings of the meeting on neurobiology of the cerebellar system*. Barcelona: University of Barcelona, 1988.
3. Balaban CD. Central neurotoxic effects of intraperitoneally administered 3-acetylpyridine, harmaline and niacinamide in Sprague-Dawley and Long-Evans rats: a critical review of central 3-acetylpyridine neurotoxicity. *Brain Res Rev* 1985;9:21–42.
4. Beaudet A, Sotelo C. Synaptic remodeling of serotonin axon terminals in rat agranular cerebellum. *Brain Res* 1981;206:305–329.
5. Bishop GA, Ho RH. Substance P and serotonin immunoreactivity in the rat inferior olive. *Brain Res Bull* 1984;12:105–113.
6. Bishop GA, Ho RH. The distribution and origin of serotonin immunoreactivity in the rat cerebellum. *Brain Res* 1985;331:195–207.
7. Bishop GA, Ho RH. Cell bodies of origin of serotonin-immunoreactive afferents to the inferior olivary complex of the rat. *Brain Res* 1986;399:369–373.
8. Campbell NC, Armstrong DM. The olivocerebellar projection in the rat: an autoradiographic study. *Brain Res* 1983;275:215–233.
9. Chan-Palay V. Fine structure of labelled axons in the cerebellar cortex and nuclei of rodents and primates after intraventricular infusions with tritiated serotonin. *Anat Embryol* 1975;148:235–265.
10. Darrow EJ, Strahlendorf HK, Strahlendorf JC. Response of cerebellar Purkinje cells to serotonin and the 5-HT$_{1A}$ agonists 8-OH-DPAT and ipsapirone in vitro. *Eur J Pharmacol* 1990;175:145–153.
11. Darrow E, Strahlendorf JC, Strahlendorf HK. Extracellular magnesium concentration alters Purkinje cell responsiveness to serotonin and analogues. *Eur J Pharmacol* 1991;209:19–25.
12. Daval G, Vergé D, Becerril A, Gozlan H, Spampinato U, Hamon M. Transient expression of 5-HT$_{1A}$ receptor binding sites in some areas of the rat CNS during post-natal development. *Int J Dev Neurosci* 1987;5:171–180.
13. Davidoff M, Schulze W. Combination of the peroxydase antiperoxydase (PAP)- and avidin-biotin-peroxydase complex (ABC)-techniques: an amplification alternative in immunocytochemical staining. *Histochemistry* 1990;93:531–536.
14. El Mestikawy S, Riad M, Laporte A-M, et al. Production of specific anti-rat 5-HT$_{1A}$ receptor antibodies in rabbits injected with a synthetic peptide. *Neurosci Lett* 1990;118:189–192.
15. Gozlan H, Ponchant M, Daval G, et al. [^{125}I]Bolton-Hunter-8-methoxy-2-(N-propyl-N-propylamino)tetralin as a new selective radioligand of 5-HT$_{1A}$ sites in the rat brain. In vitro binding and autoradiographic studies. *J Pharmacol Exp Ther* 1988;244:751–759.
16. Hamon M, Emerit MB. Facteurs chimiques impliqués dans la différentiation neuronale. In: Relier JP, Laugier J, Salle BL, eds. *Médecine périnatale (foetus et nouveau-né)*. Paris: Médecine-Science-Flammarion, 1989:194–200.
17. Herken H. Functional disorders of the brain induced by synthesis of nucleotides containing 3-acetylpyridine. *Z Klin Chem Klin Biochem* 1968;6:357–366.
18. Hökfelt T, Fuxe K. Cerebellar monoamine nerve terminals, a new type of afferent fibers to the cortex cerebelli. *Exp Brain Res* 1969;9:63–72.

19. Lorden JF, McKeon TW, Baker HJ, Cox N, Walkley SU. Characterization of the rat mutant dystonic (dt): a new animal model of dystonia musculorum deformans. *J Neurosci* 1984;4:1925–1932.
20. Lorden JF, Oltmans GA, McKeon TW, Lutes J, Beales M. Decreased cerebellar 3′,5′-cyclic guanosine monophosphate levels and insensitivity to harmaline in the genetically dystonic rat (dt). *J Neurosci* 1985;5:2618–2625.
20a. Mattheissen L, Daval G, Bailly Y, Gozlan H, Hamon M, Vergé D. Quantification of 5-HT$_{1A}$ receptors in the cerebellum of normal and x-irradiated rats during postnatal development. *Neuroscience* 1992(*in press*).
21. Maura G, Carbone R, Guido M, Pestarino M, Raiteri M. 5-HT$_2$ presynaptic receptors mediate inhibition of glutamate release from cerebellar mossy fibre terminals. *Eur J Pharmacol* 1991;202:185–190.
22. Palacios JM, Dietl MM. Autoradiographic studies of serotonin receptors. In: Sanders-Bush E, ed. *The serotonin receptors*. Clifton, NJ: Humana Press, 1988:89–138.
23. Palacios JM, Waeber C, Mengod G, Pompeiano M. Molecular neuroanatomy of 5-HT receptors. In: Fozard JR, Saxena PR, eds. *Serotonin: molecular biology, receptors and functional effects*. Basel: Birkhäuser Verlag, 1991:5–20.
24. Pranzatelli MR, Gantner C, Snodgrass SR. 3-Acetylpyridine lesions and four serotonergic behavioral syndromes in the rat. *Brain Res Bull* 1987;18:159–163.
25. Radja F, Daval G, Emerit MB, Gallissot MC, Hamon M, Vergé D. Selective irreversible blockade of 5-hydroxytryptamine$_{1A}$ and 5-hydroxytryptamine$_{1C}$ receptor binding sites in the rat brain by 8-MeO-2′-chloro-PAT. A quantitative autoradiographic study. *Neuroscience* 1989;31:723–733.
26. Radja F, Laporte A-M, Daval G, Vergé D, Gozlan H, Hamon M. Autoradiography of serotonin receptor subtypes in the central nervous system. *Neurochem Int* 1991;18:1–15.
27. Sandyk R, Fisher H. Serotonin in involuntary movement disorders. *Int J Neurosci* 1988;42:185–205.
28. Shiga T, Ichikawa M, Hirata Y. Spatial and temporal pattern of postnatal proliferation of Bergmann glial cells in rat cerebellum: an autoradiographic study. *Anat Embryol* 1983;167:203–211.
29. Simantov R, Snyder SH, Oster-Granite M-L. Harmaline-induced tremor in the rat: abolition by 3-acetylpyridine destruction of the cerebellar climbing fibers. *Brain Res* 1976;114:144–151.
30. Steinbusch HWM. Distribution of serotonin-immunoreactivity in the central nervous system of the rat. Cell bodies and terminals. *Neuroscience* 1981;6:557–618.
31. Strahlendorf JC, Lee M, Strahlendorf HK. Serotonin modulates muscimol- and baclofen-elicited inhibition of cerebellar Purkinje cells. *Eur J Pharmacol* 1991;201:239–242.
32. Takeuchi Y, Kimura H, Sano Y. Immunohistochemical demonstration of serotonin-containing nerve fibers in the cerebellum. *Cell Tissue Res* 1982;226:1–12.
33. Takeuchi Y, Sano Y. Immunohistochemical demonstration of serotonin-containing nerve fibers in the inferior olivary complex of the rat, cat and monkey. *Cell Tissue Res* 1983;231:17–28.
34. Vergé D, Matthiessen L, Daval G, Bailly Y, Kia HK, Hamon M. Localization of 5-HT$_{1A}$ serotonin receptors in the cerebellum of young rats. *Neurochem Int* 1991;19:425–431.
35. Whitaker-Azmitia PM, Azmitia EC. ^{3}H-5-Hydroxytryptamine binding to brain astroglial cells: differences between intact and homogenized preparations and mature and immature cultures. *J Neurochem* 1986;46:1186–1189.
36. Whitaker-Azmitia PM, Murphy R, Azmitia EC. Stimulation of astroglial 5-HT$_{1A}$ receptors releases the serotonergic growth factor, protein S-100, and alters astroglial morphology. *Brain Res* 1990;528:155–158.
37. Whitaker-Azmitia PM, Shemer AV, Caruso J, Molino L, Azmitia EC. Role of high affinity serotonin receptors in neuronal growth. *Ann NY Acad Sci* 1990;600:315–330.
38. Wieland S, Kreider MS, McGonigle P, Lucki I. Destruction of the nucleus raphe obscurus and potentiation of serotonin-mediated behaviors following administration of the neurotoxin 3-acetylpyridine. *Brain Res* 1990;520:291–302.
39. Wieland S, Lucki I. Altered behavioral responses mediated by serotonin receptors in the genetically dystonic (dt) rat. *Brain Res Bull* 1991;26:11–16.
40. Wiklund L, Björklund A, Sjölund B. The indolaminergic innervation of the inferior olive. I. Convergence with the direct spinal afferents in the areas projecting to the cerebellar anterior lobe. *Brain Res* 1977;131:1–21.
41. Wiklund L, Descarries L, Mollgard K. Serotoninergic axon terminals in the rat dorsal accessory olive: normal ultrastructure and light microscopic demonstration of regeneration after 5,6-dihydroxytryptamine lesioning. *J Neurocytol* 1981;10:1009–1027.
42. Young WS III, Kuhar MJ. A new method for receptor autoradiography: [^{3}H]opioid receptors in rat brain. *Brain Res* 1979;179:255–270.

Serotonin, the Cerebellum, and Ataxia, edited by P. Trouillas and K. Fuxe. Raven Press, Ltd., New York © 1993.

14
Effect of Chronic 5-HT Uptake Inhibition on Serotonergic Autoregulation

Chantal Moret and Mike Briley

Neurobiology Division I, Pierre Fabre Research Center, 81106 Castres, France

Neuronal firing and neurotransmitter release regulate, at least at the presynaptic level, the activity of the brain serotonergic neuron. Somatodendritic 5-HT$_{1A}$ autoreceptors, present in the raphe nucleus, are responsible for the modulation of neuronal firing, whereas 5-HT$_{1B}$ (or 5-HT$_{1D}$ in nonrodent species) autoreceptors, localized on terminals, play a role in the control of the release of the monoamine. When administered acutely, serotonin (5-HT) uptake inhibitors reduce neuronal firing; however, after chronic administration, this effect is attenuated or completely abolished, and neuronal firing returns to control values (11). Similarly, the behavioral response mediated by somatodendritic 5-HT autoreceptors has been shown to be attenuated by repeated administration of various 5-HT uptake inhibitors (17). It has been suggested by these authors that this reduction of effect could be explained by a desensitization of 5-HT$_{1A}$ somatodendritic autoreceptors. Interestingly this adaptive change operates over a period of time comparable to the onset of the therapeutic antidepressant effect of 5-HT uptake inhibitors.

The existence of presynaptic inhibitory serotonergic autoreceptors has been demonstrated in hypothalamic synaptosomes (10) and in cerebral cortex slices (2,18). The neurotransmitter regulates its own release via a negative feedback mechanism, mediated through the activation of presynaptic inhibitory autoreceptors (for review, see ref. 26). Using the technique described in this chapter, Langer and Moret (23) found that the 5-HT agonist lysergic acid diethylamide (LSD) inhibited 5-HT release elicited by electrical stimulation, whereas the 5-HT antagonist methiothepin increased it. In addition, the reduction by LSD was antagonized by methiothepin. Using this model, Langer and Moret (23) have shown that the specific 5-HT uptake inhibitor citalopram, when given alone, has no effect on the electrically evoked release of 5-HT, although it did decrease the inhibitory effect of LSD (23). Recent results have shown that a wide variety of antidepressants, which inhibit 5-HT uptake, also decreased the inhibition by LSD (6,15,28). Presynaptic inhibition by other 5-HT agonists, 5-methoxytryptamine (15) or dihydroergocristine (27), is similarly decreased by citalopram. None of these 5-HT uptake blockers, by themselves, modified the depolarization-induced release of 5-HT.

Thus, in view of the attenuation by 5-HT uptake inhibitors of the inhibitory effect of 5-HT agonists at the level of the terminal 5-HT autoreceptors *in vitro* and the desensitization of somatodendritic 5-HT$_{1A}$ autoreceptors obtained after chronic administration of 5-HT uptake blockers, it was considered of interest to study the effect of these compounds, given chronically, on the release of 5-HT and the sensitivity of the terminal 5-HT autoreceptors.

In addition to the modulation of neuronal firing and release of 5-HT, the regulation of 5-HT synthesis is another important control mechanism. Acute administration of 5-HT uptake inhibitors has been shown to decrease 5-HT synthesis (7,8,33). In addition, there appears to be a parallel between the potency to inhibit 5-HT uptake and the ability to decrease 5-HT synthesis. We have therefore extended our study of the effect of chronic 5-HT uptake blockade to include 5-HT synthesis as well. For both release and synthesis experiments, the uptake blocker citalopram was chosen.

METHODS

In Vitro Release Studies

Male Sprague-Dawley rats (Charles River, France), weighing 240 to 260 g at the beginning of the study (330–350 g at the end), were housed singly with a 12-hr light/dark cycle at 20°C with free access to food and water. The weight of animals in the control and treated groups evolved similarly throughout the study. Citalopram hydrobromide was incorporated in the food in proportions giving a mean consumption of 50 mg/kg per day. For the first 2 weeks, 22 g of reconstituted rat chow pellets were presented to each rat each day, and this amount was increased to 23 g for the last week. Both control and treated rats consumed the total amount of the food provided. The drug was administered for 21 days. Controls were fed the same quantity of a similarly prepared diet to which no drug was added. The drug-containing diet was replaced by the control diet 24 hr before sacrifice. At the end of the period of drug administration, there was no apparent difference in the physical state between control and treated animals.

At that time, animals were decapitated and their brains immediately removed and dissected. Slices of 0.4 mm thickness from the hypothalamus were incubated for 30 min at 37°C in Krebs solution containing 0.1 µM [^{3}H]5-HT creatinine sulfate (Amersham, France; specific activity, 10–20 Ci/mmol) and bubbled with a mixture of 95% O_2-5% CO_2. The composition of the Krebs solution was as follows (millimolar concentrations): NaCl 118.0; KCl 4.7; $CaCl_2$ 1.3; $MgCl_2$ 1.2; NaH_2PO_4 1.0; $NaHCO_3$ 25.0; glucose 11.1; disodium ethylenediamine tetraacetic acid (EDTA) 0.004; and ascorbic acid 0.11. At the end of the incubation period, single slices were transferred to glass chambers and superfused with Krebs solution, which was continuously oxygenated. The temperature of the superfusate was 37°C and the rate of superfusion was 0.5 ml/min. At 60 min (S_1) and 104 min (S_2) after the onset of superfusion, each slice was stimulated for 2 min by an electrical field generated in the chamber between two platinum electrodes (3 Hz, rectangular pulses of 20 mA current strength and 2-msec duration). Collection of samples of the superfusate Krebs solution began 8 min before the first period of electrical stimulation. The samples were collected at 4-min intervals. At the end of the experiment, the slices were solubilized with 0.5 ml Soluene 100 (Packard) and the radioactivity in the superfusate samples and the slices was determined by liquid scintillation spectrometry (Packard Tricarb 4640). The first stimulation period (S_1) was used as control and LSD was added to the superfusion medium 20 min before the second stimulation period (S_2) and remained present throughout the rest of the experiment. The amount of tritium released per 4-min sample was expressed as a fraction of the tritium content of the slice at the onset of the respective collection period. The overflow of tritium induced by electrical stimulation was calculated as the total increase of radioactivity above the resting outflow obtained in the sample immediately preceding the onset of stimulation (spontaneous release Sp_1 and Sp_2).

In order to quantify the changes in stimulated overflow of tritium induced by LSD, the ratio S_2/S_1 was calculated indicating the ratio of fractional release between the second and the first period of electrical stimulation. Statistical calculations were performed using the nonparametric Wilcoxon test. The statistical comparison of curves was carried out using the two-way analysis of variance (ANOVA). The following drugs were used: *d*-LSD bitartrate (Sandoz, Basel, Switzerland) and citalopram hydrobromide (Lundbeck, Copenhagen, Denmark).

In Vivo 5-HT Synthesis Studies

The *in vivo* activity of tryptophan hydroxylase in the frontoparietal cortex was determined by measuring the accumulation of 5-hydroxytryptophan (5-HTP) during 30 min after total inhibition of aromatic amino acid decarboxylase by *m*-hydroxybenzylhydrazine (NSD 1015) (9).

Experiments were carried out on male Sprague-Dawley rats (Janvier, France) weighing 200 to 220 g. Drugs were administered orally, 1 hr before the administration of NSD 1015 (100 mg/kg i.p.). Thirty minutes later the animals were decapitated, their brains immediately removed, placed in ice, and dissected to isolate the frontoparietal cortex. Tissue (about 100 mg) was homogenized in 0.2 N $HClO_4$ containing 0.019% $Na_2S_2O_5$ and 0.038% disodium EDTA using a Polytron (setting 7 for 15 sec). The suspension was centrifuged at 14,000 g for 20 min, the supernatants decanted and an aliquot of each sample was analyzed by high performance liquid chromatography (HPLC) with electrochemical detection for the determination of 5-HTP. The HPLC system consisted of Waters pump (model 510), automatic injector (Wisp 712), and a Baseline 810 chromatography workstation. The column was a Merck 12.5-cm, 5-μm reversed phase LiChrospher C18. Electrochemical detection was performed with a Waters detector (model 460) equipped with a glassy carbon working electrode maintained at a potential of $+0.75$ V. The mobile phase, which was delivered at a flow rate of 1 ml/min, consisted of 50 mM KH_2PO_4, 0.215 mM EDTA, 2.5 mM octylsulfonic acid, and 12.5% methanol, and the pH was adjusted to 2.65 with phosphoric acid.

For chronic treatments, rats were administered citalopram hydrobromide orally twice daily at 50 mg/kg per day for 21 days. Control animals received water. After a 24-hr washout, animals received an additional acute oral administration of citalopram (0, 1, 3, and 10 mg/kg). After 1 hr, they were injected with NSD 1015 (100 mg/kg i.p.). The rest of the experiment was the same as for acute administration described above.

Doses of drugs given in the text refer to the salt as listed above.

The significance of differences between control and treated animals in acute experiments was calculated by using the Wilcoxon's test. Data from chronic treatments were statistically analyzed by Student's t test or by ANOVA followed by Bonferroni's test to compare the experimental groups with their controls.

RESULTS

In Vitro Release Studies

In hypothalamic slices from rats treated with citalopram (50 mg/kg), the release of [^{3}H]5-HT induced by the first period of electrical stimulation (S_1) was significantly increased (54%) in comparison to control animals (Table 1). The spontaneous outflow of [^{3}H]5-HT was identical in both control and treated rats. The tissue radioactivity content prior to the first stimulation was slightly but significantly en-

TABLE 1. *Effect of chronic administration with citalopram on different parameters of [^{3}H]5-HT release*

	Control rats ($n = 29$)	Treated rats ($n = 30$)	% Change
S_1	1.36 ± 0.08	2.10 ± 0.11[a]	+54
Sp_1	1.97 ± 0.03	1.89 ± 0.03	−4
Tissue tritium content (nCi)	124 ± 3	131 ± 2[b]	+6

S_1 and Sp_1 (expressed as means ± SEM of percentages of total tissue radioactivity) represent the overflow induced by the first electrical stimulation and the resting outflow just preceding it, respectively. Tissue tritium content (expressed as means ± SEM, in nanocuries) represents the amount of tissue radioactivity per slice just preceding the first stimulation. Rats were administered for 21 days citalopram in their diet (50 mg/kg per day) with 24-hr washout. n = number of individual release experiments.

[a] $p < 0.001$ (Wilcoxon's test) when compared to the corresponding value of control rats.
[b] $p < 0.05$.
Adapted from ref. 29.

hanced (6%) in animals receiving citalopram, indicating that the uptake blocker was no longer present in the tissue at the moment of the experiment since this would have caused a decrease of tritium tissue content. In citalopram-administered animals, the concentration-effect curve of the 5-HT autoreceptor agonist LSD (0.01–1 µM), added before the second period of electrical stimulation (S_2), was significantly shifted to the right as compared to control animals (Fig. 1).

In Vivo 5-HT Synthesis Studies

Citalopram, when given acutely, reduced the accumulation of 5-HTP dose dependently (Fig. 2).

After chronic administration with citalopram, the basal accumulation of 5-HTP (no acutely added citalopram) was significantly increased in the treated rats in comparison to controls (Fig. 3). Following an additional acute administration with citalopram, 5-HTP accumulation was decreased similarly in both control and treated groups (Fig. 3).

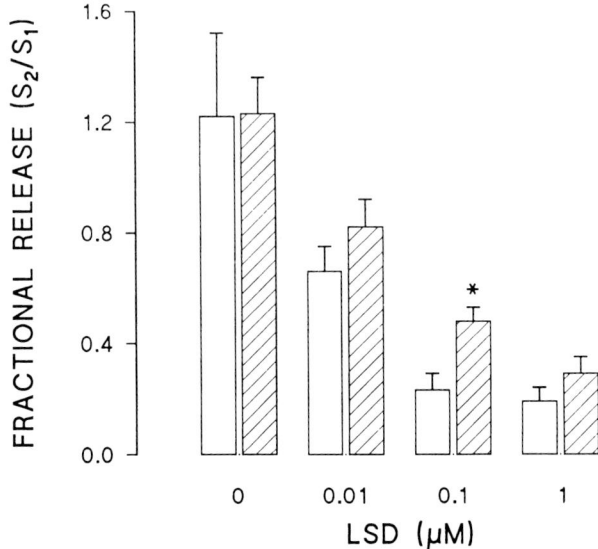

FIG. 1. Effect of repeated citalopram administration on the inhibition by LSD of electrically evoked release of [^{3}H]5-HT. Rats were administered in their diet 50 mg/kg per day citalopram with 24-hr washout. Ordinate: fraction of the total tissue radioactivity released by a 2-min period of electrical stimulation (3 Hz, 20 mA, 2 msec), expressed as the ratio S_2/S_1 obtained between the second period of stimulation in the presence of LSD (S_2) and the first control period (S_1), carried out within the same experiment. LSD was added to the superfusion medium 20 min before the second electrical stimulation. Shown are means ± SEM of at least five experiments per group. *Open* and *hatched columns* represent control and treated rats, respectively. *$p<0.02$ (Wilcoxon's test) when compared to the corresponding value in the control rats. The whole curves were significantly different (ANOVA) ($p<0.005$). (Adapted from ref. 29.)

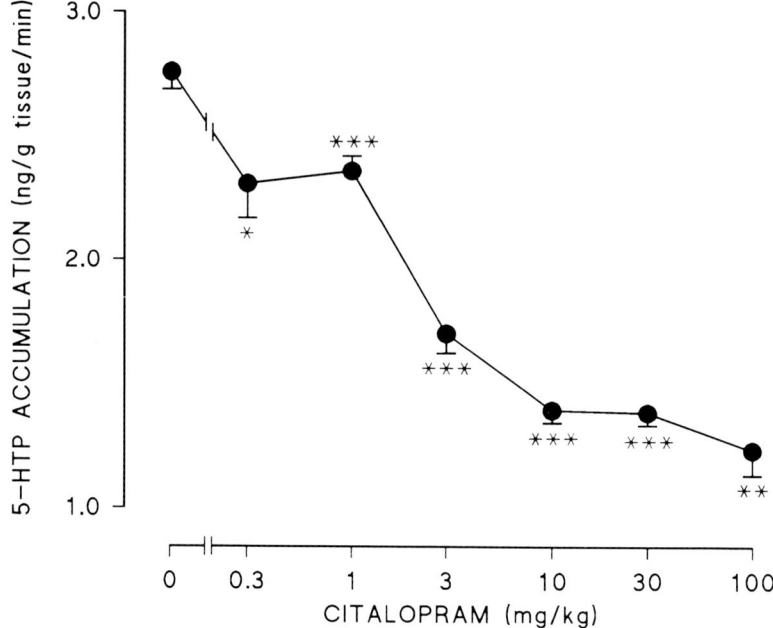

FIG. 2. Effect of citalopram on the accumulation of 5-HTP. Rats were administered citalopram orally at doses indicated in abscissa or water for control animals, and 60 min later all animals received NSD 1015 (100 mg/kg i.p.). After a further 30 min they were killed and the accumulation of 5-HTP determined in the frontoparietal cortex as described in the text. Ordinate represents the amount of 5-HTP formed over 30 min in nanograms per gram of tissue per minute. Values are means ± SEM of 4 to 21 animals. The SEM were always less than 15% of the mean values. *$p<0.05$; **$p<0.01$; ***$p<0.001$ when compared to the control value (Wilcoxon's test).

DISCUSSION

Citalopram, a clinically effective antidepressant (16,24,30), is a potent and selective 5-HT uptake blocking agent (21,22,31) that has no effect on the uptake of norepinephrine (19,21) and, after long-term administration, does not modify 5-HT$_2$ or dopamine D$_2$ or α$_1$- or β-adrenoceptors (1,22). In synaptosomes derived from rats treated acutely with citalopram, Maitre et al. (25) found an ED$_{50}$ value for 5-HT uptake inhibition of 5 mg/kg i.p. A similar value was obtained in rat platelets (25). Consequently the dose used in the present work (50 mg/kg p.o.) was sufficient to create a major reduction in the uptake of 5-HT. In rats, citalopram has a short half-life (about 3 hr), but high and fairly stable concentrations may be obtained by adding citalopram to the diet (13). A 24-hr washout period has been shown to be sufficient to reduce plasma levels to close to zero (13).

The effect of chronic administration with citalopram on both the release evoked by electrical depolarization and the sensitivity of the 5-HT autoreceptor to the agonist LSD may be satisfactorily explained by a single mechanism, namely, the syn-

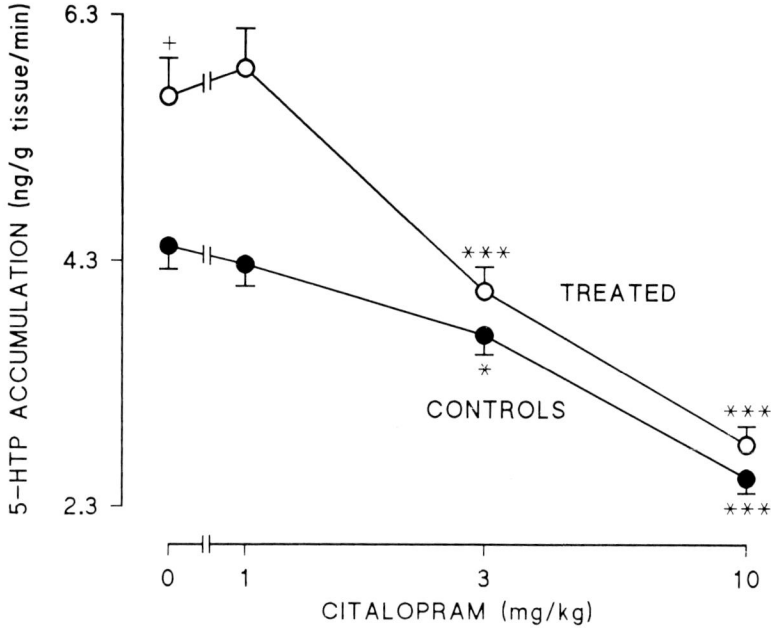

FIG. 3. Effect of a chronic administration with citalopram on the accumulation of 5-HTP. Rats were administered citalopram orally twice daily at 50 mg/kg per day for 21 days. Control rats received water. After 24 hr, they were administered citalopram orally at doses indicated in abscissa and 60 min later all animals received NSD 1015 (100 mg/kg i.p.). After a further 30 min, they were killed and accumulation of 5-HTP determined in the frontoparietal cortex as described in the text. Ordinate represents the amount of 5-HTP formed over 30 min in nanograms per gram of tissue per minute. Values are means ± SEM of 15 to 20 animals. +, $p<0.005$ when compared to the corresponding value in control rats (Student's t test). *$p<0.05$, ***$p<0.001$ when compared to the corresponding controls (ANOVA followed by Bonferroni's test).

aptic concentration of the neurotransmitter 5-HT, which is enhanced by the chronic blockade of uptake, desensitizes the 5-HT autoreceptor. The latter is thus less effective at decreasing 5-HT release through the negative feedback mechanism, which results in an increase in release at S_1. The effect is further demonstrated by the exogenous 5-HT autoreceptor agonist LSD, which acts on a less sensitive receptor with the result that the concentration-effect curve is shifted to the right. These results are compatible with electrophysiological data obtained after 14-day administration of citalopram where 5-HT neurotransmission was found to be enhanced by desensitization of both the somatodendritic and terminal 5-HT autoreceptors (11).

Similar results have been obtained in rat hypothalamic slices following long-term administration of amitriptyline (32). In rats treated with amitriptyline once daily for 21 days at 10 mg/kg i.p. with a 17-hr withdrawal, the electrically evoked overflow of [^{3}H]5-HT from hypothalamic slices was significantly increased compared to those from control rats (32). In addition, the modulatory effect of 5-HT itself or the autoreceptor antagonist methiothepin on the stimulation-induced release of [^{3}H]5-HT was completely abolished (32). Thus chronic amitriptyline appears to cause a downregulation of the terminal 5-HT autoreceptor similar to that obtained following prolonged treatment with citalopram.

Citalopram potently reduced 5-HT synthesis confirming the result already found by Carlsson and Lindqvist (8). It has been suggested by these authors that the inhibition of monoamine synthesis parallels the inhibition of monoamine uptake. Rapidly following the acute administration of a 5-HT uptake blocker, the firing of the raphe neurons is decreased (11) through the action of 5-HT on 5-HT$_{1A}$ autoreceptors. Similarly presynaptic autoreceptors situated on the serotonergic terminals are also activated by the transiently increased concentration of 5-HT and react to reduce 5-HT release and possibly synthesis. Whether the reduction in 5-HT synthesis represents an independent control system or simply reflects the rate of neuronal firing or the extent of 5-HT release remains to be determined. It is noteworthy to add here that electrical stimulation of the central serotonergic neurons increases 5-HT synthesis by activation of tryptophan hydroxylase (4,5,20).

After chronic administration with an uptake blocker, all three inhibitory effects on firing, synthesis, and release appear to be attenuated. This is presumably by desensitization (downregulation) of the respective receptors (3,11,29,33,34). This would allow the synaptic levels of the monoamine to rise with a subsequent increase in serotonergic activity, which is thought to be necessary for antidepressant action.

From the results obtained here with chronic administration with citalopram, it appears that synthesis is regulated by two independent mechanisms. The chronic presence of the compound increases basal 5-HT synthesis. This suggests that enzymatic induction occurs, due probably to chronic inhibition of the synthetic pathway. The second regulatory system that controls the inhibition of monoamine synthesis by the uptake blocker is unmodified by its chronic administration. This latter regulatory mechanism probably does not involve changes in enzyme levels since a reduction would probably require longer than 30 min. A receptor-mediated modulatory effect on the enzyme activity appears to be the most likely suggestion. It should be noted that Svensson (33) found that chronic administration with imipramine did not change the basal synthesis of 5-HT but attenuated the decrease of 5-HT synthesis following acute administration with imipramine, whereas a marked reduction of basal 5-HT synthesis was observed by Fuxe et al. (14) following long-term zimelidine treatment. The discrepancies between the various studies remain unexplained for the moment.

To what extent the control of monoamine synthesis is related to antidepressant action remains to be determined. It is, however, interesting to note that carbamazepine, a lithium-like mood stabilizer, has also been shown to decrease 5-HT synthesis (12).

In any pathology in which 5-HT is implicated, such as in depression, anxiety, obsessive compulsive disorder, and cerebellar ataxia, it is important to appreciate that the serotonergic system is highly regulated. The various regulatory mechanisms appear to be extremely potent since most "serotonergic drugs" such as antidepressants (e.g., fluoxetine), anxiolytics (e.g., buspirone), and antiobsessional drugs (e.g., clomipramine) are inactive acutely and need 3 to 6 weeks to be efficient therapeutically. It would appear that it is necessary to wait for an attenuation or desensitization of the regulatory mechanisms before the therapeutic agents are able to modify sufficiently the 5-HT system and obtain the therapeutic effect.

REFERENCES

1. Arnt J, Fredricson Overø K, Hyttel J, Olsen R. Changes in rat dopamine and serotonin function in vivo after prolonged administration of the specific 5-HT uptake inhibitor, citalopram. *Psychopharmacology* 1984;84:457–465.
2. Baumann PA, Waldmeier PC. Further evidence for negative feedback control of serotonin release in the central nervous system. *Naunyn Schmiedebergs Arch Pharmacol* 1981;317:36–43.
3. Blier P, de Montigny C, Chaput Y. Modifications of the serotonin system by antidepressant treatments: implications for the therapeutic response in major depression. *J Clin Psychopharmacol* 1987;6:24S–35S.
4. Boadle-Biber MC, Johannessen JN, Narasimhachari N, Phan T-H. Activation of tryptophan hydroxylase by stimulation of central serotonergic neurons. *Biochem Pharmacol* 1983;32:185–188.
5. Boadle-Biber MC, Johannessen JN, Narasimhachari N, Phan T-H. Tryptophan hydroxylase: increase in activity by electrical stimulation of serotonergic neurons. *Neurochem Int* 1986;8:83–92.
6. Briley M, Moret C. Modulation of 5-HT autoreceptors probably contributes to the antidepressant action of 5-HT uptake blockers. In: Briley M, Fillion G, eds. *New concepts in depression.* London: Macmillan, 1988:15–24.
7. Carlsson A. Effects of antidepressant agents on monoamine synthesis. In: *13th Symposium Medicum Hoechst, depressive disorders.* Rome, 1977:8–12.
8. Carlsson A, Lindqvist M. Effects of antidepressant agents on the synthesis of brain monoamines. *J Neural Transm* 1978;43:73–91.
9. Carlsson A, Davis JN, Kehr W, Lindqvist M, Atack CV. Simultaneous measurement of tyrosine and tryptophan hydroxylase activities in brain in vivo using an inhibitor of the aromatic amino acid decarboxylase. *Naunyn Schmiedebergs Arch Pharmacol* 1972;275:153–168.
10. Cerrito F, Raiteri M. Serotonin release is modulated by presynaptic autoreceptors. *Eur J Pharmacol* 1979;57:427–430.
11. Chaput Y, de Montigny C, Blier P. Effects of a selective 5-HT reuptake blocker, citalopram, on the sensitivity of 5-HT autoreceptors: electrophysiological studies in the rat brain. *Naunyn Schmiedebergs Arch Pharmacol* 1986;333:342–348.
12. Elphick M, Anderson SMP, Hallis KF, Grahame-Smith DG. Effects of carbamazepine on 5-hydroxytryptamine function in rodents. *Psychopharmacology* 1990;100:49–53.
13. Fredricson Overø K. Kinetics of citalopram in test animals; drug exposure in safety studies. *Prog Neuropsychopharmacol Biol Psychiatry* 1982;6:297–309.
14. Fuxe K, Ögren S-O, Agnati LF, Andersson K, Eneroth P. Effects of subchronic antidepressant drug treatment on central serotonergic mechanisms in the male rat. *Adv Biochem Psychopharmacol* 1982;31:91–107.
15. Galzin AM, Moret C, Verzier B, Langer SZ. Interaction between tricyclic and nontricyclic 5-hydroxytryptamine uptake inhibitors and the presynaptic 5-hydroxytryptamine inhibitory autoreceptors in the rat hypothalamus. *J Pharmacol Exp Ther* 1985;235:200–211.
16. Gastpar M, Gastpar G. Preliminary studies with citalopram (Lu 10–171), a specific 5-HT-reuptake inhibitor, as antidepressant. *Prog Neuropsychopharmacol Biol Psychiatry* 1982;6:319–325.
17. Goodwin GM, De Souza RJ, Green AR. Presynaptic serotonin receptor-mediated response in mice attenuated by antidepressant drugs and electroconvulsive shock. *Nature* 1985;317:531–533.
18. Göthert M, Weinheimer G. Extracellular 5-hydroxytryptamine inhibits 5-hydroxytryptamine release from rat brain cortex slices. *Naunyn Schmiedebergs Arch Pharmacol* 1979;310:93–96.
19. Hall H, Sällemark M, Wedel I. Acute effects of atypical antidepressants on various receptors in the rat brain. *Acta Pharmacol Toxicol* 1984;54:379–384.
20. Herr BE, Gallager DW, Roth RH. Tryptophan hydroxylase: activation in vivo following stimulation of central serotonergic neurons. *Biochem Pharmacol* 1975;24:2019–2023.

21. Hyttel J. Citalopram—pharmacological profile of a specific serotonin uptake inhibitor with antidepressant activity. *Prog Neuropsychopharmacol Biol Psychiatry* 1982;6:277–295.
22. Hyttel J, Fredricson Overø K, Arnt J. Biochemical effects and drug levels in rats after long-term treatment with the specific 5-HT-uptake inhibitor, citalopram. *Psychopharmacology* 1984;83:20–27.
23. Langer SZ, Moret C. Citalopram antagonizes the stimulation by lysergic acid diethylamide of presynaptic inhibitory serotonin autoreceptors in the rat hypothalamus. *J Pharmacol Exp Ther* 1982; 222:220–226.
24. Lindegaard Pedersen O, Kragh-Sørensen P, Bjerre M, Fredricson Overø K, Gram LF. Citalopram, a selective serotonin reuptake inhibitor, clinical antidepressive and long term effect—a phase II study. *Psychopharmacology* 1982;77:199–204.
25. Maitre L, Moser P, Baumann PA, Waldmeier PC. Amine uptake inhibitors: criteria of selectivity. *Acta Psychiatr Scand* 1980;61(suppl 280):97–110.
26. Moret C. Pharmacology of the serotonin autoreceptor. In: Green AR, ed. *Neuropharmacology of serotonin*. Oxford: Oxford University Press, 1985:21–49.
27. Moret C, Briley M. Dihydroergocristine-induced stimulation of the 5-HT autoreceptor in the hypothalamus of the rat. *Neuropharmacology* 1986;25:169–174.
28. Moret C, Briley M. Sensitivity of the response of 5-HT autoreceptors to drugs modifying synaptic availability of 5-HT. *Neuropharmacology* 1988;27:43–49.
29. Moret C, Briley M. Serotonin autoreceptor subsensitivity and antidepressant activity. *Eur J Pharmacol* 1990;180:351–356.
30. Øfsti E. Citalopram—a specific 5-HT-reuptake inhibitor—as an antidepressant drug: a phase II multicenter trial. *Prog Neuropsychopharmacol Biol Psychiatry* 1982;6:327–335.
31. Pawlowski L, Nowak G, Górka Z, Mazela H. Ro 11-2465 (cyan-imipramine), citalopram and their N-desmethyl metabolites: effects on the uptake of 5-hydroxytryptamine and noradrenaline in vivo and related pharmacological activities. *Psychopharmacology* 1985;86:156–163.
32. Schoups AA, De Potter WP. Species dependence of adaptations at the pre- and postsynaptic serotonergic receptors following long-term antidepressant drug treatment. *Biochem Pharmacol* 1988;37: 4451–4460.
33. Svensson TH. Attenuated feed-back inhibition of brain serotonin synthesis following chronic administration of imipramine. *Naunyn Schmiedebergs Arch Pharmacol* 1978;302:115–118.
34. Willner P. Antidepressants and serotonergic neurotransmission: an integrative review. *Psychopharmacology* 1985;85:387–404.

Serotonin, the Cerebellum,
and Ataxia, edited by
P. Trouillas and K. Fuxe.
Raven Press, Ltd., New York © 1993.

15

The Mouse 5-HT$_{1B}$ Serotonin Receptor: Cloning, Functional Expression, and Localization in Motor Control Centers

F. Saudou, L. Maroteaux, N. Amlaiky, U. Boschert, J. L. Plassat, and R. Hen

Laboratoire de Génétique Moléculaire des Eucaryotes du CNRS, INSERM U184 de Biologie Moléculaire et de Génie Génétique, Faculté de Médecine, 67085 Strasbourg, France

Serotonin (5-HT) is a neuromodulator that is involved in a variety of functions such as sleep, appetite, pain perception, and vascular contraction. This diversity of effects can be related to the fact that the serotoninergic neurons project into virtually all parts of the brain and spinal cord, although their cell bodies are concentrated in a limited area, the raphe nuclei. 5-HT activates multiple receptor subtypes that exhibit distinct pharmacological properties, signaling systems, and tissue distributions (for a review, see ref. 1). The 5-HT$_{1B}$ receptors have been identified in the rat and mouse brain where their highest density was found within the globus pallidus and the substantia nigra. However, they could not be detected in the brain of other species, including humans. These species contained instead 5-HT$_{1D}$ receptors that have a slightly different pharmacological profile but the same tissue distribution. It was therefore suggested that the 5-HT$_{1B}$ and 5-HT$_{1D}$ receptors correspond to species variants of a same receptor subtype. Both the 5-HT$_{1B}$ and the 5-HT$_{1D}$ receptors are negatively coupled with adenylate cyclase. The recent cloning of the 5-HT$_{1A}$, 5-HT$_{1C}$, and 5-HT$_2$ receptors has revealed that they belong to the large family of receptors that interact with G proteins and share a predicted seven-transmembrane domain structure (2). We have exploited the sequence homologies that exist between several members of this family to clone the gene encoding the mouse 5-HT$_{1B}$ receptor. Our results suggest that the 5-HT$_{1B}$ receptors are localized presynaptically on the terminals of striatal neurons and Purkinje cells.

MATERIALS AND METHODS

Isolation and Sequence of the 5-HT$_{1B}$ Genomic Clone

A nested PCR experiment was performed on mouse genomic DNA with the following oligonucleotides: 1, TACCTCGAGGTCGACGGTITG(C/T)TGG(C/T)TICCITT(C/T)TT; 2, AGAACTAGTGGTACCC(G/A)TIGT(G/A)TA(G/A/T)ATIA(C/T)IGG(G/A)TT; 3, AGAACTAGTGGTACCC(G/C)(T/A)(G/A)TTIAC(G/A)TAICCIA(A/G)CCA; 1 μg of DNA was annealed at 55°C and amplified at 72°C in the presence of 3 mM MgCl$_2$ for 20 cycles with primers 1 and 2, and for 20 more cycles with primers 1 and 3. The PCR products were cut with XhoI and KpnI cloned in the bluescript plasmid and sequenced. One of the deduced amino acid sequences resembled that of the RDC$_4$ receptor. The corresponding oligonucleotides were synthesized (TGGCCATGTGAAACCAGCAGGCATC; TTCCCTGGTGATGCCTATCGTAAG) and used to screen a mouse genomic library. The BglII-SacI fragment (Fig. 1) hybridizing with these two oligonucleotides was sequenced on both strands by the dideoxynucleotide technique using successive synthetic oligonucleotides.

Expression of the 5-HT$_{1B}$ Receptor in Cultured Cells

The BglII-SacI genomic fragment (Fig. 1) was inserted into the BglII and SacI sites of expression vector p513, which is a derivative of pSG5 (3) containing a multiple cloning site. The resulting recombinant was introduced into mouse NIH3T3 cells by calcium phosphate-mediated transfection, together with the recombinant pRSVneo, which encodes resistance to G418 (20 μg of 5-HT$_{1B}$ recombinant and 1 μg of pRSVneo per 10-cm dish). Transformed clones were selected in the presence of 0.5 mg/ml of G418. Isolated foci were amplified and tRNA was prepared and analyzed for expression of 5-HT$_{1B}$ mRNA. Two cell lines were selected that expressed high levels of 5-HT$_{1B}$ mRNA as determined by Northern blot analysis.

For transient expression of the 5-HT$_{1B}$ receptor, Cos-7 cells were transfected by the calcium phosphate technique with the 5-HT$_{1B}$ recombinant alone (20 μg per 10-cm dish) and analyzed 48 hr after transfection.

Radioligand Binding Assays

Membranes were prepared (4) and [^{3}H]5-HT binding assays and competition displacement experiments were performed as described in ref. 5.

cAMP Assays

Cells were seeded into 12-well plates at a density of approximately 3.10^5 cells per well, washed once with phosphate-buffered saline (PBS) and incubated for 15 min

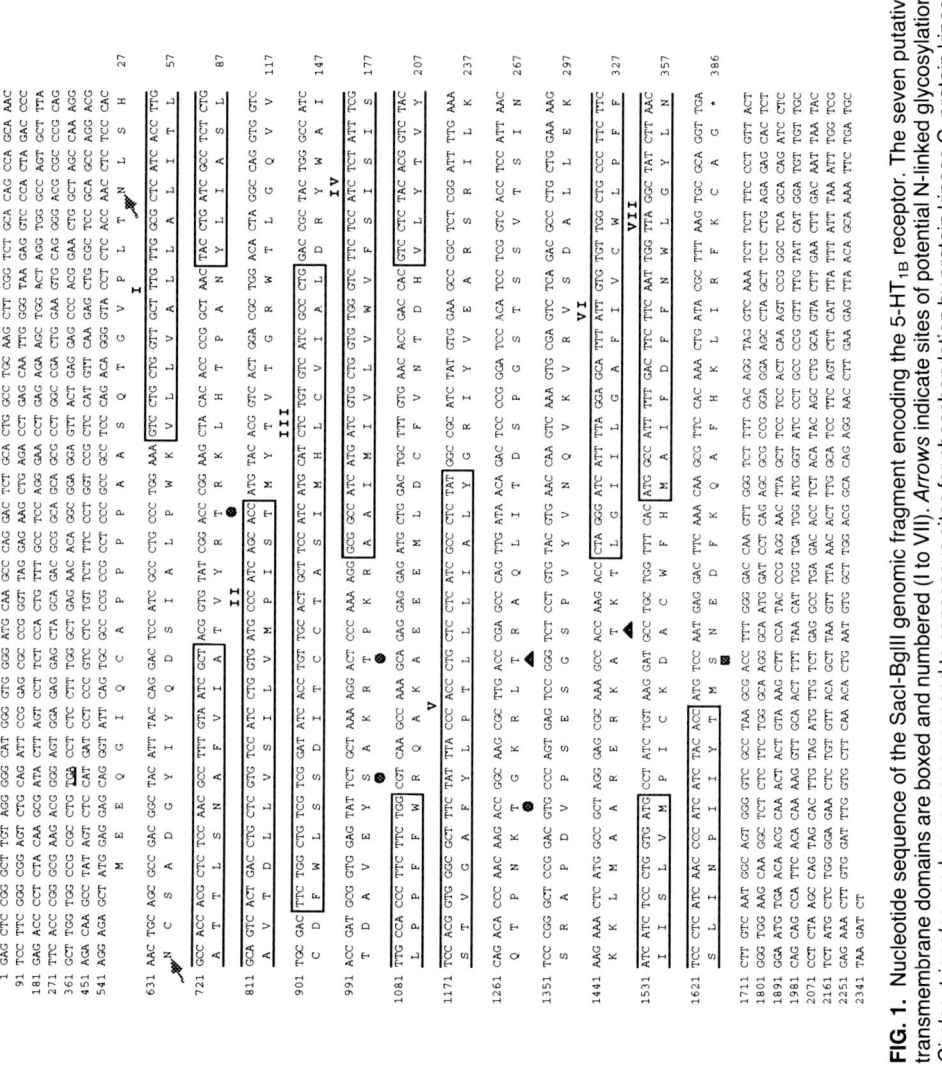

FIG. 1. Nucleotide sequence of the SacI-BglII genomic fragment encoding the 5-HT$_{1B}$ receptor. The seven putative transmembrane domains are boxed and numbered (I to VII). Arrows indicate sites of potential N-linked glycosylation. *Circles*, *triangles*, and *squares* correspond to consensus sites for phosphorylation by protein kinase C, protein kinase A, and tyrosine kinase, respectively.

at 37°C with 100 µM of isobutylmethylxanthine (IBMX) and test agents in PBS. The reaction was stopped by aspiration of the media, followed by the addition of 500 µl of ice-cold ethanol. After 2 hr at room temperature, the ethanol was collected and lyophilized. The pellet was reconstituted and cAMP was quantitated using a radioimmunoassay kit (NEN: NEK-033). The basal level of cAMP observed in the absence of drugs was about the same in all cell lines ($\approx$300 pmoles/mg of protein). Forskolin (1 µM) typically yielded a 10-fold increase in cAMP levels.

RNA Analysis

PolyA$^+$ mRNA was prepared, fractionated on 1% agarose-formaldehyde gel, and transferred to a nitrocellulose filter. The DNA probe was the BglII-SacI fragment, which was [^{32}P]-labeled by random priming and hybridized to filters at high stringency (42°C, 50% formamide, 5xSSC, 1xDenhardt's, 20 mM sodium phosphate buffer pH 6.5, 0.1% SDS, 100 µg/ml tRNA). Washings were performed at high stringency (60°C, 0.1xSSC, 0.1% SDS).

In Situ *Hybridization*

In situ hybridization was performed on cryostat sections of adult mouse brains (about 8 weeks old) as described in ref. 6. The probe used was the 5-HT$_{1B}$ BglII-SacI genomic fragment labeled by random priming with [^{35}S]ATP. Slides were exposed for 10 days.

RESULTS

Isolation of a Mouse Genomic Clone Encoding a New Member of the G Protein-Coupled Receptor Family

Sequence comparisons of G protein-coupled receptors have revealed a striking amino acid sequence conservation particularly in certain putative transmembrane domains such as domains VI and VII. We decided therefore to use degenerate oligonucleotides corresponding to these two regions to perform a series of PCR experiments on mouse genomic DNA. The resulting fragments were subcloned and sequenced. One of these fragments was used to screen a mouse genomic library. We obtained two phage recombinants that contained a 2.3 kbp long BglII-SacI fragment (Fig. 1) hybridizing with the PCR product. Sequence analysis of this fragment revealed one long open reading frame encoding a predicted protein that exhibited highest homology to the rat 5-HT$_{1A}$ serotoninergic receptor (47%) (7) and to a putative dog receptor RDC4 (59%) (8). The hydropathy analysis of this predicted protein revealed seven hydrophobic domains (numbered I to VII in Fig. 1), a feature shared by all other cloned members of the G protein-coupled receptor family. The amino-terminal end contained two putative sites for N-linked glycosylation, and the presumed cytoplasmic domains contained several consensus sites for phosphorylation by protein kinase C and A (Fig. 1).

New Receptor Has the Same Pharmacological Profile as the 5-HT$_{1B}$ Receptor

To determine whether the genomic fragment that we had isolated encoded a functional receptor, we introduced it into an eukaryotic expression vector and transfected Cos-7 cells with the resulting recombinant. Membranes of transfected cells were then assayed for their ability to bind a number of serotoninergic radioligands. While [^{125}I]LSD, [^{3}H]ketanserin, and [^{3}H]8-hydroxy-2-(di-n-propylamino)tetralin ([^{3}H]8-OH-DPAT) did not bind to these membranes, [^{3}H]5-HT displayed a single saturable binding site: $K_D = 48$ nM and $B_{max} = 19$ pmol/mg of membrane protein (not shown). In a control experiment, [^{3}H]5-HT did not bind to mock-transfected Cos-7 cells. To determine the pharmacological profile of this receptor, bound [^{3}H]5-HT was displaced with various serotoninergic drugs. These compounds displayed the following rank order of potencies: cyanopindolol>5-carboxamidotryptamine (5-CT) = RU24969>5-HT>(−)pindolol (Table 1). Ketanserin, mianserin, yohimbine, spiperone, and 8-OH-DPAT were almost inactive. This profile corresponds well with that of the rat brain 5-HT$_{1B}$ receptor (Table 1).

5-HT Inhibits Adenylate Cyclase in NIH3T3 Cells Expressing the 5-HT$_{1B}$ Receptor

To analyze the coupling of the 5-HT$_{1B}$ receptor to the second messenger machinery, we generated stable clonal cell lines expressing this receptor. In two independent cell lines expressing high levels of 5-HT$_{1B}$ mRNA, 5-HT mediated a decrease in forskolin-stimulated cAMP levels, while it had no effect on control NIH3T3 cells. This decrease in cAMP level was concentration dependent and saturable, the EC$_{50}$ for 5-HT being $1.4 \; 10^{-8}$ M (Fig. 2). Two other 5-HT$_{1B}$ agonists, 5-CT and RU24969, also induced a decrease in cAMP levels with EC$_{50}$ of 8.10^{-9} M and 5.10^{-9} M, respectively (Table 1). The effect of 5-HT could be blocked by cyanopindolol and methiothepin, which are 5-HT$_{1B}$ antagonists. The resulting EC$_{50}$ and K_I values (Table 1) are in good agreement with those we obtained in binding assays and with the values reported in rat substantia nigra for the 5-HT$_{1B}$ receptor (9). Pertussis toxin blocked the effect of 5-HT (Fig. 2), indicating that the 5-HT$_{1B}$ receptor is coupled to a pertussis toxin-sensitive G protein.

The 5-HT$_{1B}$ Receptor Is Expressed Predominantly in the Striatum and Cerebellum

Expression of 5-HT$_{1B}$ transcripts was analyzed by Northern blot and by *in situ* hybridization experiments. The Northern analysis revealed that expression was pre-

TABLE 1. Pharmacological profile of the 5-HT$_{1B}$ receptor

Drugs	Binding: pK_D'		Cyclase: pEC$_{50}$ or pK_I	
	Mouse 5-HT$_{1B}$ (Cos-7 cells)	Rat 5-HT$_{1B}$ (cortex)	Mouse 5-HT$_{1B}$ (NIH3T3 cells)	Rat 5-HT$_{1B}$ (substantia nigra)
Agonist				
5-HT	7.4 (4)	7.6	7.8 (3)	7.8
5-CT	8.0 (3)	8.3	8.1 (2)	7.9
RU24969	8.0 (3)	8.4	8.3 (2)	8.4
Antagonist				
Cyanopindolol	8.6 (3)	8.3	8.8 (3)	8.2
Methiothepin	—	7.3	8.4 (2)	8.1
(-)Pindolol	7.2 (2)	7.2	—	6.8
Mianserin	5.4 (2)	5.3	—	5.9
Ketanserin	5.2 (2)	—	—	—
Yohimbine	4.7 (2)	5.5	—	6.1
Spiperone	4.6 (2)	5.3	—	4.4
8-OH-DPAT	4.5 (2)	4.2	—	4.8

Binding data correspond to competition for [^{3}H]5-HT binding to membranes of Cos-7 cells expressing the mouse 5-HT$_{1B}$ receptor. IC$_{50}$ values required to displace 50% of [^{3}H]5-HT were determined experimentally and converted to pK_D' values according to the equation $K_D' = IC_{50}/(1 + C/K_D)$, where C is the [^{3}H]5-HT concentration (25 nM) and K_D is the equilibrium dissociation constant of [^{3}H]5-HT (48 nM). Cyclase data were obtained with an NIH3T3-derived cell line expressing the mouse 5-HT$_{1B}$ receptor. EC$_{50}$ is the concentration of agonist required to obtain a half maximal inhibition of forskolin-stimulated adenylate cyclase. The concentrations of antagonist required to inhibit the effect of 5-HT by 50% (IC$_{50}$) were determined and converted to pK_I values according to the equation $K_I = IC_{50}/(1 + C/K_D)$, where C is the 5-HT concentration (100 nM) and K_D is the EC$_{50}$ value for 5-HT (14 nM). Binding and cyclase data were compared to those reported in rat cortex and rat substantia nigra (9). Numbers in parentheses correspond to the number of independent experiments performed. The values presented are the mean of at least two independent experiments with each point performed in triplicate. Individual K_D', EC$_{50}$, and K_I values differed by less than 20%.

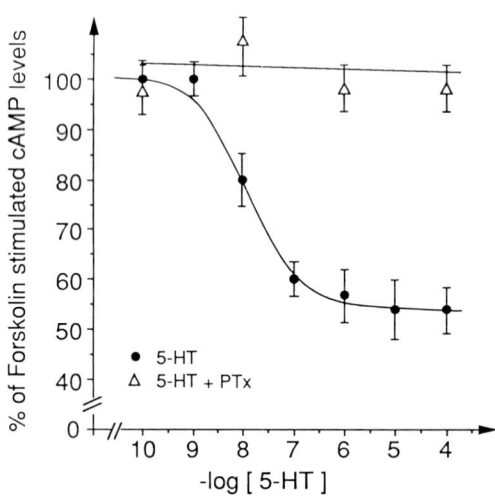

FIG. 2. 5-HT-induced decrease in cAMP levels in NIH3T3 cells expressing the 5-HT$_{1B}$ receptor. cAMP levels were expressed as a percentage of the value obtained with 1 μM for forskolin (100%). Data are the mean of three independent experiments with each point performed in triplicate. ●, 5-HT + forskolin; Δ, 5-HT + forskolin + pertussis toxin (PTx). Pertussis toxin was applied at a concentration of 100 ng/ml, 20 hr before the addition of 5-HT and forskolin.

dominant in nervous tissue. A 6-kb transcript was detected in the forebrain, hindbrain, cerebellum, and spinal cord (Fig. 3 and results not shown). To further analyze the pattern of expression of this receptor, we performed *in situ* hybridization experiments on brain sections (Fig. 4). The main sites of expression were the caudate-putamen and the Purkinje cells of the cerebellum. Weaker signals were also detected in the hippocampus, raphe nuclei, lateral septum, subthalamic nuclei, cingulate cortex, and entorhinal cortex. In a control experiment performed in the same conditions with plasmid DNA fragments instead of the 5-HT$_{1B}$ genomic fragment, no hybridization was observed.

DISCUSSION

Our binding and cyclase data indicate that the genomic clone that we have isolated encodes a functional mouse 5-HT$_{1B}$ receptor. This receptor exhibits a high degree of homology to a putative dog serotoninergic receptor RDC4 (59%) (8), which has been isolated but not characterized. However, it is unlikely that RDC4 is the dog counterpart of the mouse 5-HT$_{1B}$ receptor because, in the cases known so far, receptor subtypes exhibit an even higher degree of conservation across mammalian species, usually 85% to 95% amino acid homology. RCD4 corresponds probably to a "5-HT$_{1B}$-like" receptor.

The pattern of expression of the 5-HT$_{1B}$ mRNA indicates that a large proportion of the 5-HT$_{1B}$ receptors are located postsynaptically with respect to the afferent serotoninergic fibers originating in the raphe nuclei. Only the transcripts expressed in the raphe nuclei (Fig. 4A and B) correspond to receptors localized on the serotoninergic neurons or autoreceptors. Such autoreceptors have been proposed to modulate the release of 5-HT from the terminals of serotoninergic neurons (see ref. 1 for a review).

The main sites of expression of 5-HT$_{1B}$ mRNA are the striatum (caudate-putamen) and the Purkinje cells of the cerebellum (Fig. 4). The comparison between this

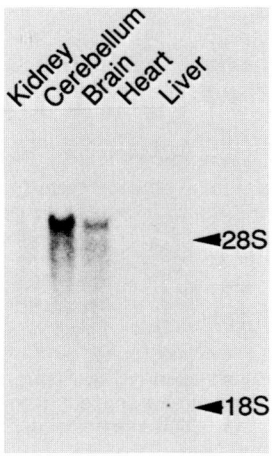

FIG. 3. Distribution of 5-HT$_{1B}$ transcripts. Northern blot analysis of polyA$^+$ RNA (5 μg) from various organs. A 6-kb RNA is detected in cerebellum and total brain and very faintly in kidney. The probe used is the [^{32}P]-labeled SacI-BglII fragment.

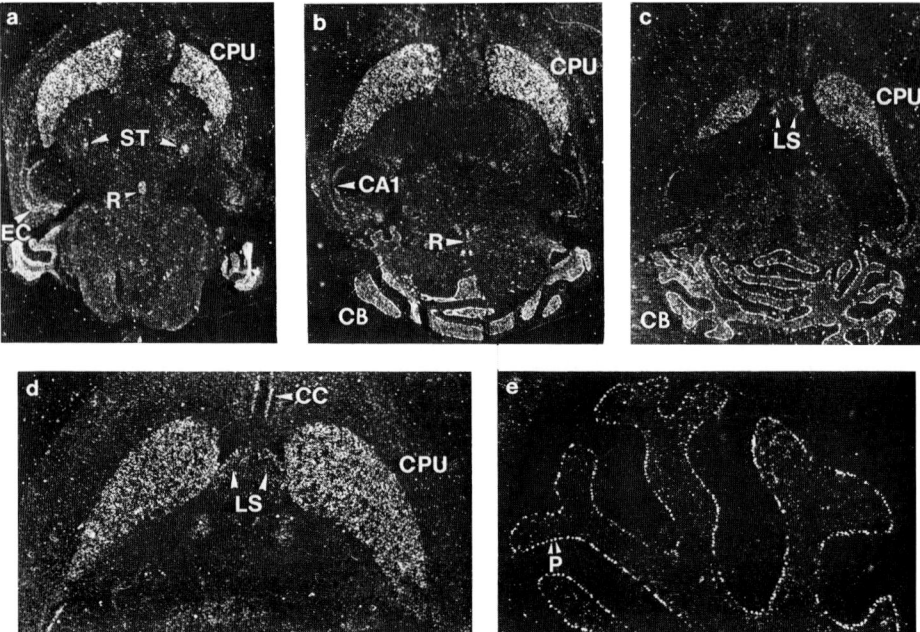

FIG. 4. *In situ* hybridization to mouse brain horizontal sections. **a–c:** Dark-field pictures of successively more dorsal sections of a whole brain (8 mm wide). **d:** 1.5 magnification (compared to a–c) of the striatal region at a depth intermediate between that of panels b and c. **e:** Fourfold magnification (compared to panels a–c) of a cerebellar region at about the same depth as c. CPU, caudate-putamen; CB, cerebellum; CC, cingulate cortex CA1, hippocampal area; EC, entorhinal cortex; LS, lateral septum; P, Purkinje cells; R, raphe nuclei; ST, subthalamic nuclei.

mRNA pattern and the pattern of the 5-HT$_{1B}$ binding sites determined by autoradiography is indicative of the pre- or postsynaptic localization of this receptor. The 5-HT$_{1B}$ binding sites were found mostly in the globus pallidus and substantia nigra (10) and to a lesser extent in the caudate-putamen. In contrast, 5-HT$_{1B}$ transcripts were detected in the caudate-putamen but not in the globus pallidus and substantia nigra. Since most efferent fibers from the caudate-putamen project to the globus pallidus and substantia nigra, it is likely that the 5-HT$_{1B}$ receptors present in the globus pallidus and substantia nigra are localized presynaptically on the terminals of projecting striatal neurons. In good agreement with this hypothesis is the observation that experimental or pathological lesions of the caudate-putamen, such as those observed in Huntington's chorea (11,12), result in a decrease in 5-HT$_{1B/1D}$ sites not only in the caudate-putamen but also in the globus pallidus and substantia nigra. The presynaptic localization of these 5-HT$_{1B}$ receptors suggests that they might modulate the release of neurotransmitters such as gamma-aminobutyric acid (GABA), substance P, or enkephalins from striatal neuron terminals. Interestingly, the dopamine D1 receptors that have been reported to stimulate GABA release in the substantia nigra (13) are also localized presynaptically on projecting striatal neurons (14). Since D1 receptors activate adenylate cyclase, while 5-HT_{1B} receptors are negatively coupled to adenylate cyclase, it is possible that these two receptors modulate GABA release in opposite ways in the substantia nigra.

The other main site of expression of 5-HT_{1B} transcripts is the Purkinje cells. 5-HT_{1B} binding sites have been detected in the deep nuclei of the cerebellum, which contain the Purkinje cell terminals (10). These 5-HT_{1B} sites could therefore correspond again to presynaptic receptors modulating GABA release from Purkinje cells.

The expression of 5-HT_{1B} receptors in the striatum, subthalamic nuclei, and cerebellum, which are brain structures involved predominantly in movement control, suggests a role for this receptor in motor function. Some experimental data, such as an increase in locomotor activity after administration of 5-HT_{1B} agonists to rats (15), support this hypothesis. It might therefore be interesting to investigate the effects of 5-HT_{1B} selective drugs in the treatment of motor disorders of the striatum and cerebellum such as Huntington's chorea and cerebellar ataxias. The availability of a cell line expressing high levels of this receptor subtype should facilitate the development of new 5-HT_{1B} agonists and antagonists. The 5-HT_{1B} genomic clone will also allow us via gene targeting techniques to produce mouse mutants and to analyze the consequences of these mutations on the physiology of the animal.

ACKNOWLEDGMENTS

We thank A. Staub and F. Ruffenach for making the oligonucleotides and D. Kauffmann and E. Rauscher for typing the manuscript. We are grateful to G. Gombos, J. de Barry, and C. Mendelsohn for valuable discussions. This work was supported by grants from CNRS, INSERM, the Association pour la recherche contre le cancer, and Rhône-Poulenc Rorer.

REFERENCES

1. Frazer A, Maayani S, Wolfe BB. *Annu Rev Pharmacol Toxicol* 1990;30:307–348.
2. Julius D. *Annu Rev Neurosci* 1991;14:335–360.
3. Green S, Isseman I, Sheer E. *Nucleic Acid Res* 1988;16:369–370.
4. Amlaiky N, Caron MG. *J Biol Chem* 1985;260:1983–1986.
5. Waeber C, Schoeffter P, Palacios JM, Hoyer D. *Naunyn Schmiedebergs Arch Pharmacol* 1989; 340:479–485.
6. Hafen E, Levine M, Garber RL, Gehring WJ. *EMBO J* 1983;2:617–623.
7. Fargin A, Raymond JR, Lohse MJ, Kolbika BK, Caron MG, Lefkowitz RJ. *Nature* 1988;335:358–360.
8. Libert F, Parmentier M, Lefort A, et al. *Science* 1989;244:569–572.
9. Shoeffter P, Hoyer D. *Naunyn Schmiedebergs Arch Pharmacol* 1989;340:285–292.
10. Pazos A, Palacios JM. *Brain Res* 1985;346:205–230.
11. Waeber C, Zhang L, Palacios JM. *Brain Res* 1990;528:197–206.
12. Waeber C, Palacios JM. *Neuroscience* 1989;32:337–347.
13. Reubi JC, Iversen L, Jessel T. *Nature* 1977;258:652–654.
14. Fremeau RT, Duncan GE, Fornaretto MG, et al. *Proc Natl Acad Sci USA* 1991;88:3772–3776.
15. Oberlander C, Demassey Y, Verdu A, van de Velde D, Bardeley C. *Eur J Pharmacol* 1987;139: 205–214.

Serotonin, the Cerebellum, and Ataxia, edited by P. Trouillas and K. Fuxe. Raven Press, Ltd., New York © 1993.

16

Multiple Actions of Serotonin on the Electrophysiology of Purkinje Cells

Howard K. Strahlendorf and Jean C. Strahlendorf

Departments of Neurology and Physiology, Texas Tech University Health Sciences Center, Lubbock, Texas 79430

The existence of a moderately dense serotonergic innervation to the cerebellar cortex and deep nuclei is now unequivocal. A number of studies using histofluorescence, autoradiography, and immunohistochemistry (3–5,24; see other chapters in this volume) have revealed the cortical serotonergic projection to consist of parallel-like fibers, diffuse meandering, varicose fibers lacking specific synaptic appositions, and a plexus of serotonergic fibers investing the Purkinje cell (PC) layer. Using the combined techniques of retrograde transport of horseradish peroxidase (HRP) with the peroxidase-antiperoxidase (PAP) reaction, Bishop and Ho (3) reported that serotonin (5-HT)-positive fibers were located in the PC layer and formed a moderately dense plexus immediately subjacent to PC bodies, extending upward to circumscribe individual Purkinje soma. It has been suggested that nonsynaptic transmission does not code for rapid, phasic information; it may represent an intermediate mode of communication whose function may be regulatory, modulating background neuronal activity (4). Thus, 5-HT may function to set, bias, or fine-tune membrane conductances of PCs to augment or depress the output of the cerebellar cortex.

The classical view that a neurotransmitter acts to change the excitability of a target cell by simply increasing or decreasing the polarization of the resting neuronal membrane has undergone significant revision in recent years. Biogenic amines such as norepinephrine (NE) and 5-HT are now known to subtly affect voltage-dependent ionic currents active at or near the resting potential. These currents are several orders of magnitude less than those affected by more traditional neurotransmitters such as glutamate and glycine and play a critical role in determining the characteristics and pattern of cell firing. Thus actions of these biogenic amines can profoundly influence the input-output relationships of these neurons and are best described as neuromodulation. Moreover, existence of both convergence and divergence in the action of neurotransmitters (neuromodulators) can result in remarkable diversity in neuronal signaling. For example, recent studies on the action of neuromodulators on hippocampal pyramidal cells indicate that different membrane receptors that use either the same or different coupling mechanisms and second messengers converge onto the same ion channel (1,16). Multiple neurotransmitter actions may be a consequence of receptor promiscuity in which a single receptor may couple to two or more G-proteins in the same cell membrane. Conversely, virtually all neuromodulators act on more than one distinct receptor subtype coupled to different ion channels (possibly via different second messengers) on the same cell (16).

Modulation of voltage-dependent currents allows fine control of various aspects of cell excitability via multiple mechanisms. For example, in hippocampal neurons (6), voltage-clamp analysis has revealed separate and possibly simultaneous effects of 5-HT on three distinct ionic currents, mediated by at least two receptor subtypes, that are dependent on agonist concentrations. Two of these actions result in increased cell excitability, while the other decreases excitability. Similar complexities of action of 5-HT undoubtedly exist in other areas of the nervous system such as the cerebellum.

The characteristic firing pattern of PCs *in vivo* consists of trains of rapid simple spikes, arising presumably from afferent volleys on the parallel fibers, interrupted periodically by complex spikes induced by climbing fiber input. *In vitro* recordings from PCs grown in culture (9) or from slices (7,8,10,11,13,14,19) reveal, in the absence of any afferent input, spontaneous rhythmic pacemaker-like activity consisting of somatic Na^+ spikes and dendritic Ca^{2+} spikes. Many PCs also exhibit oscillatory or cyclic firing in which trains of Na^+ and Ca^{2+} spikes lasting 10 to 20 sec are interrupted by quiescent periods lasting equally as long, whereas more hyperpolarized cells display no spontaneous activity until depolarized by, for example, intracellular current injection. In addition to the voltage-dependent Na^+ and K^+ (delayed rectifier) currents responsible for the fast Na^+ action potentials, the following currents exist in PCs and collectively determine the overall spectrum of spontaneous activity: a high-threshold Ca^{2+} current (Ca^{2+}-dependent action potential, and activation of Ca^{2+}-dependent K^+ [$I_{k,Ca}$]); a noninactivating Ca^{2+} current (Ca^{2+}-dependent plateau potential); a low-threshold Ca^{2+} current (spontaneous pacemaker potentials and activation of $I_{k,Ca}$ partially functioning at rest); a noninactivating Na^+ current (Na^+-dependent plateau potential); Ca^{2+}-activated K^+ currents (action potential repolarization, fast afterhyperpolarization following an action potential); a transient K^+ current similar to I_A described in other cells (determinant of interspike interval); an inward rectifying nonselective cationic current activated by hyperpolarization and similar to I_Q and I_h that also may have a small $I_{k,Ca}$ component at rest (contributes to the low resting potential and cell excitability) and voltage-independent Na^+ and K^+ currents active of rest (leak currents) (7–11,13,14,19). Thus, PCs present a host of membrane ionic currents that can conceivably serve as targets for putative neuromodulators such as 5-HT.

ACTIONS OF 5-HT ON PURKINJE CELLS

Extracellular Recordings

The function of the raphe projection to the cat cerebellum was examined by electrical activation of cells in the raphe centralis inferior (20). This manipulation predominantly produced inhibition preceded occasionally by a period of entrainment or excitation and, in some instances, only excitation. Therefore, electrical activation of neurons in the vicinity of the raphe centralis inferior elicited both excitatory and inhibitory responses of cerebellar PCs.

Subsequent studies in our laboratory were designed to determine the effects of iontophoretically applied 5-HT and purported 5-HT antagonists on spontaneously discharging PCs (21). It was shown that in rats 5-HT elicited one of three effects: inhibition (62% of cells), transient inhibition followed by excitation, termed biphasic (27% of cells), or excitation only (11% of cells). We have sought to identify which 5-HT receptor subtypes are responsible for the direct effects of 5-HT on PCs either *in situ* or *in vitro* using the cerebellar slice technique. Three findings have allowed us to conclude that involvement of $5-HT_2$ receptors in mediating the actions of 5-HT on PCs is insignificant: (i) the inability to detect any antagonist action of ketanserin on the direct effects of 5-HT; (ii) the inactivity of the selective $5-HT_2$ agonist 1-(2,5-dimethoxy-4-iodophenyl)-2-aminopropane (DOI), and (iii) evidence showing negligible $5-HT_2$ receptor binding in the cerebellar cortex (17). We have shown that inhibition is mimicked by specific $5-HT_{1A}$ agonists, 8-hydroxy-2-(di-n-propylamino)tetralin (8-OH-DPAT) and ipsapirone. Iontophoretically applied 8-OH-DPAT and ipsapirone both produced significant dose-dependent inhibitions of PC discharge.

Serotonergic antagonists were administered to characterize the 5-HT receptor subtype mediating the observed responses. 5-HT-mediated inhibitions were either not affected or augmented in the presence of iontophoretic and systemic methysergide; however, the antagonist blocked or decreased 5-HT-elicited excitation and, on occasion, reversed the excitatory effect of 5-HT to inhibition. Similar results were obtained with iontophoretically applied metergoline. In contrast, iontophoretic application of spiperone attenuated 5-HT-induced depression. Spiperone blocked the inhibitory effects of 8-OH-DPAT and ipsapirone. The mixed $5-HT_{1A}/5-HT_{1B}$ selective compounds TFMPP (*m*-trifluoromethylphenylpiperazine) and 5-CT (5-carboxamidotryptamine) produced inhibitory and excitatory effects similar to those of 5-HT; the inhibitory effects were reduced by spiperone. These results suggest that 5-HT-induced inhibition of PC firing is at least partially mediated through the $5-HT_{1A}$ receptor subtype. Although 5-HT-mediated excitation is blocked by classical 5-HT antagonists, we have failed to mimic excitation with any of the available 5-HT selective ligands.

The spontaneous discharge rate of PCs apparently is one factor that predisposes a PC to a particular effect of 5-HT. Specifically, cells that responded to 5-HT with an increase in firing rate had a consistently slower predrug firing frequency (40 Hz) than those cells that were suppressed by 5-HT (51 Hz). We have shown that with increasing firing rates the proportion of cells excited by 5-HT decreased, and the proportion of cells depressed increased. Furthermore, a statistically significant correlation between the spontaneous discharge rates of cells displaying excitation and the percentage of increase in the number of spikes per second in response to 5-HT was evident (21). These results strongly suggest that the overall qualitative effect of 5-HT is to set PCs at a preferred firing rate. One hypothesis is that PCs have excitatory and inhibitory receptors for 5-HT and that neuronal responses to iontophoretically applied 5-HT are a consequence of the interaction of 5-HT with multiple receptors. The relationship between excitatory and inhibitory receptors is determined by the firing rate of the neuron; slow discharge rates favor the functional dominance of excitatory receptors, whereas higher rates favor the activation of inhibitory receptors. Another possibility is that the effects of 5-HT may reflect an action of this amine on transmitter-activated voltage-sensitive ionic channels that are differentially sensitive to concentrations of 5-HT.

Additionally, 5-HT exerts potent modulatory effects on amino acid transmitters of the cerebellum. Increased firing in response to excitatory amino acids is blocked by 5-HT without apparent actions on baseline membrane properties or firing (12; see Chapter 17, this volume). Conversely, inhibition of firing by gamma-aminobutyric acid (GABA), muscimol, or baclofen is augmented by 5-HT in a manner inconsistent with additive actions of two inhibitory compounds (22).

In summary, we have shown that 5-HT exerts a complex action on PCs consisting of excitation, inhibition, or a biphasic response (21). The direct effects of 5-HT vary from cell to cell and are correlated with the baseline firing rate (21). In addition to its direct actions, 5-HT modulates the actions of other amino acid transmitters such as glutamate and GABA. A more complete review of these studies has recently appeared (23).

Intracellular Studies

Current Clamp

We studied the effects of 5-HT in the *in vitro* cerebellar slice preparation using intracellular recordings. PCs display characteristic somatic and dendritic action potentials that occur spontaneously or following DC stimulation. With increasing distance of the recording electrode from the soma, the fast somatic Na^+ spikes are reduced in amplitude due to electrotonic spread, whereas the slow rising dendritic Ca^{2+} spikes or bursts are more prominent. Basically, we have encountered three types of PCs: (i) cells that display a hyperpolarized resting membrane potential and do not display spontaneous activity, (ii) cells that are spontaneously active and display either Na^+ or Ca^{2+} action potentials or a combination of the two, and (iii) cells displaying oscillatory activity. The average resting membrane potential of non-spiking cells was -56.6 ± 1.8 mV, and the apparent input resistance averaged 30.6 ± 4.0 MΩ. Sixty-eight percent of PCs responded to 5-HT (50–200 μM), with a hyperpolarization averaging 5.1 ± 0.7 mV (Fig. 1B). On the other hand, 5-HT depolarized 32% of PCs by an average of 6.0 ± 1.9 mV (Fig. 1A). In these cells, effects on apparent input resistance were variable, with increases and decreases observed for both directions of polarizations. Qualitatively, these results correlate with our previously reported effects of 5-HT on the extracellularly recorded firing rate of PCs.

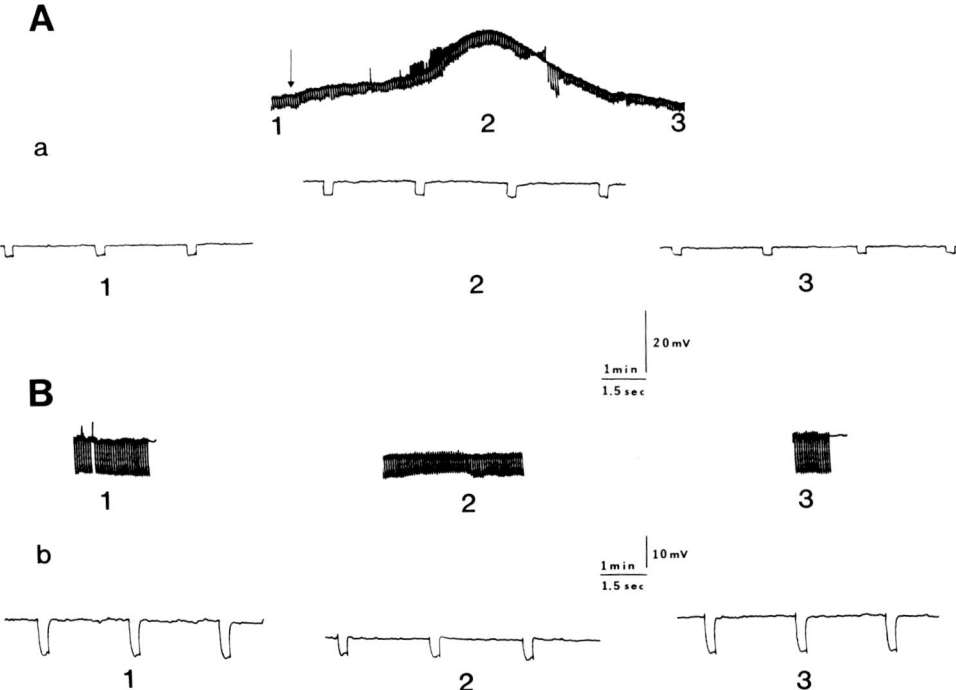

FIG. 1. 5-HT depolarizes and hyperpolarizes PCs. **A:** 5-HT, 200 μM applied by a droplet at the *arrow*, elicited a slowly developing depolarization of 18 mV accompanied by an increase in apparent input resistance as measured by 0.25 nA hyperpolarizing current injection. Spontaneous action potentials appeared during the rising slope of depolarization. On the falling phase of the depolarization, the injected current was momentarily changed. *a*: Expanded trace of membrane response to hyperpolarizing constant current injection taken at times indicated by the numbers. 1, control; 2, during maximum depolarization, and 3, recovery following 5-HT washout. Resting membrane potential of this cell was −60 mV. **B:** 5-HT, 200 μM applied by superfusion, elicited a 7-mV hyperpolarization and a decrease in apparent input resistance as measured by 0.5 nA hyperpolarizing current injection. 1, control; 2, during maximum hyperpolarization (approximately 8 min of 5-HT superfusion), and 3, recovery (approximately 10 min after 5-HT washout). *b*: Expanded trace of membrane response to hyperpolarizing constant current pulses showing the decrease in apparent input resistance. Resting membrane potential of this cell was −53 mV.

In addition to the direct hyperpolarizing and depolarizing effects of 5-HT, we noted an additional effect of 5-HT evident during a constant current hyperpolarizing pulse. During a hyperpolarizing pulse, the depolarizing relaxation or sag is indicative of activation of an inwardly rectifying current (I_h). 5-HT consistently diminished the amplitude of the depolarizing sag, an action that would contribute in part to the inhibitory effects of 5-HT on PCs. Indeed, we have observed a decrease in action potential frequency and a clustering of action potential firing in those cells displaying a decreased depolarizing sag.

Frequently, 5-HT and the 5-HT$_1$ ligand 8-OH-DPAT induced cyclic oscillatory firing of PCs that was preceded most often by a small depolarization (Fig. 2A). The cyclic firing pattern consisted of a step-like depolarization upon which Ca^{2+} and Na^+ spikes were elicited lasting about 20 sec followed by a rapid fall in membrane potential resulting in a quiescent period of about 15 sec. We also have observed that PCs displaying spontaneous oscillatory activity were affected by 5-HT and 8-OH-DPAT. These agents either slowed the periodicity or completely stopped the cyclic firing with a concomitant small hyperpolarization (Fig. 2B). These findings are of particular interest in light of the effects of 5-HT on cyclic firing in *Aplysia* R-15 cells (2). In these neurons 5-HT elicits hyperpolarization by increasing an inwardly rectifying K^+ current. Hyperpolarization occurred because of the imperfect nature of this current, allowing outward movement of K^+ at potentials more positive than -70 mV. Thus, inwardly rectifying currents may be a preferred target current for regulating cell excitability by 5-HT.

We suspect the multiple complex effects of 5-HT result from actions on several different membrane currents in PCs, resulting in a spectrum of changes in membrane polarization and firing patterns. These effects may depend on several factors including receptor subtypes, differential sensitivity to various concentrations of 5-HT, multiple membrane and cytosolic messengers, and voltage dependency of the currents. To begin to address these possibilities, we have begun an examination of 5-HT effects on a number of conductances in PCs that play a role in determining the intrinsic firing pattern of these neurons.

Voltage Clamp

Using single electrode voltage clamp (SEVC) of PCs we have examined 5-HT actions on steady-state holding current, quasisteady-state ramps, inward rectifier (I_h), and the transient outward current (I_{to}). We compared the effects of 5-HT on holding currents of cells held at -60 mV bathed with normal artificial cerebrospinal fluid (ACSF) and ACSF containing zero mM Ca^{2+}, 0.5 μM tetrodotoxin (TTX), and 2.5 mM Ni^{2+} to determine which actions of 5-HT can be ascribed to direct postjunctional effects. We know from other extracellular studies in our lab that a similar ACSF effectively blocked synaptic transmission even without TTX. The majority of cells in which 100 μM 5-HT was applied in normal ACSF showed an inward shift in holding current accompanied in the majority of cases by an increase in instan-

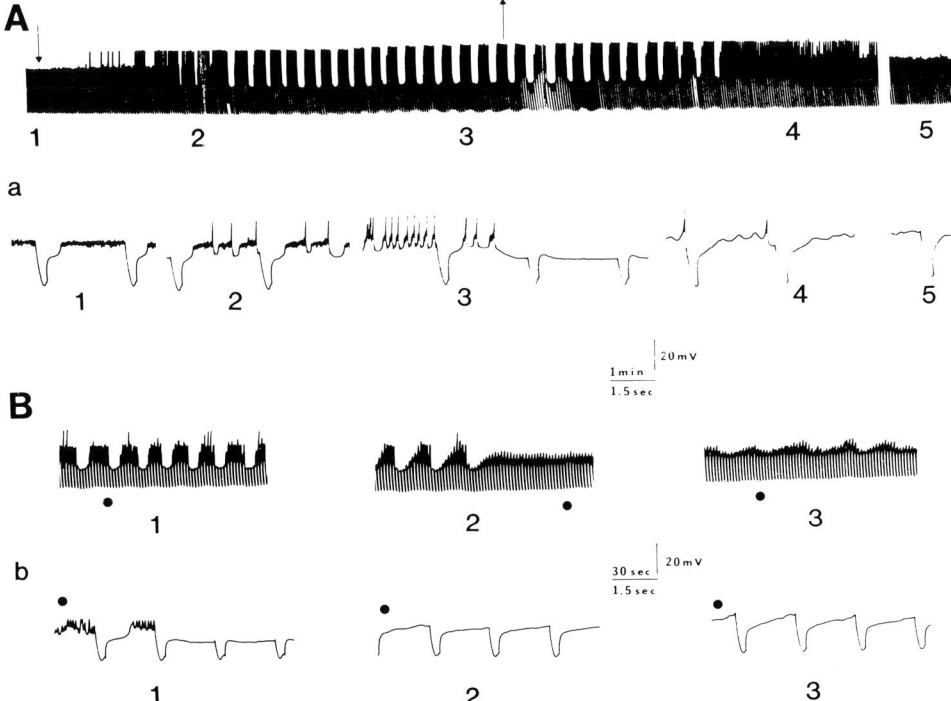

FIG. 2. 8-OH-DPAT induces and suppresses cyclic spontaneous firing of PCs. **A:** Superfusion with 100 μM 8-OH-DPAT (*downward arrow*) elicited a 2-mV depolarization with initial sodium action potentials that progressed into a regular cyclic firing pattern. When fully developed, each cycle consisted of a step-like depolarization upon which calcium and sodium spikes were elicited lasting about 20 sec followed by a rapid fall in the membrane potential resulting in a quiescent period of approximately 15 sec. Apparent input resistance was greatly reduced during the hyperpolarized valley. After turning off 8-OH-DPAT (*upward arrow*), the cyclic activity gradually subsided until the cell repolarized and all spontaneous activity ceased. 1, control; 2, the onset of spiking; 3, during the fully developed cyclic pattern; 4, beginning of recovery; and 5, recovery (approximately 20 min after turning off 8-OH-DPAT). *a:* Expanded trace of A. Note differences in apparent input resistance and calcium action potentials (truncated by the recorder frequency response). Resting membrane potential was −55 mV. Similar effects were seen with 5-HT. **B:** Superfusion with 8-OH-DPAT 50 μM stopped cyclic firing and hyperpolarized the cell by 4 mV. 1, control; 2, approximately 10 min into superfusion with 8-OH-DPAT; and 3, partial recovery (approximately 40 min after turning off 8-OH-DPAT). Apparent input resistance decreased very slightly during 8-OH-DPAT compared to the depolarized plateaus but was greater than during the hyperpolarized quiescent periods before 8-OH-DPAT. Constant current 0.5 nA hyperpolarizing pulses were passed throughout the recording. *b:* Expanded trace of B. *Solid dots* denote the times in trace B from which trace b was taken. Similar effects were seen with 5-HT.

taneous conductance. The remaining cells demonstrated an outward shift in the holding current and decreased conductance. In ACSF containing TTX and Ni^{2+} and no Ca^{2+}, PCs responded to 5-HT with an inward shift in the holding current, and in the majority of cells an increase in conductance. The remaining cells showed an outward shift in the holding current and a decrease in instantaneous conductance.

Based on these studies, we are confident that 5-HT is capable of producing multiple effects directly on target PCs in the absence of any prejunctional effects, which agree with our extracellular findings. Because similar effects of 5-HT were observed in a medium in which Na^+ and Ca^{2+} currents were removed, we speculate that the decreased inward current (outward shift) and decreased conductance may result from suppression of an inward current active at rest in some cells, e.g., I_h (see below). The other finding of a 5-HT-elicited increase in inward current with an increase in conductance may result from a small effect of 5-HT on residual cationic current; however, it is also possible that 5-HT increases a Cl^--mediated inwardly directed current when using KCl-filled electrodes.

Effects of 5-HT on quasisteady-state current voltage relationships were determined in normal ACSF, using a slow ramp voltage command (Fig. 3). Between -60 and -120 mV, 5-HT caused a voltage-dependent reduction in the steady-state inward current with an accompanying decrease in the slope conductance. The effects of 5-HT were evident at -60 mV and became increasingly larger at more hyperpolarized ranges, indicating a decreased inward rectification. Under the influence of 5-HT, the inward current was initiated at slightly more negative potentials. At potentials between -60 and -40 mV, 5-HT produced an increase in the slope conductance and outward current, although not clearly evident from the superimposed traces. These findings would suggest that 5-HT can elicit two independent voltage-sensitive effects on membrane conductance leading to a decrease in inward current and in increase in outward current. A decrease in the inward rectifier (I_h) current could explain 5-HT suppression of the inward current, whereas an augmentation of an outwardly directed K^+ current could account for the increased slope at potentials positive to -60 mV.

We have recorded and characterized the inward rectifying current I_h originally described by Crepel and Penit-Soria (7) in PCs (Fig. 4). As is evident in this figure, hyperpolarizing steps from a holding potential of -60 mV revealed a time- and voltage-dependent inward current relaxation that increased with progressively greater hyperpolarizing steps and was associated with an increased cell conductance. We examined the actions of 5-HT on the instantaneous, I_h, and steady-state currents. The I/V relations shown in Fig. 5 depict typical suppression of the steady-state and I_h currents by 5-HT and associated decrease in slope conductance. That suppression of the steady-state current is due to 5-HT suppression of the I_h current is revealed in panel C of this figure, which clearly shows a near total blockade of the I_h current. Subtracting the total I_h from the I_h in the presence of 5-HT yields 5-HT-sensitive current, which is plotted against the command potential in panel D, and reveals the voltage-dependent nature of 5-HT action. Because the steady-state I/V relationship from PCs is comprised of I_h and a Ca^{2+}-dependent K^+ conductance active at rest (7), the effect of 5-HT throughout the voltage range would suggest an action directed at both currents. Figure 6 compares the activation curve for I_h obtained in the presence of 5-HT to control. 5-HT shifted the activation curve to the left at more negative potentials and increased the slope factor. These data suggest that 5-HT-induced reduction of I_h may contribute, in part, to its inhibitory action by removing inward current present at rest and more hyperpolarized potentials.

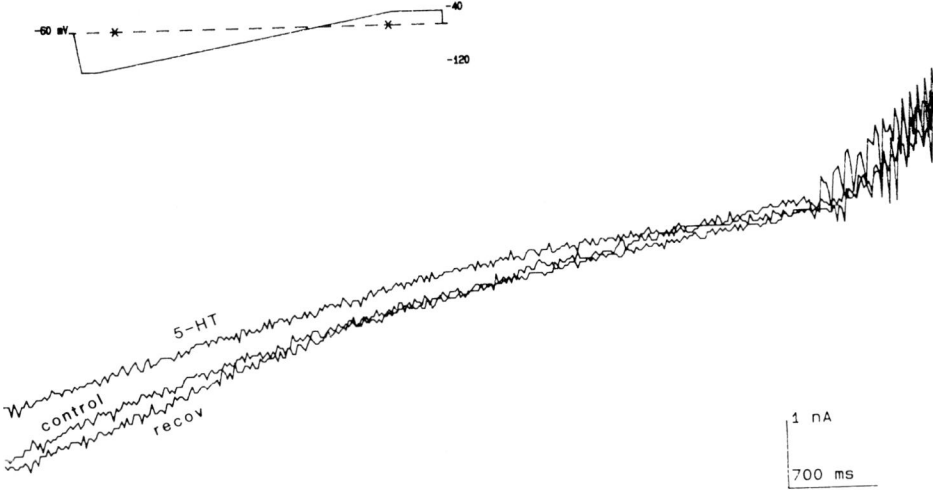

FIG. 3. Effect of 5-HT (100 μM) on quasisteady-state current. The cell was held at −60 mV, hyperpolarized to −120 mV, and then gradually depolarized to −40 mV. Between −60 and −120 mV, 5-HT caused a voltage-dependent reduction in the steady-state inward current with an accompanying decrease in the slope conductance. The effects of 5-HT were evident at −60 mV and became increasingly larger at more hyperpolarized ranges, indicating a decreased inward rectification. Under the influence of 5-HT, the inward current was initiated at slightly more negative potentials. At potential between −60 and −40 mV, 5-HT produced an increase in the slope conductance and outward current, although not clearly evident from the superimposed traces. The apparent increase in excitability, as shown by uncontrolled spiking in the presence of 5-HT, may be due to decreased space clamp conditions of distal dendrites secondary to changes in membrane conductance. These findings would suggest that 5-HT can elicit two independent voltage-sensitive effects on membrane conductance leading to a decrease in inward current and an increase in outward current. A decrease in the inward rectifier (I_h) current could explain 5-HT suppression of the inward current.

Because the existence of a hyperpolarization-activated transient outward current has only been suggested in PCs on the basis of current clamp recordings and never described using voltage clamp methods, we characterized this current utilizing criteria of voltage dependence of activation and inactivation, ionic selectivity, and pharmacologic sensitivity. Our data demonstrate that I_{to} in PCs is likely equivalent to I_A recently described in a number of excitable cells (18).

Data from voltage clamp recordings reveal that 5-HT can affect I_{to}. Figure 7 shows two sets of traces: one obtained in control conditions and the other in the presence of 10 μM 5-HT. Three reversible effects of 5-HT were noted: (i) an inward shift in the holding current, (ii) suppression of I_{to}, and (iii) suppression of the decay phase of the current. Suppression of I_{to} by 5-HT is dose dependent between concentrations of 10 nM and 50 μM. At 50 μM, an average 45% inhibition of I_{to} was noted; higher doses produced no further depression. Current clamp recordings using similar concentrations of 5-HT demonstrate an increased excitability of PCs in response to depolarizing current injections, imparting functional significance to the finding of suppression of I_{to} by 5-HT.

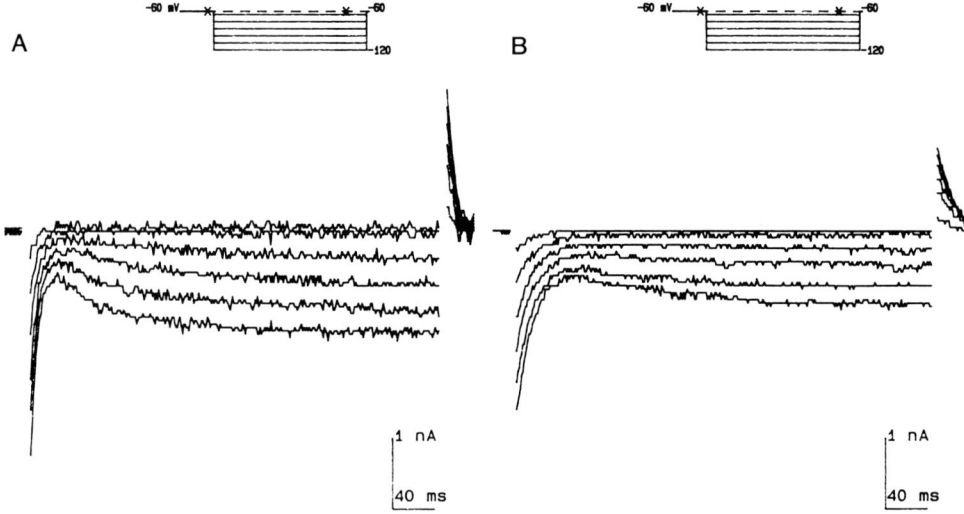

FIG. 4. 5-HT reduces an inwardly rectifying current in PCs. Families of current traces evoked by 400-msec hyperpolarizing step commands to −120 mV from a holding potential of −60 mV, as indicated above each set of traces. **A**: Control conditions; **B**, approximately 6 min after starting superfusion of 500 µM 5-HT. Note the marked suppression of the inward relaxation current at all voltage commands and minimal effect on the instantaneous current.

SUMMARY

We strongly suspect that 5-HT-elicited hyperpolarization and depolarization as observed in our current clamp recordings (and inhibition and excitation observed with extracellular recordings) are the result of complex and possible simultaneous actions by this amine on several currents that help to determine the firing pattern and output of PCs. These actions may be differentially expressed depending on the concentration of 5-HT and the voltage present across the cell membrane. These complexities of 5-HT actions on PC firing patterns and polarization are being addressed by voltage clamp methods directed at identifying the effects of 5-HT on K^+ and Ca^{2+} conductances.

Ionic conductances of PCs endow them with autorhythmic oscillatory properties. Llinas (15) recently reviewed the neurophysiology of neuronal oscillators and raised several important speculative roles for their existence. In a neuronal network, autorhythmic neurons may act as unitary oscillators (pacemakers) or as resonators (preferentially responding to certain firing frequencies). In this regard, we have shown, on the basis of extracellular recording and iontophoretic application of 5-HT, that the actions of 5-HT are dependent on the initial firing rate of the PC; slow firing cells are accelerated by 5-HT, whereas fast firing cells are slowed. Thus, 5-HT appears to set the PC at some preferred firing rate or pattern, i.e., oscillator or

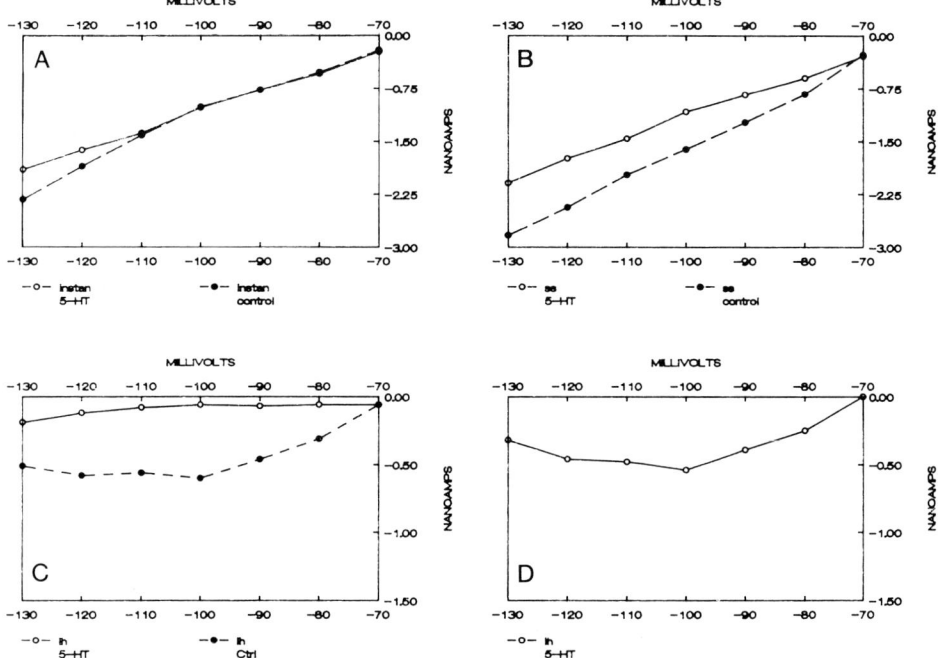

FIG. 5. The actions of 5-HT (100 μM) on the instantaneous, steady-state, and I_h currents. Instantaneous current was measured as the difference between the baseline current and the current of the end of the initial capacitance transient, and the I_h was calculated as the difference between the steady-state and instantaneous currents. The I/V relations in **B** show a suppression of the steady-state inward current by 5-HT and a decrease in slope conductance. 5-HT also decreased instantaneous current at hyperpolarizing steps negative to -110 mV (**A**), which may reflect a decrease in the background (leak) conductance. **C** shows that I_h current was nearly totally blocked by 5-HT. Subtracting the control I_h curve from that obtained in the presence of 5-HT yields the 5-HT-sensitive current, which reveals the voltage-dependent nature of the action of 5-HT (**D**).

resonator. Oscillation and resonance in the CNS may have diverse functional roles, among which are determining global functional states and timing in motor coordination. In such cases, the oscillator or resonator may provide the brain with an internal frame of reference with which to compare incoming sensory information to adjust output appropriately. In this regard, the role of presynaptic activity becomes that of initiating and shaping preprogrammed reference frames rather than creating them. Changes in this internal frame of reference, as might occur as the result of neuromodulation of intrinsic determinants of firing, could provide a means by which, over time, a new reference level is maintained for a newly acquired situation such as during motor learning. Conversely, inappropriate alterations in the internal reference frame or the inability to adjust the frame of reference as required could lead to permanent dysfunction of the system, as might occur in neurologic pathologies. Our

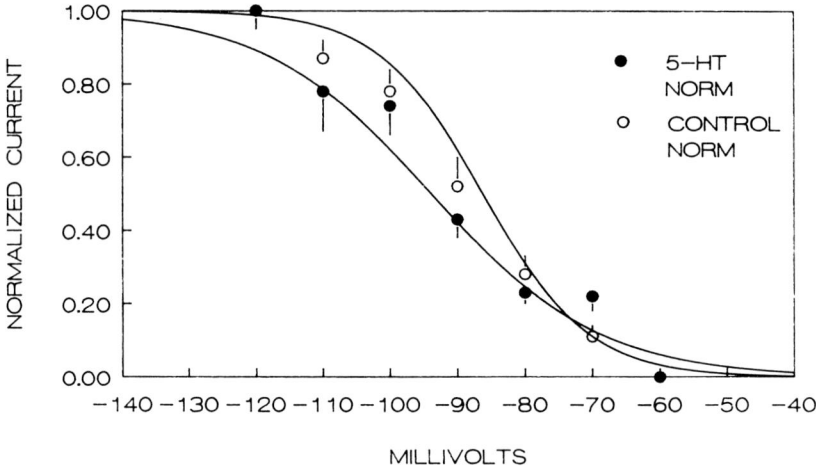

FIG. 6. Activation curve obtained by averaging the normalized I_h current from five cells. I_h was generated from holding potential set at −60 mV and applying 600-msec hyperpolarizing pulses in −10-mV increments to −120 mV. It was calculated as the difference between the instantaneous current and the steady-state inward relaxation current. Activation threshold occurred at approximately −60 mV, indicating that this current is active at rest. Fitting the raw data to the Boltzmann equation by iterative methods, the best-fit line had a half-maximal activation of approximately −86 mV with slope factor of 7.8. The general form of the Boltzmann equation is $I/I_{max} = 1/[1 + \exp(V_m − V_{0.5})/s]$, where I/I_{max} = normalized current, V_m is the membrane potential, $V_{0.5}$ is the potential to give a half-maximal value, and s is the slope factor. This current failed to reveal inactivation with command pulses up to 1,000 msec in length. The activation curve for I_h obtained in the presence of 5-HT (100 μM) was compared with control. 5-HT shifted the activation curve to the left at more negative potentials ($V_{0.5} = −91$) and increased the slope factor ($s = 11$).

data show 5-HT can either suppress or induce oscillatory firing of intracellularly recorded PCs. Based on the above discussion, this could point to a significant neuromodulatory role of 5-HT in shaping the internal frame of reference of the cerebellum, which could profoundly affect the physiology of this structure as it relates to motor coordination, motor learning, and neurologic motor disorders. It is significant therefore to determine the effects of putative neuromodulators on currents responsible for autorhythmicity of neurons.

ACKNOWLEDGMENTS

This work was supported by grants from the National Institutes of Health, the Texas Advanced Research Program, and the Tarbox Parkinson's Disease Research Institute. We extend our appreciation to all the graduate students and research associates who have contributed to this work and to Jeannie Boyd for the preparation of this manuscript.

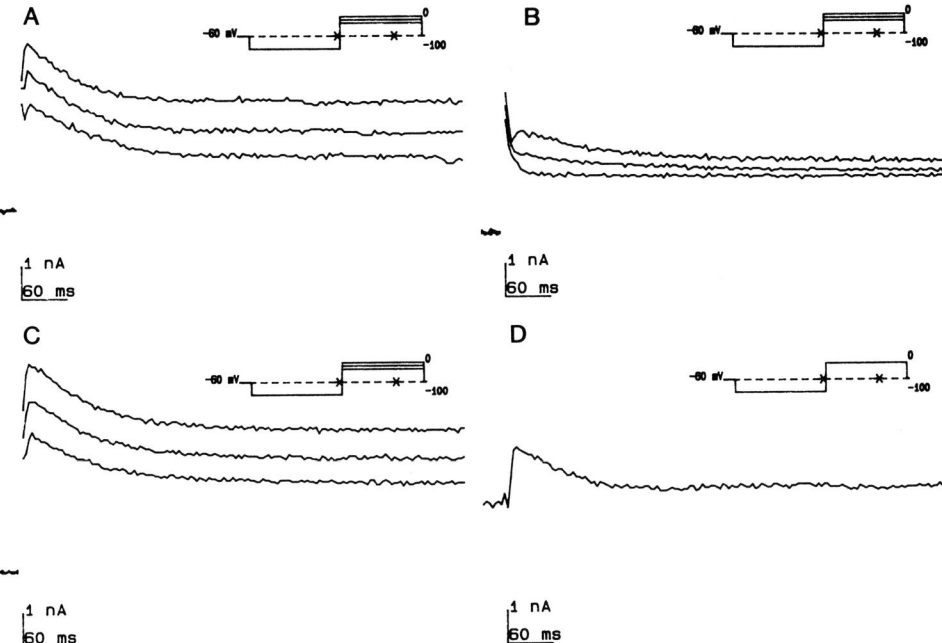

FIG. 7. 5-HT reversibly suppresses a transient outward K$^+$ current in PCs. **A** (control), **B** (5 μM 5-HT), and **C** (recovery) are families of outward currents elicited by progressively greater depolarizing commands to 0 mV following a 1-sec prepulse to -100 mV from a holding potential of -60 mV. In B, 5-HT markedly reduced I_A. Note also an increase in the inward holding current. All effects were reversed when 5-HT was removed (C). **D**: 5-HT-sensitive current from a depolarizing command to -10 mV obtained by subtracting the current in the presence of 5-HT from that in control conditions.

REFERENCES

1. Andrade R, Malenka RC, Nicoll RA. A G protein couples serotonin and GABA$_B$ receptors to the same channels in hippocampus. *Science* 1986;234:1261–1265.
2. Benson JA, Adams WB. The control of rhythmic neuronal firing. In: Kaczmarek LA, Levitan IB, eds. *Neuromodulation*. New York: Oxford Press, 1987:100–118.
3. Bishop GA, Ho RH. The distribution and origin of serotonin immunoreactivity in the rat cerebellum. *Brain Res* 1985;331:195–207.
4. Chan-Palay V. Fine structure of labelled axons in the cerebellar cortex and nuclei of rodents and primates after intraventricular infusions with tritiated serotonin. *Anat Embryo* 1975;148:235–265.
5. Chan-Palay V. Indoleamine neurons and their processes in the normal rat brain and in chronic diet-induced thiamine deficiency demonstrated by uptake of 3H-serotonin. *J Comp Neurol* 1977;176:467–494.
6. Colino A, Halliwell JV. Differential modulation of three separate K-conductances in hippocampal CAI neurons by serotonin. *Nature* 1987;328:73–77.
7. Crepel F, Penit-Soria J. Inward rectification and low threshold calcium conductance in rat cerebellar Purkinje cells. An in vitro study. *J Physiol* 1986;372:1–23.
8. Crepel F, Debono M, Flores R. β-adrenergic inhibition of rat cerebellar Purkinje cells in vitro: a voltage-clamp study. *J Physiol* 1987;383:487–498.

9. Gruol DL. Cultured cerebellar neurons: endogenous and exogenous components of Purkinje cell activity and membrane response to putative transmitters. *Brain Res* 1983;236:223–241.
10. Hounsgaard J. Pacemaker properties of mammalian Purkinje cells. *Acta Physiol Scand* 1979;106:91–92.
11. Hounsgaard J, Midtgaard J. Intrinsic determinants of firing pattern in Purkinje cells of the turtle cerebellum in vitro. *J Physiol* 1988;402:731–749.
12. Lee M, Strahlendorf JC, Strahlendorf HK. Modulatory action of serotonin on glutamate induced excitation of cerebellar Purkinje cells. *Brain Res* 1985;361:107–113.
13. Llinas R, Sugimori M. Electrophysiologic properties of in vitro Purkinje cell dendrites in mammalian cerebellar slices. *J Physiol* 1980;305:197–213.
14. Llinas R, Sugimori M. Electrophysiological properties of in vitro Purkinje cell somata in mammalian cerebellar slices. *J Physiol* 1980;305:171–195.
15. Llinas R. The intrinsic electrophysiologic properties of mammalian neurons: insights into central nervous system function. *Science* 1988;242:1654–1664.
16. Nicoll RA. The coupling of neurotransmitter receptors to ion channels in the brain. *Science* 1988;241:545–551.
17. Pazos A, Cortes R, Palacios JM. Quantitative autoradiographic mapping of serotonin receptors in the rat brain II. Serotonin-2 receptors. *Brain Res* 1985;346:231–249.
18. Rogawski MA. The A-current: how ubiquitous a feature of excitable cells is it? *Trends Neurosci* 1985;8:214–219.
19. Slater NT, McCrimmon DR, Larson-Prior LJ. Cellular properties of Purkinje cells and excitatory transmission in the isolated turtle cerebellum. *Soc Neurosci Abstr* 1988;14:1237.
20. Strahlendorf JC, Strahlendorf HK, Barnes CD. Modulation of cerebellar neuronal activity by raphe stimulation. *Brain Res* 1979;169:565–569.
21. Strahlendorf JC, Lee M, Strahlendorf HK. Effects of serotonin on cerebellar Purkinje cells are dependent on the baseline firing rate. *Exp Brain Res* 1984;56:50–58.
22. Strahlendorf JC, Lee M, Strahlendorf HK. Serotonin modulates muscimol and baclofen-elicited inhibition of cerebellar Purkinje cells. *Eur J Pharmacol* 1991;209:19–25.
23. Strahlendorf JC, Strahlendorf HK, Lee M. Electrophysiological effects of serotonin on cerebellar Purkinje cells. In: King JS, ed. *New concepts in cerebellar neurobiology*. New York: Alan R. Liss, 1987:321–347.
24. Takeuchi Y, Kimura H, Sano Y. Immunohistochemical demonstration of serotonin containing nerve fibers in the cerebellum. *Cell Tissue Res* 1982;226:1–12.

*Serotonin, the Cerebellum,
and Ataxia*, edited by
P. Trouillas and K. Fuxe.
Raven Press, Ltd., New York © 1993.

17

Differential Modulation by Serotonin of the Responses Induced by Excitatory Amino Acids in Cerebellar Nuclei Neurons and Purkinje Cells

Robert Gardette and *Francis Crepel

*INSERM U159, 75014 Paris, France;
CNRS URA 1121, Université Paris Sud, 91405 Orsay, France

In view of the importance of modulatory mechanisms in the functioning of the central nervous system, the interest in interactions between neurotransmitter substances has been rapidly growing during the past few years. As far as we know at present, neurotransmitters could be divided into two main groups. One could be called "primary acting substances" and includes neurotransmitters such as excitatory or inhibitory amino acids acting most probably essentially via "wiring transmission." The second group could be referred to as "modulatory acting substances" and comprises substances such as neuropeptides or monoamines that could act either via wiring transmission or via "volume transmission" (1,12). Obviously, some neurotransmitters can belong to both groups, depending, for instance, on the location of their site of release, close or far from postsynaptic structures (wiring versus volume transmission) and/or on the receptor subtype involved in the physiological response: ligand-gated ion channel, subclasses of receptors coupled to different G protein families, and second messenger systems (primary versus modulatory acting substances).

Serotonin (5-HT) in the cerebellum may be considered as an example of such a dual substance. Indeed, on the one hand, serotoninergic terminals in the cerebellum have been shown to be located either solely at the level of the deep cerebellar nuclei and the granular layer, as in the cat (20) or in the entire cerebellum including the molecular layer, as in the rat (4,18,35) suggesting that the physiological effects of the monoamine on Purkinje cells (PCs) could imply both wiring and volume transmission. On the other hand, 5-HT could also act via the activation of the different

5-HT receptor subtypes characterized in the cerebellum (see Chapter 12, this volume) leading either to a direct effect on the spontaneous firing of PCs and deep cerebellar nuclei neurons (DCNs) or to a modulatory effect on the responses of these cells to amino acids, as suggested by experiments with 5-HT$_{1A}$ agonists or antagonists (10; Chapter 6, this volume).

We also know that excitatory amino acid (EAA)-mediated transmission is of primary importance in the functioning of the cerebellum. Indeed, the two main afferents to PCs, the parallel (PFs) and the climbing fibers (CFs) are likely to use glutamate and aspartate, respectively, as neurotransmitters (8,19). Similarly, although definitive data on this problem are not yet available, it is most probable that part of the excitatory effect of the mossy fibers (MFs), the other main afferent system to the cerebellum, on granular cells is due to the release of EAAs from these fibers since granular cells have been shown to be responsive to glutamate and aspartate (9,15). Finally, the fact that CFs directly innervate both PCs and DCNs indicates that EAAs act also at the DCN level. Thus, EAAs play a crucial role in cerebellar functions, and this is also true for 5-HT since deficits in motor control, such as ataxia, have been reported to regress partially with administration of 5-hydroxytryptophan (36).

In keeping with these comments on experimental and clinical data, this review will present the main results obtained by our group on the characterization of EEA receptors borne by PCs and DCNs, the effects of 5-HT on the spontaneous activity, and the EEA-induced responses of these cells. These experiments were undertaken to contribute to a better understanding of the role of 5-HT in the functions of the cerebellar microcircuitry, in relation with the implication of EAAs and their different receptor subtypes in cerebellar functioning.

The results described hereafter were obtained from both extra- and intracellular recordings, either in the current clamp or voltage clamp mode, of PCs and DCNs recorded from thick cerebellar slices maintained *in vitro*, a set-up allowing long, stable electrophysiological recordings and, when necessary, rapid changes of the superfusing solution. In order to compare the effects of EEAs and 5-HT on a same cell, drugs were released in the vicinity of the dendrites of the cells from adjacent barrels of a same iontophoretic electrode.

EXCITATORY AMINO ACID RECEPTORS ON DEEP CEREBELLAR NUCLEI NEURONS AND PURKINJE CELLS

Responses of DCNs and PCs to Glutamate and Aspartate

Short iontophoretic pulse applications of glutamate and aspartate in the dendritic field of DCNs elicit a transient and dose-dependent increase in the firing rate of these cells (Fig. 1A,B) (13) in relation with the appearance of an inward current in response to EEAs when cells are intracellularly recorded in the voltage clamp mode (Fig. 1C,D) (3).

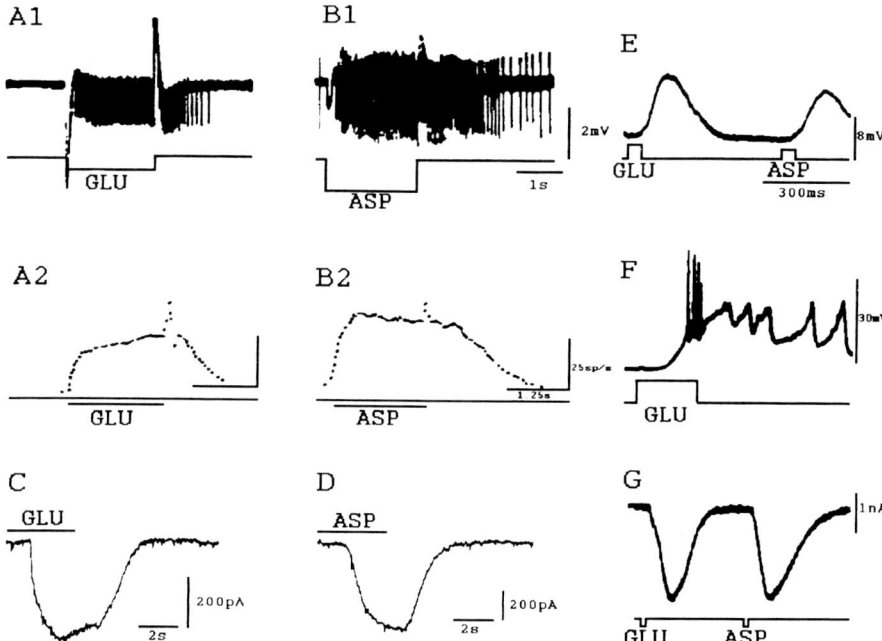

FIG. 1. Responses of DCNs and PCs to glutamate (GLU) and aspartate (ASP). **A,B**: Extracellular recordings of the responses of two DCNs to a pulse application of glutamate (A1) or aspartate (B1) and instantaneous spike frequency curves (A2,B2) derived from the above responses. **C,D**: Intracellular recordings in the voltage clamp mode of the responses induced by glutamate (C) and aspartate (D) in two other DCNs. **E–G**: Glutamate- and aspartate-induced responses in three different PCs recorded either in the current clamp mode (E,F) of the voltage clamp mode (G). (Modified from refs. 3,6,7,13.)

Similarly, iontophoretic pulse applications of glutamate or aspartate always induce excitations of PCs. When extracellularly recorded, these responses are revealed by a transient increase in the spontaneous firing frequency of the cells (5,6). When intracellularly recorded, the responses of PCs appear, in the current clamp mode, as a transient and dose-dependent depolarization, as illustrated in Fig. 1E and F (6) or, in the voltage clamp mode, as an inwardly directed current as presented on Fig. 1G (7). When this depolarization reaches threshold for spike discharge, it can induce discharge of both fast sodium and slow calcium spikes (Fig. 1F) (6,16).

Characterization of EAA Receptors Borne by DCNs and PCs

Until recently, the receptors to EAAs mediating those excitatory responses were divided into three main types: N-methyl-D-aspartate (NMDA), quisqualate, and kainate (28,37). However, recent studies have suggested that quisqualate and kainate receptors might be borne by a same molecular entity (32). We have therefore focused our study on the characterization of NMDA versus non-NMDA receptors (27) using the specific agonists NMDA and quisqualate.

Iontophoretic pulse applications of NMDA and quisqualate elicit clear-cut excitatory responses in DCNs (Fig. 2A,B), (3,13), whereas adult PCs that are always strongly excited by quisqualate (Fig. 2C,E) are usually not responsive to NMDA

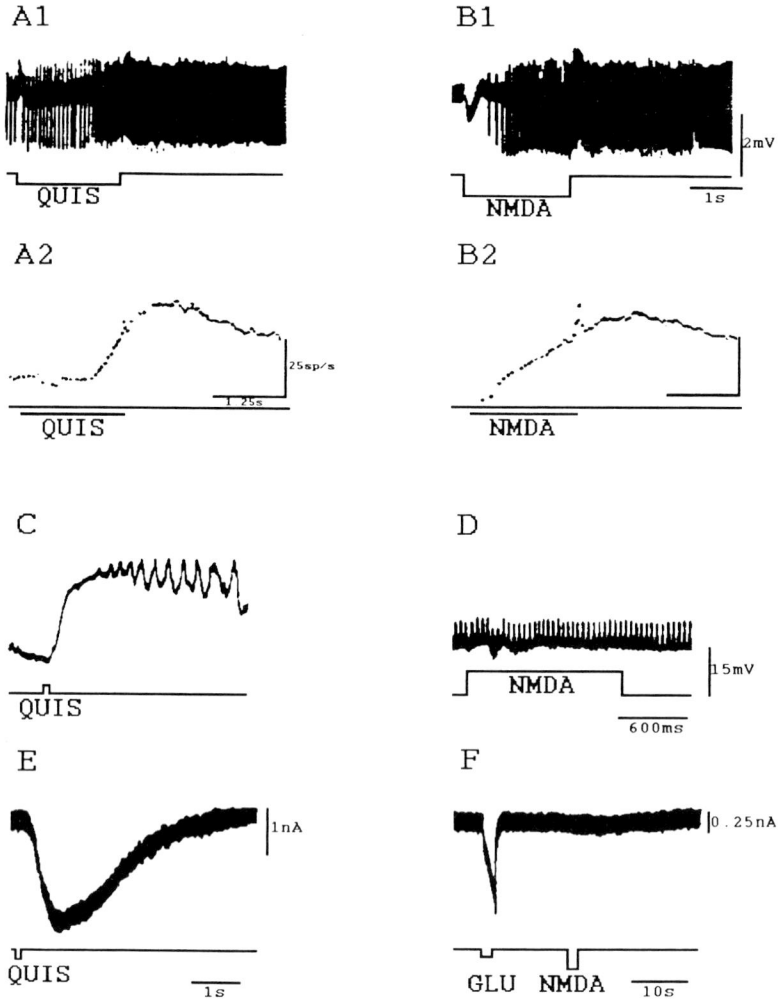

FIG. 2. Responses of DCNs and PCs to quisqualate (QUIS) and NMDA. **A,B**: Extracellular recordings of the responses of two DCNs to a pulse application of quisqualate (A1) or NMDA (B1) and instantaneous spike frequency curves (A2,B2) derived from the above responses. **C–F**: Quisqualate and NMDA-induced responses in four different PCs recorded in either the current clamp mode (C,D) or the voltage clamp mode (E,F). Note the lack of sensitivity to NMDA even when the cell is responsive to glutamate (GLU) (F). (Modified from refs. 6,7,13,21.)

(Fig. 2D,F) (6,7). Using a different preparation, the mature organotypic cultures, such a lack of sensitivity of adult PCs to NMDA has been recently confirmed by other groups (3,23). These results therefore suggest that adult PCs mainly bear non-NMDA receptors, whereas both NMDA and non-NMDA receptors are present on DCN membranes.

In keeping with these observations, 2-amino-5-phosphonovalerate (2-APV), a specific antagonist of NMDA receptors, indeed blocks totally NMDA-induced responses in DCNs, but also decreases aspartate-elicited excitations as well as, although to a lesser extent, glutamate responses (Fig. 3) (13). The response to aspartate and glutamate that persists under 2-APV can be further depressed by a subsequent addition of 6-cyano-7-nitroquinoxaline-2,3-dione (CNQX) (Fig. 3C,D) (3), thus confirming that the endogenous EAAs are mixed agonists at NMDA and non-NMDA receptors on DCNs, aspartate being more potent in activating NMDA receptors and glutamate preferentially acting via non-NMDA receptors (3,13). Conversely, 2-APV is without effect on aspartate- and glutamate-induced responses in

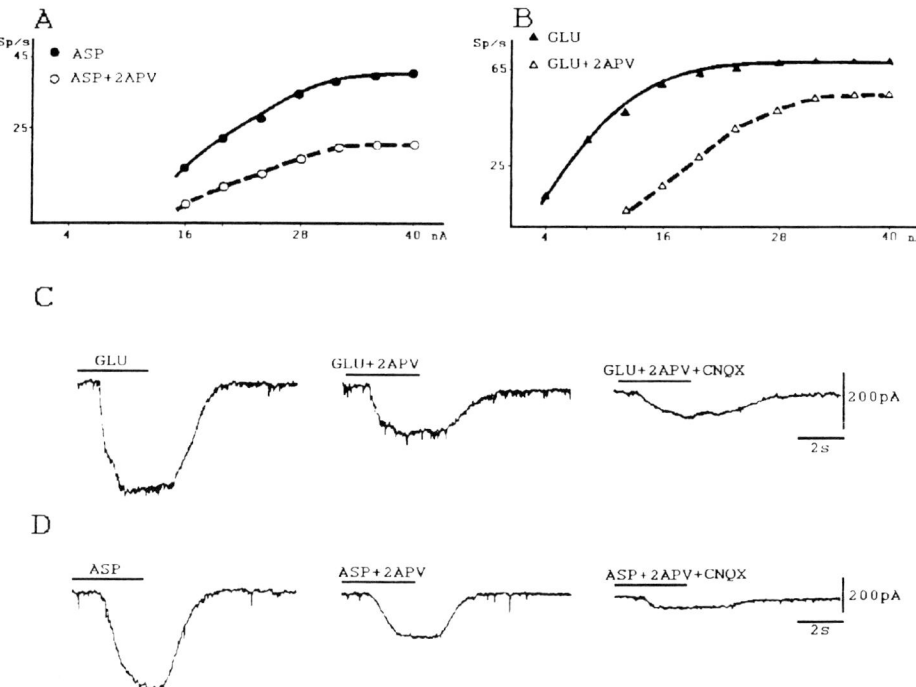

FIG. 3. Effects of the EAA receptor antagonists 2-APV and CNQX on the EAA-induced responses of DCNs. **A,B**: Effect of 2-APV on the dose-response curves obtained from extracellular recordings of two different DCNs excited by increasing doses of aspartate (ASP) (A) and glutamate (GLU) (B). **C,D**: Additive inhibitory effect of 2-APV and CNQX on whole-cell inward currents induced in two different DCNs by application of glutamate (C) and aspartate (D). (Modified from ref. 3.)

PCs, whereas those latter responses are readily blocked by CNQX (3,11,21), reinforcing the hypothesis that they are solely due to an activation of non-NMDA receptors.

Characterization of EAA Receptors Borne by Immature PCs

Interestingly enough, if adult PCs lack functional NMDA receptors, we have been able to demonstrate that PCs taken from immature rats, from birth to approximately postnatal week 3, exhibit a transient sensitivity to NMDA (11,21). Furthermore, the NMDA-induced responses of these immature PCs are indeed due to the activation of true NMDA receptors since they are insensitive to CNQX but blocked by 2-APV (21). In addition, immature PCs also respond well to iontophoretic pulse applications of glutamate (11,38), aspartate, and quisqualate (11). These data thus demonstrate that, at variance with adult PCs but comparable to DCNs, immature PCs bear both non-NMDA and NMDA receptors, these latter being transiently functional, although this has been recently challenged (24).

Finally, all the responses to EAAs described above are very likely to be due to the activation of postsynaptically located receptors since they persist even when the cells are bathed with different media containing blockers of synaptic transmission, such as tetrodotoxin, cadmium, or bicuculline (11,16,21).

EFFECTS OF 5-HT ON THE SPONTANEOUS DISCHARGE OF DEEP CEREBELLAR NUCLEI NEURONS AND PURKINJE CELLS

Steady iontophoretic applications of 5-HT elicit an increase in the spontaneous discharge of more than 90% of the recorded DCNs (14). This increase is clearly dose dependent (Fig. 4) and insensitive to methysergide bimaleate (MSD), a 5-HT antagonist preferentially acting on 5-HT_2 receptors, in contrast with what was observed on the EAA responses of the same neurons (see below).

On the contrary, and at variance with results obtained by other groups using extracellular recordings *in vivo* (33), under our experimental conditions (cerebellar slices maintained *in vitro* and intracellular recordings), the monoamine has usually no clear-cut effect on the spontaneous firing of PCs (17). Therefore, 5-HT appears to have a solely excitatory effect on the spontaneous discharge of DCNs without affecting, at least in our experimental conditions, the spontaneous firing rate of PCs.

EFFECTS OF 5-HT ON THE EXCITATORY AMINO ACID-INDUCED RESPONSES OF DEEP CEREBELLAR NUCLEI NEURONS AND PURKINJE CELLS

Deep Cerebellar Nuclei Neurons

To compare the effects of 5-HT on the extracellularly recorded responses induced in DCNs by glutamate, aspartate, quisqualate, and NMDA, four-barreled ionto-

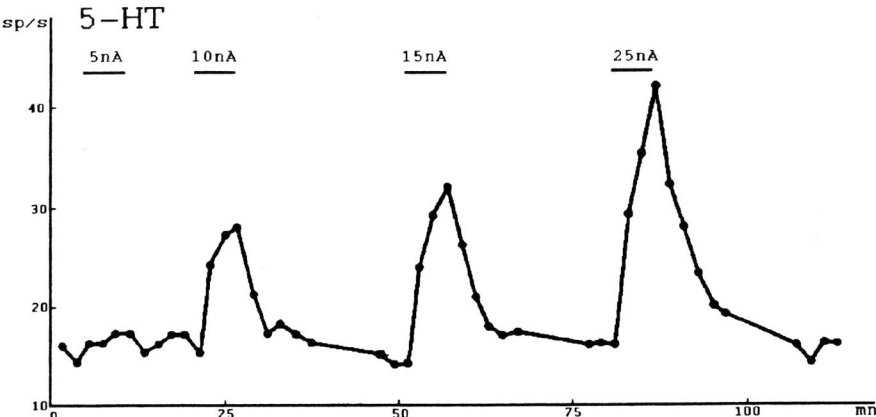

FIG. 4. Effects of 5-HT on the spontaneous discharge rate of a DCN. Note the clear-cut dose-dependent increase of the spontaneous firing of the cell in response to 5-HT. (Modified from ref. 14.)

phoretic electrodes were used throughout the experiments, one barrel being filled with NaCl for current compensation. Two other barrels were filled, respectively, with 5-HT and glutamate, whereas the last one was used to release either aspartate, NMDA, or quisqualate.

When glutamate and aspartate are paired and delivered alternately on the same nuclear neuron, the responses to EEAs, revealed by an increase in the discharge rate of the neuron as indicated before, are both diminished under a steady release of 5-HT as shown from the analysis of the instantaneous firing frequency curves of the cells, but to a different extent (Fig. 5A). This differential potency of 5-HT in antagonizing EEA-induced responses is also found when quisqualate or NMDA are paired with glutamate (Fig. 5B,C). Altogether, the maximum decrease in the responses to EEAs achieved under a steady application of 5-HT can be divided into two groups: quisqualate (54%) and glutamate (49%), on the one hand, and aspartate (32%) and NMDA (27%), on the other. These values are significantly different when they are compared from one group to another, but do not significantly differ within each group.

It must be emphasized that this decrease in the responses to EAAs is not simply due to an increase in the spontaneous discharge of the cell under 5-HT. First, in the few cells where the monoamine has no effect on the baseline firing rate, inhibition of the EAA-evoked responses is still present. Second, when cell discharge is increased by a high K^+ concentration in the bathing medium, the potency of the EAAs in exciting the neurons is not changed.

Finally, when 5-HT and MSD are simultaneously applied, the inhibitory effect of the monoamine on glutamate-elicited responses is partially antagonized, indicating that at least some of the 5-HT effect on EAA responses is mediated through the activation of MSD-sensitive 5-HT receptors, at variance with the lack of effect of MSD on the 5-HT-induced increase of the spontaneous firing of DCNs.

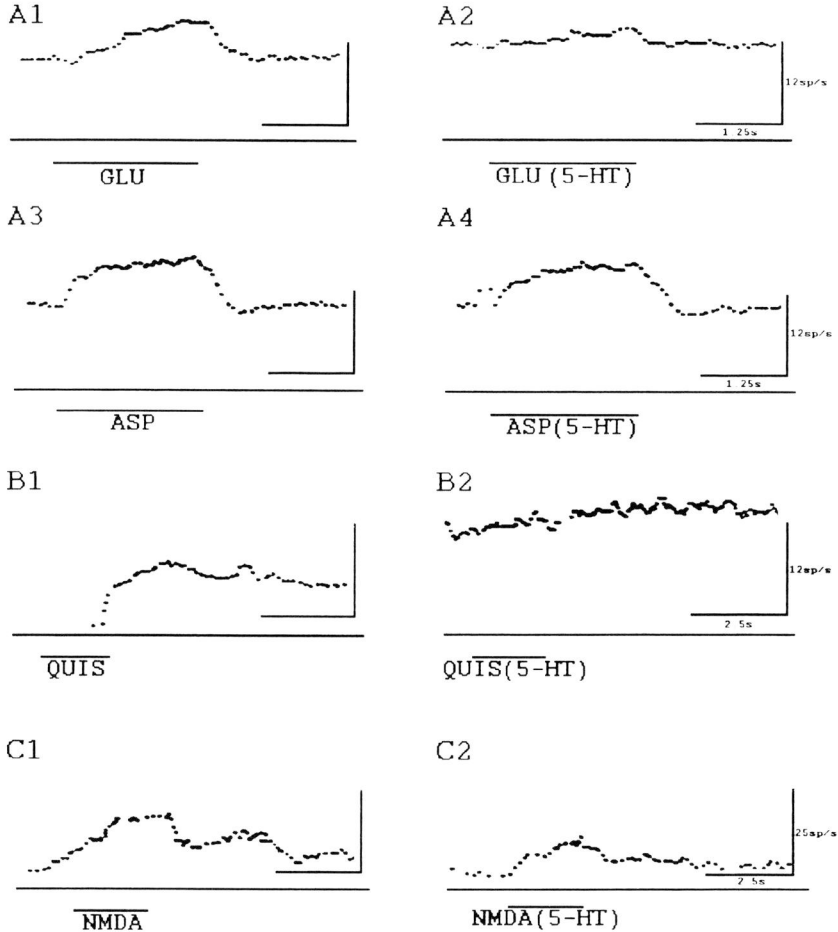

FIG. 5. Examples of the differential sensitivity to 5-HT of the EAA-induced responses in DCNs. **A**: In the same DCN, the glutamate (GLU) response (A1) is almost abolished under a steady iontophoretic application of 5-HT (A2), whereas the aspartate (ASP) response (A3) is only very slightly decreased (A4). **B**: In another DCN, the quisqualate-induced (QUIS) response (B1) is clearly decreased under a steady application of 5-HT (B2) concomitant with a marked increase in the spontaneous discharge of the cell indicated by an upward shift of the baseline of the curves. **C**: Same as in A and B but with a pulse application of NMDA in another DCN. Note the smaller inhibition of the NMDA response (C1) under 5-HT (C2) as compared with that of glutamate (A2) and quisqualate (B2) responses. (Modified from ref. 14.)

Purkinje Cells

Excluding the inefficiency of 5-HT in modifying the rate of spontaneous discharge of PCs, 5-HT acts on the EAA-elicited responses of immature PCs in the same way as on those of DCNs (17). Indeed, the mean decreases in the inward currents recorded in PCs in response to quisqualate (Fig. 6A), glutamate (Fig. 6C),

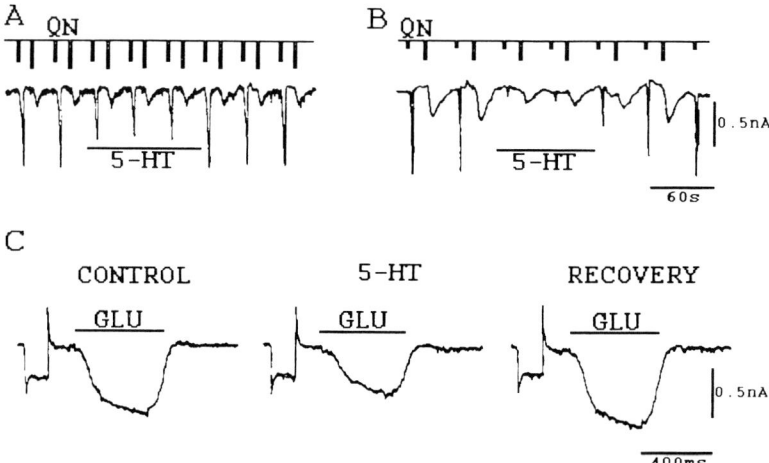

FIG. 6. Differential effects of 5-HT on the EAA-induced responses of immature PCs. **A:** Inward currents elicited in a voltage clamp recorded PC (lower trace) by quisqualate and NMDA (Q and N, pulse applications shown in A, upper trace) are differentially affected by the iontophoretic application of 5-HT. **B:** Same as in A but in a magnesium-free perfusing solution containing tetrodotoxin showing a persistence of the differential inhibitory effect of 5-HT on quisqualate and NMDA-induced responses of the same immature PC. **C:** Depression of the inward current induced by glutamate (GLU) in an immature PC by a steady iontophoretic application of 5-HT and recovery of the control response after termination of 5-HT ejection. Note the lack of effect of 5-HT on the membrane resistance of the cell as shown by the maintained value of the inward current induced by a 20-mV hyperpolarizing step before, during, and after 5-HT application. (Modified from ref. 17.)

and NMDA (Fig. 6A) are, respectively, 77%, 42.5%, and 28%. Once again, a bath application of MSD antagonizes partially the effect of 5-HT on EAA-induced firing.

Last, when synaptic transmission is blocked, the differential suppressant action of 5-HT on EAA-induced responses is still observed both for DCNs and PCs, as should be expected for a postsynaptic site of action of the drugs (see, for instance, Fig. 6B) (13,17).

On the whole, these studies indicate that 5-HT is likely to have a differential effect on NMDA and non-NMDA receptor types borne by DCNs and immature PCs.

CONCLUSION

From our results and from the observations of other groups, it is now evident that 5-HT acts as a neuromodulator for various electrical properties of cerebellar neurons. The monoamine appears to either enhance or diminish the spontaneous activity of PCs (33) and granule cells (2) and to always induce an increase in the spontaneous firing of DCNs (14). It is also a potent inhibitor of EAA-induced excitations of PCs and DCNs (14,17,22) and has complex effects on gamma-aminobutyric acid-elicited inhibitions of PCs (34). In addition to these modulations, most probably mediated via postsynaptically located receptors, 5-HT is also acting at presynaptic sites, decreasing, for instance, glutamate release from cerebellar nerve endings (25,26). Knowing that in other neurons 5-HT was reported to either facilitate or inhibit EAA-induced responses apparently depending on cell type (29–31), such a diversity of effects, including the differential modulation of NMDA versus non-NMDA receptor-mediated responses, raises the question of the mechanisms of action of the monoamine. Since it has also been shown that 5-HT receptor types can be now divided in numerous subtypes with various effector pathways (as presented, for example, in the "Receptor nomenclature supplement," *Trends in Pharmacological Sciences,* January 1991), it is highly tempting to hypothesize a correlation between the activation of a given 5-HT receptor subtype and the physiological effect of the monoamine that could also explain the variable potency of MSD in antagonizing some of the 5-HT effects in the cerebellum, while being ineffective on others. Recently, more specific agonists and antagonists for the different 5-HT receptor subtypes have been developed and are now used as tools to differentiate the subtypes involved in the responses to 5-HT. Thus, we know now that 5-HT-induced PC inhibitions are at least partially mediated by the 5-HT_{1A} receptor subtype (10) and probably the 5-HT_{1D} one (see Chapter 6, this volume), and that the effects of 5-HT on the release of endogenous glutamate appear to be dependent on the activation of both 5-HT_{1A} and 5-HT_2 receptors (26). Therefore, enlarging the battery of the pharmacological tools that are currently available appears as a promising step forward in studies devoted to 5-HT physiological actions.

REFERENCES

1. Agnati LF, Fuxe K, Zoli M, Ozini I, Toffano G, Ferraguti F. A correlation analysis of the regional distribution of enkephalin and beta-endorphin immunoreactive terminals and of opiate receptors in adult and old male rats. Evidence for the existence of two main types of communication in the central nervous system: the volume transmission and the wiring transmission. *Acta Physiol Scand* 1986;128:201–207.
2. Armstrong DL, Hay M, Terrian DM. Modulation of cerebellar granule cell activity by iontophoretic application of serotonergic agents. *Brain Res Bull* 1987;19:699–704.
3. Audinat E, Knöpfel T, Gähwiler BH. Responses to excitatory amino acids of Purkinje cells and neurones of the deep nuclei in cerebellar slice cultures. *J Physiol (Lond)* 1990;430:297–313.
4. Bishop GA, Ho RH. The distribution and origin of serotonin immunoreactivity in the rat cerebellum. *Brain Res* 1985;331:195–207.
5. Chujo T, Yamada Y, Yamamoto C. Sensitivity of Purkinje cell dendrites to glutamic acid. *Exp Brain Res* 1975;23:293–300.
6. Crepel F, Dhanjal SS, Sears TA. Effect of glutamate, aspartate and related derivatives on cerebellar Purkinje cell dendrites in the rat: an in vitro study. *J Physiol (Lond)* 1982;323:297–317.
7. Crepel F, Dupont JL, Gardette R. Voltage-clamp analysis of the effect of excitatory amino acids and derivatives on Purkinje cell dendrites in rat cerebellar slices maintained in vitro. *Brain Res* 1983; 279:311–315.
8. Cuénod M, Do K, Vollenweider F, Zollinger M, Klein A, Streit P. The puzzle of the transmitters in the climbing fibers. In: Strata P, ed. *The olivocerebellar system in motor control.* Berlin-Heidelberg: Springer-Verlag, 1989;161–176.
9. Cull-Candy SG, Howe JR, Ogden DC. Noise and single channels activated by excitatory amino acids in rat cerebellar granular neurones. *J Physiol (Lond)* 1988;400:189–222.

10. Darrow EJ, Strahlendorf HK, Strahlendorf JC. Responses of cerebellar Purkinje cells to serotonin and the 5HT$_{1A}$ agonists 8OH-DPAT and ipsapirone in vitro. *Eur J Pharmacol* 1990;175:145–153.
11. Dupont JL, Gardette R, Crepel F. Postnatal development of the chemosensitivity of rat cerebellar Purkinje cells to excitatory amino acids. An in vitro study. *Dev Brain Res* 1987;34:59–68.
12. Fuxe K, Agnati LF, Zoli M, Bjelke B, Zini I. Some aspects of the communicational and computational organization of the brain. *Acta Physiol Scand* 1989;135:203–216.
13. Gardette R, Crepel F. Chemoresponsiveness of intracerebellar nuclei neurones to L-aspartate, L-glutamate and related derivatives in rat cerebellar slices maintained in vitro. *Neuroscience* 1986;18:93–103.
14. Gardette R, Krupa M, Crepel F. Differential effects of serotonin on the spontaneous discharge and on the excitatory amino acid-induced responses of deep cerebellar nuclei neurons in rat cerebellar slices. *Neuroscience* 1987;23:491–500.
15. Garthwaite J, Brodbelt AR. Glutamate as the principal mossy fibre transmitter in rat cerebellum: pharmacological evidence. *Eur J Neurosci* 1989;2:177–180.
16. Hamon B, Crepel F, Debono MW. Voltage-dependency of the response of cerebellar Purkinje cells to excitatory amino acids. *Brain Res* 1987;419:379–382.
17. Hicks TP, Krupa M, Crepel F. Selective effects of serotonin upon excitatory amino acid-induced depolarizations of Purkinje cells in cerebellar slices from young rats. *Brain Res* 1989;492:371–376.
18. Hökfelt T, Fuxe K. Cerebellar monoamine nerve terminals, a new type of afferent fibers to the cortex cerebelli. *Exp Brain Res* 1969;9:63–72.
19. Hudson BD, Valcana T, Bean G, Timiras PS. Glutamic acid: a strong candidate as the neurotransmitter of cerebellar granule cells. *Neurochem Res* 1976;1:73–83.
20. Kerr CW, Bishop GA. Topographical organization in the origin of serotoninergic projections to different regions of the cat cerebellar cortex. *J Comp Neurol* 1991;304:502–515.
21. Krupa M, Crepel F. Transient sensitivity of rat cerebellar Purkinje cells to N-methyl-D-aspartate during development. A voltage-clamp study in in vitro slices. *Eur J Neurosci* 1990;2:312–316.
22. Lee M, Strahlendorf JC, Strahlendorf HK. Modulatory action of serotonin on glutamate-induced excitation of cerebellar Purkinje cells. *Brain Res* 1986;361:107–113.
23. Llano I, Marty A, Johnson JW, Asher P, Gähwiler BH. Patch-clamp recordings of amino acid-activated responses in "organotypic" slice cultures. *Proc Natl Acad Sci USA* 1988;85:3221–3225.
24. Llano I, Marty A, Armstrong C, Konnerth A. Synaptic- and agonist-induced excitatory currents of Purkinje cells in rat cerebellar slices. *J Physiol (Lond)* 1991;434:183–213.
25. Maura G, Ricchetti A, Raiteri M. Serotonin inhibits the depolarization-evoked release of endogenous glutamate from rat cerebellar nerve endings. *Neurosci Lett* 1986;67:218–222.
26. Maura G, Roccatagliata E, Ulivi M, Raiteri M. Serotonin-glutamate interaction in rat cerebellum: involvement of 5HT1 and 5HT2 receptors. *Eur J Pharmacol* 1988;145:31–38.
27. Mayer ML, Westbrook GL. The physiology of excitatory amino acids in the vertebrate central nervous system. *Prog Neurobiol* 1987;28:197–276.
28. McLennan H, Hicks TP, Hall JG. Receptors for the excitatory amino acids. In: DeFeudis FW, Mandel P, eds. *Amino acid neurotransmitters (Advances in biochemical psychopharmacology*, vol 29.) New York: Raven Press, 1981:213–229.
29. Murase K, Randic M, Shirasaki T, Nakagawa T, Akaike N. Serotonin suppresses N-methyl-D-aspartate responses in acutely isolated spinal dorsal horn neurons of the rat. *Brain Res* 1990;525:84–91.
30. Nedergaard S, Engberg I, Flatman JA. Serotonin facilitates NMDA responses of cat neocortical neurones. *Acta Physiol Scand* 1986;128:323–325.
31. Nedergaard S, Engberg I, Flatman JA. The modulation of excitatory amino acid responses by serotonin in the cat neocortex in vitro. *Cell Mol Neurobiol* 1987;7:367–379.
32. O'Dell TJ, Christensen BN. A voltage-clamp study of isolated stingray horizontal cell non-NMDA excitatory amino acid receptors. *J Neurophysiol* 1989;61:162–172.
33. Strahlendorf JC, Lee M, Strahlendorf HK. Effects of serotonin on cerebellar Purkinje cells are dependent on the baseline firing rate. *Exp Brain Res* 1984;56:50–58.
34. Strahlendorf JC, Lee M, Strahlendorf HK. Modulatory role of serotonin on GABA-elicited inhibition of cerebellar Purkinje cells. *Neuroscience* 1989;30:117–125.
35. Takeuchi Y, Kimura H, Sano Y. Immunohistochemical demonstration of serotonin-containing nerve fibers in the cerebellum. *Cell Tissue Res* 1982;226:1–12.
36. Trouillas P, Brudon F, Adeleine P. Improvement of cerebellar ataxia with levorotatory form of 5-hydroxytryptophan. *Arch Neurol* 1988;45:1217–1222.

37. Watkins JC. Pharmacology of excitatory amino acid transmitters. In: DeFeudis FW, Mandel P, eds. *Amino acid neurotransmitters* (*Advances in biochemical psychopharmacology*, vol 29). New York: Raven Press, 1981:205–212.
38. Woodward DJ, Hoffre BJ, Siggins GR, Bloom FE. The ontogenetic development of synaptic junctions, synaptic activation and responsiveness to neurotransmitter substances in rat cerebellar Purkinje cells. *Brain Res* 1971;34:73–97.

Serotonin, the Cerebellum,
and Ataxia, edited by
P. Trouillas and K. Fuxe.
Raven Press, Ltd., New York © 1993.

18

Modulation of Locus Coeruleus Activity by Serotoninergic Afferents

Michel Buda, Hideo Akaoka, *Gary Aston-Jones, Paul Charléty, Karima Chergui, Guy Chouvet, and †Pierre-Hervé Luppi

*INSERM U171, CNRS URA 1195, Centre Hospitalier Lyon Sud, F-69310 Pierre-Bénite, France; *Division of Behavioral Neurobiology, Department of Mental Health Sciences, Hahnemann University, Philadelphia, Pennsylvania; †Département de Médecine Expérimentale, INSERM U52, Université Claude Bernard, 69008 Lyon, France*

In addition to its specific intrinsic connections, the cerebellar cortex also receives diffuse afferent fibers from two groups of brain stem nuclei, the raphe system and the locus coeruleus (LC). The raphe supplies the serotoninergic innervation to different layers of the cerebellar cortex. The noradrenergic nerve terminals present at these levels originate from the LC (17). These aminergic projections from brain stem nuclei are thought to have a widespread modulatory action on cerebellar function. The cerebellar serotoninergic innervation appears to be involved in several disorders such as cerebellar ataxia (see Chapters by Trouillas et al., this volume).

The functional importance of the monoaminergic cerebellar innervation has stimulated research concerning the mechanisms by which serotonin (5-HT) can exert its modulatory influence. Theoretically, this role may be exerted in two different fashions. 5-HT released from serotoninergic cerebellar terminals can act directly on postsynaptic cells. The cellular basis of such modulatory role has been extensively studied (7; see also Chapters 16 and 17, this volume). 5-HT can also indirectly influence cerebellar function by acting on the different sources of cerebellum afferent inputs. This may well be the case for 5-HT terminals located within the olivary complex or LC. In the latter example, 5-HT released from serotoninergic axon terminals that inpinge on the LC noradrenergic (LC-NA) neurons could exert a modulatory effect on cerebellar cells through the cerebellar noradrenergic innervation. A functional antagonistic interaction between neuronal systems containing 5-HT and norepinephrine (NE) in the brain had already been suspected in the late 1950s (9). Subsequent combined pharmacological and physiological studies have indicated that such an interaction is of importance in the control of brain activity during behavioral states such as the sleep-waking cycle (see ref. 20 for review).

In this chapter, we briefly summarize all direct and indirect data that support a role of the serotoninergic innervation in the regulation of LC-NA neurons.

SEROTONINERGIC AFFERENTS TO LOCUS COERULEUS: ANATOMICAL AND MORPHOLOGICAL STUDIES

Chemical Neuroanatomy

Substantial serotoninergic input to LC is indicated by high levels of 5-HT and 5-hydroxyindoleacetic acid (5-HIAA) in tissue samples including LC (13, 30). Specific $5-HT_1$ binding sites have also been reported to be present at this level (50). The LC area receives a dense network of 5-HT-containing fibers and terminals as demonstrated by different histological studies (see below). The dense 5-HT input to LC is also indicated by the presence of 5-HT uptake sites visualized by autoradiography (24), tryptophan hydroxylase immunoreactivity (35,49), and finally 5-HT immunoreactivity (6,45,46).

Morphological Studies

Presumed serotoninergic nerve endings have been morphologically identified in the LC area (16,24,28,35). All studies agree that these endings preferentially contact dendrites of LC neurons. In contrast, it is not clear from these ultrastructural studies whether the serotoninergic terminal fibers make synaptic contact (16,28) or not (24,35) with LC neurons. In addition, there is still some uncertainty as to whether the serotoninergic terminals contact the noradrenergic neurons directly or indirectly through interneurons as suggested by Maeda et al. (28).

Anatomical Studies

Previous anatomical studies from our and other laboratories have indicated that serotoninergic afferents to LC may arise from midbrain raphe nuclei (8,10,25,32). Afferents evidenced in these seminal works could not be demonstrated in a more recent study in which no retrogradely labeled cells were found in raphe nuclei after restricted injection of wheat germ agglutinin-conjugated horseradish peroxidase (WGA-HRP) or Fluoro-Gold (FG) into the LC (3). Following such tracer injection, only two medullary areas were shown to contain a great number of retrogradely labeled neurons: the nucleus paragigantocellularis lateralis (PGi) and dorsomedial region of the nucleus prepositus hypoglossi (PrH). However, no retrogradely labeled serotoninergic neurons could be evidenced in these areas (36). Given the high density of serotoninergic terminals within the LC, it was difficult to explain such controversial results as WGA-HRP and FG have been reported as more sensitive than other tracers available at that time.

We recently reinvestigated the origin of serotoninergic fibers within the LC by using retrograde transport of a highly sensitive, newly introduced tracer, the beta subunit of cholera toxin (CTb) (see ref. 27). Briefly, 20-μm cryostat sections were processed for CTb immunohistochemistry using diaminobenzidine (DAB)-nickel

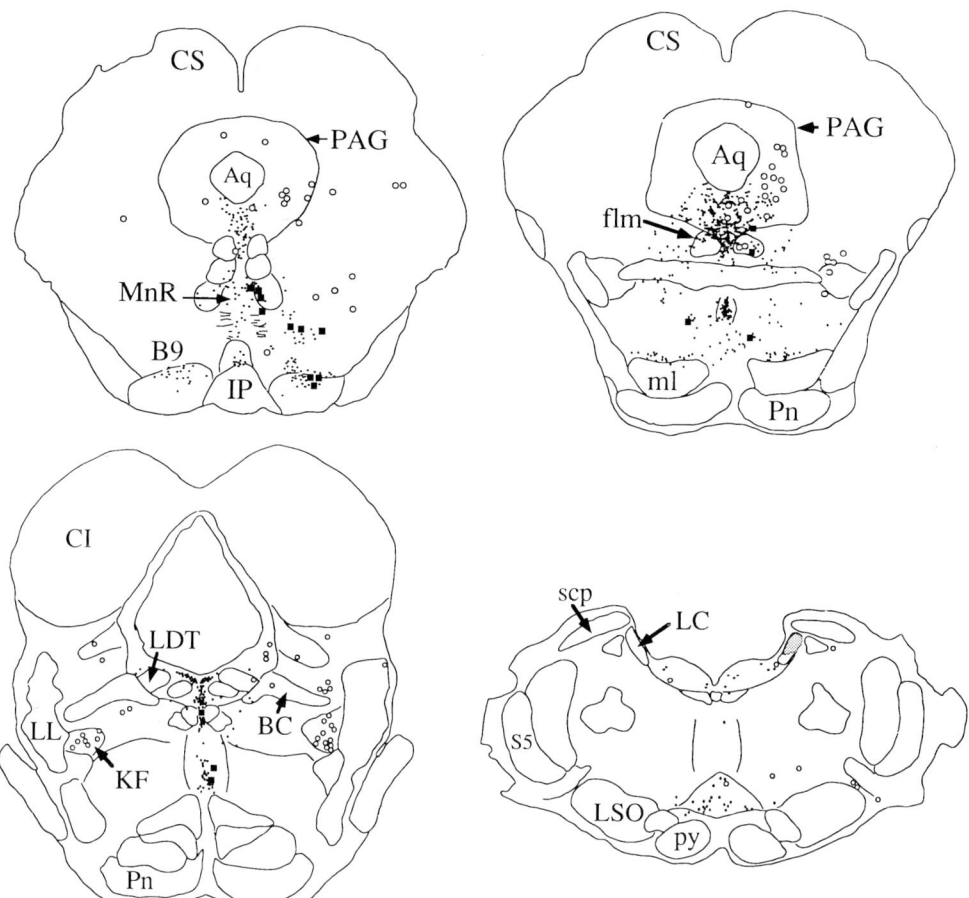

FIG. 1. Distribution of neurons retrogradely labeled with CTb following its injection into the LC. Retrogradely labeled 5-HT neurons (*filled squares*), retrogradely labeled non-5-HT neurons (*open circles*), and nonretrogradely labeled 5-HT neurons (*black dots*). Plots were drawn from sections from one representative CTb injection site (*stippling* in the last plot) that did not incorporate structures neighboring LC. CS, superior colliculus; PAG, periaqueductal gray; Aq, aqueduct; MnR, median raphe; B9, B9 serotoninergic cell group; IP, interpeduncular nucleus; flm, fascicularis longitudinalis medialis; ml, medial lemniscus; Pn, pontine nucleus; CI, inferior colliculus; LDT, laterodorsal tegmental nucleus; BC, brachium conjunctivum; LL, lateral lemniscus; KF, Kölliker-Fuse nucleus; scp, superior cerebellar peduncle; LC, locus coeruleus; S5, trigeminal nerve; LSO, lateral superior olive; py, pyramidal tract.

reaction. On the same sections, 5-HT immunoreactivity was visualized by DAB alone. Double-labeled neurons were identified as cells containing black granules of CTb over a brown, diffusely stained cytoplasm.

After CTb injection in rat LC, 5-HT double-labeled cells were consistently observed in the median raphe, the B9 serotoninergic cell group. Double-labeled neurons were also consistently found in the reticular formation localized laterally to the median raphe and inside the fascicularis longitudinalis medialis. Fewer double-labeled cells were found in the nuclei raphe dorsalis and pontis (Fig. 1). No or only occasional double-labeled cells were observed in the peri-LC area, the nucleus raphe magnus, and PGi. In contrast with some previous studies (25,28), these results suggest that the 5-HT input to the LC may originate from 5-HT pontine nuclei outside the dorsal raphe, in particular the B9 5-HT group, median raphe, and surrounding reticular formation. Our results suggest also that the 5-HT innervation is not primarily issued from the peri-LC area or medullary serotoninergic nuclei, as previously suggested (36). Further experiments are in progress to evaluate the full extent of the injected tracer, as it is possible that some of the retrogradely labeled cells represent uptake by terminals outside LC.

BIOCHEMICAL EVIDENCE FOR A CONTROL OF LC-NA ACTIVITY BY 5-HT

In this section we review some of the biochemical evidence for a serotoninergic influence on LC-NA neurons. The strategies used in the past two decades to demonstrate an influence of serotoninergic neurons on LC-NA neurons were mainly based on measuring specific metabolic changes in LC-NA neurons after manipulation of 5-HT systems. Three different approaches were used: (i) limited electrolytic lesions of the raphe nuclei; (ii) neurotoxin-specific destruction of 5-HT terminals; (iii) pharmacological inhibition of 5-HT synthesis. Finally, the resulting observations were complemented by a direct study of the 5-HT action on LC explants in culture.

Limited Electrolytic Lesions of the Raphe System

Midbrain raphe electrolytic lesions were first shown to induce changes of NE turnover in noradrenergic terminal brain areas (22). These primary observations stimulated further studies to test the hypothesis of a serotoninergic control of the synthesis of NE in the LC by fibers originating in the raphe. Electrolytic coagulation of either the nucleus raphe dorsalis, the nucleus raphe centralis, or the raphe pontis led to highly significant increases in the activity of tyrosine hydroxylase (TH), the rate-limiting enzyme of NE synthesis (33), measured from homogenates of the LC region (26,29). The elevation of TH activity observed after the single or combined lesions of the different brain stem raphe nuclei was always progressive and reversible over a 8- to 15-day period with a maximum reached 4 to 6 days after lesion. These latter studies indicated that such alteration of TH activity might be one of the mechanisms responsible for the increase in NE turnover observed in previous studies. They also revealed a long-term effect of such lesions on TH activity within the somadendritic region of LC-NA neurons. Finally, these lesion studies also revealed that only destruction of raphe nuclei leading to significant decreases in 5-HT content in the LC area was able to provoke a significant elevation in TH activity (29).

Destruction of 5-HT Terminals by Specific Neurotoxins

Intraventricular injection of 5,6-dihydroxytryptamine (5,6-DHT) provokes also a significant increase in TH activity in the LC (41). Reversal of the 5,6-DHT effect was obtained by pretreatment with chlorimipramine (a 5-HT reuptake blocker that protects 5-HT terminals against the neurotoxin). This increase was clearly shown to be correlated with a decrease in 5-HT content of the LC at various doses of 5,6-DHT and protection of the serotoninergic fibers against this neurotoxin by pretreatment with different 5-HT uptake inhibitors (21,31). This observation strongly suggested that 5-HT terminals could play an important role in the control of LC metabolic activity. Furthermore, the involvement of the 5-HT fibers present within the LC complex was reasonably accepted in view of the fact that local injection of 5,6-DHT directly into the LC was also followed by significant increases in TH activity in this structure (37).

Studies with intracerebroventricular injections of 5,6-DHT revealed also that the alterations of TH activity were accompanied by alterations in dopamine-β-hydroxylase activity, the enzyme that catalyzes the transformation of dopamine into NE and that is specifically localized within noradrenergic (or adrenergic) neurons. In contrast, activities of other enzymes involved in catecholamine metabolism such as DOPA-decarboxylase or monoamine oxidase, but also present within other types of neurons, were not altered (21). Such selectivity in enzyme regulation ressembles the one observed in the transsynaptic induction of TH in the peripheral sympathetic nervous system (47).

Pharmacologically Induced Depletion of Brain 5-HT Content

Administration of parachlorophenylalanine (PCPA), a specific depletor of brain 5-HT, leads to a significant increase in TH activity in the LC area. Repeated treatment with this drug (300 mg/kg daily) was necessary to significantly alter TH activity. Daily injections of the drug for 3 to 4 days were necessary to induce prolonged significant decreases in 5-HT levels of the LC area and parallel increases in TH activity (Fig. 2). Maximum elevation in enzyme activity occurred several days (at day 4 after the last of a series of four successive daily injections of PCPA) after 5-HT had reached its minimum level (13). When LC-5-HT levels were restored to normal by pretreatment with 5-hydroxytryptophan (5-HTP) (the direct precursor of 5-HT), the increase in TH activity was greatly reduced. Altogether these results provide additional evidence for a role of 5-HT in the regulation of NE synthesis within LC neurons.

Role of Serotoninergic Fibers in the Regulation of TH Within LC-NA Neurons

The above results clearly show that all situations leading to the inactivation of the 5-HT system provoke an increase in TH activity within the LC. The pattern of TH

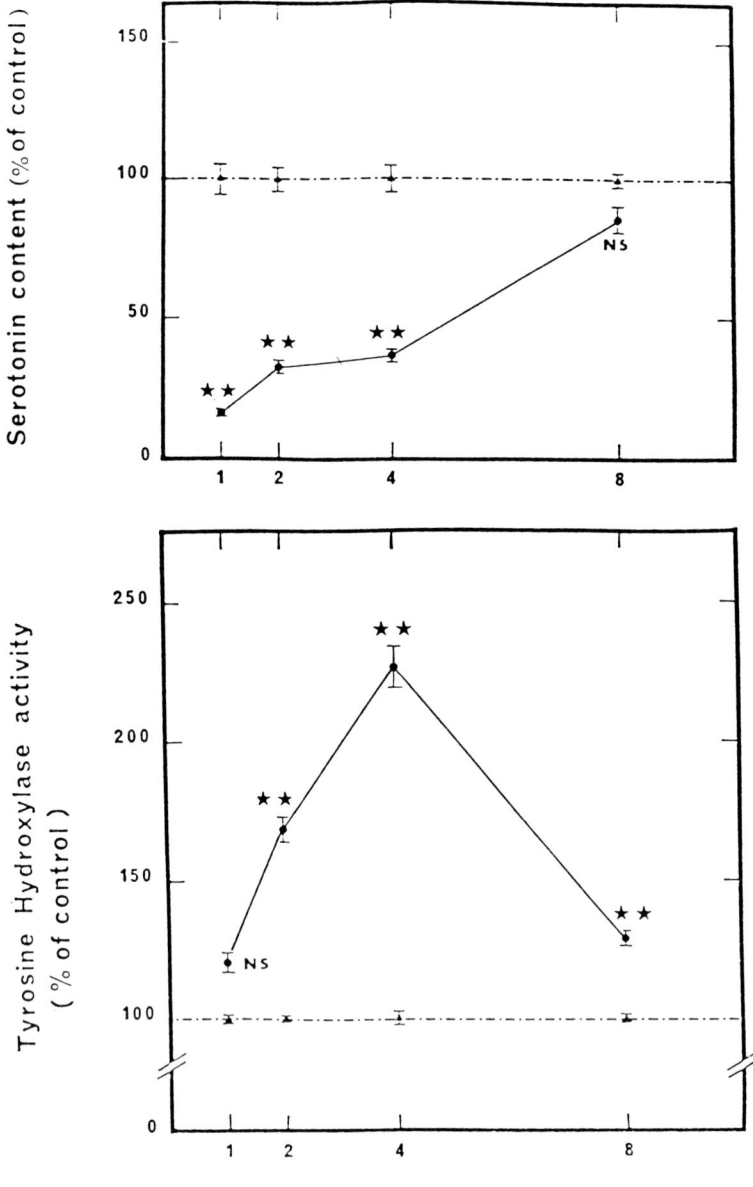

FIG. 2. TH activity and 5-HT content in the rat LC at various days after successive injections of PCPA (once daily, 300 mg/kg i.p.). Each point represents means ± SEM of 9 to 12 animals. Each control value represents five to six rats. For each point, changes in TH activity and 5-HT content are normalized to the corresponding control value (horizontal 100% line). NS, not significant; $p > 0.05$; **, significant at $p < 0.001$.

activation in the different experimental conditions studied is always about the same: the enzyme activation occurs over an 8- to 15-day period, with a maximum at day 4 after the end of the specific treatment, and this activation is reversible. Immunotitration studies of LC homogenates with increased TH activity had revealed that TH elevation resulted from the accumulation of TH molecules (29). Furthermore, studies in 5,6-DHT treated animals have also shown increased specific TH-mRNA associated with increased TH activity (Fig. 3). These results support the contention that inactivation of the 5-HT system alters TH enzyme protein synthesis within LC-NA neurons.

The mechanisms of the regulation of LC-NA TH synthesis by 5-HT were further studied *in vitro* with culture explants of newborn LC. A decrease in TH activity was observed as early as 24 hr after 5-HT was added to the culture medium. This effect was dose dependent and reversible over a long-term period (several days after 5-HT removal from the culture medium). The effect of 5-HT was suppressed with equimolar concentrations of 5-HT receptor antagonists such as metergoline or methiothepin (MTT) (Fig. 4). The action of 5-HT was not additive to that of inhibitors of protein synthesis, suggesting that the regulation of TH activity by 5-HT may involve protein synthesis (14). Thus, these *in vitro* studies corroborate the *in vivo* results and favor the hypothesis that 5-HT released from fibers present around LC-NA neurons may regulate TH synthesis and activity through specific serotoninergic receptors.

In conclusion, the biochemical data reviewed here clearly demonstrate the role of 5-HT in the regulation of LC neurons. The main point revealed in these studies is that 5-HT action occurs on a long-term basis, most probably involving both membrane and genomic processes.

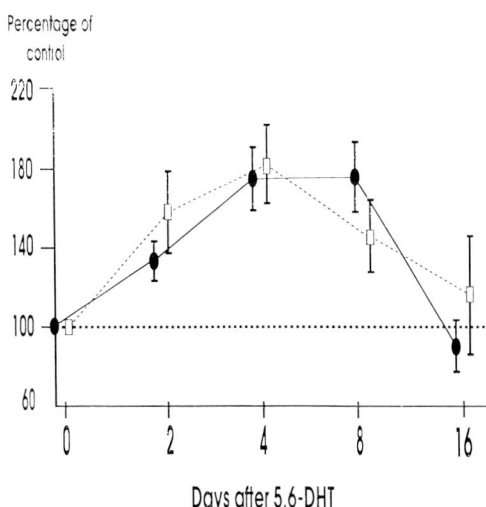

FIG. 3. TH activity (●) and mRNA levels (□) in the LC at various days following an i.c.v. injection of 50 mg of 5,6-DHT. The results (means ± SEM of 7 to 15 independent experiments) are expressed as a percentage of the corresponding values in appropriate vehicle-injected rats sacrificed at the same posttreatment time.

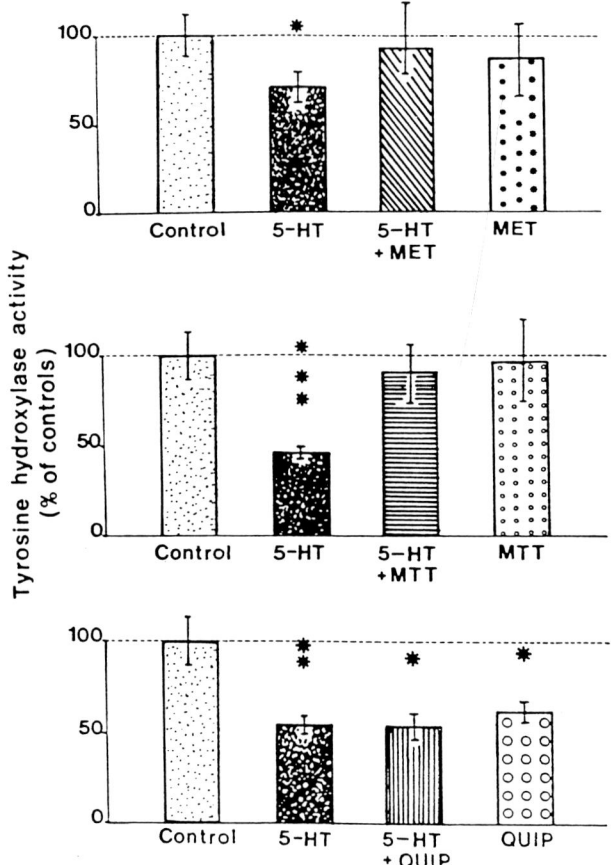

FIG. 4. Effect of different serotoninergic drugs on the 5-HT-induced decrease in TH activity in LC explants. Seven-day-old cultures of LC explants were treated with 5-HT alone, a combination of 5-HT plus metergoline (MET, 10^{-5} M), MTT (10^{-5} M) quipazine (QUIP, 10^{-5} M), or by the drug alone. TH activity was expressed as a percentage of the value in control explants. Data are means ± SEM (bars) values from four to seven experiments. Control TH activity was 95.7, 85.1, and 76.2 pmol of DOPA/10 min/explant for the experiments with MET, MTT, and QUIP, respectively. Values that are significantly different compared with controls are indicated: *$p<0.05$; **$p<0.01$; ***$p<0.001$. Comparison of 5-HT/5-HT+MET was not significant, but comparison of 5-HT/5-HT+MTT was significant ($p<0.001$).

ELECTROPHYSIOLOGICAL STUDIES

Despite the functional implications of serotoninergic innervation of LC, little is known about the role of 5-HT in electrical activity of LC neurons. If the increase of LC activity after depletion of 5-HT by PCPA (15) is consistent with the biochemical changes within the LC, as reviewed herein, sertraline, a selective serotoninergic uptake blocker, has no effect on the spontaneous firing of these neurons (48). Systemic administration of 5-HT$_2$ or hallucinogenic (1,38) serotoninergic agonists inhibit the tonic discharge rate of LC neurons, whereas 5-HT$_1$ agonists tend to increase the tonic activity (42). Paradoxically, 5-HT$_2$ or hallucinogenic serotoninergic agonists, while decreasing tonic discharge rate, increase the excitability of LC neurons in response to sensory stimuli (38). Segal (43) reported an inhibition of the basal discharge rate and a decrease in the responsiveness of these cells to noxious stimuli by direct microapplication of 5-HT into LC. We have reexamined the electrophysiological effects of 5-HT on LC single cell activity *in vivo*, in particular the interactions between 5-HT and excitatory amino acids (EAAs), which have been suggested to play an important role in the adaptation of LC discharge in responses to physiological changes (4).

Single cell extracellular recordings of LC neurons combined with microiontophoretic techniques were performed on halothane-anesthetized rats as previously described (5,11,12). To improve recording quality, a glass microelectrode was glued alongside the multibarrel ejection pipette so that the recording tip extended 15 to 20 µm beyond the multibarrel tip. LC neurons were identified online according to criteria described elsewhere in detail (5). For quantitative analysis, the firing rates of each cell were determined for two periods of 10 sec before and during each pulse of iontophoretic application of glutamate (Glu). Values obtained from three consecutive Glu pulses were used to calculate for each cell the mean basal firing rate and mean firing rate during the Glu pulse. The Glu-induced responses were determined as the mean firing rate during Glu minus the mean basal rate. A serotoninergic substance was then continuously coiontophoresed with pulsed Glu, and the effects of each substance tested were expressed as a percentage of the Glu-evoked response before any application of serotoninergic compound. Data are expressed as the mean ± SEM.

Effect of 5-HT on Spontaneous and Evoked Activity of LC Neurons

The spontaneous firing rate of LC neurons recorded with compound iontophoretic pipettes containing Glu ranged from 0.4 to 7.5 spike/sec, with an average value of 2.3 ± 0.1 spike/sec ($n = 247$) (5,11). Iontophoretic application of 5-HT only produced inconsistent effects on basal discharge rate of LC neurons. In agreement with a previous study in urethane-anesthetized rats (43), the majority of LC neurons were weakly inhibited (51 of 109 cells). 5-HT had no effect on 49 neurons and excited nine remaining cells. Overall, basal activity of LC neurons was reduced 14 ± 2% by iontophoretic 5-HT ($n = 109$). Such weak effect is not due to the iontophoretic techniques used, as putative transmitters other than 5-HT yielded pronounced and consistent effects on basal LC discharge. Indeed, iontophoretic application of NE (23 of 25 cells), gamma-aminobutyric acid (GABA) (13 of 13), or glycine (15 of 15) potently inhibited LC neuronal discharge. Also, iontophoretic Glu or acetylcholine (ACh) consistently and reproducibly activated LC neurons (201 of 211 and 22 of 25 cells, respectively).

Despite the inconsistent effects of 5-HT on LC basal discharge, 5-HT potently decreased excitatory responses of LC neurons evoked by iontophoretic Glu. As shown in Fig. 5, 5-HT reduced Glu-induced excitation by $43 \pm 4\%$ ($n = 109$), while having little or no effect on the basal activity of the same neurons. Note that this attenuation of Glu-induced activation by 5-HT was independent of its effects on basal activity, and Glu-evoked responses were not entirely blocked, even by increasing 5-HT ejection current. Such a decrease of Glu-induced excitation by iontophoretic 5-HT is not an artifact of the iontophoretic technique used. Control iontophoresis through a side barrel containing physiological saline solution was never able to attenuate excitation induced by Glu, even with current greater than that used for 5-HT. In addition, results obtained by pressure application of 5-HT through the same barrel used for iontophoresis closely resembled those found for iontophoretic 5-HT. Contrary to 5-HT, NE decreased basal LC activity, but not excitatory responses to Glu or ACh (Fig. 5). 5-HT acts specifically on LC excitation induced by Glu, as activation of the same neurons produced by ACh was not affected by intracoerulear 5-HT. Iontophoretic as well as pressure applications of 5-HT were unable to decrease excitatory responses of LC neurons to iontophoretic ACh (Fig. 5, five of six and four of five neurons, respectively).

Subtypes of 5-HT Receptors Involved in the Attenuation of Glu-Evoked Responses

The effect of 5-HT on Glu-evoked excitation of LC neurons is specific to 5-HT receptors, as their antagonists methysergide (MTS) or MTT significantly reduced the effect of 5-HT on Glu-induced response (Fig. 6). Next, the receptor subtypes involved in the reduction of Glu-evoked activation of LC neurons by 5-HT were more precisely characterized. Given the number of functional subtypes of 5-HT receptors and the relative difficulty to obtain specific agonists or antagonists suitable for iontophoretic use (i.e., high concentration generally required), we studied the possible implication of $5-HT_1$ and $5-HT_2$ receptor subtypes. The effect of 5-HT could be mimicked by the $5-HT_1$ agonist RU 24969 ($n = 11$, Fig. 7). Furthermore, the $5-HT_{1A}$ agonists 8-hydroxy-2-(di-n-propylamino)tetralin (8-OH-DPAT) ($n = 16$) and buspirone ($n = 27$), but not the $5-HT_{1B}$ agonist m-trifluoromethylphenylpiperazine (TFMPP) ($n = 13$), reduced the magnitude of Glu-evoked excitation (Fig. 7). In contrast, the $5-HT_2$ antagonist ketanserin failed to reverse, and the $5-HT_2$ agonist 1-(2,5-dimethoxy-4-iodophenyl)-2-aminopropane (DOI), failed to mimic, the effect of 5-HT on Glu-induced activation (Fig. 7, $n = 8$ and 6, respectively). As iontophoretic applications of ketanserin or TFMPP have been shown to be effective in other brain areas (23,44), our results indicate that 5-HT acts at $5-HT_{1A}$ receptors to attenuate the excitation of LC neurons induced by Glu.

Attenuation of Opiate Withdrawal-Induced Activation of LC Neurons by Enhanced 5-HT Neurotransmission

The specific interaction between 5-HT and Glu suggests that 5-HT modulates the responsiveness of LC neurons to afferent inputs, rather than increasing or decreas-

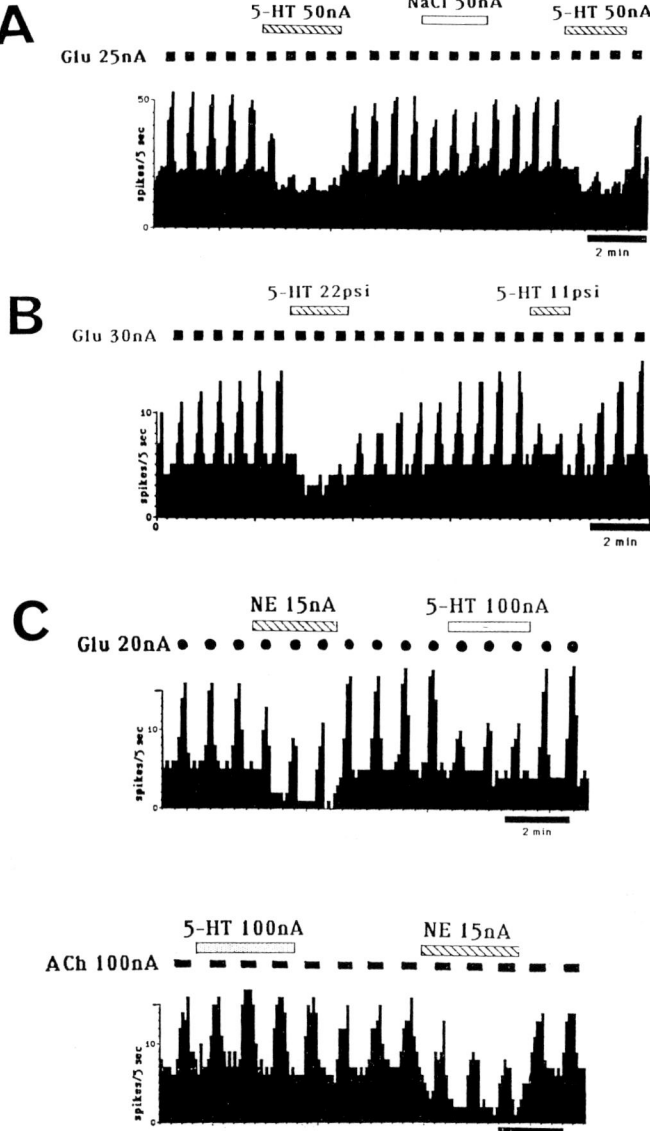

FIG. 5. Computer-generated integrated activity-time histograms revealing interactions of 5-HT and Glu on LC discharge. **A**: Iontophoretic pulses of Glu (applied at *solid bars*) activate a typical LC neuron. Coiontophoresis of 5-HT (applied at *hatched bars*), but not of saline (applied at *open bar*) attenuates Glu response but has little effect on basal discharge. **B**: 5-HT applied by pressure (at *stippled bars*) attenuates responses to iontophoretic Glu (applied at solid bars), mimicking effect of iontophoretic 5-HT. Note the slow recovery after 5-HT application. **C**: Comparison of norepinephrine NE and 5-HT effects on responses to Glu and ACh for the same LC neuron. NE applied with a long pulse of low current (at *hatched bars*) inhibits basal activity but leaves responses evoked by Glu (applied at *solid circles, upper trace*) or ACh (applied at *solid bars, lower trace*) intact. In contrast, 5-HT applied in long pulses (at *open bars*) does not affect basal discharge rate, but attenuates responses to Glu (*upper trace*). Note that, although responses to Glu are attenuated by 5-HT, responses of the same LC neuron to ACh remain intact during application of 5-HT (*lower trace*). Ordinates, number of spikes per 5 sec; abcissas, time (calibration bars = 2 min).

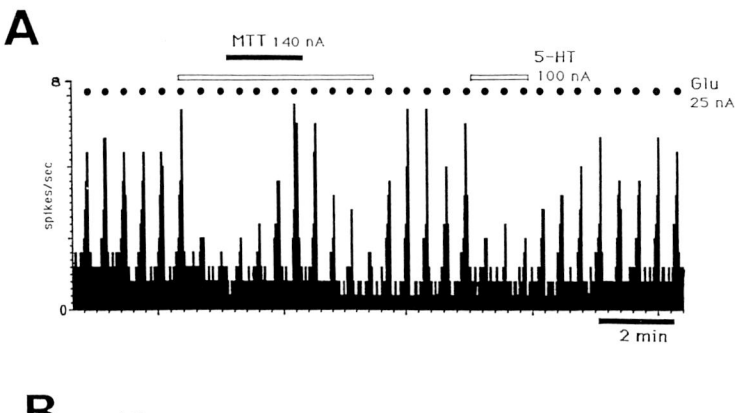

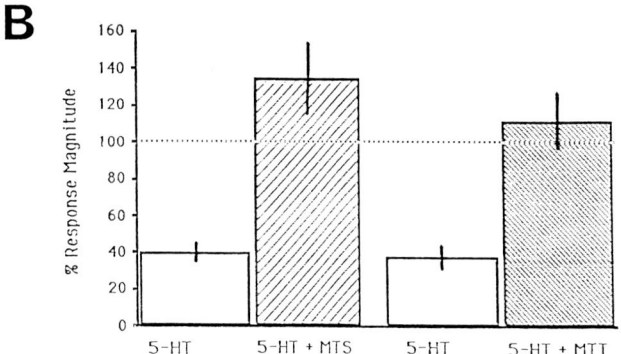

FIG. 6. Antagonists of 5-HT receptors attenuate effects of 5-HT on LC neurons. **A**: Attenuation of the response magnitude to iontophoretically applied Glu (at *solid circles*) by 5-HT (at *open bars*) is reversed by coiontophoresis of MTT (at *solid bar*). Ordinates, spikes per second; abcissas, time. Calibration bar = 2 min. **B**: Effects of coiontophoresis of MTS and MTT on attenuation of the response magnitude to Glu by 5-HT. The response magnitude under 5-HT, 5-HT + MTS, and 5-HT + MTT was calculated for each cell as percentage of the response magnitude for Glu alone on the same cell (baseline response magnitude, 100). Results are expressed as means ± SEM. Both MTS ($n=6$) and MTT ($n=4$) antagonized the effect of 5-HT on responses to Glu: the response magnitude observed with 5-HT plus the antagonist is significantly ($p<0.05$) greater than the Glu response magnitude observed with 5-HT alone.

ing their tonic impulse activity. In particular, 5-HT may attenuate excitatory responses mediated by EAA afferents, such as electrical stimulation of the rear footpad (4), bladder distention (34), or opiate withdrawal (2,39). Here we show that the hyperactivity of LC neurons during opiate withdrawal is attenuated by agents that increase 5-HT neurotransmission. Such a finding is of significant clinical interest as the LC-NA system has been proposed to play an important role in the expression of autonomic or psychological aversive symptoms during opiate withdrawal (40). Experiments were performed on halothane-anesthetized rats after 6 days of chronic

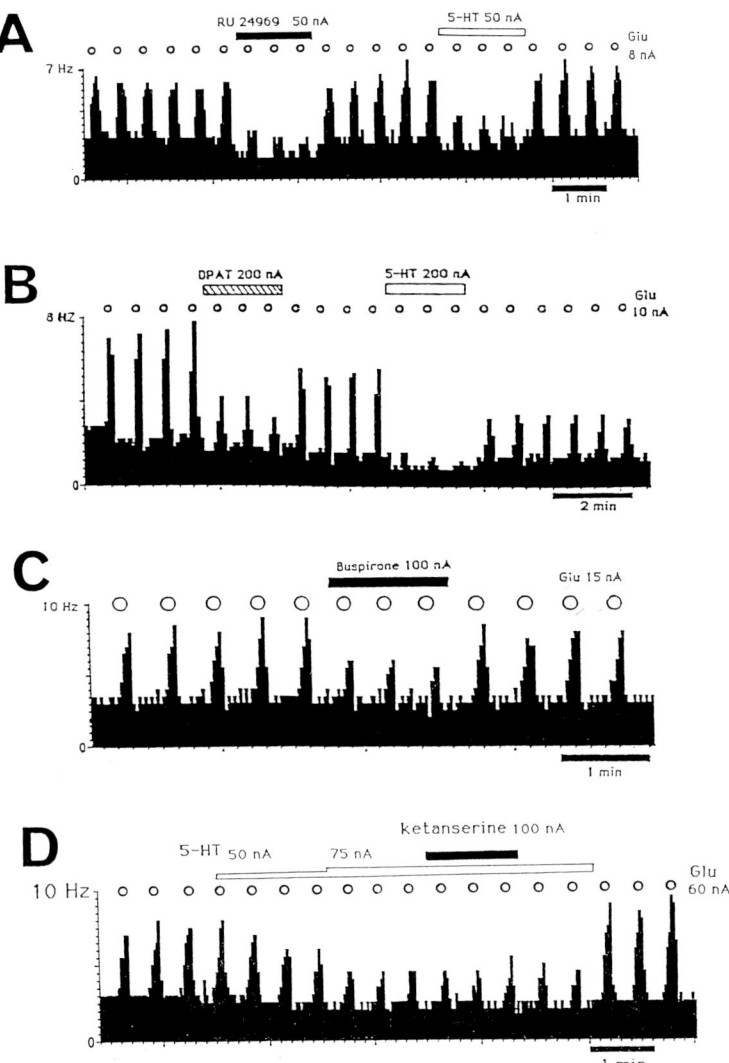

FIG. 7. Effects of 5-HT and related drugs on responses of LC neurons to iontophoretic Glu. **A:** Ionotophoretic application of the 5-HT$_1$ agonist RU24969 (*solid bar*) mimics the effect of 5-HT (*open bar*) on Glu-evoked (*open circles*) responses. **B,C:** The same phenomenon is observed with iontophoretic application of the 5-HT$_{1A}$ agonists 8-OH-DPAT (B, at *hatched bar*) and buspirone (C, at *solid bar*). **D:** The decrease of Glu-evoked excitations induced by iontophoretic 5-HT is not affected by coiontophoresis of the 5-HT$_2$ antagonist ketanserin (at *solid bar*). Ordinates, LC neurons firing frequency in hertz; abcissas, time (calibration bars = 1 min, except in B, 2 min).

administration of morphine as previously described (2). In all chronically treated rats, LC neurons exhibited the characteristic increase of their activity upon morphine withdrawal, pharmacologically precipitated by intravenous injection of the opiate antagonist naloxone (0.1 mg/kg, one injection per animal, $n=78$). We pooled data from all LC neurons sampled during the 10- to 30-min period postnaloxone to compare mean firing rates postwithdrawal obtained following different pharmacological treatments.

As shown in Fig. 8, d-fenfluramine (2 mg/kg i.v.), a 5-HT releaser/uptake blocker (18), potently reduced the magnitude of activation produced by opiate withdrawal. The mean firing rate of LC neurons during opiate withdrawal (10- to 30-min period postnaloxone) was strongly reduced by d-fenfluramine treatment, from 3.9 ± 0.4 to 2.1 ± 0.4 spikes/sec ($n = 14$ and 5, respectively). d-Fenfluramine seems to act via endogenous 5-HT systems (at least partly), as its depletion prior to opiate withdrawal considerably reduced the effectiveness of this drug: in PCPA-treated animals, the firing rate during opiate withdrawal after d-fenfluramine was significantly greater than in nontreated rats (3.5 ± 0.2 vs 2.1 ± 1 spikes/sec, $n = 8$ and 5, respectively). Possible implication of endogenous 5-HT is further indicated by the effectiveness of the two 5-HT uptake blockers fluoxetine (4 mg/kg i.v., $n=6$) or sertraline (3 mg/kg i.p., $n=5$), associated or not with prior treatment with 5-HTP

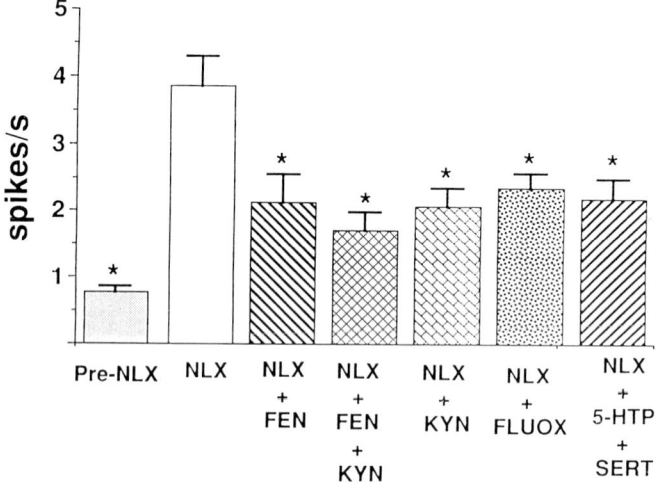

FIG. 8. Relative effectiveness of different treatments to attenuate LC hyperactivity induced by opiate withdrawal. Treatments that enhance 5-HT neurotransmission, or i.c.v. kynurenate (KYN) reduced the withdrawal-induced LC hyperactivity to a very similar level, about 2 spikes per second. But the effects of EAA antagonism and elevated serotoninergic transmission were not additive, as the combined treatment with d-fenfluramine (FEN) and KYN was not more effective than each one of these drugs administered alone. Note also that 5-HTP treatment alone did not affect the magnitude of opiate withdrawal-induced LC activation. SERT, sertraline; NLX, naloxone; FLUOX, fluoxetine.

29. McRae-Degueurce A, Bérod A, et al. Alterations in tyrosine hydroxylase activity elicited by raphe nuclei lesions in the rat locus coeruleus: evidence for the involvement of serotonin afferents. *Brain Res* 1982;235:285–301.
30. McRae-Degueurce A, Milon H. Serotonin and dopaminergic afferents to the rat locus coeruleus: biochemical study after lesioning of the ventral mesencephalic tegmental-A10 region and the raphe dorsalis. *Brain Res* 1983;263:344–347.
31. McRae-Degueurce A, Pujol JF. Correlation between the increase in tyrosine hydroxylase activity and the decrease in serotonin content in the rat locus coeruleus after 5,6-dihydroxytryptamine. *Eur J Pharmacol* 1979;59:131–135.
32. Morgane PJ, Jacobs MS. Raphe projections to the locus coeruleus in the rat. *Brain Res Bull* 1979;4:519–534.
33. Nagatsu T, Levitt M, Udenfriend S. Tyrosine hydroxylase: the initial step in norepinephrine biosynthesis. *J Biol Chem* 1964;238:2910–2917.
34. Page ME, Akaoka H, Valentino RJ. Bladder distention activates noradrenergic locus coeruleus neurons by an excitatory amino acid mechanism (*submitted*).
35. Pickel VM, Joh TH, Reis DJ. A serotoninergic innervation of noradrenergic neurons in nucleus locus coeruleus: demonstration by immunocytochemical localization of the transmitter specific enzymes tyrosine and tryptophan hydroxylase. *Brain Res* 1977;131:197–214.
36. Pieribone VA, Van Bockstaele E, Shipley MT, Aston-Jones G. Serotoninergic innervation of rat locus coeruleus derives from non-raphe brain areas. *Soc Neurosci Abstr* 1989.
37. Pujol JF, Keane P, McRae-Degueurce A, Lewis BD, Renaud B. Biochemical evidence for serotoninergic control of the locus coeruleus. In: Garattini JF, Pujol JF, Samanin R, eds. *Interactions between putative neurotransmitters in the brain.* New York: Raven Press, 1978:401–410.
38. Rasmussen K, Aghajanian GK. Effect of hallucinogens on spontaneous and sensory-evoked locus coeruleus unit activity in the rat: reversal by selective 5-HT2 antagonists. *Brain Res* 1986;385:395–400.
39. Rasmussen K, Aghajanian GK. Withdrawal-induced activation of locus coeruleus neurons in opiate-dependent rats: attenuation by lesions of the nucleus paragigantocellularis. *Brain Res* 1989;505:346–350.
40. Redmond DE Jr, Krystal JH. Multiple mechanisms of withdrawal from opioid drugs. *Annu Rev Neurol* 1984;7:443–478.
41. Renaud B, Buda M, Lewis BD, Pujol JF. Effects of 5,6-dihydroxytryptamine on tyrosine hydroxylase activity in central catecholaminergic neurons of the rat. *Biochem Pharmacol* 1975;24:1739–1742.
42. Sanghera MK, German DC. The effects of benzodiazepine and non-benzodiazepine anxiolytics on locus coeruleus unit activity. *J Neural Transm* 1983;57:267–279.
43. Segal M. Serotoninergic innervation of the locus coeruleus from the dorsal raphe and its action on responses to noxious stimuli. *J Physiol* 1979;286:401–415.
44. Sprouse JS, Aghajanian GK. Electrophysiological responses of serotoninergic dorsal raphe neurons to 5-HT 1A and 5-HT 1B agonists. *Synapse* 1987;1:3–9.
45. Steinbush HWM. Distribution of serotonin immunoreactivity in the central nervous system of the rat: cells bodies and terminals. *Neuroscience* 1981;6:557–618.
46. Steinbush HWM. Serotonin immunoreactivity neurons and their projections in the CNS. In: Björklund A, Hökfelt T, Kuhar MJ, eds. *Classical transmitters and transmitter receptors in the CNS*, part II. Amsterdam: Elsevier, 1984:68–125.
47. Thoenen H, Otten V, Schwab M. Orthograde and retrograde signals for the regulation of neuronal gene expression: the peripheral sympathetic nervous system as a model. In: Schmidt FO, Warden FG, eds. *The Neurosciences*, fourth study program. Cambridge, MA: MIT Press, 1979:911–928.
48. Valentino RJ, Curtis AL, Parris DG, Wehby G. Antidepressant actions on brain noradrenergic neurons. *J Pharmacol Exp Ther* 1990;253:833–840.
49. Weissman D, Belin M-F, Aguera M, et al. Immunohistochemistry of tryptophan hydroxylase in the rat brain. *Neuroscience* 1987;23:291–304.
50. Weissmann-Nanopoulos D, Mach E, Magre J, Demassey Y, Pujol JF. Evidence for the localisation of 5-HT 1A binding sites on serotonin containing neurons in the raphe dorsalis and raphe centralis nuclei of the rat brain. *Neurochem Int* 1985;7:1061–1072.

(100 mg/kg i.p.), to attenuate the magnitude of naloxone-induced hyperactivity of LC neurons (Fig. 8). Finally, the 5-HT agents tested herein may act by reducing the influence of EAA inputs to LC, as blockade of EAA receptors (i.c.v. kynurenate, 0.5 μmol) was no more effective in decreasing withdrawal-induced LC hyperactivity, following enhancement of 5-HT neurotransmission by d-fenfluramine. As shown in Fig. 8, after treatments with d-fenfluramine or kynurenate alone, as well as after their combined treatment, the mean firing rates of LC neurons post-naloxone were very similar (2.2 ± 0.3, 2.1 ± 0.3, and 1.7 ± 0.3 spikes/sec, $n = 12$, 6, and 5, respectively). As the clinical effectiveness of clonidine, an α_2 agonist, in relieving some of autonomic and behavioral symptoms (40) is thought to be due in large part to its attenuation of LC hyperactivity, the same symptoms may be also relieved by the 5-HT agents tested herein, which we have shown to reduce withdrawal-induced LC hyperactivity.

CONCLUSION

All the observations presented shed some light on the mechanisms governing the balance between two important monoaminergic systems in the brain. All anatomical, biochemical, pharmacological, and electrophysiological observations summarized in this review converge to demonstrate a modulatory influence of 5-HT on LC-NA neuron activity. There is strong evidence that the serotoninergic terminal fibers present in the LC area are the anatomical support of such an interaction. It is not yet clear whether this influence is direct or indirect on LC-NA cells or indirect on afferent neurons. A very interesting point that emerges from these studies is that the action of 5-HT on LC neurons does not seem to be limited to the regulation of their electrical activity but may also extend to the control of the synthesis of the rate-limiting enzyme in NE synthesis. Clearly then, 5-HT influence extends from membrane to genome.

The importance of such an interaction has already been suspected concerning the regulation of normal brain activity. However, this interaction has also been thought to be involved in the genesis of psychiatric disorders including depression and anxiety. Finally, we propose this balance to also be an important factor in neurologic disorders such as cerebellar ataxia, which involve specific monoaminergic pathways to cerebellum.

REFERENCES

1. Aghajanian GK. Mescaline and LSD facilitate the activation of locus coeruleus neurons by peripheral stimuli. *Brain Res* 1980;186:492–498.
2. Akaoka H, Aston-Jones G. Opiate withdrawal-induced hyperactivity of locus coeruleus neurons is substantially mediated by augmented excitatory amino acid input. *J Neurosci* 1991;11:3830–3839.
3. Aston-Jones G, Ennis M, Pieribone V, Nickell WT, Shipley MT. The brain nucleus locus coeruleus: restricted afferent control of a broad efferent network. *Science* 1986;234:734–737.
4. Aston-Jones G, Shipley MT, Chouvet G, et al. Afferent regulation of locus coeruleus neurons: anatomy, physiology and pharmacology. *Prog Brain Res* 1991;88:47–75.

5. Aston-Jones G, Akaoka H, Charléty P, Chouvet G. Serotonin selectively attenuates the glutamate-evoked activation of noradrenergic locus coeruleus neurons. *J Neurosci* 1991;11:760–769.
6. Aston-Jones G, Shipley MT, Ennis M, Williams JT, Pieribone V. Restricted afferent control of locus coeruleus neurons revealed by anatomical physiological, and pharmacological studies. In: Heal DJ, Marsden CA, eds. *The pharmacology of noradrenaline in the central nervous system.* Oxford: Oxford University Press, 1990:187–247.
7. Bloom FE. General features of chemically identified neurons. In: Björklund A, Hökfelt T, eds. *Handbook of chemical neuroanatomy: classical neurotransmitters in the CNS,* vol 2, part I. Amsterdam: Elsevier, 1984:1–22.
8. Bobillier P, Petitjean F, Salvert D, Ligier M, Seguin S. Differential projection of the nucleus raphe dorsalis and raphe centralis as revealed by autoradiography. *Brain Res* 1975;85:205–210.
9. Brodie B, Shore P. A concept for a role of serotonin and norepinephrine as chemical mediators in the brain. *Ann NY Acad Sci* 1957;66:631–642.
10. Cedarbaum JM, Aghajanian GK. Afferent projections to the rat locus coeruleus as determined by a retrograde tracing technique. *J Comp Neurol* 1978;178:1–16.
11. Charléty P, Aston-Jones G, Akaoka H, Buda M, Chouvet G. 5-HT decreases glutamate-evoked activation of locus coeruleus neurons through 5-HT 1A receptors. *C R Acad Sci Paris* 1991;312:421–426.
12. Chouvet G, Akaoka H, Aston-Jones G. Serotonin selectively decreases glutamate-induced excitation of locus coeruleus neurons. *C R Acad Sci Paris* 1988;306:339–344.
13. Crespi F, Buda M, McRae-Degueurce A, Pujol JF. Alteration of tyrosine hydroxylase activity in the locus coeruleus after administration of p-chlorophenylalanine. *Brain Res* 1980;191:501–509.
14. Devau G, Multon MF, Pujol JF, Buda M. Inhibition of tyrosine hydroxylase activity by serotonin in explants of newborn rats locus coeruleus. *J Neurochem* 1987;49:665–670.
15. Ferron A. Modified coeruleo-cortical noradrenergic neurotransmission after serotonin depletion by PCPA: electrophysiological studies in the rat. *Synapse* 1988;2:532–536.
16. Groves PM, Wilson CJ. Monoaminergic presynaptic axons and dendrites in the rat locus coeruleus seen in reconstructions of serial sections. *J Comp Neurol* 1980;193:853–862.
17. Hökfelt T, Fuxe K. Cerebellar monoamine nerve terminals, a new type of afferent fibers to the cortex cerebelli. *Exp Brain Res* 1969;9:63–72.
18. Invernizzi R, Berettera C, Garattini S, Samanin R. D- and L-isomers of fenfluramine differ markedly in their interaction with brain serotonin and catecholamines in the rat. *Eur J Pharmacol* 1986;120:9–15.
19. Jacobs BL. Locus coeruleus neuronal activity in behaving animals. In: Heal DJ, Marsden CA, eds. *The pharmacology of noradrenaline in the central nervous system.* Oxford: Oxford University Press, 1990:248–265.
20. Jouvet M. The role of monoamines and acetylcholine-containing neurons in the regulation of the sleep-waking cycle. In: Adrian RH, et al., eds. *Neurophysiology and neurochemistry of sleep and wakefulness. (Review of physiology,* vol 64). Berlin: Springer-Verlag, 1972:166–307.
21. Keane P, McRae-Degueurce A, Renaud B, Crespi F, Pujol JF. Alterations in tyrosine hydroxylase and dopamine-beta-hydroxylase activity in the locus coeruleus after 5,6 dihydroxytryptamine. *Neurosci Lett* 1978;8:143–150.
22. Kostowski W. Brain noradrenaline, depression and anti-depressant drugs: facts and hypothesis. *Trends Pharmacol Sci* 1981;2:314–317.
23. Lakoski JM, Aghajanian GK. Effects of ketanserin on neuronal responses to serotonin in the prefrontal cortex, lateral geniculate and dorsal raphe nucleus. *Neuropharmacology* 1985;24:265–273.
24. Léger L, Descarries L. Serotonin nerve terminals in the locus coeruleus of adult rat: a radioautographic study. *Brain Res* 1978;145:1–13.
25. Léger L, McRae-Degueurce A, Pujol JF. Origine de l'innervation sérotoninergique du locus coeruleus chez le rat. *C R Acad Sci Paris* 1980;290:807–810.
26. Lewis BD, Renaud B, Buda M, Pujol JF. Time course variations in tyrosine hydroxylase activity in the rat locus coeruleus after electrolytic destruction of the nuclei raphe dorsalis or centralis. *Brain Res* 1976;108:339–349.
27. Luppi P-H, Fort P, Jouvet M. Iontophoretic application of unconjugated cholera toxin b subunit (CTb) combined with immunohistochemistry of neurochemical substances: a method for transmitter identification of retrogradely labeled neurons. *Brain Res* 1990;534:209–224.
28. Maeda T, Kojima Y, Arai R, et al. Monoaminergic interaction in the central nervous system: a morphological analysis in the locus coeruleus of the rat. *Comp Biochem Physiol* 1991;98C:193–201.

19

Effects of Harmaline on Serotonergic Neurotransmission

*†M. Weiss, *P. Blier, and *C. de Montigny

*Neurobiological Psychiatry Unit, Department of Psychiatry,
McGill University, Montreal, Quebec, Canada H3A 1A1;
†Laboratoire de Pharmacodynamie, Faculté de Pharmacie, F-13385 Marseille, France

Harmaline, an indolic monoamine oxidase inhibitor (MAOI) of type A (12,15), produces an activation of the CNS, inducing hallucinations and producing a generalized tremor at 8 to 12 Hz. The involvement of the olivocerebellar system in this harmaline-induced motor disturbance has been well documented (10,19).

At the brain stem level, the olivocerebellar system and the bulbar reticular formation were shown to be involved in the genesis of harmaline-induced tremor. Lesion experiments have demonstrated that the rhythmic activity induced by harmaline in the vestibular and bulbar reticular nuclei (gigantocellularis, paramedian, and lateral reticular nuclei) was initiated neither from the spinal cord nor structures rostral to the pons. In cerebellectomized animals, the inferior olive was the only structure that still showed a rhythmic activity following harmaline administration.

Moreover, as shown in the diagrammatic representation of the olivocerebellofastigiobulbar system (Fig. 1A), Purkinje cells in the cerebellar cortex were found to be driven by rhythmic discharges of the inferior olive neurons through the olivocerebellar climbing fiber pathway. The subsequent rhythmic complex spike discharge of Purkinje cells in turn evoked a rhythmic firing of fastigial, lateral vestibular, and bulbar reticular neurons. Moreover, from simultaneous recordings of cerebellar and brain stem neurons after harmaline administration (Fig. 1B), a precise time relationship between the rhythmic activity recorded at these different levels was observed supporting such a mechanism of signal transfer along the olivocerebellobulbar system. Contralateral olivary activities (lower traces) were recorded simultaneously with a Purkinje cell complex spike activity (1), a fastigial neuron activity (2), and a bulbar reticular neuron activity (3). The Purkinje and olivary neurons fire in a synchronized manner, and the rhythmic activity stops and resumes at the same time in both structures (Fig. 1B-1). Each rhythmic discharge in the olivocerebellar system is followed by a silent period in the activity of fastigial neurons (Fig. 1B-2), with a latency of about 5 to 10 msec, compatible with an

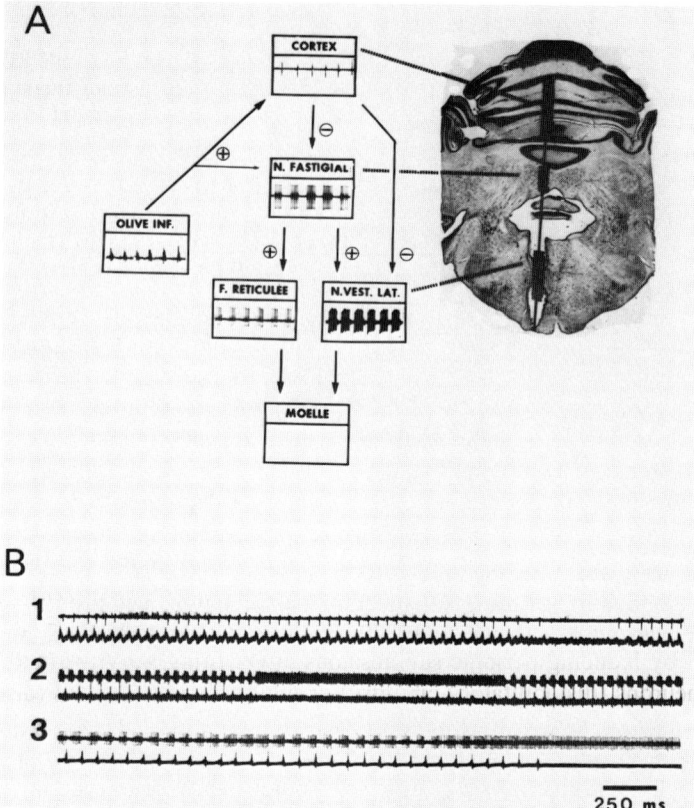

FIG. 1. Harmaline-induced rhythmic activity in the olivocerebellobulbospinal system. **A**: Olivocerebellofastigiobulbar system involved in the production of the harmaline-induced tremor. *Hatched* portions of microelectrode track on histological slice (*right*) correspond to sites where rhythmic activity was recorded. **B**: Simultaneous recordings from cerebellar and brain stem neurons under harmaline: Contralateral olivary activity (*lower traces*) is recorded simultaneously with Purkinje cell complex spike activity (*upper trace*, recording 1), fastigial neuron activity (*upper trace*, recording 2), and bulbar reticular neuron activity (*upper trace*, recording 3).

inhibition of fastigial activity through the olivo-Purkinje-fastigial pathway. Finally, good synchrony can be observed between the activity of fastigial (Fig. 1B-2) and reticular (Fig. 1B-3) units when considering the olivary cell discharge as the timing reference. In Fig. 1B (traces 2 and 3), it can be seen that the fastigial and the bulbar reticular units discharge tonically during the olivocerebellar pauses.

This suggests that each climbing fiber response results in a direct inhibition of fastigial neurons followed by a period of disinhibition, with a corresponding sequence of disfacilitation and excitation of the target neurons in the brain stem. These findings are fully consistent with the description of Ito et al. (17,18) of the mechanism of the signal transfer in the cerebellofastigiobulbar pathway.

At the spinal level, the time correlations observed (35,36) from simultaneous recordings of rhythmic activities of Purkinje cells (extracellular recordings) and spinal neurons (intracellular recordings) suggest that two distinct mechanisms are involved in the transfer of rhythmic signals to spinal motoneurons (Fig. 2). In this figure typical recordings are used to illustrate the operation of this model. When considering cerebellar discharge as a timing reference for tremorogenic events occurring at the different levels of the olivocerebellobulbospinal system, the fact that the rhythmic activity of bulbar and spinal interneurons stops and resumes at approximately the same time indicates the excitatory nature of their linkage. The sustained discharge of spinal interneurons, corresponding to a tonic firing of bulbar reticular units during the Purkinje cell pause, supports this contention. On the other hand, the time relationship observed between cerebellar Purkinje cell discharge and spinal motoneuron activity suggests that tremorogenic supraspinal influences might act on motoneurons through two distinct mechanisms. Each cerebellar complex spike discharge, which results in a periodic suppression of interneuron tonic activity, coincides with the onset of either a hyperpolarization or depolarization of motoneuron membranes. Moreover, the sustained discharge of spinal interneurons, during the occasional Purkinje cell pauses of long duration corresponds, respectively, to a maximal depolarization or a sustained hyperpolarization of motoneurons.

These results suggest that tremorogenic supraspinal influences act, at the spinal cord level, by inducing periodic suppressions of the firing activity of either excitatory interneurons (disfacilitatory circuitry) or inhibitory interneurons (disinhibitory circuitry), as shown in Fig. 2. The disfacilitatory or disinhibitory nature of the subsequent membrane potential changes of motoneurons was assessed by means of intracellular current ejections, according to Coombs and Eccles criteria (7,8).

Hence, harmaline induces a rhythmic activation of the olivocerebellar system, which was shown to be responsible for the tremor. The mechanism whereby harmaline triggers a rhythmic firing of olivary neurons remains unknown. Most likely, harmaline would facilitate the intrinsic tendency of olivary cells to fire in a synchronous manner due to the synaptic organization of the inferior olivary nucleus (23,24) (see Fig. 3). One of the mechanisms proposed for this activation is the suppression by harmaline of a tonic inhibitory influence acting on the inferior olive (16,29,39). This inhibitory influence might be serotonergic in nature (30,40). The structural analogy presented by harmaline with serotonin (5-HT) and the affinity of harmaline for 5-HT receptors (13) support this hypothesis. As 5-HT-containing neurons are known to be principally located in the brain stem raphe nuclei (9), recordings from dorsal raphe 5-HT neurons were performed to assess the effect of harmaline administration on their firing activity (37). Figure 3 illustrates the electrophysiological paradigm used to assess the effect of harmaline on 5-HT neurotransmission.

As shown in Fig. 4-1, systemic administration of harmaline (40 mg/kg i.p.) suppressed, with a latency of about 3 min, the firing activity of dorsal raphe 5-HT neurons, as do lysergic acid diethylamide (LSD) (26) and selective 5-HT$_{1A}$ agonists such as gepirone, buspirone and tandospirone (3,14) as well as MAOI (1).

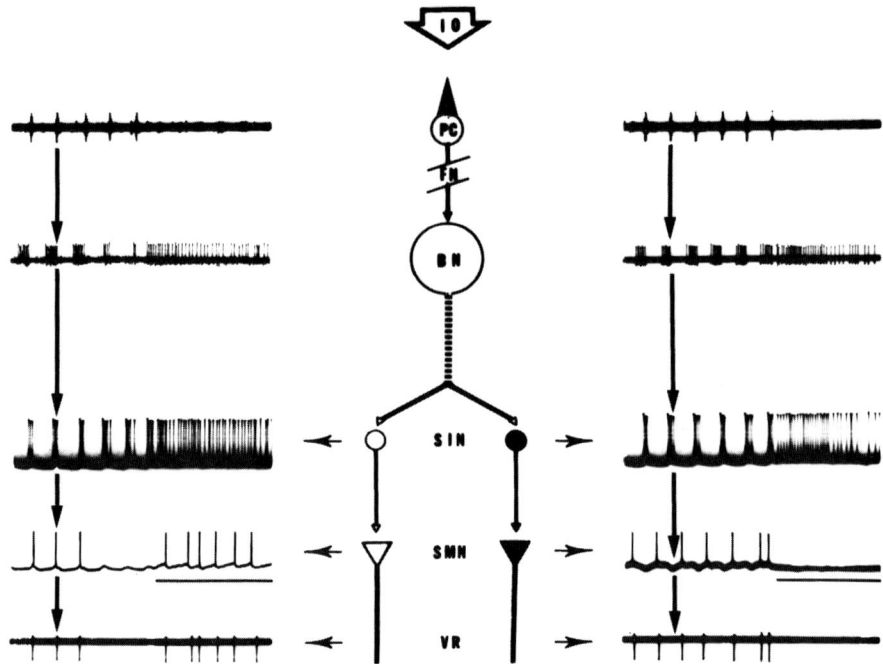

FIG. 2. Tremorogenic olivocerebellobulbar influences acting on spinal neurons (from ref. 36). *Left* (white neurons): disfacilitatory circuitry. *Right* (black neurons): disinhibitory circuitry. IO, inferior olivary nucleus; PC, cerebellar Purkinje cells; FN, fastigial nucleus; BN, bulbar nuclei where rhythmic activity was recorded (lateral vestibular, gigantocellularis, paramedian, and lateral reticular nuclei); SIN, spinal interneurons; SMN, spinal motoneurons; VR, motor axons in spinoventral roots. Typical recordings are used to illustrate the operation of the model. Rhythmic activities presented by olivary and fastigial neurons are not illustrated. Cerebellar discharge (PC) is considered as the timing reference for tremorogenic events occurring at the bulbar (BN) and spinal (SIN, SMN, VR) levels. Time relation between Purkinje cell and bulbar discharge from ref. 10. Time relation between Purkinje cell and spinal neurons from ref. 36.

Besides a MAOI-related mechanism by which harmaline could induce indirectly an activation of somatodendritic 5-HT_{1A} receptors, through an increment of 5-HT levels in dorsal raphe, this suppressive effect of harmaline on the firing activity of dorsal raphe neurons might be due to a direct agonistic action on these 5-HT_{1A} autoreceptors. To determine whether harmaline activates the 5-HT_{1A} receptors, we undertook to examine the effect of microiontophoretic applications of harmaline on CA3 dorsal hippocampus pyramidal neurons, mainly for the following two reasons: first, autoradiographic studies have shown this brain region to be enriched in 5-HT_{1A} binding sites (25); second, 5-HT receptors mediating the hyperpolarizing response of these neurons to 5-HT have been well characterized to be of the 5-HT_{1A} subtype (2,28), as is the case for the somatodendritic 5-HT autoreceptor.

As shown by the integrated firing rate histogram of the dorsal hippocampus pyramidal neuron presented in Fig. 5, the microiontophoretic application of harmaline

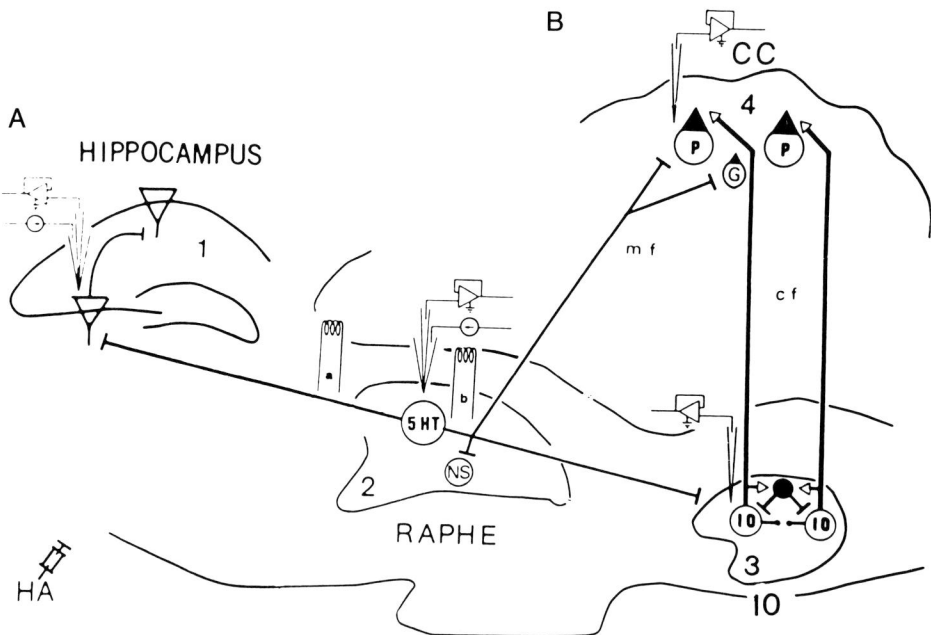

FIG. 3. Electrophysiological paradigm used to assess the effects of harmaline on 5-HT neurotransmission in raphe-hippocampal and raphe-olivocerebellar systems. Excitatory actions (⇒); inhibitory actions (-|). **A**: Raphe-hippocampal system. *1*, Responsiveness of CA3 dorsal hippocampus pyramidal neurons to microiontophoretic application of 5-HT and harmaline (see Fig. 5). *2*, Responsiveness of dorsal 5-HT raphe neurons to microiontophoretic application of 5-HT and harmaline (experiments in progress). Interactions between 5-HT neurons and nonserotonergic cells (NS) were studied (37). The effects of systemic administration of harmaline on the firing activity of dorsal raphe 5-HT neurons (see Fig. 4-1) and the responsiveness of hippocampus postsynaptic neurons (see Fig. 6A) to microiontophoretic applications of 5-HT were assessed. **B**: Raphe-olivocerebellar system. *3*, Structural organization of the inferior olivary (IO) nucleus: recurrent collaterals of inferior olivary neurons project on inhibitory olivary interneurons (black neuron). Ephaptic connections (→ ←). *4*, Cerebellar cortex (CC), P, Purkinje cells; G, Golgi neurons and other non-Purkinje cells; mf, mossy fibers generating simple spike responses of Purkinje cells; cf, climbing fibers, generating complex spike discharges in Purkinje cells. The effects of an intraperitoneal administration of harmaline on the firing activity of dorsal raphe 5-HT neurons (see Fig. 4-1) and the neuronal activities in the olivocerebellar system (see Fig. 4-2) were studied. The effects of an electrical stimulation of the serotonergic system (a and b) on the firing activity of dorsal hippocampus pyramidal neurons (see Fig. 8) and olivocerebellar neurons (see Fig. 9) were assessed prior to and following harmaline administration.

onto dorsal hippocampus pyramidal neurons suppressed their firing activity, thus mimicking the effect of 5-HT. However, harmaline was much less potent than 5-HT when taking into account the concentrations of drugs (20 mM for harmaline vs 0.5 mM for 5-HT) and the currents (30 nA of harmaline vs 5 nA of 5-HT) required to obtain a clear suppressant effect.

The first possibility to account for this weak effect of harmaline, contrasting with the potent suppressive effect of 5-HT on the firing activity of the dorsal hippo-

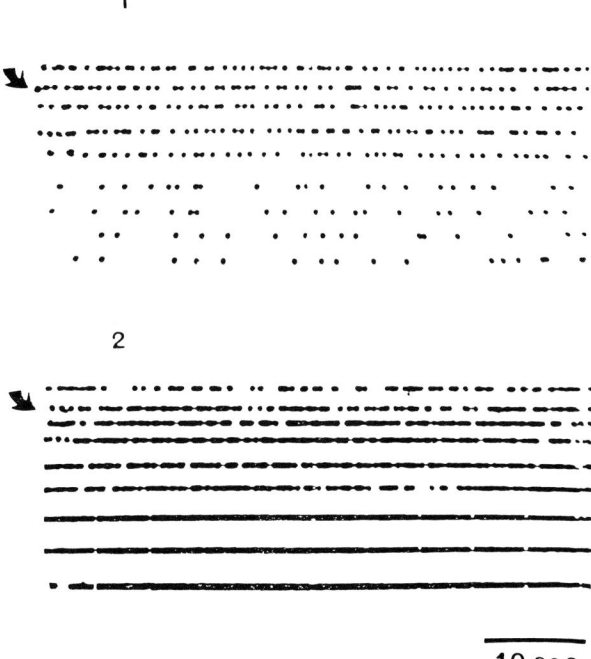

FIG. 4. Comparison of the effects of harmaline on a 5-HT dorsal raphe neuron (1) and on a non-Purkinje cerebellar cell (2). Dot raster displays of raphe (1) and cerebellar (2) cell discharges. The recordings are continuous. Each dot in the rasters corresponds to a neuronal discharge. *Curved arrows* in 1 and 2 indicate the time of harmaline administration. The time base applies to both traces.

campus pyramidal neurons, is that harmaline might act as a partial agonist on the dorsal hippocampus 5-HT$_{1A}$ receptors, as suggested for several other 5-HT$_{1A}$ agonists by Sprouse and Aghajanian (31,32).

In an attempt to determine if harmaline acted as a partial agonist on postsynaptic 5-HT$_{1A}$ receptors as do gepirone (4), tandospirone (14), and flesinoxan (11), the effects of its systemic administration and its microiontophoretic application on the responsiveness of dorsal hippocampus pyramidal neurons to 5-HT were tested. Neither its intraperitoneal injection nor its concomitant microiontophoretic application reduced the effect of microiontophoretically applied 5-HT (Fig. 6). Hence, the later result indicates that harmaline does not act as a partial agonist at postsynaptic 5-HT$_{1A}$ receptors, since the microiontophoretic application of such partial agonists (e.g., gepirone, tandospirone, and flesinoxan) readily blocks the effect of the concomitant application of 5-HT (4,11,14).

These observations might nevertheless be consistent with the possibility that harmaline acts as a full, although weak, agonist on the postsynaptic 5-HT$_{1A}$ receptors. To verify this hypothesis, we used the buspirone analog BMY-7378, a potent

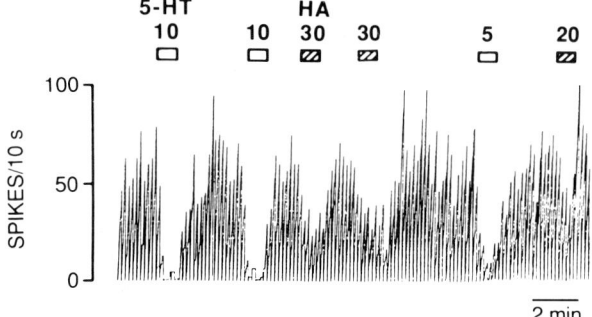

FIG. 5. Integrated firing rate histogram of a dorsal hippocampus pyramidal neuron showing the effects of the microiontophoretic application of 5-HT (0.5 mM) and harmaline (HA) (20 mM). The microiontophoretic currents used are given in nanoamperes. The neuron was activated with an ejection current of 10 nA of acetylcholine. All ejection currents are positive.

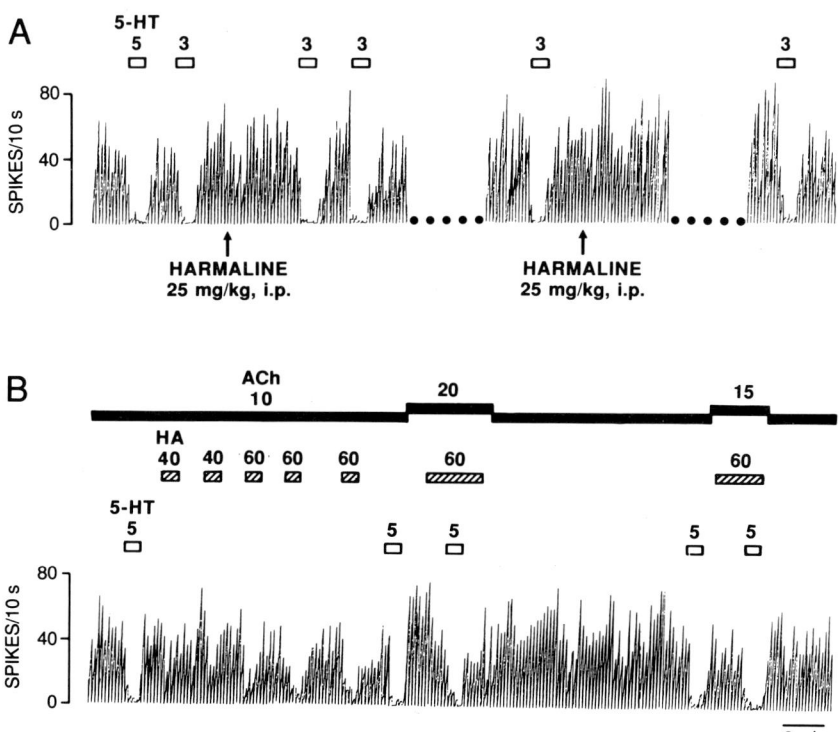

FIG. 6. Integrated firing rate histograms of two CA3 dorsal hippocampus pyramidal neurons showing the effect of systemic (**A**) and microiontophoretic (**B**) administration of harmaline (HA) on the suppressant effect of microiontophoretically applied 5-HT. The histogram in A is discontinuous (*dots* indicate time intervals of 5 min). The current of acetylcholine (ACh) used to activate neuron A was 10 nA. Histograms in B show the effectiveness of the microiontophoretic application of 5-HT before, during, and after the concurrent application of harmaline.

$5-HT_{1A}$ antagonist (41), which was shown by Chaput and de Montigny (6) to readily suppress the effect of 5-HT and 8-hydroxy-2-(d-n-propylamino)tetralin (8-OH-DPAT) on dorsal hippocampus pyramidal neurons. As shown in Fig. 7, BMY-7378 failed to antagonize the harmaline-induced suppression of the firing activity of dorsal hippocampus pyramidal neurons. These results indicate that harmaline does not produce its suppressant effect via the activation of $5-HT_{1A}$ receptors.

Whatever the exact mechanism by which harmaline could interact with serotonergic neurotransmission, the balance between its suppressant effect on the firing activity of dorsal raphe 5-HT neurons following its acute systemic administration, and its weak suppressant effect at the postsynaptic level, could result in a decrease of a serotonergic inhibitory input on target neurons.

Although at the hippocampal level, harmaline administration did not modify the discharge rate of pyramidal neurons, this assumption is nevertheless supported by the enhanced rate of discharge of cortical cerebellar neurons, simple spike discharges of non-Purkinje cells as well as Purkinje cell complex spike discharges, concomitant to decreased firing activity of dorsal raphe 5-HT neurons following the systemic administration of harmaline (40 mg/kg i.p.), as illustrated in Fig. 4.

To test the effect of harmaline on 5-HT neurotransmission, electrical stimulation experiments on the 5-HT pathways were performed to determine their effects on the hippocampus and cerebellum cell discharges. The effects of a repetitive stimulation of 5-HT pathways on hippocampus pyramidal cell discharges and Purkinje cell activities in the cerebellar cortex were assessed prior to and following harmaline administration.

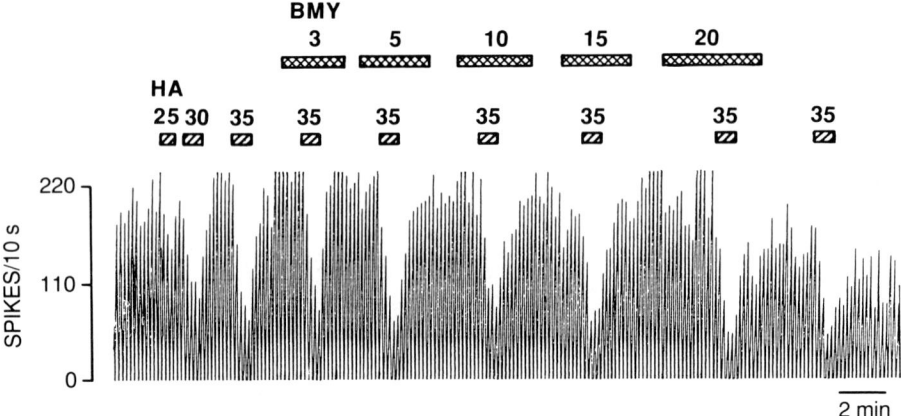

FIG. 7. Integrated firing rate histogram of a dorsal hippocampus pyramidal neuron showing the effect of microiontophoretic applications of BMY 7378 (5 mM) with increasing currents on the suppressant effects of microiontophoretically applied harmaline (20 mM). A constant current of acetylcholine (0.2 nA) was used to activate the neuron.

The suppressant effect of the stimulation of the 5-HT pathway on the firing activity of dorsal hippocampus pyramidal neurons has been well documented to be mediated by 5-HT. In particular, it is blocked by the 5-HT$_{1A}$ antagonist BMY-7378 (6). The effects of such stimulations prior to and following harmaline administration are illustrated in Fig. 8. The administration of harmaline reduced the effectiveness of

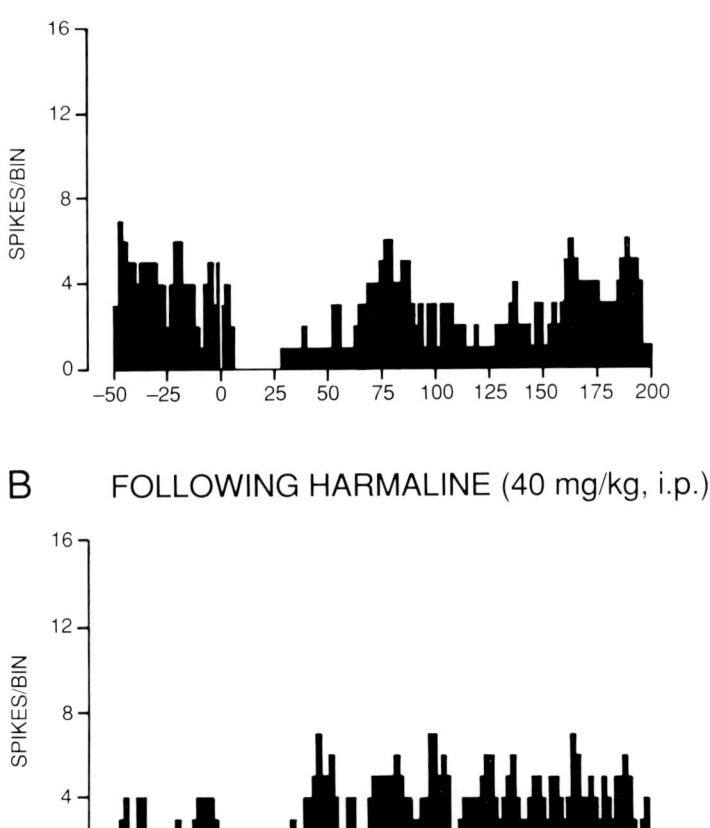

FIG. 8. Peristimulus time histograms (PSTH) obtained from the same CA3 hippocampal pyramidal neuron showing the effect of the stimulation of the 5-HT pathway prior to (**A**) and following (**B**) the administration of harmaline. Each PSTH was constructed from 150 stimuli of 0.5 msec delivered at 1 Hz with an intensity of 300 µA. Bin width is 2 msec. The stimulation pulse is delivered at time 0.

the stimulation. The ratio of the inhibitory effect of stimulation S2 (following harmaline) over S1 (prior to harmaline) was 0.67 (mean value from six rats), i.e., its efficacy was reduced by one-third. A direct antagonistic action of harmaline on postsynaptic 5-HT receptors, resulting in a blockade of the effect of endogenous 5-HT released by the stimulation, can be ruled out on the basis of the microiontophoretic experiments reported above. The possibility that the reduced effectiveness of the stimulation might be due to the activation of terminal 5-HT autoreceptors by increased levels of endogenous 5-HT resulting from MAO inhibition by harmaline can be excluded from the observation that acute administration of pargyline does not modify the effectiveness of the stimulation (20). An agonistic action of harmaline on 5-HT$_{1B}$ autoreceptors located on serotonergic terminals (34), resulting in a decrease in the amount of 5-HT released per impulse, remains to be tested using 5-HT$_{1B}$ antagonists such as methiothepin.

At the cerebellar level, midbrain raphe stimulation (10 Hz for 3 sec) was demonstrated to produce a long duration (5–10 msec) suppression of all cerebellar activities (38), including simple spike firing, as already demonstrated by Strahlendorf et al. (33), as well as complex spike discharge of Purkinje cells (Fig. 9-1). As shown in this illustration (from ref. 38), the five successive trains of stimulations were still effective after harmaline administration (Fig. 9-2). However, a decrease in the effectiveness of the stimulation to suppress the complex spike discharges, as it seems to be the case here, might be masked by the harmaline-induced enhancement of the complex spike discharge frequency of Purkinje cells (from 1 to 7 Hz), and by the concomitant disappearance of the simple spike firing, due to the prolonged refractory period (up to 100 msec) of the Purkinje cell membrane following each complex spike discharge.

In conclusion, the results of the microiontophoretic experiments reported here do not support the hypothesis of a direct interaction of harmaline with 5-HT$_{1A}$ receptors as the mechanism responsible for the release of an inhibitory control exerted on target cells. Mechanisms whereby harmaline would modify serotonergic neurotransmission remain to be elucidated. A direct agonistic interaction of harmaline with 5-HT$_{1B}$ terminal autoreceptors remains a possibility to be tested.

As another mechanism, a possible inhibitory interaction of harmaline with GABA$_A$-benzodiazepine receptors, which were shown by Lista et al. (20–22) to enhance the 5-HT release, has been suggested by Robertson (27) on the basis of radioligand binding data (displacement of [^{3}H]flunitrazepam by harmaline) and the antagonistic effect of diazepam on the harmaline-induced tremor. According to this model, harmaline might displace an endogenous ligand whose role would be to facilitate GABA neurotranmission. Testing of this hypothesis is now in progress in our laboratory.

ACKNOWLEDGMENTS

We wish to thank Drs. P. Pisano-Crevat and A. Vaille for their collaboration, M. Boulay for his assistance with the electronics, L. Caille for computer programing, G. Filosi for the illustrations, and H. Cameron for her secretarial assistance.

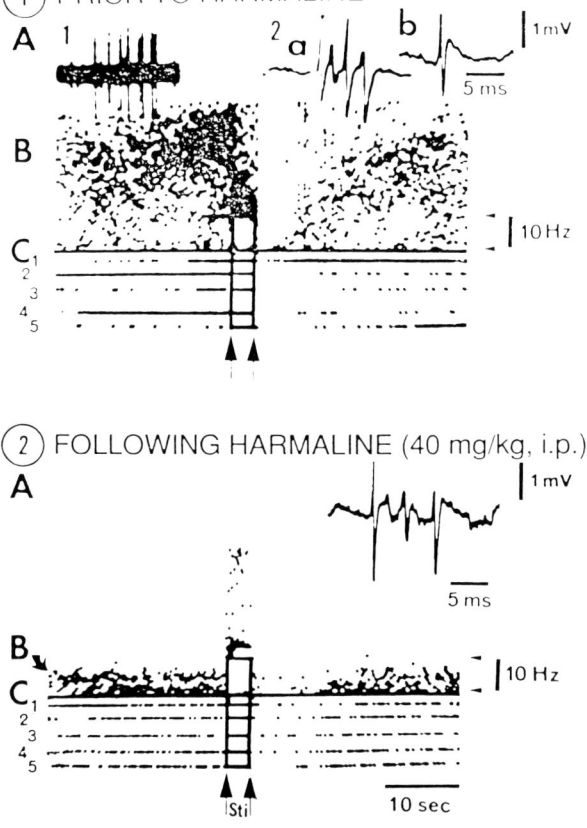

FIG. 9. Suppressive effect of raphe stimulation on Purkinje cell discharge before (①) and after (②) harmaline administration (modified from ref. 38). ①: A, analogical trace corresponding to the first 15 sec of cell discharge (trace 1 of raster C). A-1: Rate per second; time calibration of A-1 is indicated at the bottom of the figure. A-2: Typical waveforms of a complex spike discharge (a) and simple spike discharge (b) of a Purkinje cell. ②: A, same cell 10 min after harmaline administration. Note the total disappearance of simple spike discharge after drug administration. B: Superposed sweeps of the instantaneous frequency plot of the cell discharge on the 250-sec activity recorded in C. Curved arrow in B indicates the level of the harmaline-induced rhythmic discharge at about 7 Hz. C: Dot raster display of cell discharge. The five successive traces (1–5) are continuous. Each dot in the raster corresponds to a neuronal discharge. The neuron exhibited both complex and simple spikes prior to harmaline, but only complex spikes following harmaline administration.

REFERENCES

1. Aghajanian GK, Graham AW, Sheard MH. Serotonin-containing neurons in brain: depression of firing by monoamine oxidase inhibitors. *Science* 1970;169:1100–1102.
2. Andrade R, Nicoll RA. Pharmacologically distinct actions of serotonin on single pyramidal neurones of the rat hippocampus recorded in vitro. *J Physiol (Lond)* 1987;394:99–124.
3. Blier P, de Montigny C. Modification of 5-HT neuron properties by sustained administration of the 5-HT$_{1A}$ agonist gepirone: electrophysiological studies in the rat brain. *Synapse* 1987;1:470–480.

4. Blier P, de Montigny C. Differential effect of gepirone on pre- and postsynaptic receptors: single-cell recording studies. *J Clin Psychopharmacol* 1990;10(suppl 3):13S–20S.
5. Blier P, de Montigny C, Azzaro AJ. Effect of repeated amiflamine administration on serotonergic and noradrenergic neurotransmission: electrophysiological studies in the rat CNS. *Naunyn Schmiedebergs Arch Pharmacol* 1986;334:253–260.
6. Chaput Y, de Montigny C. Effects of the 5-HT$_1$ receptor antagonist, BMY 7378, on 5-HT neurotransmission: electrophysiological studies in the rat CNS. *J Pharmacol Exp Ther* 1988;246:359–370.
7. Coombs JS, Eccles JC, Fatt P. The specific ionic conductances and the ionic movements across the motoneural membrane that produce the inhibitory post-synaptic potential. *J Physiol (Lond)* 1955;130:326–373.
8. Coombs JS, Eccles JC, Fatt P. Excitatory synaptic action in motoneurones. *J Physiol (Lond)* 1955;130:374–395.
9. Dahlström A, Fuxe K. Evidence for the existence of monoamine-containing neurons in the central nervous system. I. Demonstration of monoamines in the cell bodies of brain stem neurons. *Acta Physiol Scand* 1964;62(suppl 232):1–55.
10. de Montigny C, Lamarre Y. Rhythmic activity induced by harmaline in the olivo-cerebello-bulbar system of the cat. *Brain Res* 1973;53:81–95.
11. de Montigny C, Ortemann C, Blier P. Effect of the 5-HT$_{1A}$ agonist flesinoxan on the 5-HT system: electrophysiological studies in the rat CNS. *Soc Neurosci Abstr* 1991;17:82.1.
12. Fuller RW, Wong CJ, Hemrick-Luecke SK. MD 240928 and harmaline: opposite selectivity in antagonism of the inactivation of types A and B monoamine oxidase by pargyline in mice. *Life Sci* 1986;38:409–412.
13. Glennon RA. Serotonin receptor interactions of harmaline and several related β-carbolines. *Life Sci* 1981;29:861–865.
14. Godbout R, Chaput Y, Blier P, de Montigny C. Tandospirone and its metabolite, 1-(2-pyrimidinyl)-piperazine (1-PP): I. Effects of acute and long-term tandospirone on serotonin neurotransmission. *Neuropharmacology* 1991;30:679–690.
15. Hamon M, Pichat L. ^{3}H-harmaline: a useful tool for studying MAO-A. In: Tipton KF, Dostert P, Strolin-Benedetti M, eds. *Monoamine oxidase and disease—prospects for therapy with reversible inhibitors*. New York: Academic Press, 1984:63–72.
16. Headley PM, Lodge O, Duggan AW. Drug induced rhythmical activity in the inferior olivary complex of the rat. *Brain Res* 1976;101:461–478.
17. Ito M, Udo M, Mano N, Kawai N. Synaptic action of the fastigio-bulbar impulses upon neurones in the medullary reticular formation and vestibular nuclei. *Exp Brain Res* 1970;11:29–47.
18. Ito M, Yoshida M, Obata K, Kawai N, Udo M. Inhibitory control of intra-cerebellar nuclei by the Purkinje cell axons. *Exp Brain Res* 1970;10:64–80.
19. Lamarre Y, de Montigny C, Dumont M, Weiss M. Harmaline-induced rhythmic activity of cerebellar and lower brain stem neurones. *Brain Res* 1971;32:246–250.
20. Lista A, Blier P, de Montigny C. The benzodiazepine receptor inverse agonist DMCM decreases serotonergic transmission in rat hippocampus: an in vivo electrophysiological study. *Synapse* 1990;6:175–178.
21. Lista A, Blier P, de Montigny C. GABA$_A$-benzodiazepine receptors modulate 5-HT release: in vivo electrophysiological studies in the rat hippocampus. *Ann NY Acad Sci* 1990;604:622–625.
22. Lista A, Blier P, de Montigny C. Benzodiazepine receptors modulate 5-HT neurotransmission in the rat dorsal hippocampus: in vivo electrophysiological evidence. *J Pharmacol Exp Ther* 1990;254:318–323.
23. Llinas R, Volkind RA. The olivo-cerebellar system: functional properties as revealed by harmaline-induced tremor. *Exp Brain Res* 1973;18:69–87.
24. Llinas R, Baker R, Sotelo C. Electrotonic coupling between neurons in cat inferior olive. *J Neurophysiol* 1974;37:560–571.
25. Marcinkiewicz M, Vergé D, Gozlan H, Pichat L, Hamon M. Autoradiographic evidence for the heterogeneity of 5-HT$_1$ sites in the rat brain. *Brain Res* 1984;291:159–163.
26. Martial J, de Montigny C, St-Laurent J, Quirion R. LSD ou lysergide: pharmacologie et mécanismes d'action. *Psychotropes* 1988;4:7–11.
27. Robertson HA. Harmaline-induced tremor: the benzodiazepine receptor as a site of action. *Eur J Pharmacol* 1980;67:129–132.
28. Segal M, Azmitia EC, Whitaker-Azmitia PM. Physiological effects of selective 5-HT$_{1A}$ and 5-HT$_{1B}$ ligands in rat hippocampus: comparison to 5-HT. *Brain Res* 1989;502:67–74.

29. Sjölund B, Björklund A, Wiklund L. The indoleaminergic innervation of the inferior olive, part 2: relation to harmaline induced tremor. *Brain Res* 1977;131:23-37.
30. Sjölund B, Wiklund L, Björklund A. Functional role of serotoninergic innervation of the inferior olivary cells. In: Courville J, de Montigny C, Lamarre Y, eds. *The inferior olivary nucleus: anatomy and physiology*. New York: Raven Press, 1980:163-168.
31. Sprouse JS, Aghajanian GK. Electrophysiological responses of serotoninergic dorsal raphe neurons to 5-HT_{1A} and 5-HT_{1B} agonists. *Synapse* 1987;1:3-9.
32. Sprouse JS, Aghajanian GK. Responses of hippocampal pyramidal cells to putative serotonin 5-HT_{1A} and 5-HT_{1B} agonists: a comparative study with dorsal raphe neurons. *Neuropharmacology* 1988;27:707-715.
33. Strahlendorf JC, Strahlendorf HK, Lee M. Electrophysiological effects of serotonin on cerebellar Purkinje cells. In: *New concepts in cerebellar neurobiology*. New York: Alan R. Liss, 1987:321-347.
34. Vergé D, Daval G, Patey A, Gozlan A. El Mestikawy S, Hamon M. Presynaptic 5-HT autoreceptors on serotonergic cell bodies and/or dendrites but not terminals are of the 5-HT_{1A} subtype. *Eur J Pharmacol* 1985;113:463-464.
35. Weiss M. Influence du système olivo-cérebello-bulbaire sur les neurones moteurs de la moelle lombaire chez le chat après administration d'harmaline. *Arch Ital Biol* 1978;116:1-15.
36. Weiss M. Rhythmic activity of spinal interneurones in harmaline-treated cats. A model for olivo-cerebellar influence at the spinal level. *J Neurol Sci* 1982;54:341-348.
37. Weiss M, Pellet J. Raphe-cerebellum interactions. I. Effects of cerebellar stimulation and harmaline administration on single unit activity of midbrain raphe neurons in the rats. *Exp Brain Res* 1982;48:163-170.
38. Weiss M, Pellet J. Raphe-cerebellum interactions. II. Effects of midbrain raphe stimulation and harmaline administration on single unit activity of cerebellar neurons in the rats. *Exp Brain Res* 1982;48:171-176.
39. Wiklund L, Sjölund B, Björklund A. Serotoninergic innervation of the inferior olive: involvement in tremor mechanisms. *Neurosci Lett* 1978;1:55.
40. Wiklund L, Sjölund B, Björklund A. Morphological and functional studies on the serotoninergic innervation of the inferior olive. *J Physiol (Paris)* 1981;77:183-186.
41. Yocca FD, Hyslop DK, Smith DW, Maayani S. BMY 7378, a buspirone analog with high affinity, selectivity, and low intrinsic activity at the 5-HT_{1A} receptor in rat and guinea pig hippocampal membranes. *Eur J Pharmacol* 1987;137:293-294.

Serotonin, the Cerebellum, and Ataxia, edited by
P. Trouillas and K. Fuxe.
Raven Press, Ltd., New York © 1993.

20

3-Acetylpyridine and Thiamine Deficiency-Induced Cerebellar Models and the Pathophysiology of Ataxia

Andreas Plaitakis

Department of Neurology, Mount Sinai School of Medicine, New York, New York 10029

THE CEREBELLUM AND ITS DYSFUNCTION: HISTORICAL BACKGROUND

The Greek physician Herophilus (335-200 B.C.), known as the father of anatomy, is generally credited for first describing the human cerebellum. Its function, however, remained obscure until about two millennia later when Luigi Rolando (1773–1831), on the basis of ablation experiments, first suggested that the cerebellum is involved in motor control. Following these original observations, extensive experimental studies utilizing ablation techniques, along with subsequently developed stimulation methods, have unequivocally established a major role for the cerebellum in many aspects of motor coordination.

While this basic work was laying the foundation for understanding the physiologic function of the cerebellum, reports began to appear over a century ago indicating that disorders exist in humans that are characterized pathologically by selective degeneration and atrophy of the cerebellum and its connections and clinically by disturbed motor coordination or ataxia. These observations not only have helped us to understand clinicopathological correlations, but they have also stimulated further interest in basic cerebellar research.

Rapid progress toward understanding the anatomy and connectivity of the cerebellum occurred during the past few decades following the description of the cerebellar cellular systems by Ramon y Cajal, which markedly facilitated the study of the physiologic processes at the neuronal and synaptic levels. In recent years the introduction of new tools and experimental procedures, such as animal models, tissue culture techniques, immunocytochemical methods, neuroimaging applications, and molecular biology approaches, has furthered our understanding of the cerebellum and its functions. However, despite these advances the pathophysiology of ataxia or disordered cerebellar function remains to be understood better.

It is well known that the cerebellum is particularly sensitive to a variety of metabolic insults such as hypoxia, hypoglycemia, heavy metal and other intoxications, nutritional deficiencies, and inborn errors of amino acid, lipid, purine, and carbohydrate metabolism. Moreover, viral agents, endocrinopathies, and autoimmune processes often affect the cerebellum selectively. The reasons for this selective cerebellar vulnerability have not been fully understood. Elucidation of these mechanisms will undoubtedly help us to understand ataxia and develop rational treatments for this disorder.

ANIMAL MODELS AND THE PATHOPHYSIOLOGY OF ATAXIA

The study of animal models for ataxia has proven useful for understanding human cerebellar disorders. This is particularly true for those produced by nutritional deficiencies, specific neurotoxins, transmissible agents, and genetic mutations. Of the neurotoxic agents, two pyridine compounds, 3-acetylpyridine (3-AP) and 1-methyl-4-phenyl-1,2,3,6-tetrahydropyridine (MPTP), are capable of lesioning the inferior olivary nucleus and the substantia nigra, respectively, and as such, they have been used extensively for producing models for olivopontocerebellar atrophy (OPCA) and Parkinson's disease.

The first part of the present investigations was based on the biological effects of 3-AP, which, acting as a nicotinamide antagonist, leads to synthesis of abnormal nucleotides in the brain that affect oxidation-reduction processes. These studies led to the detection of glutamate dehydrogenase (GDH) deficiency and abnormal metabolism of neuroexcitatory amino acids in patients with ataxic disorders and suggested glutamatergic neuroexcitotoxic mechanisms in the pathogenesis of these disorders. A similar strategy, based on the mode of action of MPTP, has been also used lately to detect a defect in mitochondrial oxidative metabolism in patients with Parkinson's disease.

The second part of our investigations on ataxia is based on animal models induced by thiamine antimetabolites and/or nutritional deficiency of this vitamin. Thiamine is known to play a major role in carbohydrate and energy metabolism serving as coenzyme of important oxidoreductases (dehydrogenases). These studies revealed alterations in neuroexcitotoxic amino acids and the serotonergic system of the brain. These data, taken together with recent studies showing that similar serotonergic abnormalities occur in animals exposed to neuroexcitotoxic compounds, suggest that excitotoxin-induced brain serotonergic alterations play a role in the pathogenesis of ataxia.

THE 3-ACETYLPYRIDINE MODEL

Over two decades ago, Herken (1) presented a thorough review of the investigative efforts of his time that led to the elucidation of the biological events responsible for 3-AP neurotoxicity. It had been well established by then that parenteral adminis-

TABLE 1. Pattern of neuronal degeneration in 3-AP intoxication and OPCA

CNS region	3-AP[a]	OPCA
Inferior olives	+ + + +	+ + + +
Cranial nerve nuclei		
IX, X	+ + +	+ to + + +
XII	+ + +	+ to + + +
VII	+	0 to + +
Pons	+	+ to + + +
Substantia nigra	+	0 to + +
Spinal cord	0	0 to + +

[a] The number of plus signs indicates the degree of neuronal degeneration ranging from 0 (no involvement) to + + + + (marked destruction of neurons of the region). The pattern of neuronal degeneration induced experimentally by 3-AP is based on the observations of Desclin and Escubi (2).
From ref. 69.

tration of this compound to rats (80 mg/kg body weight) induces an acute encephalopathic state characterized by seizures and abnormal motor behavior. Under these conditions affected animals often succumb to the acute encephalopathy (within hours to a few days following exposure to the toxic agent), but those surviving manifest long-lasting coordination disturbances (cerebellar ataxia).

Early in these investigations it was shown that 3-AP acts as a nicotinamide antimetabolite displacing the vitamin from the nicotinamide adenyldinucleotide (NAD[P]) system to form abnormal nucleotides in animal tissues. Brain microsomes containing high nucleosidase activity were shown to incorporate 3-AP into the nicotinamide adenine dinucleotide phosphate (NADP) synthesizing 3-AP adenine dinucleotide phosphate (3-APADP) in amounts greater than those of the normal nucleotide (NADP). Also the brains of animals exposed to 3-AP were found to contain high levels of 3-APADP (1). It was further shown that in the presence of 3-APADP(H), the catalytic activity of NADP-dependent dehydrogenases was altered causing abnormalities in oxidation-reduction (hydrogen transfer) processes (1).

As described above, animals that survive the acute encephalopathy induced by 3-AP show a long-lasting equilibrium disorder (ataxia). The underlying mechanism of this ataxia remained uncertain until Desclin and Escubi (2) convincingly showed that degeneration of the inferior olivary cells and lower cranial cell nuclei occur consistently in these animals (2). Other central nervous system regions, such as areas of the pons and substantia nigra, also show neuropathologic alterations, but these are less consistent than the above changes (Table 1).

Partial GDH Deficiency in OPCA

While reviewing the histopathologic changes induced by 3-AP we became aware that the pattern of these alterations was quite similar to that found in patients with a particular form of cerebellar degeneration known by the descriptive pathologic term

OPCA (Table 1). This disorder is often genetically transmitted, although it can also occur sporadically. We then considered that the neuronal systems that degenerate in both the animal model and the human disease may be selectively vulnerable to a common biochemical factor. Since 3-AP toxicity is mediated through inhibition of NADP(H)-dependent oxidoreductases, the possibility was further raised that patients with OPCA may be genetically deficient in one of these oxidoreductases.

We tested this hypothesis by measuring several NADP(H)-requiring enzymes in homogenates of cultured skin fibroblasts from a 19-year-old patient with a progressive cerebellar and extrapyramidal syndrome consistent with OPCA (3). Results revealed a selective deficiency of the NAD(P)-requiring enzyme GDH (3). The defect persisted after several passages of the cultured cells and was also present at different concentrations of the enzyme's substrate. Leukocytes isolated from the peripheral blood of this patient also showed reduced GDH activity (3).

Since these original observations, reports from 12 different laboratories have appeared in the literature (4–20a). They all describe significant GDH reductions in leukocytes, platelets, and cultured skin fibroblasts of patients with late-onset neurodegenerative disorders consistent with OPCA and other multiple-system atrophies. The majority of these patients manifested a combination of cerebellar, extrapyramidal, bulbar, and motor neuronal deficits, whereas others were atypical in their clinical presentation (6,13,16). Many of these cases occurred sporadically but others were familial. Those occurring in families affected primarily siblings, and no clear evidence was found for a vertical transmission of the genetic trait. However, some investigators have reported GDH abnormalities in OPCA patients from dominant pedigrees (9–11,21).

The molecular basis of these enzyme changes has not, as yet, been fully characterized. Early studies (6) using crude tissue homogenates suggested the presence of at least two distinct forms of GDH activity in human tissues designated "soluble-heat stable" and "particulate-heat labile" (6). Studies in patients with partial GDH deficiency revealed that the enzyme defect was limited to one of these forms (6,12, 20a), thus suggesting that they are under different genetic control.

Characterization of human brain GDH has been facilitated by the development of a highly efficient purification method that has permitted the isolation of substantial amounts of the human enzyme in a homogeneous form (21). Electrophoretic analysis of GDH purified from human brain with the use of a nonequilibrium, pH gradient, two-dimensional polyacrylamide gel electrophoresis technique (21) revealed that the human enzyme consists of four major isoproteins (designated GDH 1, 2, 3, and 4) differing in their charge and size (Fig. 1). In normal controls, the relative abundance and the molecular mass of these isoproteins followed the order 1>2>3>4.

Using these techniques, GDH has been purified to homogeneity from cerebellar tissue obtained at autopsy from a few OPCA patients and controls and analyzed by the high resolution electrophoretic technique indicated above (21). These studies showed that the cerebellar enzyme of a patient with the childhood-onset variant of OPCA associated with retinal degeneration was distinctly different from that of

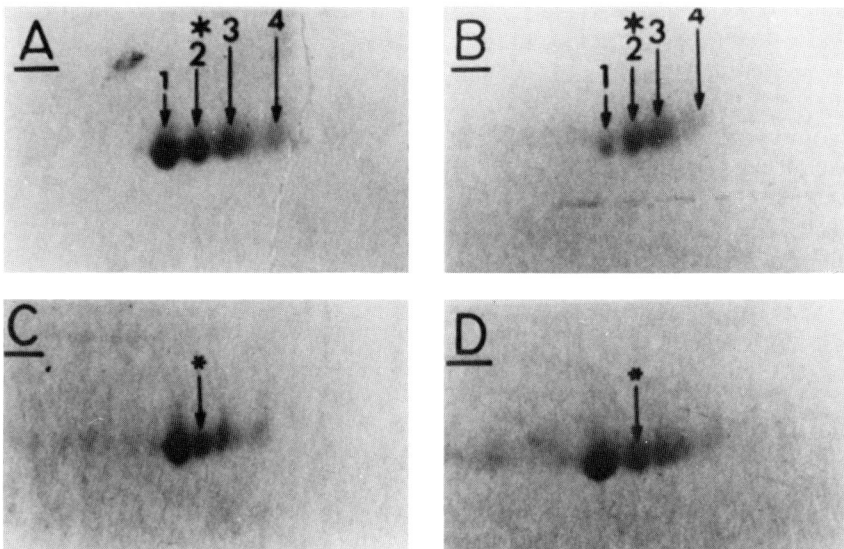

FIG. 1. Isoproteins of GDH purified to homogeneity from cerebellar autopsy tissue and analyzed by two-dimensional nonequilibrium pH gradient electrophoresis (21). **A**: Neurologically normal subject who died of an acute myocardial infarction. **B**: Patient with non-HLA linked form of dominant OPCA associated with retinal degeneration, slowed saccades, myoclonus, amyotrophy, and peripheral neuropathy. **C,D**: Patients from the HLA-linked Schut-Haymaker kindred (non-GDH deficient). *Asterisk* indicates ^{35}S-labeled GDH synthesized by Hep G2 cells. The labeled enzyme was immunoprecipitated from cell lysates and mixed (in trace amounts) with the purified human brain GDH. Its position, in relation to the four brain GDH isoproteins (comigration with the GDH isoprotein 2) was revealed by autoradiography of the slab gel. GDH isoprotein 1, which is more abundant than other GDH isoproteins in the cerebellum of normal and disease controls is markedly reduced in the patient with the variant of dominant OPCA with retinal degeneration. (Data are from ref. 21.)

neurologically normal controls as well as patients with Parkinson's disease, amyotrophic lateral sclerosis, and the Schut-Haymaker OPCA (non-GDH deficient) (21) (Fig. 1). Thus, GDH isoprotein 1, which in nonneurologic and neurologic controls was found to be more abundant than the other GDH isoproteins, was markedly reduced in this patient (Fig. 1).

GDH activity was reduced in the soluble brain fraction of this patient. Moreover, the soluble GDH showed altered kinetic properties with the K_m for the enzyme's substrates α-ketoglutarate, glutamate, NADH, and NADPH being significantly increased (by three- to fivefold) (21). As such, these data revealed that the altered electrophoretic pattern of this patient's enzyme is associated with abnormal catalytic properties and function.

Additional progress has been achieved in recent years toward the molecular characterization of human GDH following the cloning of cDNAs encoding for human GDH (22). This has permitted the detection of multiple GDH-specific mRNAs and genes in human tissues as well as the existence of two loci for human GDH on chromosomes 10 and X, respectively (23). Further studies currently in progress aim at characterizing these genes and their products in health and disease and determining the molecular basis of the phenotypic polymorphism encountered in patients with GDH deficiency. Definite proof for the presence of GDH gene mutation(s) requires the demonstration of an abnormal DNA sequence. The advent of the polymerase chain reaction and the characterization of the structure of the GDH-specific human genes will undoubtedly permit rapid progress toward this direction in the near future.

Pathogenesis of GDH-Deficient Cerebellar Degeneration

Because GDH plays a central role in glutamate metabolism and because the neuroexcitotoxic potentials of glutamate have been well established (24), detection of GDH deficiency was the first observation that linked a genetic molecular defect to mechanisms of neuroexcitotoxicity (25). There is ample evidence that glutamate serves as the major excitatory transmitter in mammalian brain (26). The amino acid is thought to be released at nerve endings during neurotransmission to act on postsynaptic receptors. This neurotransmitter action is then terminated by uptake primarily into the surrounding glial cells (27) where it can be oxidized by GHD to α-ketoglutarate or be aminated to glutamine by glutamine synthetase.

Additional studies on GDH-deficient patients revealed significant increases in the plasma levels of glutamate and decreases in the concentration of α-ketoglutarate, thus indicating a partial metabolic block of glutamate oxidation (25,28). Moreover, oral loading with monosodium glutamate resulted in excessive accumulation of glutamate in the plasma (25,28). In contrast, glutamate levels were markedly reduced in brain tissue obtained at autopsy from such patients (21). Aspartate levels were also reduced, although to a lesser extent than glutamate concentrations (21). Other investigators have also reported altered glutamate and/or aspartate levels in brain tissues as well as in the plasma and urine of patients with cerebellar degenerative disorders (29,30).

Since most free glutamate in nervous tissue is intracellular and plasma levels may reflect concentrations present in the extracellular fluids, the above data showing that glutamate levels are elevated in plasma and decreased in neural tissues suggest that an altered distribution of glutamate occurs between its intracellular and extracellular pools. These changes may be related to the strategic localization and function of this enzyme in glutamatergic pathways as described below.

Recent immunocytochemical studies by Aoki et al. (31) showed that, under conditions expected to reveal the membrane-bound form of the enzyme, GDH immunoreactivity was markedly enriched in CNS regions receiving putative glutamatergic innervation (glutamatergic receptive areas). In these regions the enzyme has been shown to be localized in glial processes (31) and thought to play a role in synaptic glutamate detoxification. In view of these considerations, dysfunction of GDH may impair the ability of the glial cells to metabolize transmitter glutamate, which could

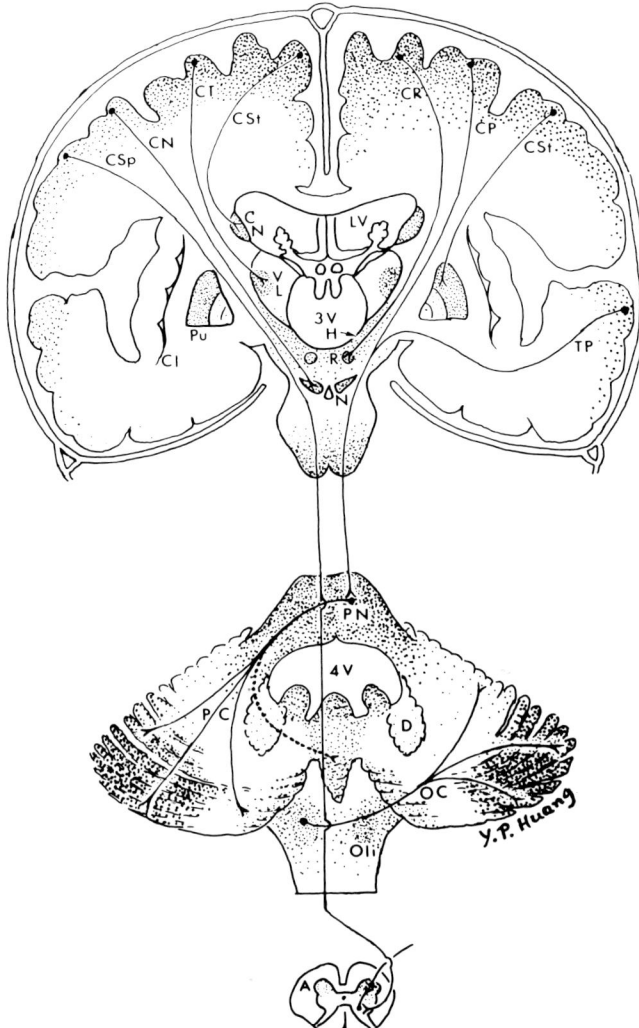

FIG. 2. Putative glutamatergic fiber systems of the brain in relation to morphologic alterations occurring in GDH-deficient OPCA. Areas *coarsely dotted* are thought to receive glutamatergic innervation as described by Huang and Plaitakis (32). These glutamatergic receptive regions correspond to rat brain areas shown by Aoki et al. (31) to be particularly rich in GDH immunoreactivity. Degenerative changes involving many of these regions have been revealed by computed tomography and magnetic resonance imaging in GDH-deficient OPCA patients (32). Putative glutamatergic tracks are labeled: CN, corticonigral; CP, corticopontine; CR, corticorubral; CSt, corticostriatal; CT, corticothalamic; OC, olivocerebellar; PC, pontocerebellar; Pu, putamen; C_N, caudate nucleus; 4V, fourth ventricle; 3V, third ventricle; D, dentate nucleus; Oli, inferior olive; H, hypothalamus; TP, temporopontine fibers; CSp, corticospinal track; N, substantia nigra; R, red nucleus; LV, lateral nucleus; A, anterior horns.

then accumulate in excessive amounts at the synaptic cleft and cause degeneration of the postsynaptic neurons according to the neuroexcitotoxic hypothesis (25). As shown in Fig. 2, patients with GDH deficiency indeed show a topographic distribution pattern of brain lesions that is compatible with the selective degeneration of glutamatergic postsynaptic neurons (32).

If this neuroexcitotoxic hypothesis is correct, one would expect to find in this disorder a selective disappearance of postsynaptic neurons bearing glutamate receptors. To investigate this possibility, the binding of L-glutamate was measured in cerebellar cortical tissue obtained at autopsy from OPCA patients. Results revealed that L-glutamate binding was markedly decreased in these patients without a change in the affinities and the pharmacologic properties of the binding sites (33). Moreover, autoradiographic studies (34–36) showed significant decreases in the quisqualate type of glutamate receptor present primarily in the molecular layer of the cerebellar cortex. These changes were, however, found not only in patients with the GDH-deficient form of OPCA but also in patients with other types of this disease, thus suggesting glutamatergic neuroexcitotoxic mechanisms as a common way to neurodegeneration in these disorders.

THE THIAMINE-DEFICIENT MODEL

It has been well established that acute thiamine deficiency (TD) in humans can cause a specific clinical syndrome, known as Wernicke's encephalopathy, which is characterized by cerebellar ataxia, ophthalmoplegia, global confusion, and sometimes by vasomotor and thermoregulatory disturbances (37). Some patients surviving the acute encephalopathy develop a characteristic amnestic syndrome known as Korsakoff's psychosis. Accordingly, some authors refer to the neurologic complications of TD collectively as Wernicke-Korsakoff syndrome (37). Specific regions of the brain stem, cerebellum, thalamus, and hypothalamus have been shown to be histologically affected in such patients (37). Similar clinical manifestations and brain pathologic changes have also been described in various species of experimental animals made thiamine deficient either by a diet lacking this vitamin or the use of thiamine antimetabolites (38).

Most of the thiamine present in cells occurs as thiamine pyrophosphate, which serves as the coenzyme for enzymes responsible for (i) decarboxylation of α-keto acids and (ii) the formation and degradation of α-ketols. These enzymes are of particular importance for carbohydrate and energy metabolism. In addition to its coenzyme role, thiamine is also thought to play a role in the function of excitable membranes, but this has been poorly understood.

Our work sought to elucidate the biological consequences of thiamine deprivation as they relate to brain dysfunction in deficiency states. Previous studies, which explored the activity of thiamine-dependent enzymes in TD, produced conflicting results (39,40). Moreover, when significant reductions in the thiamine-dependent enzymes were found, the magnitude of these changes was perhaps not sufficient to explain brain dysfunction (39,40).

It is, however, possible that changes of greater magnitude may occur in vulnerable neuronal populations due to their particular metabolic requirements, and such changes may be difficult to detect in whole-tissue homogenates. It is also possible that certain subcellular systems, such as synaptic terminals, which have high metabolic activity and consequently high requirements for thiamine, may also be selectively susceptible to TD. Previous morphologic studies had indeed suggested that nerve terminals and presynaptic boutons are affected early in TD (41). These considerations led us to explore the effect of TD in synaptic transmission by studying the high affinity uptake and release systems as well as the metabolism of selected putative transmitters in the brain of thiamine-deficient animals.

Production of Acute TD

Rats were made thiamine deficient either chronically by placing them on a thiamine-deficient diet or acutely by the use of a thiamine-deficient diet and the supplemental administration of pyrithiamine (PT) (0.5 mg/kg per day) (42). This thiamine antimetabolite has been shown to cross the blood-brain barrier and cause a rapid depletion of brain thiamine. Controls were pair-fed animals maintained on a thiamine-deficient diet supplemented by thiamine (42).

The animals treated chronically with a thiamine-deficient diet developed anorexia and weight loss after 2 to 3 weeks and behavioral manifestations such as gait ataxia, piloerection, hypothermia, and stimulus-sensitive convulsions after 6 to 9 weeks on the diet. On the other hand, the animals treated with PT developed anorexia and weight loss by days 8 to 10 and early neurologic deficits such as ataxic gait and a tendency to walk backward by days 11 to 12 on PT treatment. More dramatic behavioral changes such as stimulus-sensitive convulsions with opisthotonus, rotation, abnormal body posturing, weakness, hypothermia, and piloerection occurred by days 13 to 14. The animals deteriorated rapidly afterward. Marked weakness, loss of righting reflex, shallow respiration, loose bowel, erection, and a sharp drop in body temperature occurred prior to the animals' death. Because the behavioral changes in the PT-treated animals developed within a predictable period of time and with less variability in the time of onset and mode of evolution as compared to the animals treated with a thiamine-deficient diet alone, most of our experiments were done with the use of PT.

Uptake and Release of Putative Neurotransmitters by Brain Synaptosomes: Selective Impairment of Serotonin Uptake

Crude mitochondrial-synaptosomal fractions were prepared by differential centrifugation of homogenates from various brain regions of thiamine-deficient and control animals (42). After preincubation of these synaptosomes for 5 min, the following radioactive neurotransmitters were added, giving a final concentration within the range of the high-affinity uptake system for each of them: norepinephrine 6.8×10^{-8} M, serotonin (5-HT) 3.7×10^{-8} M, choline 5.9×10^{-8} M, gamma-aminobutyric acid (GABA) 5.72×10^{-8} M, glutamic and aspartic acid 10^{-5} to 10^{-6} M, glycine 1.2×10^{-7} M, or taurine 6×10^{-6} M. The K^+-stimulated release of these putative neurotransmitters was studied in these synaptosomal preparations as previously described (42).

Results revealed that the high-affinity uptake of 5-HT by the synaptosomal preparations isolated from the cerebellum of the thiamine-deficient animals was selectively decreased (by 40%; $p<0.01$) as compared to that of pair-fed controls (Fig. 3). In the PT-treated animals, the decrease in 5-HT uptake correlated with the appearance of neurologic symptoms. Synaptosomal preparations isolated from the hypothalamus of the thiamine-deficient animals also showed decreased 5-HT uptake (by 20%), but these changes were not statistically significant. On the other hand, no changes were found in the 5-HT uptake by synaptosomes isolated from the telencephalon of the experimental animals. The K^+-stimulated release of 5-HT from cerebellar synaptosomes was not altered in the thiamine-deficient animals.

Kinetic analysis of 5-HT uptake by cerebellar synaptosomes in thiamine-deficient animals revealed that both the V_{max} and the K_m decreased (to 50% and 60% of control, respectively) (Fig. 3A), indicating an alteration both in the number of serotonergic synaptosomes and the affinity of 5-HT uptake. Administration of thiamine to animals with acute deficiency reversed the neurologic symptoms and decreased 5-HT uptake to almost normal (Fig. 3B). The decrease in 5-HT uptake was selective because the uptake of other putative transmitters was not affected except for the uptake of glutamate and aspartate, which was significantly increased in synaptosomal preparations isolated from the cerebellum of PT-treated animals with early neurologic symptoms (43).

5-HT Metabolism in the Brain of Thiamine-Deficient Animals

Since the high-affinity uptake for 5-HT was found to be selectively affected in TD, we examined the concentration of 5-HT, its precursor tryptophan, and its main metabolite 5-hydroxyindoleacetic acid (5-HIAA) in various brain regions of animals with acute TD. Results revealed that the concentration of 5-HIAA increased significantly in all seven brain regions studied. In contrast the levels of 5-HT and its precursor tryptophan were not significantly altered (44,45).

To determine the mechanism(s) responsible for the increased brain levels of 5-HIAA, 5-HT turnover rates were determined by two different techniques. The first method was based on measuring the rate of 5-HT accumulation following the administration of the monoamine oxidase inhibitor pargyline and the second by the rate of [^{14}C]5-HIAA formation following intracisternal administration of [^{14}C]5-HT. In addition, the rate of disappearance of the intracisternally administered [^{14}C]5-HIAA was used for estimating the rate of transport of this metabolite of 5-HT from the brain (45).

Results obtained with the use of both methods revealed that 5-HT turnover rates increased significantly in all brain regions studied of thiamine-deficient animals as

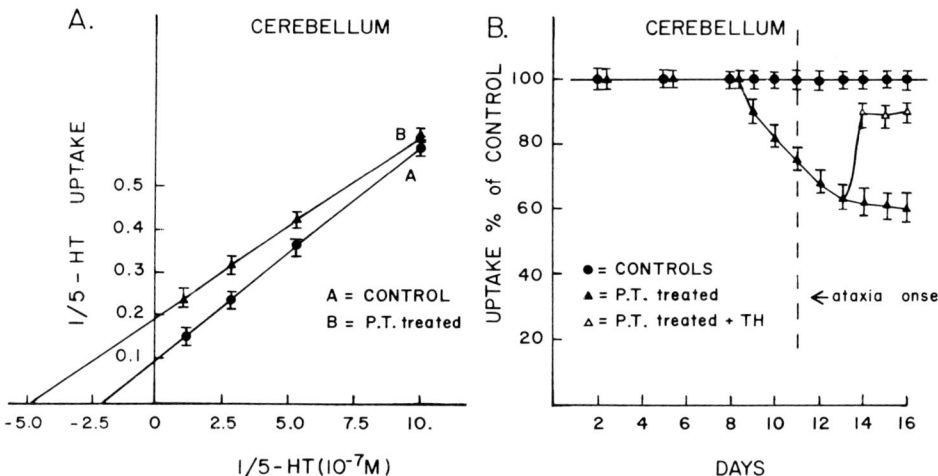

FIG. 3. A: Reciprocals of [^{3}H]5-HT concentration and its uptake by cerebellar synaptosomes of control and PT-treated rats. 5-HT uptake is defined as 10^4 dpm per milligram protein per 10 min. The points represent mean values ± SD from triplicate determinations. **B:** Effect of TD on 5-HT uptake by cerebellar synaptosomes during the course of acute TD induced by a thiamine-deficient diet and supplemental administration of PT. Each point is the average ± SD of triplicate determinations. After 12 days, some of the thiamine-deficient animals were taken off PT and administered thiamine subcutaneously (10 mg/100 g body weight). (From ref. 42.)

compared to controls, with the greatest changes occurring in the cerebellum of these animals (45). Moreover, the increased 5-HT turnover, as determined by the rate of [^{14}C]5-HIAA formation from [^{14}C]5-HT, correlated with regional thiamine turnover rates (Table 2) (46) and susceptibility to TD. In addition, studies employing intracisternal injections of [^{14}C]5-HIAA showed that part of the increase in the 5-HIAA levels described above was due to impaired transport of the compound from the brain (45).

Additional studies (47,48), utilizing autoradiography after intraventricular infusion of tritiated 5-HT, revealed a marked loss of 5-HT uptake by serotonergic axons throughout the brain with relative preservation of the subependymal serotonergic plexus. In addition, the visualized 5-HT axons showed a dystrophic appearance both in the cerebellum and other regions of the brain (47,48). In the cerebellum, serotonergic systems thought to be involved in synaptic transmission (serotonergic mossy and parallel fibers) were markedly affected, whereas those considered to be nonsynaptic (independent fibers) were relatively preserved (47). Hence, these findings may account for the different K_m for 5-HT uptake found in the thiamine-deficient animals (Fig. 3A).

These data accord modern concepts about the cerebellar serotonergic system, which is thought to consist of: (i) classical wiring (synaptic) transmission and (ii) volume transmission. The latter seems to utilize extracellular fluid as a pathway for electrical and chemical communication (49). As such, the above findings suggest

TABLE 2.

	Effect of TD on 5-HT turnover in rat brain ($[^{14}C]$5-HIAA/$[^{14}C]$5-HT)			Thiamine content and turnover rates in rat brain[a]	
	Control	Treated	% Increase	Thiamine levels	Turnover rate
Cerebellum	1.02	1.88[b]	84	4.37 ± 0.07	0.55
Medulla-pons	1.41	2.27[c]	60	2.90 ± 0.14	0.54
Hypothalamus	0.97	1.66[c]	71	2.86 ± 0.12	0.36
Midbrain	1.53	2.50[c]	63	3.10 ± 0.11	0.29
Striatum	3.83	4.26	11	3.32 ± 0.15	0.27
Cortex	1.40	1.46	4	2.61 ± 0.15	0.16

[a]Data from ref. 46.
5-HT turnover rates were determined by the rate of $[^{14}C]$5-HIAA formation following intracisternal administration of $[^{14}C]$5-HT. Animals were made thiamine deficient by the use of a thiamine-deficient diet and the supplemental administration of PT as described in the text. $[^{14}C]$5-HT (1 μCi in 25 μl of aqueous ascorbic acid) was injected prior to sacrifice. $[^{14}C]$5-HT and $[^{14}C]$5-HIAA were isolated and radioactivity was measured. Each value is the mean + SE of five rats.
[b]$p<0.05$.
[c]$p<0.01$.
Data are from ref. 45.

that TD may impair the cerebellar function by affecting the serotonergic synaptic system while sparing the volume 5-HT transmission.

Amino Acid Alterations in the Brains of Thiamine-Deficient Animals

Free amino acid levels were measured in three brain regions (cerebral cortex, medulla-pons, and cerebellum) at different stages of acute TD induced by PT treatment. Results showed that the levels of aspartate decreased significantly in all brain regions studied (43) (Fig. 4). In the medulla-pons and cerebellum (but not the cerebral cortex), a significant decrease in aspartate occurred just prior to the onset of clinical symptoms (day 10 of PT treatment). The decline in aspartate levels continued during the symptomatic stage of TD, as shown in Fig. 4. By day 14, when animals were severely affected, the greatest decreases occurred in the medulla-pons (36% of control) and cerebellum (55% of control), whereas the cerebral cortex showed less change (78–75% of control).

Glutamate levels showed small, but significant, decreases in the medulla-pons only (88–82% of control) in symptomatic animals (12–14 days of TD). In contrast, glutamine levels increased significantly in all three brain regions of PT-treated animals with acute symptoms of TD (Fig. 4). In addition, there was a small but significant decrease in the levels of serine in PT-treated rats. Other amino acids did not change significantly except for GABA as described below. Treatment with thiamine completely reversed all these amino acid changes and this correlated with the clinical improvement of these animals (4).

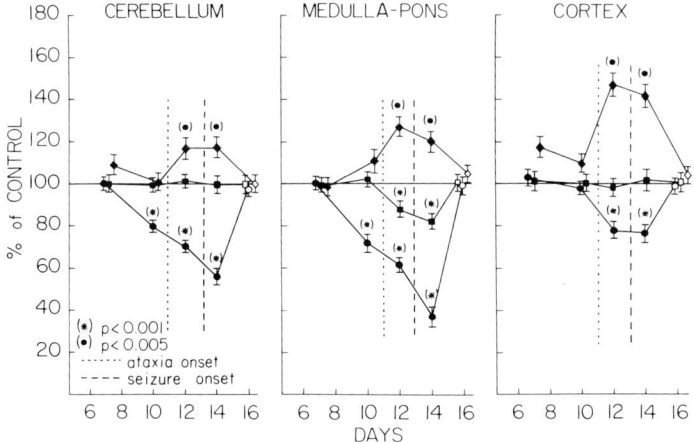

FIG. 4. Effect of TD on amino acid levels in three brain regions of rat and subsequent effects of thiamine therapy. Animals were made thiamine deficient acutely by the use of a thiamine-deficient diet and the supplemental administration of PT as described in the text. On day 14 some of the deficient animals (*open symbols*) were taken off PT and administered thiamine subcutaneously (10 mg/100 g body weight daily). Aspartate (●), glutamate (■), glutamine (♦). (From ref. 43.)

Alterations in Other Neurotransmitters

Determination of choline and acetylcholine levels in various brain regions of PT-treated rats revealed a significant decrease in the levels of acetylcholine (72% of control) but not in the levels of choline in the striatum of these animals (50). However, acetylcholine and choline levels remained unchanged in the hypothalamus, cerebral cortex, cerebellum, and medulla-pons of the deficient rats. GABA levels also showed a small but significant decrease (87% of control) in the striatum but not other CNS areas of these animals. Last, the levels of cyclic GMP were found to be significantly decreased (39% of control) in the cerebellum of PT-treated rats (50).

Pathophysiologic Considerations

Neurotransmitter Amino Acids

The mechanism(s) by which TD leads to brain amino acid alterations is not readily apparent. As described above, the levels of aspartate (and in some regions glutamate) decreased significantly, whereas the levels of glutamine increased in the same brain areas. Since thiamine is known to serve as coenzyme of pyruvate and α-ketoglutarate dehydrogenase, two key enzymes involved in the Krebs cycle, it is possible that these changes may result from a metabolic block of the oxidation of pyruvate and α-ketoglutarate in brain.

It is, however, difficult to reconcile this explanation with the results of enzymatic assays showing that the activities of these enzymes remain normal or near normal in animals with early TD. Also, labeling studies have so far failed to show a metabolic block within the Krebs cycle (oxidation of α-ketoglutarate), as suggested by some authors (51). In this regard, Gaitonde et al. (52) found decreased metabolism of [U-^{14}C]glucose and presented evidence for a defect in glycolysis at the hexokinase level. We have also found a decreased metabolism of [^{14}C]glucose into amino acids in regional areas of PT-treated rats (53). However, under these conditions the labeling of aspartate, glutamate, glutamine, and GABA from [^{3}H]acetate was unaffected. Since [^{14}C]glucose labels primarily the neuronal compartment, and [^{3}H]acetate the glial compartment, these data suggest that the metabolic consequences of TD are directed primarily against neurons. We found no differences in the ratio of labeled glutamate to labeled aspartate, and, as such, a metabolic block at the α-ketoglutarate level seems unlikely.

Hakim (54) has shown that prior to the appearance of clinical signs of TD cerebral blood flow increases significantly (up to 200% of control) in brain regions that are vulnerable to TD. The same structures then experience a significant rise in local cerebral glucose utilization (LCGU) and focal acidosis despite a persisting hyperperfusion. In the late stage of TD, inhomogeneous perfusion and declining LCGU were detected. These changes were thought to be identical to those occurring in cerebral ischemia (54).

In the cerebral ischemia model, which has been studied extensively, the above metabolic changes have been shown to be associated with significant increases in the extracellular glutamate concentrations (55), whereas the intracellular content of this amino acid declines significantly (56). Decreased energy metabolism is thought to be responsible for these changes since cellular processes that are responsible for maintaining a high intracellular-extracellular gradient for these amino acids are energy dependent. There is evidence that the high levels of extracellular glutamate mediate the neuronal degeneration that occurs in ischemia since it can be attenuated by glutamate receptor blockers.

Similar mechanisms may also be responsible for the aspartate and glutamate alterations that occur in the brain in TD. Since most free aspartate and glutamate present in cerebral tissue are intracellular (the extracellular levels are extremely small), the decline in the levels of these compounds, as shown to occur in the brain in TD, reflects decreases in the intracellular pools of these amino acids. This may result from: (i) an increased release of these compounds from the nerve terminals, (ii) leakage through the nerve cell membrane, and/or (iii) decreased intracellular synthesis.

Although measurement of extracellular levels by the microdialysis technique (as done in the cerebral ischemia model) is required to confirm the above hypothesis, data already exist in support of this possibility, indicating that neuroexcitotoxic mechanisms are responsible for the neurodegenerative processes of TD (57,58). It can, thus, be further speculated that in areas vulnerable to TD, the enhanced excitatory transmission leads to increased neuronal activity, which may in turn be responsible for the rise in cerebral blood flow and LCGU reported by Hakim (54) as well as the findings of McCandles (59), who showed that the high-energy phosphates are paradoxically increased in the brain of thiamine-deficient animals.

Serotonergic Alterations

As described above, the 5-HT high-affinity uptake was found to be decreased in TD. This was associated with morphologic changes of serotonergic axons as visualized by autoradiography. In addition, the 5-HT turnover rates increased significantly, and this correlated with the regional vulnerability seen in TD. The serotonergic neurons, however, did not appear to be lost in TD because the brain levels of 5-HT remained normal or even increased in some regions. Crespi and Jouvet (60) have also shown that indoleamine histofluorescence was increased in the raphe nucleus of thiamine-deficient animals. Similar alterations in both 5-HT turnover and morphologic appearance of serotonergic axons have been recently shown to be induced by potent neuroexcitotoxic amino acid analogues (61) (Fig. 5–7). Hence, it seems quite likely that the alterations in neuroexcitotoxic amino acids are responsible for the serotonergic changes that occur in TD.

The "Biochemical Lesion" in TD

Ever since Peters in 1936 (62) first suggested that a "biochemical lesion" occurs in the brain prior to the development of the permanent pathologic changes induced by TD, the nature of this lesion remains elusive. On the basis of these observations and the considerations presented above, we propose the following working hypotheses: (i) The brain is a highly heterogeneous structure composed of different cellular and subcellular systems with particular metabolic requirements and needs for thiamine. (ii) Cells and/or subcellular structures with high thiamine turnover are depleted early in thiamine deprivation and these may include synaptic terminals that are normally sites of high metabolic activity. (iii) In TD, energy metabolism may fail in these structures, impairing the ability of neurons to maintain high intracellular/extracellular gradients for neuroexcitatory amino acids. (iv) Increased extracellular (synaptic) concentrations of these amino acids may then occur, mediating the biochemical and morphologic alterations of serotonergic neurons as well as the neurodegenerative processes found in the brain in TD.

Malfunction of brain neurotransmitter systems, including serotonergic transmission and excitatory transmission mediated by amino acids, may underlie the neurologic manifestations of TD. The finding that cyclic GMP levels were altered in the cerebellum supports this possibility. Cyclic GMP is thought to function as a second messenger in the cerebellum, being modulated by the excitatory amino acids glutamate and aspartate (63) and a serotonergic pathway (50). In addition, alterations in

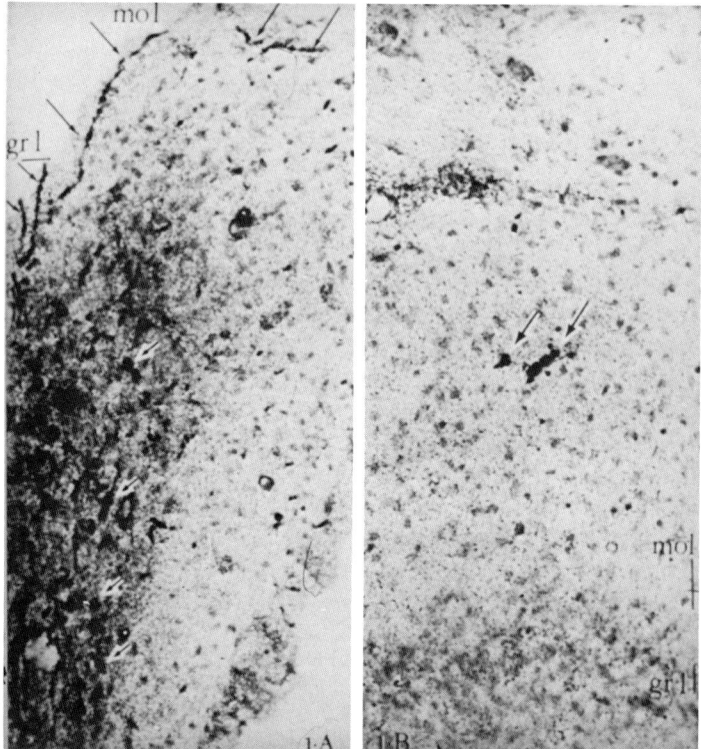

FIG. 5. A: Autoradiograph showing labeled 5-HT axons in the cerebellar cortex of a control animal. *Large arrows* indicate mossy fiber rosettes in the granular layer (gr 1). In the molecular layer (mol) long varicose fibers are labeled (*small arrows*). Also, small labeled boutons are seen in both the granular and molecular layers. **B**: Autoradiograph of a section through the cerebellar cortex of a thiamine-deficient rat. Labeled dystrophic serotonergic axons (*arrows*) are seen in the molecular layer. The granular layer shows paucity of labeled mossy fibers. (From ref. 47.)

cholinergic and GABAergic mechanisms appear to occur in other brain regions such as the basal ganglia, and these may contribute to brain dysfunction in TD.

Correlation with Neurologic Manifestations

As already mentioned, the clinical manifestations of acute TD in humans include cerebellar ataxia, ophthalmoplegia, global confusion, recent memory loss, confabulation, thermoregulatory disturbances, and weight loss. In contrast to the often occurring severe loss of recent memory, long-term memory and previously acquired skills are relatively preserved in the Wernicke-Korsakoff syndrome. In the rat additional manifestations include piloerection, stimulus-sensitive myoclonus, opisthotonus, and muricide behavior.

The selective involvement of the cerebellar 5-HT synaptic fibers, shown in the above studies (42), may lead to impairment of fine synaptic control in the cerebellar

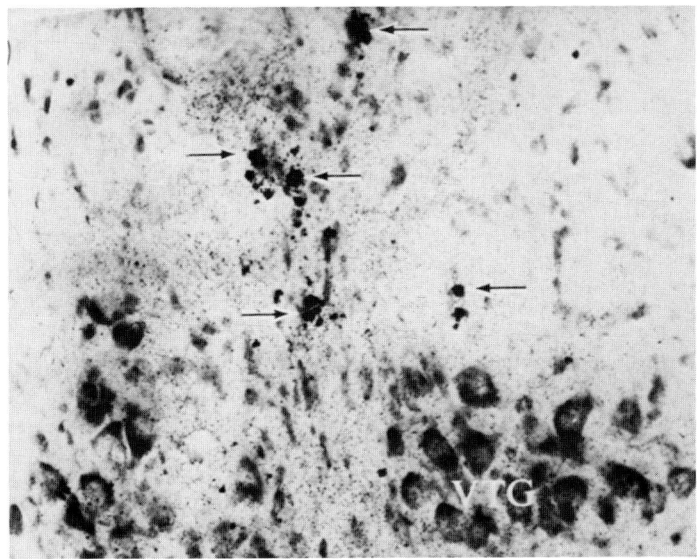

FIG. 6. Autoradiograph showing labeled dystrophic 5-HT axons (*arrows*) in the raphe superior centralis nucleus of a thiamine-deficient animal. VTG, ventral tegmental nucleus of Von Gudden. (From ref. 48.)

cortex (replacement with the diffuse volume transmission?) with resultant cerebellar dysfunction (ataxia) (42,50). A role for serotonergic mechanisms in the pathogenesis of ataxia is supported by the beneficial therapeutic responses obtained with the

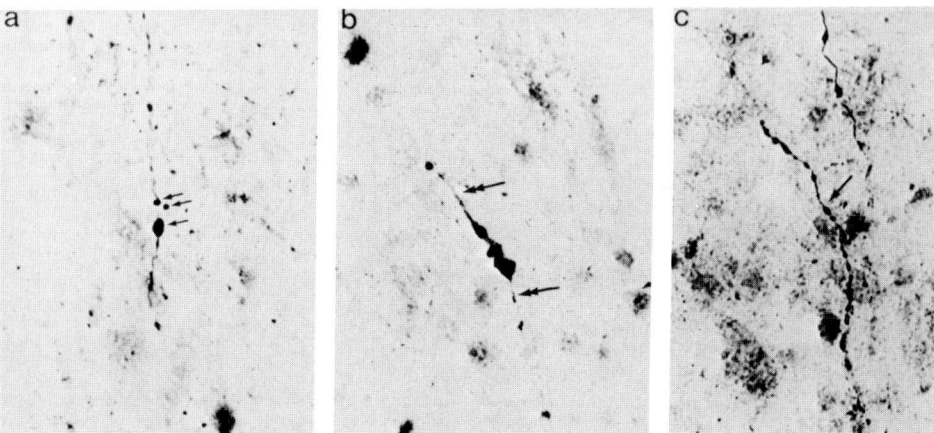

FIG. 7. a–c: Autoradiographs showing axonal changes of 5-HT positive fibers in the regio superio of the hippocampal formation 4 days after local injection of quinolinic acid. **a:** Lesioned area. Note large droplets (*arrows*) in an axon. **b:** Lesioned area: large swelling of an affected axon (*double arrows*). **c:** Adjacent to lesioned area: note numerous varicosities found in a 5-HT pontine axon. (From ref. 61.)

use of 5-HT precursors in patients with ataxia and/or myoclonus (64–66). Interestingly, the aspect of cerebellar ataxia that was found to be particularly sensitive to 5-HT precursors relate predominantly to midline dysfunction (disturbances of stance and gait). TD is known to affect primarily these cerebellar functions (37).

With respect to other manifestations of TD, Crespi and Jouvet (60) have shown sleep cycle disturbances in thiamine-deficient animals and attributed them to serotonergic alterations. Onodera et al. (67) showed that muricide behavior in thiamine-deficient rats could be modified by agents acting on the brain serotonergic system.

Last, the characteristic mental disturbances of TD encephalopathy, involving primarily the recent memory (including the ability of the patient to acquire new experiences and be aware of the events of daily life), may reflect brain serotonergic malfunction. There is evidence that serotonergic neurons play a key role in processes related to recent memory function, while long-term memory seems to require protein synthesis (68). It is, thus, tempting to speculate that the recent memory disturbances seen in patients with the Wernicke-Korsakoff syndrome relate to a selective involvement of brain serotonergic neurons, while the long-term memories, stored via the synthesis of protein, are not affected in this syndrome.

ACKNOWLEDGMENTS

Supported by NIH grants NS16871 and 5-MO1-RR00071, Division of Research Resources, General Clinical Research Center Branch.

REFERENCES

1. Herken H. Functional disorders of the brain induced by synthesis of nucleotides containing 3-acetylpyridine. *Z Klin Chem* 1968;6:635–637.
2. Desclin JC, Escubi J. Effects of 3-acetylpyridine on the central nervous system of the rat as demonstrated by silver methods. *Brain Res* 1974;77:349–364.
3. Plaitakis A, Nicklas WJ, Desnick RJ. Glutamate dehydrogenase deficiency in three patients with spinocerebellar syndrome. *Ann Neurol* 1980;7:297–303.
4. Yamaguchi T, Hayashi K, Murakami H, et al. Glutamate dehydrogenase deficiency in spinocerebellar degenerations. *Neurochem Res* 1982;7:627–636.
5. Duvoisin RC, Chokroverty S, Lepore F, Nicklas WJ. Glutamate dehydrogenase deficiency in patients with olivopontocerebellar atrophy. *Neurology* 1983;33:1322–1326.
6. Plaitakis A, Berl S, Yahr MD. Neurological disorders associated with deficiency of glutamate dehydrogenase. *Ann Neurol* 1984;15:144–153.
7. Plaitakis A. Abnormal glutamate metabolism of neuroexcitatory amino acids in olivopontocerebellar atrophy. In: Duvoisin RC, Plaitakis A, eds. *The olivopontocerebellar atrophies. (Advances in Neurology*, vol 41). New York: Raven Press, 1984:225–243.
8. Chokroverty S, Duvoisin RC, Sacheo R, et al. Neurophysiologic study of olivopontocerebellar atrophy with or without glutamate dehydrogenase deficiency. *Neurology* 1985;35:652–659.
9. Sorbi S, Tonini S, Giannini E, et al. Abnormal platelet glutamate dehydrogenase activity and activation in dominant and non-dominant olivopontocerebellar atrophy. *Ann Neurol* 1986;19:239–245.
10. Sorbi S, Piacetini S, Fani C, et al. Abnormalities of mitochondrial enzymes in hereditary ataxias. *Acta Neurol Scand* 1989;80:103–110.
11. Finocchiaro G, Taroni F, Di Donato S. Glutamate dehydrogenase in olivopontocerebellar atrophies: leukocytes, fibroblasts, and muscle mitochondria. *Neurology* 1986;36:550–553.

12. Konagaya Y, Konagaya M, Takayanagi T. Glutamate dehydrogenase and its isozyme activity in olivopontocerebellar atrophy. *J Neurol Sci* 1986;74:231–236.
13. Aubby D, Saggu HK, Jenner P, et al. Leukocyte glutamate dehydrogenase activity in patients with degenerative neurological disorders. *J Neurol Neurosurg Psychiatry* 1988;51:893–902.
14. Orsi L, Bertolotto A, Bringolio F, et al. Glutamate dehydrogenase (GDH) deficiency in different types of progressive hereditary cerebellar ataxia. *Acta Neurol Scand* 1988;78:394–400.
15. Kajiyama K, Ueno S, Tatsumi T, et al. Decreased glutamate dehydrogenase protein in spinocerebellar degeneration. *J Neurol Neurosurg Psychiatry* 1988;51:1078–1080.
16. Duvoisin RC, Nicklas WJ, Ritchie V, et al. Low leukocyte glutamate dehydrogenase activity does not correlate with a particular type of multiple system atrophy. *J Neurol Neurosurg Psychiatry* 1988;51:1508–1511.
17. Tatsumi C, Yorifuji S, Takahashi M, Tarui S. Decreased viability of skin fibroblasts from patients with glutamate dehydrogenase deficiency. *Neurology* 1989;39:541–542.
18. Kostic VS, Mojsilivic LJ, and Stojanovic M. Degenerative neurological disorders associated with deficiency of glutamate dehydrogenase. *J Neurol* 1989;236:111–114.
19. Iwattsuji K, Nakamura S, Kameyama M. Lymphocyte glutamate dehydrogenase activity in normal aging and neurological diseases. *Gerontology* 1989;35:218–224.
20. Kaakola S, Marnela K-M, Oja SS, et al. Leukocyte glutamate dehydrogenase and CSF amino acids in alate onset ataxias. *Acta Neurol Scand* 1990;82:225–229.
20a. Abe T, Ishiguto S, Saito H, et al. Partially deficient glutamate dehydrogenase activity and attenuated oscillatory potentials in patients with spinocerebellar degeneration. *Invest Ophthalmol Vis Sci* 1992;33:447–452.
21. Hussain MM, Zannis V, Plaitakis A. Characterization of glutamate dehydrogenase isoproteins purified from the cerebellum of normal subjects and patients with degenerative neurological disorders, and from human neoplastic cell lines. *J Biol Chem* 1989;264:20730–20735.
22. Maurothalassitis G, Tzimagiorgis G, Mitsialis A, et al. Isolation and characterization of cDNA clones encoding human liver glutamate dehydrogenase: evidence for a small gene family. *Proc Natl Acad Sci USA* 1988;85:3494–3498.
23. Jung KY, Warter S, Rumpler Y. Assignment of the GDH loci to human chromosomes 10q23 and Xq24 by in situ hybridization. *Ann Genet* 1989;32:109–110.
24. Olney JW. Excitatory amino acids and neuropsychiatric disorders. *Biol Psychiatry* 1989;26:505–525.
25. Plaitakis A, Berl S, Yahr MD. Abnormal glutamate metabolism in adult-onset degenerative neurological disorder. *Science* 1982;216:193–196.
26. Fonnum F. Glutamate: a neurotransmitter in mammalian brain. *J Neurochem* 1984;42:1–11.
27. Balcar VJ, Borg J, Mandel P. High affinity uptake of L-glutamate and L-aspartate by glial cells. *J Neurochem* 1977;27–28.
28. Plaitakis A, Berl S. Oral glutamate loading in disorders with spinocerebellar and extrapyramidal involvement: effect on plasma glutamate, aspartate and taurine. *J Neural Transm* 1983(suppl 19):65–74.
29. Perry TL. Four biochemically different types of dominantly inherited olivopontocerebellar atrophy. In: Duvoisin RC, Plaitakis A, eds. *The olivopontocerebellar atrophies* (Advances in Neurology, vol 41). New York: Raven Press, 1984:205–216.
30. Sawada M, Seriu N, Udaka F, et al. Cerebellar ataxia with glutamic aciduria. *Acta Neurol Scand* 1991;84:70–72.
31. Aoki C, Milner TA, Rex Sheu K-FR, et al. Regional distribution of astrocytes with intense immunoreactivity for glutamate dehydrogenase in rat brain: implications for neuroglia interactions in glutamate transmission. *J Neurosci* 1987;7:2214–2231.
32. Huang YP, Plaitakis A. Morphological changes in olivopontocerebellar atrophy in computed tomography and comments on its pathogenesis. In: Duvoisin RC, Plaitakis A, eds. *The olivopontocerebellar atrophies* (Advances in Neurology, vol 41). New York: Raven Press, 1984:39–81.
33. Tsiotos P, Plaitakis A, Mitsakos A, et al. L-glutamate binding sites of normal and atrophic human cerebellum. *Brain Res* 1989;481:87–96.
34. Hatziefthimiou A, Mitsakos A, Mitsaki E, et al. Quantitative autoradiographic study of L-glutamate binding studies in normal and atrophic human cerebellum. *J Neurosci Res* 1991;28:367–375.
35. Albin RL, Gilman S. Autoradiographic localization of inhibitory and excitatory amino acid transmitter receptors in human normal and olivopontocerebellar atrophy cerebellum. *Brain Res* 1990;522:37–45.

36. Macowiec RL, Albin RL, Cha JJ, et al. Two types of quisqualate receptor are reduced in human OPCA cerebellar cortex. *Brain Res* 1990;523:309–312.
37. Victor M, Adams RD, Collins GH. The Wernicke-Korsakoff syndrome: a clinical and pathologic study of 245 patients, 82 with post-mortem examination. *Contemp Neurol Ser* 1971;7:1–206.
38. Plaitakis A, Nicklas WJ, Berl S. Thiamine deficiency: selective impairment of the cerebellar serotoninergic system. *Neurology* 1978;28:691–698.
39. Dreyfus PM. Thiamine deficiency encephalopathy: thoughts on its pathogenesis. In: Gubler CJ, Fujiwara M, Dreyfus PM, eds. *Thiamine*. New York: Wiley, 1976:229–239.
40. Gubler CL. Biochemical changes in thiamine deficiencies. In: Gubler CJ, Fujiwara M, Dreyfus PM, eds. *Thiamine*. New York: Wiley, 1976:121–141.
41. Pena CE, Felter. Ultrastructural changes of the lateral vestibular nucleus in acute experimental thiamine deficiency. *Z Neurol* 1973;204:263–280.
42. Plaitakis A, Nicklas WJ, Berl S. Thiamine deficiency: selective impairment of the cerebellar serotonergic system. *Neurology* 1978;28:691–698.
43. Plaitakis A, Nicklas WJ, Berl S. Alterations in uptake and metabolism of aspartate and glutamate in brain of thiamine deficient animals. *Brain Res* 1979;171:489–502.
44. Plaitakis A, Van Woert MH, Hwang EC, Berl S. The effect of acute thiamine deficiency on brain tryptophan, serotonin and 5-hydroxylindoleacetic acid. *J Neurochem* 1978;31:1087–1089.
45. Van Woert MH, Plaitakis A, Hwang EC, Berl S. Effect of thiamine deficiency on brain serotonin turnover. *Brain Res* 1979;179:103–110.
46. Rindi G, Patrini G, Comincioli V, Reggiani C. Thiamine turnover rate in some areas of rat brain and liver: a preliminary note. *Experientia* 1979;35:498–499.
47. Chan-Palay V, Plaitakis A, Nicklas WJ, Berl S. Autoradiographic demonstration of loss of labeled indoleamine axons in the cerebellum of chronic diet-induced thiamine deficiency. *Brain Res* 1977;138:380–384.
48. Chan-Palay V. Indoleamine neurons and their processes in normal and in chronic diet-induced thiamine deficiency demonstrated by uptake of ^{3}H-serotonin. *J Comp Neurol* 1977;176:467–494.
49. Fuxe K, Agnati L. Volume transmission in the brain: novel mechanisms for neural transmission. *Adv Neurosci* 1991;1:1–624.
50. Plaitakis A, Hwang EC, Van Woert MH, et al. Effect of thiamine deficiency on brain neurotransmitter systems. *Ann NY Acad Sci* 1982;378:367–381.
51. Butterworth R. Cerebral thiamine-dependent enzyme changes in experimental Wernicke's encephalopathy. *Metab Brain Dis* 1986;3:165–175.
52. Gaitonde MK, Fayein NA, Johnson AL. Decreased metabolism in vivo of glucose into amino acids of the brain of thiamine deficient rats after treatment with pyrithiamine. *J Neurochem* 1975;24:1215–1223.
53. Plaitakis A, Nicklas WJ, Berl S. B_1 deficiency: ^{14}C-glucose, ^{3}H-acetate and $NaH^{14}CO_3$ flux into the brain amino acids. *Trans Am Soc Neurochem* 1980;11:122.
54. Hakim AM. Effect of thiamine deficiency and its reversal on cerebral blood flow in the rat. Observations on the phenomena of hyperperfusion, "no reflow," and delayed hypoperfusion. *J Cereb Blood Flow Metab* 1986;6:79–85.
55. Benevensite H, Drejer J, Schonsboe A, Diemer NH. Elevation of extracellular concentrations of glutamate and aspartate in rat hippocampus during transient cerebral ischemia monitored by intracerebral microdialysis. *J Neurochem* 1984;43:1369–1374.
56. Erecinska M, Nelson D, Wilson DF, et al. Neurotransmitter amino acids in the CNS. 1. Regional changes in amino acid levels in rat brain during ischemia and re-perfusion. *Brain Res* 1984;304:9–22.
57. Armstrong-James M, Ross DT, Chen F, Ebner FF. The effect of thiamine deficiency on the structure and physiology of the rat forebrain. *Metab Brain Dis* 1988;3:91–124.
58. Langlais PJ, Mair RG. Protective effects of the glutamate antagonist MK-801 on pyrithiamine-induced lesions and amino acid changes in rat brain. *J Neurosci* 1990;10:1664–1674.
59. McCandles DW. Energy metabolism in the lateral vestibular nucleus in pyrithiamine-induced thiamine deficiency. *Ann NY Acad Sci* 1982;378:355–364.
60. Crespi F, Jouvet. Sleep and indoleamine alterations induced by thiamine deficiency. *Brain Res* 1982;248:275–283.
61. Aldinio C, Mazzari S, Toffano G, et al. Effects of intracerebral injections of quinolinic acid on serotonergic neurons in the rat brain. *Brain Res* 1985;341:57–65.
62. Peters RA. The biochemical lesion in vitamin B_1 deficiency: application of modern biochemical analysis in its diagnosis. *Lancet* 1936;230:1161–1165.

63. Roberts PJ, Foster GA. Pharmacology of excitatory amino acid receptors mediating the stimulation of rat cerebellar cyclic GMP levels in vitro. *Life Sci* 1980;27:215–221.
64. Trouillas P. Regression of cerebellar syndrome with long-term administration of 5-HTP or the combination of 5-HT-benzerizide. *Ital J Neurol Sci* 1984;5:253–266.
65. Van Woert MH, Rosenbaum D, Howieson et al. Long-term therapy of myoclonus and other neurological disorders with L-5-hydroxytryptophan and carbidopa. *N Engl J Med* 1977;296:70–75.
66. Plaitakis A. Modulation of monoaminergic and amino acid transmission as a means for therapeutic intervention in ataxia. *Can J Neurol Sci* (*in press*).
67. Onodera K, Kisara K, Ogura Y. Effect of 5-hydroxytryptophan on muricide response induced by thiamine deficiency. *Arch Int Pharmacodyn* 1979;240:220–227.
68. Kandell ER. Cellular mechanisms of learning and the biological basis of individuality. In: Kande ER, Schwartz JH, Jessel TM, eds. *Principles of neural sciences*. New York: Elsevier, 1991:1009–1030.
69. Plaitakis A. Abnormal metabolism of neuroexcitatory amino acids in olivopontocerebellar atrophy. In: Duvoisin RC, Plaitakis A, eds. *The olivopontocerebellar atrophies* (*Advances in Neurology*, vol 41). New York: Raven Press, 1984:225–243.

*Serotonin, the Cerebellum,
and Ataxia*, edited by
P. Trouillas and K. Fuxe.
Raven Press, Ltd., New York © 1993.

21

Collateral Sprouting of Cerebellar Climbing Fibers After Subtotal Lesions of the Inferior Olive

L. Wiklund, *F. Rossi, *P. Strata, and †J. J. L. van der Want

*Laboratoire de Physiologie Nerveuse, CNRS, 91190 Gif-sur-Yvette, France;
*Department of Human Anatomy and Physiology, 10125 Turin, Italy;
†Netherlands Ophthalmic Research Institute, 1100 AC Amsterdam, The Netherlands*

Climbing fibers originate in the inferior olive and synapse directly with Purkinje cells in the cerebellar cortex. Each Purkinje cell receives a single climbing fiber. The individual climbing fiber forms an extensive terminal arborization with numerous synaptic boutons on the dendrites of the Purkinje cell and represents a powerful excitatory input to the Purkinje cell (for review, ref. 4).

Specific parts of the olivary subnuclei project to distinct sagittal zones of the cerebellum, and within these the climbing fiber input is organized in narrow microzones. These microzones have specific receptive fields, and it has been suggested that they constitute the basic functional units of cerebellar circuitry controlling specific motor functions (2). Identified microzones are 100 to 300 µm wide and more than a millimeter long, but the theoretical limit would be zones consisting of a single row of Purkinje cells (5). Recently, we demonstrated that subtotal lesions of the inferior olive result in collateral sprouting of surviving climbing fibers that extend their field of innervation to large numbers of Purkinje cells (6–8). This plasticity may have implications for cerebellar function in certain pathological conditions.

METHODS

Rats received intraperitoneal injections of 3-acetylpyridine (3-AP), which resulted in the degeneration of 90% to 99% of the olivary neurons. Survival times ranged from 3 days to 1 year. Climbing fibers were visualized with the anterograde Phaseolus vulgaris leukoagglutinin (PHA-L) technique. PHA-L lectin was injected electrophoretically into the inferior olive, and rats survived for 5 to 7 days before perfusion fixation. Labeled nerve fibers were detected with sensitive immunocytochemical techniques at light and electron microscopic levels. In some experiments, anti-CarpII parvalbumin antibody was used as selective marker of Purkinje cell somas and dendrites. Climbing fiber arborizations were analyzed on serial sections and camera lucida reconstructions, and quantified with simple computer analysis. (For a detailed account of the methods used, see refs. 7,8.)

NORMAL CLIMBING FIBERS

Climbing fibers originate in the inferior olive, and these olivocerebellar axons cross the midline, traverse the brain stem, and join the inferior cerebellar peduncle, which they follow to the cerebellum. Arriving in the deep cerebellar white matter, bundles of olivary axons run toward different parts of the cerebellar cortex. In the cortex, the axons cross the granular layer to reach their target Purkinje cells on which they form extensive terminal arborizations, which are denoted climbing fibers. The individual climbing fiber forms a few synaptic boutons on the Purkinje cell soma, and its smooth main stalk ascends along the Purkinje cell dendrites into the molecular layer and gives rise to numerous fine varicose fibers, which synapse on "dendritic thorns" of the proximal dendrites of the Purkinje cell. Due to the orientation of the Purkinje cell dendritic tree, the climbing fiber arborization is typically fan-like and oriented in the parasagittal plane. Climbing fibers do not reach the spiny branchlets of the Purkinje cell, on which the parallel fibers synapse.

SPROUTING OF LESIONED CLIMBING FIBERS

After 3-AP lesioning, the number of neurons in the inferior olives was reduced by 90% to 99%, and the numbers of visualized climbing fibers were correspondingly decreased. The few surviving climbing fibers in the molecular layer did not, however, show any signs of degeneration.

As soon as 3 to 7 days after lesioning, the surviving climbing fibers showed signs of sprouting. Newly formed fibers extended from any level of the climbing fiber arborization in the molecular layer, but sprouting was never observed from olivocerebellar axons traversing the granular layer or white matter. The newly formed sprouts seemed to grow haphazardly in any direction through the molecular layer. After some distance the smooth sprouted fibers gave rise to new terminal arborizations of varicose fibers, which grew along denervated Purkinje cell dendrites and occasionally around the soma. After shorter survival times the newly formed arborizations only covered part of the neighboring Purkinje cell dendritic trees, growing toward the pial surface and/or the soma to cover the reinnervated Purkinje cells. After 1 to 2 months (Fig. 1), sprouted climbing fibers often formed complete terminal arborizations around some reinnervated Purkinje cells, but the sprouting process had continued to engage even larger numbers of denervated Purkinje cells, the result

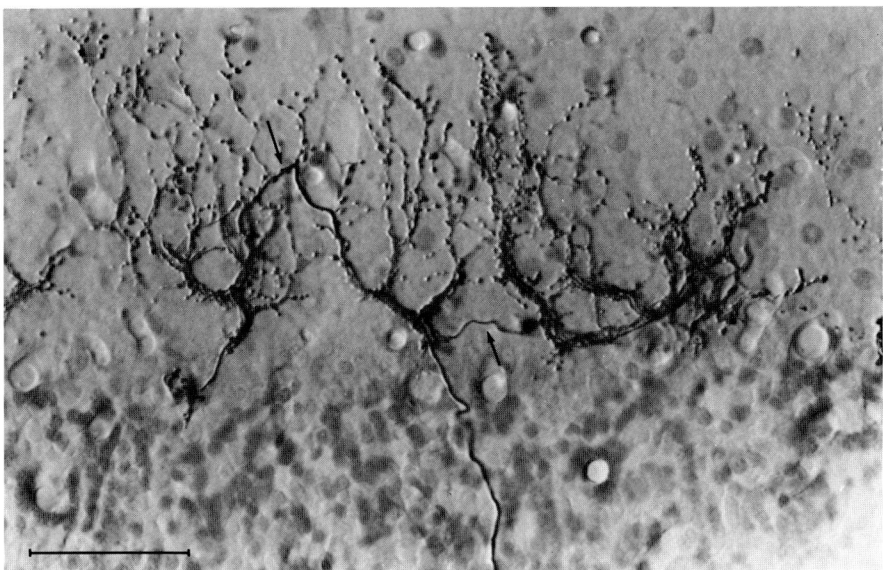

FIG. 1. Light microscopic micrograph of a PHA-L-labeled climbing fiber demonstrating extensive sprouting 1 year after 3-AP lesioning of the inferior olive. On this parasagittal section, the olivocerebellar axon can be seen traversing the granular layer to reach the Purkinje cell it originally innervated, on which it forms an extensive climbing fiber arborization. Two sprouts (*arrows*) grow out from the parent arborization and form new climbing fiber arborizations around neighboring Purkinje cells. Bar 50 μm. (Modified from ref. 7.)

being that some Purkinje cells were well reinnervated while others were contacted by just a few varicose terminals (Fig. 2).

Electron microscopic analysis showed that the newly formed climbing fibers formed synaptic junctions on dendritic thorns of proximal Purkinje cell dendrites (Figs. 3 and 4). Hence, the appearance and distribution of newly formed synapses were very similar to normal climbing fiber innervation.

The collateral sprouting and growth process of climbing fibers continued for at least 2 months. Even after 6 months and 1 year survival, no regression or retraction of newly formed climbing fiber arborizations was noted, indicating that a permanent reinnervation had been established. The reinnervation process resulted in clusters of Purkinje cells contacted by the same sprouted climbing fiber. These clusters extended for several hundred micrometers, and it was estimated that surviving climbing fibers may extend their domain of innervation 5 to 10 times (Fig. 2).

DISCUSSION

The presented experiments have shown that cerebellar climbing fibers possess a considerable plastic capacity. After subtotal lesions of the inferior olive, surviving

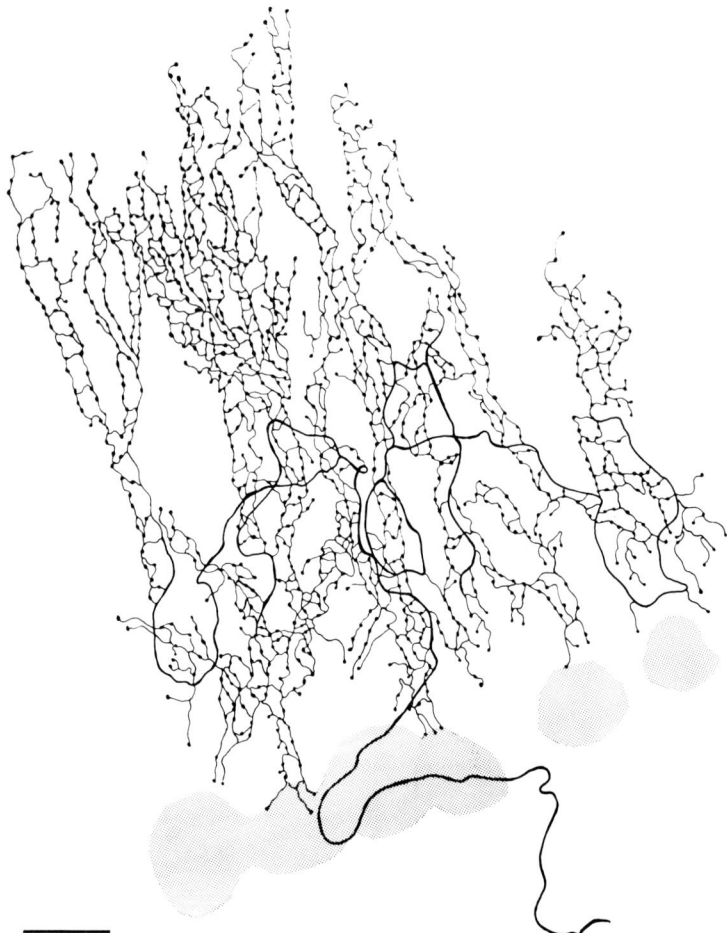

FIG. 2. Camera lucida drawing that partly reconstructs a cluster of climbing fiber arborizations emanating from a single sprouted climbing fiber. Purkinje cell somata are indicated by *dotted areas*. On this frontal section, the Purkinje cell dendritic tree and climbing fiber arborizations are seen "in profile," i.e., as thin vertically oriented sheaths of terminals. It can be estimated from the drawing that the climbing fiber has sprouted to reinnervate five neighboring Purkinje cells. Bar 25 μm.

climbing fibers send out new fibers, which extend for considerable distances through the molecular layer, and reinnervate many neighboring Purkinje cells. The newly formed climbing fiber arborizations form normal looking synapses on the appropriate part of Purkinje cell dendrites, and from the work of Benedetti and Strata (1) it can be concluded that they are electrophysiologically functional.

This process of collateral sprouting and reinnervation has several interesting implications. It provides a convenient model for the study of neuron-target interactions (8). Since surviving climbing fibers extend their domain of innervation several fold, it is likely that the growth of climbing fibers is stimulated by a trophic influence

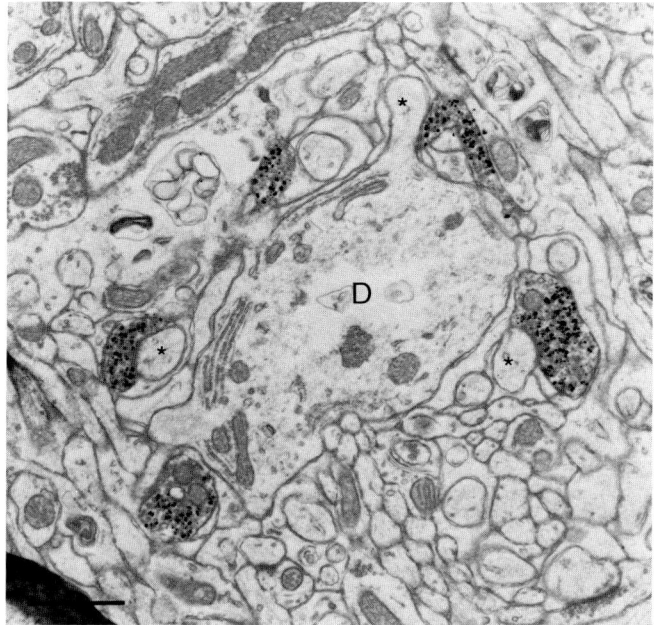

FIG. 3. Electron micrograph of PHA-L-labeled sprouted climbing fiber boutons surrounding a Purkinje cell dendrite (D). The immunocytochemcial labeling appears as granular precipitate of high electron density. The newly formed climbing fiber boutons synapse with dendritic thorns (*) emanating from the dendritic shaft. Bar 1 μm.

exerted by denervated Purkinje cells. The nature of this trophic influence remains to be identified.

Plasticity of neuronal connections and reinnervation in the central nervous system are often viewed as a means of repair and reestablishment of lost connections, which contributes to the restoration or improvement of function in injured neuronal networks. According to this view, collateral sprouting of climbing fibers would serve to reestablish climbing fiber control over denervated Purkinje cells, and therefore improve the olivocerebellar modulatory influence over cerebellar circuitry (3). Contrary to this view, it may be argued that collateral sprouting of climbing fibers may be detrimental to cerebellar function. As noted at the beginning of this chapter, the olivocerebellar climbing fiber system is organized in narrow, sagittally arranged microzones, and it has been suggested that these constitute the functional subunits of the cerebellum (2). Collateral sprouting of climbing fibers for hundreds of micrometers would, if the process does not respect the boundaries of microzones, disturb this proposed functional organization of cerebellar circuitry. Climbing fiber collateral sprouting could, therefore, decrease the precision of cerebellar function. On the other hand, it may be that the cerebellar circuitry may be reprogrammed to function with a modified zonal organization. Specific experiments are needed to determine the functional consequences of climbing fiber collateral sprouting.

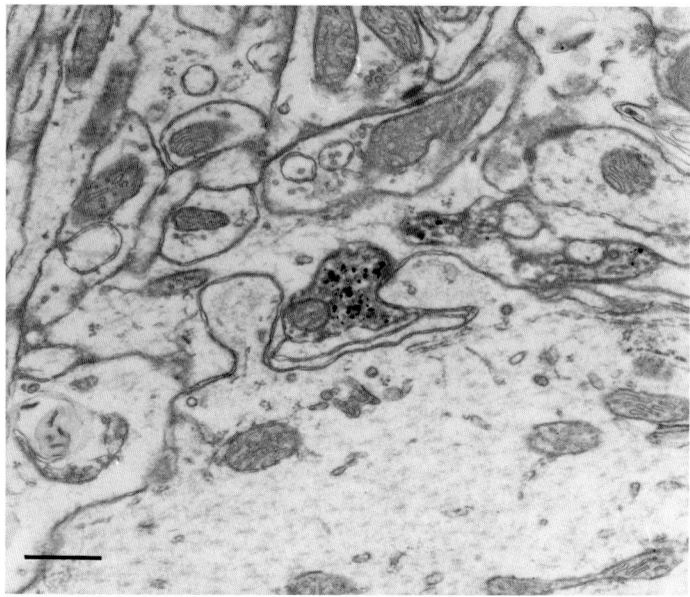

FIG. 4. Higher magnification of a labeled sprouted climbing fiber bouton that forms a synapse with a dendritic thorn. A neighboring dendritic thorn is unoccupied. Bar 0.5 μm.

It is unknown whether climbing fiber plasticity and collateral sprouting play a role in clinical phenomena. It seems plausible, however, that such remodeling of climbing fiber connections may occur in syndromes like hereditary ataxias, which involve neuronal loss in the inferior olives.

REFERENCES

1. Benedetti F, Strata P. Functional synaptogenesis in the cerebellar cortex after inferior olive lesion. In: Bonavita N, Piccoli F, eds. *Biological aspects of neuron activity*. Padova: Fidia Biomedical Information, 97–107.
2. Ekerot C-F, Garwicz M, Schouenborg J. Topography and nociceptive fields of climbing fibres projecting to the cerebellar anterior lobe in the cat. *J Physiol (in press)*.
3. Ekerot C-F, Kano M. Long term depression of parallel fibre synapses following stimulation of climbing fibres. *Brain Res* 1985;342:357–360.
4. Ito M. *The cerebellum and neuronal control*. New York: Raven Press, 1984.
5. Oscarsson O. Functional units of the cerebellum sagittal zones and microzones. *Trends Neurosci* 1979;2:143–145.
6. Rossi F, Wiklund L, van der Want JJL, Strata P. Climbing fibre plasticity in the cerebellum of the adult rat. *Eur J Neurosci* 1989;1:543–547.
7. Rossi F, Wiklund L, van der Want JJL, Strata P. Reinnervation of cerebellar Purkinje cells by climbing fibres surviving a subtotal lesion of the inferior olive in the adult rat. I. Development of new collateral branches and terminal plexuses. *J Comp Neurol* 1991;308:513–535.
8. Rossi F, van der Want JJL, Wiklund L, Strata P. Reinnervation of cerebellar Purkinje cells by climbing fibres surviving a subtotal lesion of the inferior olive in the adult rat. II. Synaptic organization of reinnervated Purkinje cells. *J Comp Neurol* 1991;308:536–554.

*Serotonin, the Cerebellum,
and Ataxia*, edited by
P. Trouillas and K. Fuxe.
Raven Press, Ltd., New York © 1993.

22

Cerebellar Monoamines in the "Purkinje Cell Degeneration" Mutant Mouse

B. Ghetti, L. C. Triarhou, and R. W. Fuller

*Laboratory of Cellular and Molecular Neuropathology,
Department of Pathology, Indiana University School of Medicine,
and Eli Lilly Research Laboratories, Indianapolis, Indiana 46202-5120*

In human degenerative disorders of the central nervous system (CNS), the reaction of central monoaminergic (MA) systems to the loss of their target neurons has been studied by neurochemical methods, whereas the underlying structural alterations of these systems are relatively less well understood. Correlative neurochemical and morphological studies in experimental animals can offer valuable insights into the response of MA systems to degeneration.

In degenerative conditions due to genetic or nongenetic causes, neuronal loss is usually the most evident manifestation associated with CNS dysfunction. A distinct feature of nervous systems is that the selective loss of a neuronal population, regardless of cause, may initiate a cascade of regressive changes in pre- and postsynaptic neuronal systems.

One way to investigate neuronal loss and its consequences experimentally is by using laboratory mice with genetic mutations that lead to selective neuronal death. By using such animals, one can choose the temporal stages of the various degenerations to study, while in human neurodegenerative diseases, and particularly in the cerebellar heredoataxias, it is usually difficult to establish whether an observed atrophy or loss (or both) of a particular neuronal group is *primary* (i.e., due to a genetic effect) or *secondary* (i.e., due to transsynaptic degeneration).

In neurological mutant mice one can recognize two orders of degenerative phenomena: (i) a primary loss of neurons that are programmed to degenerate through a more or less direct action of the mutant allele and (ii) a secondary (or transsynaptic) neuronal response that is in most cases characterized by degeneration or atrophy of cells pre- or postsynaptic to the neurons-targets of the mutation. The survival of MA systems appears not to be highly dependent on the integrity of the target neurons.

In this chapter we present an overview of studies carried out in the "Purkinje cell degeneration" (*pcd*) mutant mouse, with particular emphasis on the changes that occur in MA systems. In this mutant, a progressive degeneration of cerebellar Purkinje cells begins on postnatal day 17 and is complete by day 45 (1,2). In addition to the genetically determined Purkinje cell loss, death of granule cells, which is probably transneuronal, also takes place (3,4). Thus, the *pcd* mutant provides a model in which the fate of cerebellar MA fibers can be studied after the complete loss of a major target of both norepinephrine (NE) and serotonin (5-HT) systems (i.e., the Purkinje cells), and the partial loss of another neuronal target (i.e., the granule cells).

The MA innervation of the cerebellar cortex comprises NE and 5-HT fibers (5–7). The origin of the NE innervation of the cerebellar cortex lies in neurons of the dorsal part of the nucleus locus coeruleus and also in neurons of the fields A5 and A7 and of the nucleus subcoeruleus (8–11). Electron microscopic and physiological studies have provided evidence that the Purkinje cells constitute a target for NE fibers (8).

The origin of 5-HT afferents lies in neurons of the dorsal raphe nuclei of the pons and the medullary and pontine reticular formation (12,13). Purkinje cells constitute one cerebellar neuron type that is innervated by raphe 5-HT neurons. Granule cells are also innervated by 5-HT afferents. 5-HT-containing axons are distributed throughout the cerebellar cortex, as evidenced by immunocytochemistry (13,14), and have been described to be in apposition with Purkinje cell and granule cell dendrites and basket, stellate, and Golgi neurons, as well as parallel fibers (12, 15,16).

GENETICALLY DETERMINED DEGENERATION OF PURKINJE CELLS IN THE *pcd* MUTANT

A genetically determined loss of virtually all Purkinje cells takes place in *pcd* mice during the period that follows the maturation of the cerebellum, i.e., between 17 and 45 days of age (1,2). This mutant was named based on its neuropathological phenotype. The *pcd* allele is recessive and has been localized to mouse chromosome 13 (17).

In the cerebellum of 17-day-old *pcd* mutant mice, Purkinje cells appear to have a normal morphology, except that a metachromatic mass consisting of polyribosomes is present in the basal pole of the perikaryon; following that stage, Purkinje cell somata and dendrites undergo dark degeneration and cytoplasmic shrinkage (Fig. 1A).

At 23 days of age, the degenerative process of Purkinje cells has advanced and cell debris is found in the molecular and Purkinje cell layers, as well as in the granule cell layer and the deep cerebellar nuclei, resulting from the fragmentation of dendrites, perikarya, and Purkinje axon terminals. Some surviving Purkinje cells are still seen.

The loss of Purkinje cells in *pcd* mutants progresses rapidly. It is estimated that

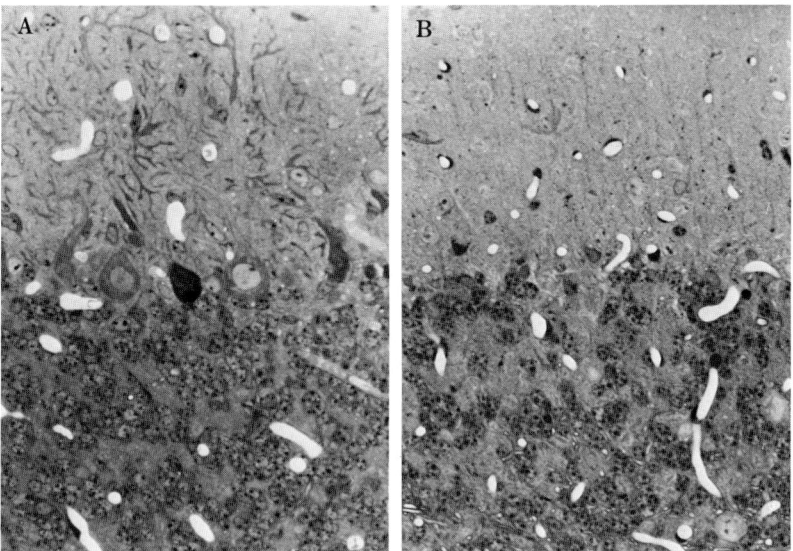

FIG. 1. Semithin sections of *pcd* cerebellum during (**A**) and following (**B**) the completion of degeneration of Purkinje cells in the cerebellar cortex.

about 25% to 50% of Purkinje cells have already degenerated by postnatal days 22 to 24 (1). The loss of Purkinje cells takes place in clusters, in such a way that remaining Purkinje cells are organized in parasagittal bands at the coronal plane with a symmetrical disposition relative to the midline (18). Eventually (i.e., after 45–50 days of age), more than 99% of the Purkinje cells disappear and the *pcd* cerebellum becomes devoid of immunoreactivity for specific Purkinje cell protein markers, such as calcium-binding protein, polypeptide PEP-19, and cyclic GMP-dependent protein kinase (18–20). In histological preparations one can see cell debris throughout the molecular, Purkinje, and granule cell layers, as well as in the subcortical white matter and the deep cerebellar nuclei. At later ages (6 months and beyond), a remarkable atrophy of the cerebellar cortex is observed. The cortex essentially consists only of molecular and granule cell layers (Fig. 1B). The overall size of the cerebellum is substantially reduced; the average change in weight of fixed cerebella is from 41 mg at 23 days to 22 mg at 300 days, in contrast to normal mouse cerebellum, which is about 55 to 60 mg (21).

SEQUENCE AND EXTENT OF DEGENERATIVE EVENTS IN THE CEREBELLAR CIRCUITRY

Among neuronal populations that project to Purkinje cells, 49% of neurons in the inferior olivary complex are lost between 17 and 300 days of age; a loss of 18% is evident by day 23 (22). Further, a 90% loss of granule cells is observed between 3 and 20 months of age (4). Among neuronal populations that are postsynaptic to Purkinje cells, 21% of neurons in the deep cerebellar nuclei are lost by 10 months of age (21). Neurochemically, a 48% loss of glutamate and a 55% loss of aspartate—the putative neurotransmitters of granule cells and inferior olivary neurons, respectively—are found (24). Cerebellar content of NE and 5-HT remains unchanged, but their metabolism is decreased after 6 months of age (25–27).

The extent, pattern, and timing of degeneration, along with a comparative analysis of data from other cerebellar mutants characterized by Purkinje cell deficits, support the notion that all of these changes are probably secondary to the loss of Purkinje cells. In general, transneuronal losses proceed at a slower rate than losses resulting fom a direct genetic effect.

SEQUENCE AND EXTENT OF DEGENERATIVE EVENTS IN CEREBELLAR MONOAMINES

Norepinephrine System

Purkinje cell degeneration mutant mice were examined during the course of Purkinje cell death and at 3, 5, 6, 9, and 12 months of age (28). Glyoxylic acid fluorescence histochemistry for catecholamines was used to determine the modality of response of NE fibers to the profound structural alterations of the cerebellar cortex.

In the mouse, histofluorescent NE fibers form linear and tortuous profiles through the granule cell layer, form pericellular arrays alongside Purkinje cell somata, and branch into radially and longitudinally oriented chains of varicosities (Fig. 2A).

In the mutants, a progressive increase in the density of NE varicosities accompanies the progressive shrinkage of the molecular layer (Fig. 2B); this is most conspicuous at 6 to 12 months of age, when the molecular layer is depleted both of Purkinje cell dendrites and parallel fibers. NE fibers in these zones form dense parallel bundles of varicose profiles; their density reaches about 600% of normal at 9 to 12 months of age. The progressive increase in the density of NE variscosities in the molecular layer of mutant mice is most likely due to the altered geometry of the cerebellar cortex and not to newly sprouted fibers. It appears that the state of health of the environment surrounding the NE fibers in the cerebellar cortex has little influence on their anatomical integrity.

5-HT System

In normal mice, 5-HT immunoreactive fibers are distributed to all cerebellar lobules (Fig. 3A), with an anterior to posterior preference gradient. While all cortical layers receive 5-HT immunoreactive fibers, their density appears higher in the granule cell layer.

Following the degeneration of Purkinje cells in *pcd* mutant mice, 5-HT-immunoreactive fibers survive and become compressed in a lesser volume of tissue, which results from the cerebellar atrophy, thus giving the appearance of a higher

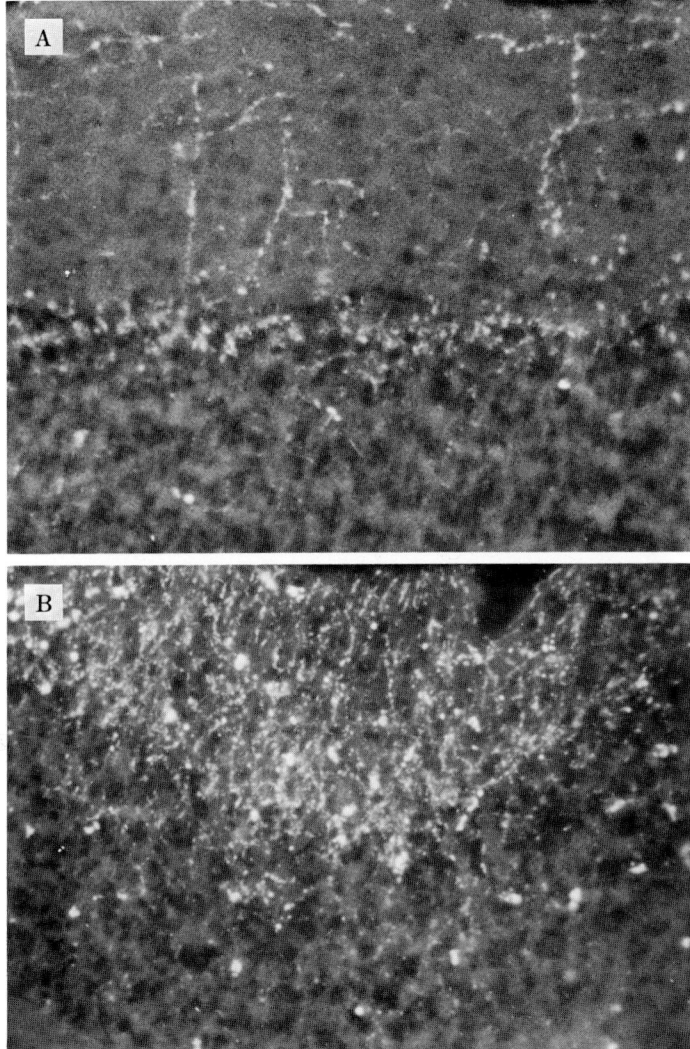

FIG. 2. Catecholamine histofluorescence in the cerebellar cortex of normal (**A**) and *pcd* mutant (**B**) mouse. Note the higher density of fibers in the mutant.

fiber density than normal (Fig. 3B). As with NE fibers, it appears that the survival of 5-HT axons in the cerebellum is not influenced by the death of Purkinje and granule cells.

Ultrastructure of Monoamine-Containing Nerve Terminals

Fixation of tissue with potassium permanganate has been used to demonstrate small granular vesicles in MA nerve terminals, including both catecholamines and

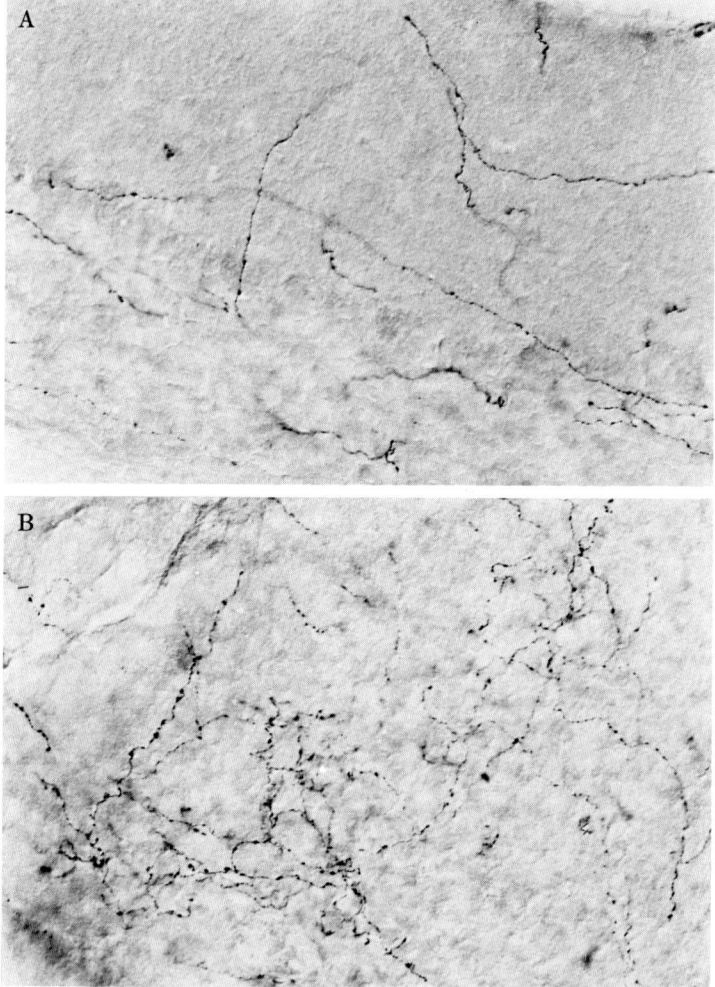

FIG. 3. Immunocytochemistry with anti-5-HT antiserum in the cerebellar cortex of normal (**A**) and *pcd* mutant (**B**) mouse. Note the higher density of fibers in the mutant.

indoleamines. In control mice, MA nerve terminals are found mainly in apposition with Purkinje cell dendrites. One MA nerve terminal is found in an area of molecular layer of approximately 4,000 μm^2 or larger.

After the degeneration of Purkinje cells in *pcd* mutant mice, MA terminals can still be seen in the cerebellar cortex by electron microscopy, and with a higher incidence: at 45 days of age, the average incidence of MA nerve terminals in the molecular layer of the declive and tuber vermis is one every 1,310 μm^2; at 3 months, one every 840 μm^2; at 6 months, one every 690 μm^2; at 9 months, one every 360 μm^2; and at 1 year of age, one every 290 μm^2. MA nerve terminals are ensheathed by astroglial processes in most of the instances (Fig. 4A and B). They are also apposed to boutons that contain agranular vesicles, and to stellate cells in the molecular layer. Synaptic specializations in the form of thickening of the synaptic membranes are not observed in either control or mutant mice.

The survival of MA axons following loss of their target cells might be attributed to the lack of an intimate adhesion to their target elements, to a possible functional interaction with the glia, or to the integrity of the extracerebellar terminal fields of the MA axon collaterals (29).

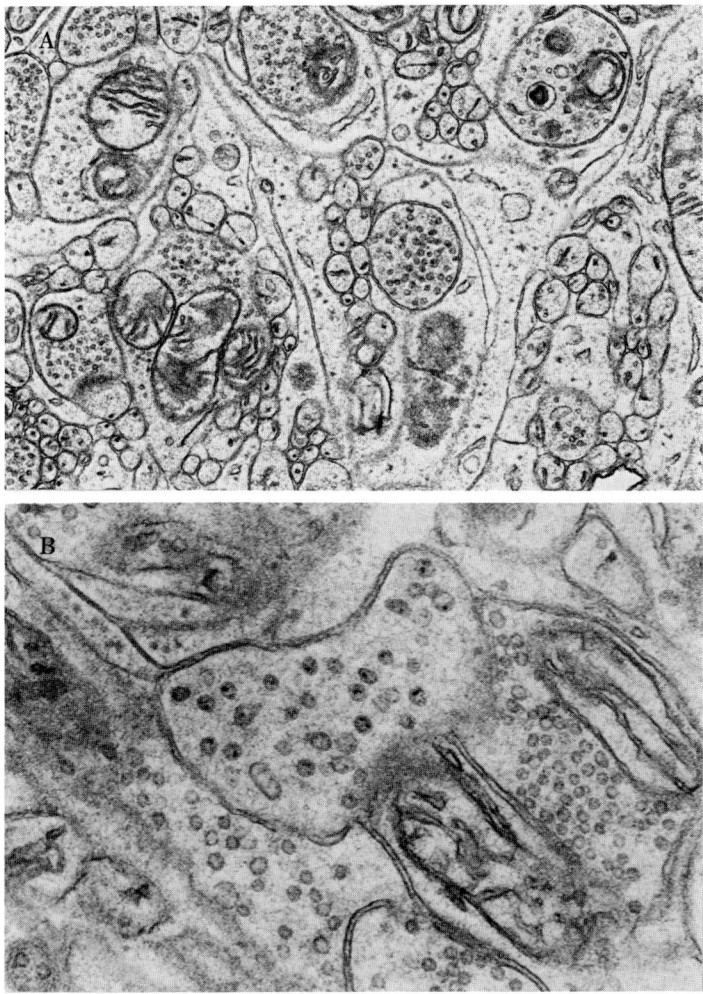

FIG. 4. Electron microscopy of cerebellar cortex of *pcd* mutant mice after tissue fixation with potassium permanganate to demonstrate dense-core vesicles in monoamine-containing nerve terminals (**A,B**). Severe astroglial reaction is seen in A.

NEUROCHEMICAL CHANGES

The degeneration of Purkinje cells induces several sets of neurochemical changes, namely, (a) loss of molecules contained in Purkinje cells, (b) modifications in glial markers, and (c) changes involving molecules contained in cells that degenerate or atrophy consequently to Purkinje cell loss.

Norepinephrine

At 25 to 280 days of age, no significant changes in NE content (pmol/cerebellum) were detected during or after Purkinje cell degeneration (25). However, since degeneration led to a reduction in cerebellar weight, NE concentration was increased in *pcd* mutants. These neurochemical data, in agreement with the fluorescence histochemical results, indicate that in spite of the loss of a major postsynaptic target, the cerebellar NE input remains stable.

NE metabolism was also studied in brain regions of *pcd* mutants (26). The purpose of those studies was to determine if Purkinje cell loss is followed by an alteration of cerebellar NE turnover. The concentration of NE and of its major metabolite in mouse brain, 3-methoxy-4-hydroxy-phenylglycol (MHPG), were measured by liquid chromatography with electrochemical detection. The concentration of MHPG and the ratio of the concentrations of MHPG over NE (MHPG/NE) were taken as indices of NE turnover. Although the cerebellar content of NE in *pcd* mice did not differ from controls, MHPG and the MHPG/NE ratio were slightly decreased in 3-month-old, and more so in 6- and 9-month-old mutants compared to controls. The content of MHPG or the MHPG/NE ratio was not decreased in younger mutants, 22 or 45 days old. The accumulation of L-DOPA (3,4-dihydroxyphenylalanine) after administration of NSD 1015 to inhibit aromatic L-amino acid decarboxylase was measured as an index of NE synthesis. The accumulation of L-DOPA in *pcd* cerebellum was, respectively, decreased to 69%, 53%, and 37% of control values at 3, 6, and 12 months; it did not change in the brain stem, while it was slightly decreased in the hypothalamus. MHPG content and concentration and the MHPG/NE ratio did not change in the brain stem. In the hypothalamus, NE concentration and content were slightly increased in *pcd* mice at all ages, and the MHPG/NE ratio was decreased in 6- and 9-month-old mice. It summary, although NE axons in the cerebellum are maintained in *pcd* mice after Purkinje cell degeneration, NE turnover is decreased, suggesting that the synthesis and release of neurotransmitter does not continue at normal rates at stages concomitant with the absence of target cells.

5-HT

The content and turnover of 5-HT were determined in the cerebellum of *pcd* mutant mice at 3 to 15 months of age. The content of 5-HT did not decrease in *pcd* mouse cerebellum but tended to increase slightly after 7 months. The ratio of 5-hydroxyindoleacetic acid (5-HIAA) to 5-HT was significantly decreased in cerebellum at 7 to 15 months but not at 3 or 6 months. The decrease in this ratio is indicative of decreased 5-HT turnover. Similar changes were not seen in the brain stem or hypothalamus in mice up to 14 months old, but slight decreases were observed at 15 months. Another index of turnover, the accumulation of 5-HIAA after administration of probenecid to block its efflux from brain, was decreased by 46% in 7-month-old *pcd* mice in the cerebellum, but not in the brain stem or hypothalamus. The decrease in 5-HT turnover in the cerebellum of *pcd* mutant mice occurs subsequently to and perhaps owing to the loss of the target Purkinje and granule cells.

CONCLUDING REMARKS

We have examined and quantified anatomical and neurochemical events related to Purkinje cell loss in the *pcd* neurological mutant mouse, with particular attention to the impact of cell loss on pre- and postsynaptic neuronal groups. We have found that the persistence of MA presynaptic axons following Purkinje cell degeneration markedly contrasts with the severity of response of non-MA presynaptic axons.

Purkinje cells of the cerebellar cortex are integral elements of a "point-to-point system" (30). Point-to-point systems are those in which each nerve cell contacts no more than a few target neurons. In contrast, the cerebellar MA system is part of a "global" system (30). Global systems are those in which a few nerve cells innervate very extensive terminal domains. As we have shown, loss of Purkinje cells triggers profound transneuronal regressive changes in inferior olivary neurons and granule cells. On the contrary, MA systems do not undergo regressive changes in spite of the progressive separation from their targets.

In addition to the differences in connectivity of point-to-point systems versus global systems, other factors may play a role in the survival of MA axons following target loss: (i) the lack of synaptic contacts between MA terminals and target cells protects the presynaptic MA terminals from structural damage, when target neurons degenerate and (ii) the diffuse innervation that MA neurons provide throughout the CNS makes these axons resistant to injuries occurring in discrete areas.

REFERENCES

1. Mullen RJ, Eicher EM, Sidman RL. Purkinje cell degeneration, a new neurological mutation in the mouse. *Proc Natl Acad Sci USA* 1976;73:208–212.
2. Landis SC, Mullen RJ. The development and degeneration of Purkinje cells in pcd mutant mice. *J Comp Neurol* 1978;177:125–144.
3. Ghetti B, Alyea CJ, Muller J. Studies on the Purkinje cell degeneration (pcd) mutant: primary pathology and transneuronal changes. *J Neuropathol Exp Neurol* 1978;37:617.
4. Triarhou LC, Norton J, Alyea C, Ghetti B. A quantitative study of the granule cells in the Purkinje cell degeneration (pcd) mutant. *Ann Neurol* 1985;18:146.
5. Andén N-E, Fuxe K, Ungerstedt U. Monoamine pathways to the cerebellum and cerebral cortex. *Experientia* 1967;23:838–839.

6. Fuxe K. The distribution of monoamine terminals in the central nervous system. *Acta Physiol Scand* 1965;64(suppl 247):37–120.
7. Hökfelt T, Fuxe K. Cerebellar monoamine nerve terminals, a new type of afferent fibers to the cortex cerebelli. *Exp Brain Res* 1969;9:63–72.
8. Hoffer BJ, Siggins GR, Oliver AP, Bloom FE. Activation of the pathway from locus coeruleus to rat cerebellar Purkinje neurons: pharmacological evidence of noradrenergic central inhibition. *J Pharmacol Exp Ther* 1973;184:553–569.
9. Olson L, Fuxe K. On the projections from the locus coeruleus noradrenaline neurons: the cerebellar innervation. *Brain Res* 1971;28:165–171.
10. Pasquier DA, Gold MA, Jacobowitz DM. Noradrenergic perikarya (A5–A7, subcoeruleus) projections to the rat cerebellum. *Brain Res* 1980;196:270–275.
11. Tohyama M. Comparative anatomy of cerebellar catecholamine innervations from teleosts to mammals. *J Hirnforsch* 1976;17:43–60.
12. Chan-Palay V. Fine structure of labelled axons in the cerebellar cortex and nuclei of rodents and primates after intraventricular infusions with tritiated serotonin. *Anat Embryol* 1975;148:235–265.
13. Bishop GA, Ho RH. The distribution and origin of serotonin immunoreactivity in the rat cerebellum. *Brain Res* 1985;331:195–207.
14. Takeuchi Y, Kimura H, Sano Y. Immunohistochemical demonstration of serotonin-containing nerve fibers in the cerebellum. *Cell Tissue Res* 1982;226:1–12.
15. Sotelo C, Beaudet A. Influence of experimentally induced agranularity on the synaptogenesis of serotonin nerve terminals in rat cerebellar cortex. *Proc R Soc Lond [Biol]* 1979;206:133–138.
16. Chan-Palay V. *Cerebellar dentate nucleus.* Berlin: Springer-Verlag, 1977;390–454.
17. Green MC. *Genetic strains and variants of the laboratory mouse.* Stuttgart/New York: Gustav-Fischer-Verlag, 1981.
18. Wassef M, Sotelo C, Cholley B, Brehier A, Thomasset M. Cerebellar mutations affecting the postnatal survival of Purkinje cells in the mouse disclose a longitudinal pattern of differentially sensitive cells. *Dev Biol* 1987;124:379–389.
19. Chang AC, Triarhou LC, Alyea CJ, Low WC, Ghetti B. Developmental expression of polypeptide PEP-19 in cerebellar cell suspensions transplanted into the cerebellum of pcd mutant mice. *Exp Brain Res* 1989;76:639–645.
20. Wassef M, Simons J, Tappaz ML, Sotelo C. Non-Purkinje cell GABAergic innervation of the deep cerebellar nuclei: a quantitative immunocytochemical study in C57BL and in Purkinje cell degeneration mutant mice. *Brain Res* 1986;399:125–135.
21. Triarhou LC, Norton J, Ghetti B. Anterograde transsynaptic degeneration in the deep cerebellar nuclei of Purkinje cell degeneration (pcd) mutant mice. *Exp Brain Res* 1987;66:577–588.
22. Ghetti B, Norton J, Triarhou LC. Nerve cell atrophy and loss in the inferior olivary complex of "Purkinje cell degeneration" mutant mice. *J Comp Neurol* 1987;260:409–422.
23. Triarhou LC, Ghetti B. Stabilisation of neurone number in the inferior olivary complex of aged "Purkinje cell degeneration" mutant mice. *Acta Neuropathol* 1991;81:597–602.
24. McBride WJ, Ghetti B. Changes in the contents of glutamate and GABA in the cerebellar vermis and hemispheres of the Purkinje cell degeneration (pcd) mutant. *Neurochem Res* 1988;13:121–125.
25. Ghetti B, Fuller RW, Sawyer BD, Hemrick-Luecke SK, Schmidt MJ. Purkinje cell loss and the noradrenergic system in the cerebellum of pcd mutant mice. *Brain Res Bull* 1981;7:711–714.
26. Ghetti B, Perry KW, Fuller RW. Norepinephrine metabolism in the cerebellum of the Purkinje cell degeneration (pcd) mutant mouse. *Neurochem Int* 1987;10:39–47.
27. Ghetti B, Perry KW, Fuller RW. Serotonin concentration and turnover in cerebellum and other brain regions of pcd mutant mice. *Brain Res* 1988;458:367–371.
28. Felten DL, Felten SY, Perry KW, Fuller RW, Nurnberger JI Sr, Ghetti B. Noradrenergic innervation of the cerebellar cortex in normal and in Purkinje cell degeneration mutant mice: evidence for long-term survival following loss of the two major cerebellar cortical neuronal populations. *Neuroscience* 1986;18:783–793.
29. Triarhou LC, Ghetti B. Monoaminergic nerve terminals in the cerebellar cortex of Purkinje cell degeneration mutant mice: fine structural integrity and modification of cellular environs following loss of Purkinje and granule cells. *Neuroscience* 1986;18:795–807.
30. Sotelo C, Alvarado-Mallart RM. Growth and differentiation of cerebellar suspensions transplanted into the adult cerebellum of mice with heredodegenerative ataxia. *Proc Natl Acad Sci USA* 1986;83:1135–1139.

23

L-5-Hydroxytryptophan, Serotonin, and Brain Protein Synthesis

Patrick Lepetit, *Monique Touret, Eric Grange, Nadine Gay, and Pierre Bobillier

*Groupe de Neuroanatomie Fonctionnelle, CNRS URA 1195, Laboratoire d'Anatomie Pathologique, Faculté de Médecine Alexis Carrel, 69372 Lyon, France; *INSERM U52, CNRS URA 1195, Département de Médecine Expérimentale, Université Claude Bernard, 69008 Lyon, France*

In vivo, L-5-hydroxytryptophan (L-5-HTP) is the intermediate product in the biosynthetic pathway in which serotonin (5-HT) is formed from the amino acid tryptophan. Hence, the systemic administration of L-5-HTP is a method widely used in neurobiology to increase the brain levels of 5-HT (11,13) and reverse the effects of decreased brain 5-HT level found after the administration of *p*-chlorophenylalanine (p-CPA), a well-known inhibitor of tryptophan hydroxylase (6). L-5-HTP is also used in the treatment of affective disorders and certain types of myoclonus, involuntary movement disorders (14), and cerebellar ataxia.

Previous studies by Weiss et al. (15,16) have shown that the administration of a large dose of L-5-HTP in developing rats induces whole brain polysome dissociation, an effect that reflects protein synthesis inhibition. This effect of L-5-HTP was dependent on the conversion of this compound to 5-HT because it was prevented by pretreatment with L-aromatic amino acid decarboxylase inhibitor (15) and by the 5-HT antagonists methysergide and cyproheptadine (16). *In vitro* studies by Hemminki (4) have also indicated that 5-HT markedly inhibits neuronal protein and RNA synthesis. In addition, the intracranial injection of 5-HT has been shown to inhibit cerebral protein synthesis *in vivo* (2). Taken together, the results of these previous studies have indicated the possibility of an inhibitory role for 5-HT in the control of brain protein synthesis. Since L-5-HTP is widely used as a precursor of 5-HT in both basic research and the treatment of a variety of clinical disorders, it was of interest to investigate *in vivo* whether the systemic administration of L-5-HTP in intact or p-CPA-treated rats inhibits protein synthesis either in the brain as a whole or in selected areas. Therefore, we have estimated local rates of brain protein synthesis in freely moving rats by quantitative autoradiographic measurement of the incorporation of methionine into brain proteins (10); on the second day after a single intravenous injection of p-CPA (280 mg/kg) and 40 min after either the sequential or independent intravenous administration of L-5-HTP (60 mg/kg). Previous reports of the results have been presented (8,9).

Local cerebral rates of methionine incorporation into proteins were examined in 60 brain nuclei, covering the main anatomical and functional regions of the brain. L-5-HTP induced general decreases in the rates of plasma methionine incorporation into brain proteins (mean % effect: 50% compared to controls). The restoration of 5-HT synthesis by the administration of L-5-HTP in p-CPA-treated rats induced more marked decreases in the rate of methionine incorporation (mean % effect: 70% compared to rats treated only with p-CPA).

The administration of L-5-HTP reduced the rate of methionine incorporation in all the brain areas examined. For example, in the cerebellum (granular layer), raphe dorsalis, locus coeruleus, pontine and lateral reticular formation, pontine nuclei, and red nucleus, protein synthesis was reduced (% effect ± SEM) by $50 \pm 3\%$, $51 \pm 3\%$, $54 \pm 9\%$, $51 \pm 10\%$, $46 \pm 5\%$, $44 \pm 3\%$, and $55 \pm 9\%$, respectively (9). The uniformity of the inhibition of brain protein synthesis by L-5-HTP in spite of important differences in serotonergic innervation and binding sites density indicates that the importance of the inhibition of protein synthesis does not depend on the importance of the normal 5-HT innervation. The fact that L-5-HTP induces marked decreases in protein synthesis of brain areas that do not receive major 5-HT innervation is consistent with the homogeneous rise in regional brain 5-HT concentrations found 1 hr after the administration of 50 mg/kg L-5-HTP (13) and may be attributed to the unspecific localization of L-5-HTP decarboxylation sites. L-5-HTP is an amino acid that could directly affect protein synthesis by competing with natural amino acids at the level of the blood-brain barrier and amino acylation of RNAs. However, the inhibition of brain protein synthesis by L-5-HTP is unlikely to be due to restricted brain uptake of methionine. Control experiments in a separate group showed no change in brain concentration of methionine 1 hr after the administration of the same dose of L-5-HTP in intact rats (9). Furthermore, the low brain levels of L-5-HTP usually found after L-5-HTP loading (11,12) are somewhat consistent with the hypothesis that L-5-HTP may directly compete with the amino acylation of tRNAs. In addition, Weiss et al. (15) showed that treatment with an aromatic amino acid decarboxylase inhibitor prevents the dissociation of brain polysomes normally induced by the administration of L-5-HTP (200 mg/kg) to immature rats. These results indicate that L-5-HTP may have little direct effect on brain protein synthesis at the dose level used in the present study (60 mg/kg). Thus, the inhibition of methionine incorporation after L-5-HTP, taken in conjunction with the inhibition of neuronal protein and RNA synthesis by 5-HT, previously demonstrated *in vitro* (4), support the hypothesis of an inhibitory effect of elevated 5-HT levels on brain protein synthesis.

Considering the structural and functional capacities of proteins and the slow turnover of the majority of brain proteins (7), it is expected that the rapid changes in protein synthesis following L-5-HTP reflects the initiation of longer term neurochemical changes that may have delayed functional expression. Indeed, 5-HT has been involved in the regulation of long-term processes such as neuronal development (17), neurite outgrowth and synaptogenesis (3), memory consolidation (2), and long-term changes in electrophysiologic properties of *Aplysia* neurons (1). All these long-term processes are dependent on changes in protein metabolism; however, the nature of the specific proteins involved in these processes has been determined only in neuronal systems much simpler than mammalian brain (1).

The overall inhibition of brain protein synthesis by L-5-HTP and 5-HT does not exclude the possibility of selective increases in the synthesis of specific proteins (1). For example, the selective destruction of the central serotonergic system by 5,7-dihydroxytryptamine has been shown to cause both increases and decreases in the concentration of individual proteins in the hippocampus and parietal cortex of rats (5).

While the precise mechanism of the 5-HT-induced inhibition of brain protein synthesis has not yet been established, it is thought to be mediated by the activation of 5-HT receptors (16) and presumably involves second messengers such as adenosine $3',5'$-monophosphate (1) and transmembrane ion fluxes.

There remains the question whether the changes in brain protein synthesis induced by L-5-HTP are involved in the therapeutic effects of this compound. If we consider that the administration of an appropriate dose of L-5-HTP increases brain 5-HT concentration within a few hours and that the improvement of depressive or neurological symptoms requires several weeks or month, it is likely that L-5-HTP induces long-term processes involving changes in protein synthesis. The first possibility would be that 5-HT directly inhibits or induces the synthesis of specific brain proteins involved in the pathologic process. The second possibility would be that L-5-HTP restores indirectly some brain metabolic alterations through either changes in the neuroendocrine status (i.e., steroids, growth and thyroid hormones) or increased release of trophic factors (i.e., protein S-100) by glial cells (18). Our current work is therefore focusing on the characterization of the individual proteins involved in the metabolic response to increased brain 5-HT content.

REFERENCES

1. Eskin A, Garcia KS, Byrne JH. Information storage in the nervous system of Aplysia: specific proteins affected by serotonin and cAMP. *Proc Natl Acad Sci USA* 1989;86:2458–2462.
2. Essman WB. Age dependent effects of 5-hydroxytryptamine upon memory consolidation and cerebral protein synthesis. *Pharmac Biochem Behav* 1973;1:7–14.
3. Haydon PG, McCobb DP, Kater SB. Serotonin selectively inhibits growth cone motility and synaptogenesis of specific identified neurons. *Science* 1984;226:561–564.
4. Hemminki K. Effects of added substances on RNA and protein synthesis in immature neurons. *J Neurochem* 1973;20:373–378.
5. Heydorn WE, Creed GJ, Nguyen KQ, Jacobowitz DM. Effect of 5,7-dihydroxytryptamine on the concentration of individual proteins in different areas of the rat brain. *Brain Res* 1986;368:193–196.
6. Koe BK, Weissman A. p-Chlorophenylalanine: a specific depletor of brain serotonin. *J Pharmacol Exp Ther* 1966;154:499–516.
7. Lajtha A, Dunlop D. Turnover of protein in the nervous system. *Life Sci* 1981;29:755–767.
8. Lepetit P, Touret M, Grange E, Gay N, Bobillier P. Decreased protein synthesis in hypothalamic

nuclei following L-5-hydroxytryptophan in intact and p-chlorophenylanine pretreated rats. *Neurosci Lett* 1991;122:218–220.
9. Lepetit P, Touret M, Grange E, Gay N, Bobillier P. Inhibition of methionine incorporation into brain proteins after the systemic administration of p-chlorophenylalanine and L-5-hydroxytryptophan. *Eur J Pharmacol* 1991;209:207–212.
10. Lestage P, Gonon M, Lepetit P, et al. An in vivo kinetic model with L-^{35}S-methionine for the determination of local cerebral rates of methionine incorporation into protein in the rat. *J Neurochem* 1987;48:352–363.
11. Löscher W, Pagliusi SR, Müller F. L-5-hydroxytryptophan: correlation between anticonvulsant effect and increases in level of 5-hydroxyindoles in plasma and brain. *Neuropharmacology* 1984;23: 1041–1048.
12. Moir ATB, Eccleston DJ. The effect of precursor loading on the cerebral metabolism of 5-hydroxyindoles. *J Neurochem* 1968;15:1093–1108.
13. Okada F, Saito Y, Fujieda T, Yamashita I. Monoamine changes in the brain of rats injected with L-5-hydroxytryptophan. *Nature* 1972;238:355–356.
14. Sandyk R, Fisher H. Serotonin in involuntary movement disorders. *Int J Neuroscience* 1988;42: 185–205.
15. Weiss BF, Wurtman RJ, Munro HN. Disaggregation of brain polysomes by L-5-hydroxytryptophan: mediation by serotonin. *Life Sci* 1973;13:411–416.
16. Weiss BF, Liebschutz JL, Wurtman RJ, Munro HN. Participation of dopamine- and serotonin-receptors in the disaggregation of brain polysomes by L-DOPA and L-5HTP. *J Neurochem* 1975;24: 1191–1195.
17. Whitaker-Azmitia PM, Azmitia EC. Stimulation of astroglial serotonin receptors produces media which regulates development of serotonergic neurons. *Brain Res* 1989;497:80–85.
18. Whitaker-Azmitia PM, Murphy R, Azmitia EC. Stimulation of astroglial 5-HT$_{1A}$ receptors releases the serotonergic growth factor, protein S-100, and alters astroglial morphology. *Brain Res* 1990; 528:155–158.

*Serotonin, the Cerebellum,
and Ataxia*, edited by
P. Trouillas and K. Fuxe.
Raven Press, Ltd., New York © 1993.

24

Serotonergic CSF Abnormalities in Human Acquired and Genetic Ataxias

P. Trouillas, N. Charles, *B. Renaud, *N. Eynard, and †P. Adeleine

*Neurology Service and Ataxia Research Center, Alexis Carrel Faculty of Medicine, Neurological Hospital and Claude Bernard University, 69003 Lyon, France; *Laboratoire de Neuropharmacologie Biochimique, Service de Biologie, Hôpital Neurologique, 69003 Lyon, France; †Biostatistical Unit, Faculté Alexis Carrel, Laboratoire d'Informatique des Hospices Civils de Lyon, 69003 Lyon, France*

Determination of the metabolites of neurotransmitters in cerebrospinal fluid (CSF) is considered a valid method to study pathological processes (1,2). 5-Hydroxyindoleacetic acid (5-HIAA), the major metabolite of serotonin, and homovanillic acid (HVA), the main metabolite of dopamine, derive principally from the central nervous system (3,4). Abnormalities of these metabolites in ataxias might provide valuable information on the serotonergic and dopaminergic systems of the patients.

The experimental model of thiamine deprivation has shown that the serotonergic cerebellar system is selectively affected in animals (5,6). Specific neurochemical abnormalities have been observed including impaired synaptosomal serotonergic uptake (6,7) and elevation of the 5-HIAA cerebellar content (8). A relationship between ataxia and serotonergic abnormalities has been suggested (7).

In the heredoataxic *pcd* mice, Ghetti et al. (9) showed low 5-HIAA cerebellar values and a cerebellar reduction of the serotonin turnover with the probenecid test. In the "reeler mouse," Oshugi et al. (10) reported a markedly increased value of serotonin and 5-HIAA in the cerebellum.

To date, there is no study in humans that shows a clear relationship between cerebellar ataxia and CSF monoamine abnormalities. In this respect, cortical cerebellar ataxia is a highly interesting human genetic model of pure cerebellar ataxia and may allow valid correlations to be made between metabolic abnormalities and ataxia. Human deficiency-alcoholic states are known to include ataxias and thiamine deficiency (11,12), comparable with experimental models.

We present here the first monoaminergic turnover studies in cerebellar cortical ataxia and deficiency alcoholic ataxia, together with 14 cases of typical Friedreich's ataxia.

METHODS

Protocol of the Probenecid Test

The tests were performed while the patients were free of any psychotropic or other drugs for at least 10 days. Two lumbar punctures (LP), 24 hr apart, were carried out at 14:30. On day 1, the patients were asked to remain in bed from 6:30 until 14:30, at which time the first LP was performed. On day 2, the protocol was the same as on day 1, but prior to the second LP, the patients were given an intravenous infusion of probenecid (75 mg/kg body weight) starting at 6:30 and lasting for about 5 hr. Two milliliters of CSF were obtained at each LP. After routine cytochemical determinations, the supernatant was stored at $-40°C$ until analysis, usually performed within 2 weeks.

Measurement of CSF 5-HIAA and HVA by Liquid Chromatography and Electrochemical Detection

HVA and 5-HIAA were determined on 10 µl of CSF supernatant using reversed-phase high performance liquid chromatography coupled with electrochemical detection (HPLC-ED) as described previously (13). CSF levels of probenecid were determined on 10 µl of CSF supernatant by HPLC coupled with ultraviolet (UV) detection (13).

Since the probenecid concentrations vary over a large range, the ratios increase of monoamines after probenecid test/probenecid were calculated to allow better comparison of the results between patients (14). These ratios were called delta 5-HIAA/prob and delta HVA/prob. They reflect the serotonergic and dopaminergic turnover.

PATIENTS

Probenecid tests were performed in 40 subjects. Eight subjects were controls free of any neurological peripheral or central disease (mean age: 43.5 years).

Nine patients had cortical cerebral atrophy, either autosomal dominant (ADCA type III according to Harding [15]) or sporadic; the mean age of onset was 48 years. All patients underwent magnetic resonance imaging (MRI). The selection of the patients was done with great care. Clinically the cerebellar ataxia was pure and mainly static. No patient had pontine atrophy at MRI: all suspected cases of olivopontocerebellar atrophy were discarded. The patients had only an atrophy of the anterior lobe, particularly marked in the vermis.

Nine patients had a deficiency state with or without alcoholism, with chronic anorexia, chronic food deficiency, and a thiamine level lower than 70 nmol/l (normal: 70–130 nmol/liter); the ataxic symptoms had lasted for at least 6 months (mean age 44 years).

Fourteen patients had typical Friedreich's ataxia (mean age: 29 years), selected using criteria more severe than those of Geoffroy et al. (16): all cases had myocardiopathy at echocardiography; linkage to chromosome 9 had been established in all the cases presented (17). In three Friedreich patients treated with 16 mg/kg per day of D,L-5-HTP for 12 months, probenecid tests were performed before and after treatment.

RESULTS

Controls

Table 1 gives baseline CSF values of the monoamines and delta monoamine/prob ratios.

Correlation studies disclosed that there was a clear link between 5-HIAA and HVA values ($r = 0.80$, $p = 0.01$) and also a clear correlation between baseline 5-HIAA values and delta 5-HIAA/prob ($r = -0.88$, $p = 0.01$). There was no correlation between HVA baseline values and delta 5-HIAA/prob. Thus, in normal subjects, it was observed that the serotonergic turnover is correlated with the 5-HIAA baseline values.

Cortical Cerebellar Atrophy

The main finding is the existence of significantly decreased values of 5-HIAA (Table 1, Fig. 1). However, when the turnover was studied, there was a strong, statistically significant tendency toward an increased serotonergic turnover (Table 1, Fig. 2). HVA baseline values and HVA turnover were similar to those of 5-HIAA and significantly so (Table 1, Figs. 3 and 4).

Correlation studies indicated that there was no more link between baseline 5-HIAA values and baseline HVA values, while the correlation between delta 5-HIAA/prob and 5-HIAA values was also abolished. So, this condition is characterized by a statistical independence of the serotonergic turnover and 5-HIAA baseline values.

TABLE 1. *Mean values ± SEM of baseline metabolite values and the ratio of increase of metabolite/probenecid in the different ataxia groups*

Group	No.	5-HIAA (nmol/liter)	Ratio delta 5-HIAA/prob	HVA (nmol/liter)	Ratio delta HVA/prob
Controls	8	124.2 ± 20	6.8 ± 0.9	236.1 ± 36.6	7.1 ± 0.5
Cerebellar cortical atrophy	9	69.1 ± 7.3[a]	12.1 ± 2[a]	99.3 ± 7.9[a]	15.9 ± 3.4[a]
Friedreich's ataxia	14	88.7 ± 9.7[b,c]	10.1 ± 1.5[c]	97.4 ± 8.8[a]	17.6 ± 2.4[a]
Deficiency-alcoholic	9	143.2 ± 31.3	9.5 ± 1.8	128.4 ± 19[a]	9.9 ± 2.7

[a] Significant at $p < 0.05$.
[b] Nearly significant $0.05 < p < 0.09$.
[c] $n = 13$; one missing datum.

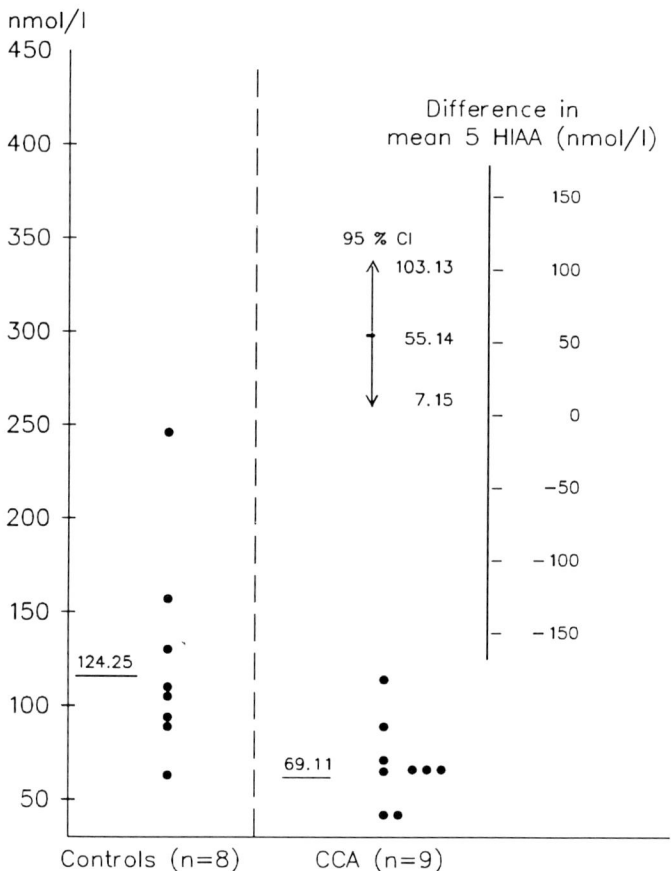

FIG. 1. 5-HIAA values in eight controls and nine cortical cerebellar atrophy patients with mean levels of 124.25 and 69.11 nmol/l, respectively. The difference between the sample means is shown to the right together with the 95% confidence interval from 7.15 to 103.13 nmol/l.

Deficiency-Alcoholic Ataxia

These patients presented a trend to an elevation of baseline 5-HIAA values (Table 1, Fig. 5), contrasting with significantly diminished HVA values (Table 1).

The probenecid test demonstrated a slight trend to an elevation of the serotonergic turnover (Table 1, Fig. 6).

Correlation studies revealed that a significant link had appeared between the serotonergic turnover and the HVA turnover ($r = 0.88$, $p < 0.01$).

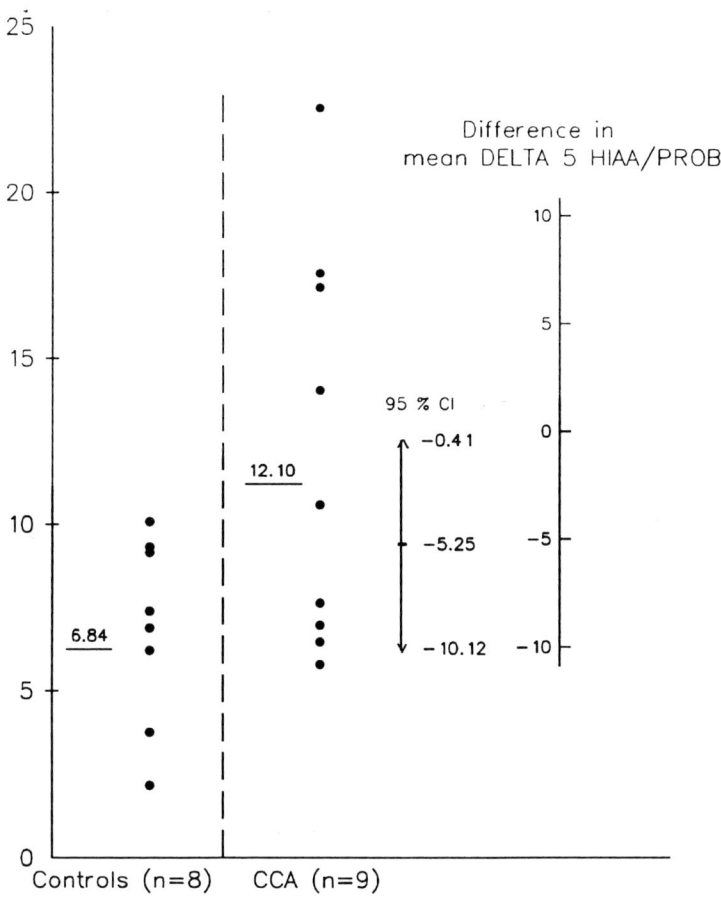

FIG. 2. Delta 5-HIAA/prob ratio in eight controls and nine cortical cerebellar atrophy patients with mean levels of 6.84 and 12.10, respectively. The difference between the sample means is shown to the right together with the 95% confidence interval from −10.12 to −0.41.

Friedreich's Ataxia

Baseline values showed nearly significantly diminished values of 5-HIAA (Table 1, Fig. 5).

The probenecid results indicated that the serotonergic turnover was increased (Fig. 6), but not significantly, while the HVA turnover was significantly elevated (Table 1). Correlation studies revealed that the baseline values of 5-HIAA and HVA were no longer linked, while the correlation between 5-HIAA baseline values and delta 5-HIAA/prob was also abolished. Conversely, an abnormal link had appeared between the increase in the HVA turnover and the increase in the serotonergic turnover ($r = .084$, $p < 0.01$).

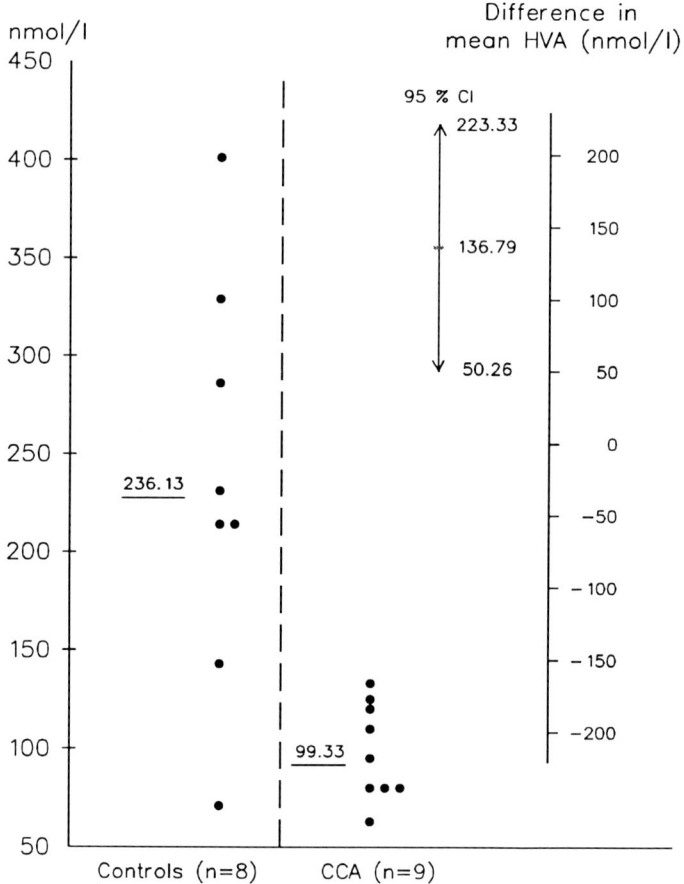

FIG. 3. HVA values in eight controls and nine cortical cerebellar atrophy patients with mean levels of 236.13 and 99.33, respectively. The difference between the sample means is shown to the right together with the 95% confidence interval from 50.26 to 223.33.

In the three patients receiving 5-HTP, a clear increase in 5-HIAA values and 5-HIAA turnover was observed (Table 2). Except in one case, the HVA values and HVA turnover were also augmented.

DISCUSSION

General Findings

A particularly clear and significant serotonergic abnormality is the low mean 5-HIAA value in cerebellar cortical atrophy. This serotonergic impairment in a pure

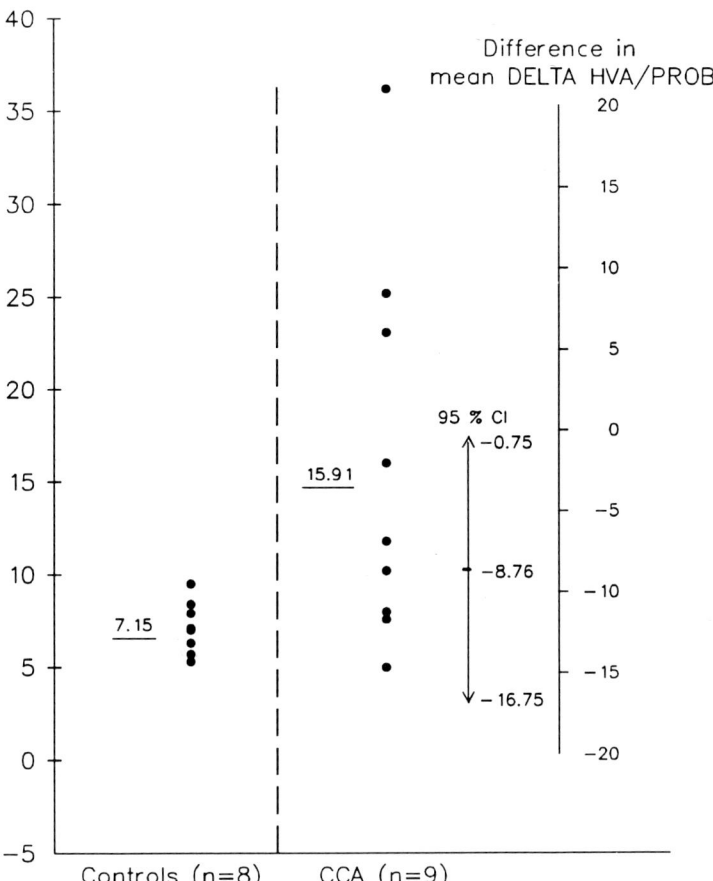

FIG. 4. Delta HVA/prob ratio in eight controls and nine cortical cerebellar atrophy patients with mean levels of 7.15 and 15.91, respectively. The difference between the sample means is shown to the right together with the 95% confidence interval from −16.75 to −0.75.

ataxia must be emphasized. It is interesting to note that there is a similar trend in Friedreich's ataxia.

A significant decrease in baseline HVA values is observed in the three groups, with an increased dopaminergic turnover in the two groups of genetic ataxias.

It remains to be determined if these neurochemical abnormalities are specifically related to ataxia.

This puzzling biochemical syndrome might be called the monoaminergic paradigm of ataxia.

Yet if one considers, as Agren et al. (18), that 5-HIAA "controls" HVA and that

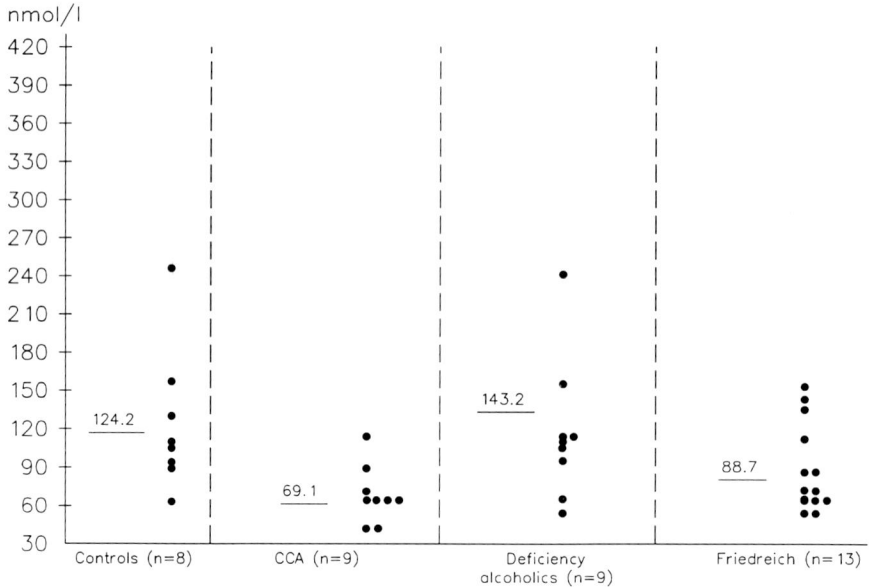

FIG. 5. Comparative representation of 5-HIAA values in the CSF of controls, cortical cerebellar atrophy patients (CCA), Friedreich's ataxia patients, and deficiency-alcoholic ataxia patients.

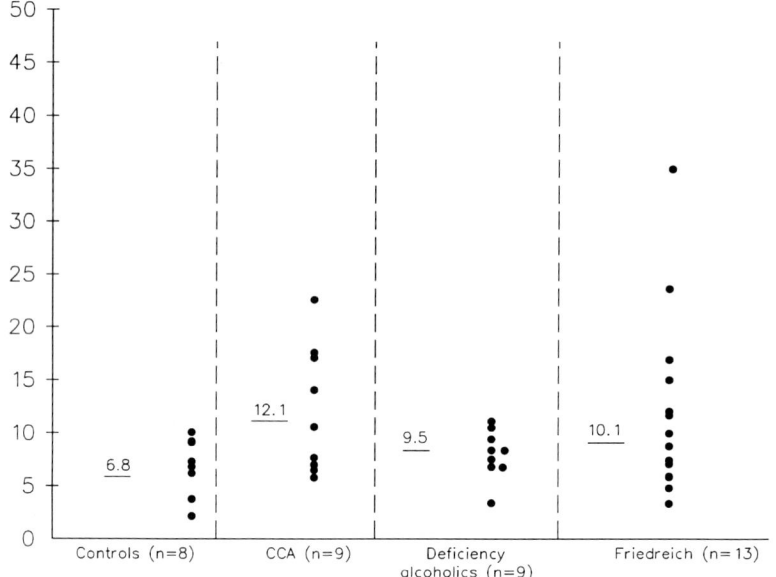

FIG. 6. Comparative representation of delta 5-HIAA/prob ratios in controls, cortical cerebellar atrophy patients (CCA), Friedreich's ataxia patients, and deficiency-alcoholic ataxia patients.

TABLE 2. *Metabolite values and ratios of increase of metabolite/probenecid in three Friedreich's ataxia patients before and after 12 months of a D,L-5-HTP (16 mg/kg per day)*

	Before 5-HTP				After 5-HTP			
Patients	5-HIAA (nmol/ liter)	Delta 5-HIAA/ prob	HVA (nmol/ liter)	Delta HVA/ prob	5-HIAA (nmol/ liter)	Delta 5-HIAA/ prob	HVA (nmol/ liter)	Delta HVA/ prob
1	54	3.3	113	9.5	167	14.5	148	10.4
2	153	5.9	149	16.7	452	8.4	105	2.1
3	135	4.8	120	12.7	130	34.9	116	20.9

serotonin turnover has a regulatory action on dopamine turnover, the serotonergic abnormalities might be primary, while the dopaminergic abnormalities might be only consequences.

These data would explain the fact that a serotonin precursor like L-5-HTP is sometimes successful in pure cerebellar ataxia, while L-Dopa administration has no particular effect (Trouillas, *unpublished*).

Cerebellar Cortical Atrophy and Serotonergic Impairment

To our knowledge, low 5-HIAA values in the CSF of patients with cerebellar cortical atrophy have never been mentioned. This particular serotonergic disturbance includes a paradoxical increase in the serotonergic turnover.

These complex abnormalities might involve a primary attack of the serotonergic system with compensatory increased serotonin synthesis. In cases with short evolution in these series, the serotonergic turnover was considerably increased; conversely, after 10 years of evolution, the serotonergic turnover tended to be normal or even low. These data might explain the disappearance of the statistical link between baseline 5-HIAA values and the serotonergic turnover.

Another hypothesis is that a complex serotonergic disorder includes both an increased efflux of 5-HIAA and an increase in the serotonergic turnover.

However, the hypothesis of a serotonergic primary attack might be more valid, because it is in keeping with the good pharmacological results especially obtained in cortical cerebellar atrophies with 5-HTP or L-5-HTP (19–22). A primary deficit is compatible with long-term replacement therapy. Patients with cortical cerebellar atrophy are able to take the drug for several years just like patients with Parkinson's disease with Dopa administration.

The syndrome including low HVA values and increased HVA turnover is mysterious and may indicate that the attack also involves the dopaminergic system biochemically. Alterations of the nigrostriatal system are not known in this disease. The dopaminergic abnormalities might merely reflect a functional variation of the dopaminergic system under an abnormal serotonergic control.

Friedreich's Ataxia and Monoaminergic Disturbances

The monoaminergic disturbances in Friedreich's ataxia are very much like that of cortical cerebellar atrophy. All the trends are in the same direction. The decrease in 5-HIAA baseline values is almost significant. The serotonergic impairment appears milder than in cerebellar cortical atrophy.

These low 5-HIAA values might account for the fairly good results observed at the beginning of the disease with L-5-HTP treatment (19–23). The abnormal link between the exaggeration of HVA turnover and that of 5-HIAA turnover might again indicate a functional link between the two metabolisms, rather than actual dopaminergic lesions.

It is known, from positron emission tomography studies, that there is an exaggerated metabolism of the brain in Friedreich's ataxia, especially in the striatum (24). This striatal activity might be related to the enhanced dopaminergic turnover.

Deficiency-Alcoholic Ataxias

The trend to an increase in 5-HIAA values is found only in this type of ataxia and can be compared with the serotonergic experimental thiamine-deficiency syndromes (7,8) where 5-HIAA is increased in the central nervous system.

This might be explained, as in the experimental syndrome, both by an impaired efflux of 5-HIAA from the brain (and/or CSF) and by an increase in the serotonergic cerebellar synthesis.

The increased serotonergic turnover might itself be explained, according to Plaitakis et al. (8), by a defect in the vesicular storage mechanism for serotonin, which would expose it to an enhanced catabolism. A compensatory increased synthesis rate, to maintain normal steady-state levels of serotonin, might then take place. The primary deficit might be that of a serotonin binding protein (25) on serotonergic neurons.

It is important to remark that direct effects of alcohol on the serotonergic metabolism are similar to those of thiamine deprivation. In the mouse, Tabakoff et al. (26) showed that single or chronic administration of ethanol provoked an increase in the brain levels of 5-HIAA. In brain, Tabakoff et al. (27) reported that ethanol inhibits, in acute experiments, the transport of 5-HIAA from the subarachnoid space.

In regard to the decreased HVA values in our patients, a direct ethanol effect might be implied, since a dopaminergic hypoactivity has been forwarded in ethanol-treated animals (28,29). It has also been shown that ethanol abolishes the dopamine release from synaptosomal fractions of the striatum (30).

CONCLUSION

In a pure human cerebellar ataxia, cerebellar cortical atrophy, a significant decrease in CSF 5-HIAA values is observed. These data are consistent with the serotonergic hypothesis of ataxia and the good pharmacological results of L-5-HTP observed in this specific group of patients.

In Friedreich's ataxia, a serotonergic impairment is also observed but is less marked than in cerebellar atrophy.

In deficiency-alcoholic patients, serotonergic abnormalities are comparable to those of experimental thiamine-deficiency models.

ACKNOWLEDGMENT

We thank Mrs. Paquelet and Mrs. Canova for their excellent assistance in the realization of this manuscript.

REFERENCES

1. Anderson H, Roos B. 5-Hydroxyindoleacetic acid in cerebrospinal fluid of hydrocephalic children. *Acta Pediatr Scand* 1969;58:601–608.
2. Bowers MB, Gerbode FA. Relationships of monoamine metabolites in human cerebrospinal fluid to age. *Nature* 1968;1256.
3. Bartholini G, Tissot R, Pletscher A. Brain capillaries as a source of homovanillic acid in the cerebrospinal fluid. *Brain Res* 1971;27:163–168.
4. Ecleston D, Ashcroft GW, Moir ATB, et al. A comparison of 5-hydroxyindoles in various regions of dog brain and cerebrospinal fluid. *J Neurochem* 1968;15:947–957.
5. Chan-Palay V, Plaitakis A, Nicklas N, Berl S. Autoradiographic demonstration of loss of labeled indoleamine axons of the cerebellum in chronic diet-induced thiamine deficiency. *Brain Res* 1977;138:380–384.
6. Plaitakis A, Van Woert MH, Hwang EC, Berl S. The effect of acute thiamine deficiency on brain tryptophan, serotonin, and 5-hydroxyindoleacetic acid. *J Neurochem* 1978;31:1087–1089.
7. Plaitakis A, Nicklas JN, Berl S. Thiamine deficiency: selective impairment of the cerebellar serotonergic system. *Neurology* 1978;28:691–698.
8. Plaitakis A, Hwang EC, Van Woert H, Szilagui PA, Berl S. Effect of thiamine deficiency on brain neurotransmitter systems. *Ann NY Acad Sci* 1982;367–381.
9. Ghetti B, Perry KW, Fuller RW. Serotonin concentration and turnover in cerebellum and other brain regions of pcd mutant mice. *Brain Res* 1988;457:367–371.
10. Oshugi K, Adachi K, Andoc K. Serotonin metabolism in the CNS in cerebellar ataxia mice. *Experientia* 1986;42:1245–1247.
11. Victor M, Adams RD. On the etiology of the alcoholic neurologic disease with special references to the role of nutrition. *Am J Clin Nutr* 1961;9:379–397.
12. Victor M, Adams RD, Collins GH. The Wernicke-Korsakoff syndrome: a clinical and pathological study of 245 patients with post mortem examination. *Contemp Neurol Ser* 1981;7:1–206.
13. Gagnieu MG, Menouni-Foray V, Guardiola P, Quincy CI, Renaud B. Liquid chromatographic determination of homovanillic acid, 5-hydroxy indoleacetic acid and probenecid levels in human cerebrospinal fluid during probenecid test. *Clin Chim Acta* 1984;139:1–12.
14. Davis KL, Fauler KF, Hollister LE, Barchas JD, Berger PA. Physostigmine induced alteration of dopamine metabolites in CSF of normal subjects. In: Usdin E, Snyder SH, eds. *Frontiers in catecholamine research*. New York: Pergamon Press, 1973:1122–1124.
15. Harding AE. The clinical features and classification of the autosomal dominant cerebellar ataxias: a study of eleven families including descendents of the "Drew family of Walworth." *Brain* 1982;105:1–28.
16. Geoffroy G, Barbeau A, Breton G, Lemieux G, Aube M, Leger C. Clinical description and roentgenologic evaluation of patients with Friedreich's ataxia. *J Can Sci Neurol* 1976;3:279–286.
17. Fujita R, Trouillas P, Agid Y, Seck A, Tommas-Davenas C, Driesel A. Confirmation of linkage of Friedreich's ataxia to chromosome 9 and identification of a new closely linked marker. *Genomics* 1989;4:110–111.

18. Agren H, Mefford IN, Rudorfer MU, Linnoila M, Potter N. Interacting neurotransmitter systems. A non-experimental approach to the 5HIAA-HVA correlation in human CSF. *J Psychiatr Res* 1986; 20:175–193.
19. Trouillas P, Garde A, Robert JM, Adeleine P, Bard J, Brudon F. Régression du syndrome cérébelleux sous administration à long terme de L-5-HTP ou de l'association 5HTP-bensérazide: 25 observations quantifiées et traitées par ordinateur. *Rev Neurol* 1980;12:891.
20. Trouillas P, Garde A, Robert JM, Adeleine P. Régression de l'ataxie cérébelleuse humaine sous administration à long terme de 5-hydroxytryptophane. *C R Acad Sci* 1981;292:119–122.
21. Trouillas P, Garde A, Robert JM, Renaud B, Adeleine P, Bard J, Brudon F. Régression du syndrome cérébelleux sous administration à long terme de L-5-HTP ou de l'association 5HTP-bensérazide: vingt-six observations quantifiées et traitées par ordinateur. *Rev Neurol* 1982;5:415–435.
22. Trouillas P, Brudon F, Adeleine P. Improvement of cerebellar ataxia with levorotatory form of 5-hydroxytryptophan. *Arch Neurol* 1988;45:1217–1222.
23. Wessel K, Diener HC, Dichgans J. Long loop reflexes and postural ataxia: follow up with and treatment by 5-HTP in patients with Friedreich ataxia. In: Amblard V, Berthoz A, Clarac F, eds. *Posture and gait. Development, adaptation and modulation.* Amsterdam: Elsevier, 1988:237–244.
24. Gilman S, Junk L, Marker DS, Koeppe RA, Kluin KJ. Cerebral glucose hypermetabolism in Friedreich ataxia detected with positron emission tomography. *Ann Neurol* 1990;28:750–757.
25. Tamir H, Gerson MD. Storage of serotonin binding protein in synaptic vesicles. *J Neurochem* 1979;33:35–44.
26. Tabakoff B, Ritzmann RF, Boggan NO. Inhibition of the transport of 5-hydroxyindoleacetic acid from brain by ethanol. *J Neurochem* 1975;24:1043–1051.
27. Tabakoff B, Bulat MM, Anderson RA. Ethanol inhibition of transport of 5-hydroxyindoleacetic acid from cerebrospinal fluid. *Nature* 1975;254:708–710.
28. Hoffman PL, Tabakoff B. Alteration in dopamine sensitivity by chronic ethanol treatment. *Nature* 1977;268:551–553.
29. Rabin RA, Wolfe BB, Dibner MD, Zahniser NR, Merchoir C, Molinoff PB. Effects of ethanol administration and withdrawal on neurotransmitter receptor systems in C57 mice. *J Pharmacol Exp Ther* 1980;213:491–496.
30. Mullin MJ, Ferko AP. Alterations in dopaminergic function after subacute ethanol administration. *J Pharmacol Exp Ther* 1983;225:694–698.

Serotonin, the Cerebellum, and Ataxia, edited by
P. Trouillas and K. Fuxe.
Raven Press, Ltd., New York © 1993.

25

The Serotonergic Hypothesis of Cerebellar Ataxia and Its Pharmacological Consequences

Paul Trouillas

Neurology Service and Ataxia Research Center, Alexis Carrel Faculty of Medicine, Neurological Hospital and Claude Bernard University, 69003 Lyon, France

Cerebellar ataxia is a complex disorder, involving several elementary motor control dysfunctions of trunk, limbs, and phonation, as well as tonus abnormalities.

Multiple types of neurons in the cerebellum and the brain stem are involved in the neurophysiology of cerebellar functions. Some forms of ataxias might be due to multiple destructions of this neuronal circuitry with specific electrophysiological deficits. For such disorders, a neuropharmacology of ataxia would hardly be possible.

Yet, if there were major neurotransmitter systems for the whole cerebellum and related ganglia, there might be ataxias due to a clear neurochemical origin and the possibility of a logical neuropharmacology.

In 1980, we put forward the serotonergic hypothesis for cerebellar ataxia, postulating that the deficit of this indoleamine played a key role in the generation of cerebellar ataxia (1,2). The rationale was based on the physiological effects of serotonin (5-HT) on Purkinje cells and the existence of the raphe-olivocerebellar system delivering 5-HT to multiple precerebellar and cerebellar targets.

We could show that 5-hydroxytryptophan (5-HTP), a precursor of 5-HT, was able to induce a significant regression of several aspects of human ataxias (1–4) and that the levorotatory form of 5-HTP was the biologically active form of the molecule (1,5).

Because norepinephrine is also a cerebellar neurotransmitter, a noradrenergic hypothesis for ataxia might also be proposed, but we have not yet found data in favor of such a theory.

A detailed review of the physiological, anatomical, and pharmacological data in favor of the serotonergic hypothesis is presented here.

NEUROPHYSIOLOGICAL DATA

From a physiological point of view, Purkinje cells of the cerebellar cortex appear to be major target cells for 5-HT. Bloom et al. (6), showed that the monoamine had mainly an inhibiting action on these cells.

Strahlendorf et al. (7–9) revealed diverse and complex effects of 5-HT on Purkinje cells, including inhibition, excitation, and biphasic responses. They discovered that actions of 5-HT were also dependent on the initial firing rate of the Purkinje cell: slow-firing cells were accelerated, while fast-firing cells were slowed. Strahlendorf et al. (10) postulated that 5-HT may set the Purkinje cells to a preferred firing rate, thus being a stabilizing neuromodulator. Raphe stimulation induced an inhibition of Purkinje and fastigial cells, which was diminished by 5-HT antagonists.

Gardette et al. (11) showed that 5-HT was able to enhance the spontaneous firing of the cells of the deep cerebellar nuclei. When studying the excitatory responses of two excitatory amino acids (glutamate and aspartate) on Purkinje cells and deep cerebellar nuclei neurons, Gardette and Crepel (Chapter 17, this volume) showed that 5-HT was also able to decrease these responses. Since this effect was maintained in the presence of tetrodotoxin (TTX) and in low-calcium medium, a postsynaptic site of action was probable. As this effect was observed at doses at which there was no direct effect on cerebellar neurons, it was suggested that the receptors in question were different from those involved in the direct effects.

The experimental cerebellar harmaline syndrome appeared to be clearly related to 5-HT. This indolic monoamine-oxidase inhibitor (MAOI) of type A, a 5-HT analogue, was shown to induce rhythmic activity of cerebellar and lower brain stem neurons (12,13), activating the cerebellar cortex through climbing fibers (14). The drug was shown to suppress the firing of dorsal raphe neurons (15). Sjölund et al. (16) were able to demonstrate specific relationships between harmaline tremor and the serotonergic innervation of the inferior olivary nucleus. They postulated a normal inhibitory serotonergic input in the inferior olive, blocking the oscillatory activity of olivary neurons. The harmaline tremor and the oscillatory activities have been shown to be suppressed by 5-HTP administered systemically (17).

Is there an ataxia related to the harmaline tremor and is this ataxia corrected by 5-HTP? This point is not well documented. One could assume that such a considerable cerebellar dysfunction should provoke, besides the tremor, disturbances of equilibrium and movements.

The hypothesis of cerebellar and olivary serotonergic receptors was formulated on the basis of anatomical studies (18,19) and of neurophysiological experiments (20–24). Palacios et al. (Chapter 12, this volume) were able to demonstrate the existence of 5-HT_{1B} serotonergic receptors, particularly in the molecular layer of the posterior vermis, and higher densities of 5-HT_{1B} and 5-HT_{1C} receptors in the cerebellar deep nuclei. The inferior olivary nucleus showed intermediate levels of 5-HT_{1B} receptors and 5-HT_2 receptor transcripts. In the mouse, Saudou et al. (Chapter 15, this volume) could clone a functional 5-HT_{1B} receptor. The main sites of expression of the 5-HT_{1B} mRNA were the striatum and the Purkinje cells of the cerebellum. It is postulated that these 5-HT_{1B} receptors are localized presynaptically on the terminals of Purkinje cells and that they might modulate the release of neurotransmitters such as gamma-aminobutyric acid (GABA).

Raiteri et al. (25) showed that the endogenous release of glutamate by rat cerebellar slices was potently inhibited by the stimulation of both 5-HT_{1A}-like and 5-HT_2 receptors. The 5-HT_{1A}-like presynaptic receptors appear to be localized on glutamergic terminals originating from climbing and parallel fibers, while the presynaptic 5-HT_2 receptors were located on mossy fiber terminals (Chapter 11). Thus, serotonergic afferents seem to undergo a potent physiological control of the postsynaptic effects of the glutamergic cerebellar afferents.

The indoleamine therefore seems to have direct modulating effects on olivary and Purkinje cells and deep cellular nuclei neurons. It has also indirect modulating effects on the presynaptic delivery of glutamate, the postsynaptic effect of glutamate, and also probably the presynaptic release of GABA. Finally, 5-HT has numerous effects on multiple neurochemical cerebellar targets and deeply influences the cerebellar physiological function.

ANATOMICAL DATA: THE RAPHE-OLIVOCEREBELLAR SYSTEM

In 1969, Hökfelt and Fuxe (26) described serotonergic and noradrenergic afferent fibers to the cortex of the cerebellum. Fuxe et al. (27) later mentioned that the perikarya might be located in the midbrain raphe nuclei B6 and B7. Shinnar et al. (28) demonstrated that horseradish peroxidase (HRP) injected in lobules VI and VII retrogradely labeled the rostral pole of the raphe magnus, raphe pontis, and raphe centralis superior. HRP injected in the cat's flocculus retrogradely labeled the raphe dorsalis and raphe centralis superior and inferior (29). Batini et al. (30) showed that raphe pallidus was also related to lobule VII. Bobillier et al. (31) demonstrated that the serotonergic fibers emerge from the ventral border of the centralis superior and reach the cerebellum by the brachium pontis.

In the original work of Hökfelt and Fuxe (26) in the rat, the serotonergic afferents were observed mainly in the molecular layer of the cerebellum, especially in the anterior lobe. The serotonin (5-HT) nerve terminals were fine and varicose fibers. They ran mainly in the transverse plan of the folium, parallel to the surface.

Chan-Palay (18,19,32,33) gave an extensive description of the cerebellar serotonergic system, using intraventricular infusion of labeled 5-HT. Autoradiography of the cerebellar cortex showed a vast plexus of labeled indoleamine axons, including three systems: (i) mossy fiber rosettes in the granular layer, (ii) parallel fiber-like axons in the molecular layer, and (iii) a diffuse branching plexus distributed to all layers. All the deep cerebellar nuclei, dentate, interpositus, and fastigius are richly innervated.

Chan-Palay stressed the heterogeneity of connections of this system. It includes classical synaptic contacts with dendrites of granule cells and cerebellar cortical interneurons. Nonsynaptic terminals are also observed, probably delivering the neurotransmitter by neurohumoral dispersion.

The existence of the raphe-cerebellar serotonergic system was confirmed by Beaudet and Sotelo (34). Bishop et al. (35) showed that there is a distinct bundle of serotonergic axons in the brachium conjunctivum in the opossum. They found that the densest distribution of 5-HT took place at the Purkinje cell-granule cell border. Takeuchi et al. (36) studied the system in primates and showed that the serotonergic innervation was still present in the molecular layer of the cerebellum and the cerebellar nuclei.

Purkinje cells are undoubtedly target cells for the serotonergic system at the level of their dendrites. However, according to Takeuchi et al. (36), there is no morphological evidence that serotonergic neurons of the brain stem directly terminate on the somata of Purkinje cells.

Serotonergic terminals also exist in the inferior olive and are particularly dense in the dorsal accessory and the medial accessory nuclei (16,37). In the monkey, Takeuchi et al. (36) found a particularly dense serotonergic innervation in the caudal medial accessory olive, the lateral portion of the dorsal accessory olive, and the dorsal and lateral lamellae of the principal olive. Remarkably, the serotonergic terminals are mainly present in those olivary zones receiving direct spinal afferences (37) that project selectively onto the anterior lobe. The involvement of this 5-HT-regulated spino-olivo-vermis system in postural equilibrium seems obvious.

In humans, the existence of the cerebellar serotonergic system is highly probable, but difficult to prove, probably because there has been no previous pharmacological manipulation, as in animals. Yet the existence of raphe serotonergic neurons has been fully demonstrated (Chapters 2 and 4, this volume).

5-HT IN ANIMAL AND HUMAN MODELS OF ATAXIA

Serotonergic Impairment in Experimental Thiamine-Deficiency Models

In 1977, Chan-Palay et al. (32) showed autoradiographically a loss of labeled serotonergic axons in the cerebellum of thiamine-deprived rats, affecting the mossy fiber system and the parallel fiber-like neurons. Serotonergic terminals to the inferior olive were also affected.

The selectivity of the biochemical impairment of the serotonergic system was underlined by Plaitakis et al. (38,39). They were able to show a decrease of serotonergic synaptosomal uptake in affected animals. This abnormality was correlated with the onset of ataxia. Plaitakis et al. (40) demonstrated later that serotonergic abnormalities also included an exaggeration of the cerebellar 5-HT turnover and an elevation of cerebellar 5-hydroxyindoleacetic acid (5-HIAA).

On an experimental basis, a possible relationship between the serotonergic abnormalities and ataxia had been postulated by Chan-Palay (33) and Plaitakis et al. (39).

It is important to note that the selective reduction of 5-HT uptake might be due to primary midbrain lesions. Kuhar et al. (41) had shown in 1972 that raphe lesions were able to induce a selective reduction of 5-HT synaptosomal uptake in the forebrains of rats.

5-HT and Murine Ataxic Mutants

In *pcd* mutant mice, Ghetti et al. (42) showed a decrease of the 5-HT turnover and low 5-HIAA values in the late stages of the disease. Probenecid tests showed a specifically cerebellar reduction of the 5-HT turnover. In the mice, the terminal fields of the 5-HT axons were markedly reduced, due to the virtually complete Purkinje cell loss, and the subsequent loss of 90% of the granule cells, the olivary neurons also being affected. Although the noradrenergic terminals remain intact the norepinephrine turnover is also decreased (43).

Oshugi et al. (44) showed that tryptophan hydroxylase was significantly reduced in the "reeler mouse," while 5-HIAA and 5-HT values were markedly increased. Specifically cerebellar high 5-HT and 5-HIAA values were also observed in "staggerer" and "weaver" mice.

Human Deficiency-Alcoholic Syndromes

In this volume, we mention in a series of nine deficiency-alcoholic ataxic patients a particular biochemical syndrome involving serotonergic metabolism specifically (Chapter 24). In the CSF, baseline 5-HIAA values were found to be high and the probenecid-induced 5-HIAA variations were also increased, but not significantly so. Thus, this serotonergic syndrome is comparable to the syndrome described in thiamine-deprived animals by Plaitakis (40). Elevated baseline 5-HIAA values seem to indicate an impaired efflux of 5-HIAA, while probenecid-induced values might indicate an exaggeration of the 5-HT turnover, as in thiamine-deprived animals.

Human Heredoataxias

Cerebellar values of 5-HT and 5-HIAA are not known in heredoataxias, while there is a reduction of the cerebellar norepinephrine values in olivopontocerebellar atrophy (OPCA) (45). 5-HT abnormalities in the CSF of cerebellar atrophies and Friedreich's ataxia have not been mentioned (46).

In the CSF of cerebellar cortical atrophies, we found significantly decreased baseline values of 5-HIAA (Chapter 24). With the probenecid test, we were able to show that there is a strong tendency toward an increase in the 5-HT turnover. The syndrome might involve a primary serotonergic impairment with a compensatory increased turnover of 5-HT.

Monoaminergic abnormalities of Freidreich's ataxia were in the same direction as those of cortical cerebellar atrophy, with a lesser degree of serotonergic impairment.

Human Primary 5-HT Metabolism Abnormalities and Ataxia

In 1956, Baron et al. (47) described a hereditary disease characterized by fluctuating cerebellar ataxia associated with abnormal tryptophan metabolism.

In 1959, Southren et al. (48) reported the case of a 49-year-old woman with hyperserotoninemia and a clinical syndrome including hypertension, flushes, and ataxia. 5-HIAA values were normal in urine indicating an abnormal pathway in metabolizing endogenous 5-HT. A functional deficiency of brain-tissue 5-HT was suspected. Improvement in ataxia by diphenylhydantoin was observed together with the normalization of serotoninemia. Reserpine provided an aggravation of ataxia and mental disturbances.

PHARMACOLOGICAL DATA

On the basis of the serotonergic hypothesis of ataxia, in 1977 we treated a first patient with cerebellar ataxia due to a deficient regimen, using 500 mg of D,L-5-HTP. A film was made showing the dramatic regression of the static ataxia. Particularly striking was the disappearance of the anteroposterior rapid sway in 2 weeks.

Twenty-six patients were then gathered, with diseases such as Friedreich's ataxia, late cerebellar cortical atrophy, OPCA, and postsurgical injuries. In 1980 (1–4), with accurate quantitative evaluation, we were able to show that D,L-5-HTP at the dose of 16 mg/kg per day was regularly and partially active on cerebellar ataxia of different conditions. Friedreich's ataxia was undoubtedly sensitive at the beginning of its evolution, but the degenerative process continued. Several cases of cortical cerebellar atrophies were clearly sensitive.

The levorotatory form of 5-HTP was shown to be the active form of the molecule (1,5). The effect was particularly observed on static performance and speech. Kinetic performance was more irregularly influenced, but could be partially L-5-HTP sensitive (Fig. 1). A considerable increase of the CSF 5-HT turnover was demonstrated in treated patients (4).

The effect of 5-HTP in cerebellar ataxia was confirmed by Rascol et al. (49). Wessel et al. (50), with accurate posturographic measures, showed a long-term effect in Friedreich's ataxia. They have confirmed their observations (Chapter 27). We were able to confirm by posturography the "L-5-HTP phenomenon" of improvement of static ataxia, particularly in cerebellar cortical atrophy patients (Fig. 2).

In 1988, in a double-blind study including 30 patients, we (5) could confirm that the levorotatory form of the molecule was definitely the biologically active form. Improvement of cortical cerebellar atrophies was confirmed. Again, static and speech performance was found to be particularly sensitive. Yet we could observe the clear phenomenon of L-5-HTP resistance in several conditions (51).

In Tables 1 and 2, we present the results of a 10 mg/kg per day regimen of L-5-HTP for 6 months, with a qualitative evaluation of the response, to give an over-

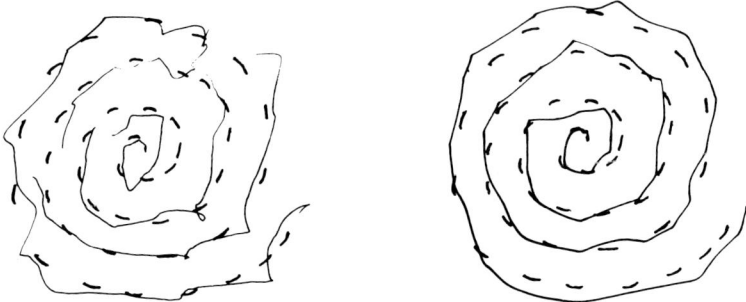

FIG. 1. Improvement of kinetic performance after 4 months of an L-5-HTP 10 mg/kg per day regimen in a patient with sporadic pure cerebellar cortical atrophy.

view of L-5-HTP sensitivity and L-5-HTP resistance among the different causative forms of ataxia. OPCA is not regularly sensitive; dominant forms of OPCA are resistant in our experience. Machado-Joseph disease is definitely resistant. Conversely, the genetic dominant forms of cerebellar cortical atrophies are regularly sensitive. Marinesco-Sjögren syndrome appeared to be slightly sensitive. Massive postinfectious (viral) atrophy of the cerebellum was regularly resistant. Ataxia in multiple sclerosis, when the disease is stabilized by an azathropine regimen, is regularly sensitive.

Small brain stem infarcts with chronic ataxia may be L-5-HTP sensitive. In a patient with pure static ataxia, we observed only a small dorsal mesencephalic infarct in the territory of the superior cerebellar artery (Fig. 3). This syndrome was clearly and quickly sensitive to L-5-HTP, at the dose of 300 mg per day. We realized that the lesion might involve mesencephalic serotonergic neurons, especially those of nucleus raphe dorsalis or their projections to the brachium conjunctivum

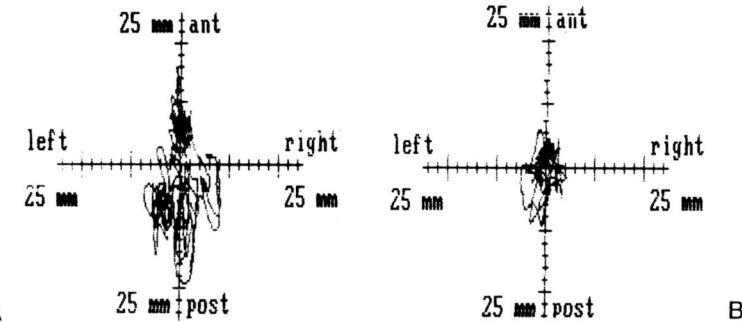

FIG. 2. The L-5-HTP phenomenon. Improvement in static performance assessed by posturography 4 months after an L-5-HTP 10 mg/kg per day regimen in the same patient as in Fig. 1. **A**: Before treatment; **B**, after treatment.

TABLE 1. L-5-HTP sensitivity in different types of genetic ataxias

Type of ataxia	Number of cases	L-5-HTP sensitivity		
		Speech	Static	Kinetic
Cortical cerebellar atrophy				
Autosomal dominant (Harding, 1982, type III)	2	+	+	+
Sporadic early and late onset	6	+	+	+
OPCA				
Early onset sporadic, purely cerebellar	2	+	+	+
Late onset sporadic, purely cerebellar	2	±	±	0
Autosomal dominant, Schut-Haymaker type	2	0	0	0
Early onset sporadic with spinal and peripheral involvement	2	0	0	0
Machado-Joseph disease	2	0	0	0
Marinesco-Sjögren syndrome	1	+	+	+
Friedreich's ataxia				
Stance still possible	6	+	+	+
Stance lost	6	±	±	0

(Kopp et al., Figs. 10 and 11, this volume). Bishop et al. (35) demonstrated a serotonergic raphe-cerebellar bundle in the brachium conjunctivum. Therefore, the lesion might induce a serotonergic disconnection between the upper brain stem raphe neurons and the anterior lobe of the cerebellum. The integrity of Purkinje cells might account for the quick effect induced by the neurotransmitter replacement. This particular neurochemical model of serotonergic disconnection may explain the good results observed in ataxias following small brain stem infarcts located on raphe-cerebellar or reticulo-cerebellar serotonergic pathways.

Drug doses and the utilization of a decarboxylase inhibitor are important to get significant results in routine therapy. Intolerance problems have been mentioned:

TABLE 2. L-5-HTP sensitivity in different types of acquired ataxias

Type of ataxia	Number of cases	L-5-HTP sensitivity		
		Speech	Static	Kinetic
Vinylchloride intoxication with cortical cerebellar atrophy	1	+	+	+
Toluene intoxication with cortical cerebellar atrophy	1	+	+	+
Trichlorethylene intoxication with cortical cerebellar atrophy	1	+	+	+
Alcoholic cerebellar atrophy	4	Nonevaluable, sometimes +		
Postinfectious (viral) cerebellar atrophy	1	0	0	0
Cerebellar and brain stem infarcts with static ataxia	2	+	+	+
Brain stem hemorrhage	1	0	0	0
Paraneoplastic cerebellar atrophy	1	0	0	0
Posttraumatic cerebellar ataxia	1	0	0	0
Sarcoidosis with cerebellar ataxia	1	0	+	+

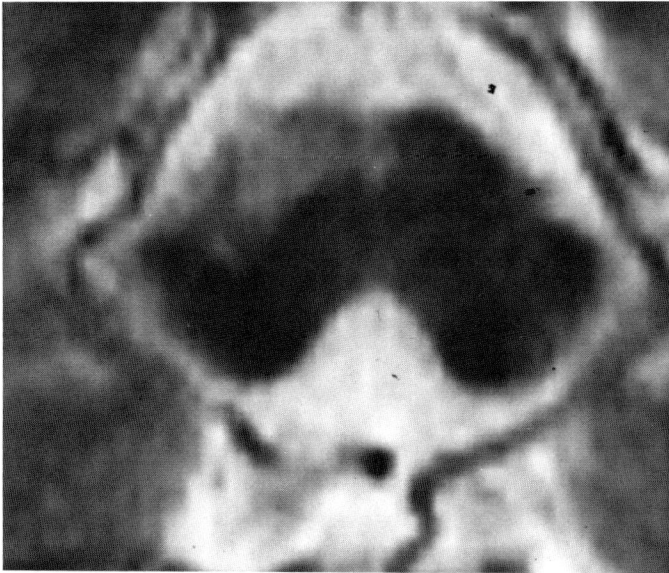

FIG. 3. Nucleus raphe dorsalis, ataxia, and possible serotonergic disconnection. This 74-year-old patient had a purely static ataxia, well and quickly improved by L-5-HTP 5 mg/kg per day. The only detectable lesion on magnetic resonance imaging was this mediodorsal mesencephalic infarct, possibly involving serotonergic neurons. The lesion might interrupt the raphe-cerebellar bundle between the nucleus raphe dorsalis and brachium conjunctivum.

diarrhea, nausea, vomiting, and sleepiness. The digestive symptoms are very rare when a decarboxylase inhibitor is added. High doses may be administered: in cerebellar cortical atrophies, doses of 16 mg/kg per day of L-5-HTP (i.e., 1,000 mg/day) can be safely administered for years with a decarboxylase inhibitor. To reach such a regimen safely, a progressive increasing of the doses of L-5-HTP and of the decarboxylase inhibitor is necessary. Benserazide must not be used before the age of 22 because of metaphyseal growth disturbances.

CONCLUSIONS

These data might bring about a reconsideration of the understanding of cerebellar ataxia itself. In the mechanism of many ataxias, conventional deficits of myelinated fibers and ongoing effector devices might not be the origin of cerebellar dysfunction. An important aspect of ataxia might be related to a long-term neurotransmitter deficit due to anatomic "serotonergic disconnection" (multiple sclerosis, lacunes) or to alterations of the neurotransmitter metabolism, primary or secondary. The chronic lack of 5-HT seems to play a key role in the creation of the syndrome.

The volume transmission of the indoleamine, according to the concept of Fuxe and Agnati (52), might then be insufficient to maintain the physiological activity of the multiple target cells, olivary neurons, Purkinje cells, and cerebellar nuclei neurons. Complex glutamate and/or GABA dysfunctions would then occur.

Thus, the replacement of 5-HT, especially when Purkinje cells are intact, might restore a sufficient volume transmission of 5-HT and progressively suppress the neurophysiological and/or neurochemical abnormalities.

In case of serious destruction of target cells in the cerebellar cortex, cerebellar nuclei, and/or in olivary nuclei, or in case of massive destruction of the serotonergic receptors in these structures, ataxia might be partially or completely L-5-HTP resistant. This might be the case in massive postinfectious cerebellar disorders and severe degenerations like those in OPCA.

L-5-HTP resistance might also be due to the existence of ataxias of other neurochemical origins. In this regard, the hypotheses of "noradrenergic ataxias" and "glutamergic ataxias" may also be made.

However the phenomenon of L-5-HTP resistance should not cast doubt on the concept of the therapeutic value of L-5-HTP. For when the neuropharmacology of cerebellar ataxia is examined, one realizes that few molecules have been proposed: thyrotropin-releasing hormone, sodium valproate, propranolol, physostigmine, and choline. None has shown a clear-cut benefit.

After nearly 15 years of experience, it can be underlined that the serotonergic hypothesis of ataxia has led to the imperfect, but first real treatment of cerebellar ataxia.

REFERENCES

1. Trouillas P, Garde A, Robert JM, et al. Régression du syndrome cérébelleux sous administration à long terme du L-5HTP ou de l'association 5-HTP-bensérazide: vingt-cinq observations quantifées et traitées par ordinateur. *Rev Neurol* 1980;12:891.
2. Trouillas P, Garde A, Robert JM, Adeleine P. Régression de l'ataxie cérébelleuse humaine sous administration à long terme de 5-hydroxytryptophane. *C R Acad Sci* 1981;292:119–122.
3. Trouillas P, Garde A. Regression of cerebellar ataxia with long-term 5-HTP therapy assessed by computerized data processing. In: *Abstracts of the 12th World Congress of Neurology, Kyoto, Japan, September 20–25, 1981*. Princeton, NJ: Excerpta Medica International Congress Series 548, 1981:382.
4. Trouillas P, Garde A, Robert JM, et al. Régression du syndrome cérébelleux sous administration à long terme de 5-HTP ou de l'association 5-HTP-benzérazide: vingt-six observations quantifiées et traitées par ordinateur. *Rev Neurol* 1982;5:415–435.
5. Trouillas P, Brudon F, Adeleine P. Improvement of cerebellar ataxia with levorotary form of 5-hydroxytryptophan. A double-blind study with quantified data processing. *Arch Neurol* 1988;45:1217–1222.
6. Bloom FC, Hoffer BJ, Siggins GR, Barker JL, Nicoll RA. Effects of serotonin on central neurons: microiontophoretic administration. Federation Proceedings 1972;31:97–106.
7. Strahlendorf JC, Lee M, Strahlendorf HK. Effects of serotonin on cerebellar Purkinje cells are dependent on the baseline firing rate. *Exp Brain Res* 1984;56:50–59.
8. Strahlendorf JC, Strahlendorf HK, Lee M. Enhancement of cerebellar Purkinje cell complex discharge activity by microiontophoretic serotonin. *Exp Brain Res* 1986;61:614–624.
9. Lee M, Strahlendorf JC, Strahlendorf HK. Picrotoxin but not bicuculline antagonizes 5-hydroxytryptamine-induced inhibition of cerebellar Purkinje neurons. *Exp Neurol* 1987;97:577–591.
10. Strahlendorf JC, Strahlendorf HK, Barnes CD. Modulation of cerebellar neuronal activity by raphe stimulation. *Brain Res* 1979;169:565–569.

11. Gardette R, Krupa M, Crepel F. Differential effects of serotonin on the spontaneous discharge and on the excitatory aminoacid-induced responses of deep cerebellar nuclei neurons in rat cerebellar slices. *Neuroscience* 1987;23:491–500.
12. Ahmed A, Taylor NRW. The analysis of drug-induced tremor in mice. *Br J Pharmacol* 1959;14:350–354.
13. Lamarre Y, De Montigny C, Dumont M, Weiss M. Harmaline-induced activity of cerebellar and lower brain stem neurones. *Brain Res* 1971;32:248–250.
14. De Montigny C, Lamarre Y. Rhythmic activity induced by harmaline in the olivo-cerebellar-bulbar-system of the cat. *Brain Res* 1973;53:82–95.
15. Weiss M, Pellet J. Raphe-cerebellum interactions. I. Effects of cerebellar stimulation and harmaline administration on single unit activity of midbrain raphe neurons in the rats. *Exp Brain Res* 1982;48:163–170.
16. Sjölund B, Björklund A, Wiklund L. The indolaminergic innervation of the inferior olive. 2. Relation to harmaline induced tumor. *Brain Res* 1977;131:23–37.
17. Bowman NC, Osuide G. Interaction between the effects of tremor and harmaline and other drugs in chicks. *Eur J Pharmacol* 1968;3:106–111.
18. Chan-Palay V. Fine structure of labeled axons in the cerebellar cortex and nuclei of rodents and primates after intraventricular infusions with tritiated serotonin. *Anat Embryol* 1975;148:235–265.
19. Chan-Palay V. *Cerebellar dentate nucleus: organization, cytology and transmitters.* New York: Springer-Verlag, 1977.
20. Tsang D, Lai G. Accumulation of cyclic adenosine 3'5-monophosphate in human cerebellar cortex slices: effects of monoamine receptor agonists and antagonists. *Brain Res* 1978;140:307–313.
21. Headley PM, Lodge D. Studies on field potentials and on single cells in the inferior olivary complex of the rat. *Brain Res* 1976;101:445–459.
22. Darrow J, Strahlendorf HK, Strahlendorf JC. Response of cerebellar Purkinje cells to serotonin and the 5-HT1A agonist 8-OH-DPAT and ipsa in vitro. *Eur J Pharmacol* 1990;175:145–153.
23. Darrow E, Strahlendorf JC, Strahlendorf HK. Extracellular magnesium alters responsiveness to serotonin and analogues. *Eur J Pharmacol* 1991;201:239–242.
24. Strahlendorf JC, Lee M, Strahlendorf HK. Serotonin modulates muscimol and baclofen-elicited inhibition of cerebellar Purkinje cells. *Eur J Pharmacol* 1991;201:239–242.
25. Raiteri M, Maura G, Bonanno G, Pittaluga A. Differential pharmacology and function of two 5-HT1 receptors modulating transmitter release in rat cerebellum. *J Pharmacol Exp Ther* 1986;237:644–648.
26. Hökfelt T, Fuxe K. Cerebellar monoamine nerve terminals, a new type of afferent fibers to the cortex cerebelli. *Exp Brain Res* 1969;9:63–72.
27. Fuxe K, Jonsson G. Further mapping of cerebral 5-hydroxytryptamine neurons: studies with the neurotoxic dihydroxytryptamines. In: *Advances in biochemical psychopharmacology.* New York: Raven Press, 1974:1–12.
28. Shinnar S, Maciewicz RJ, Shofer RJ. A raphe projection to cat cerebellar cortex. *Brain Res* 1975;97:139–143.
29. Sato Y, Kanasaki T, Karashi K. Afferent projections from the brainstem to the floccular three zones in cats. II. Mossy fiber projections. *Brain Res* 1983;272:37–48.
30. Batini C, Corvisier J, Hardy O. Projections des noyaux réticulaires bulbaires et des noyaux du raphé sur les lobules VI et VII du cortex cérébelleux du chat. *C R Acad Sci* 1977;284:1805–1806.
31. Bobillier P, Seguin S, Petitjean F, Salvert D, Touret M, Jouvet M. The raphe nuclei of the cat brain stem: a topographical atlas of their afferent projections as revealed by autoradiography. *Brain Res* 1976;113:449–486.
32. Chan-Palay V, Plaitakis A, Nicklas N, Berl S. Autoradiographic demonstration of loss of labeled indoleamine axons of the cerebellum in chronic diet-induced thiamine deficiency. *Brain Res* 1977;138:380–384.
33. Chan-Palay V. Indoleamine neurons and their processes in the normal rat brain and in chronic diet-induced thiamine deficiency, demonstrated by 3H-serotonin. *J Comp Neurol* 1979;176:467–494.
34. Beaudet A, Sotelo C. Synaptic remodeling of serotonin axon terminals in rat agranular cerebellum. *Brain Res* 1981;206:305–329.
35. Bishop GA, Ho RH, King JS. Localization of serotonin immunoreactivity in the opossum cerebellum. *J Comp Neurol* 1985;235:301–321.
36. Takeuchi Y, Kimura H, Sano Y. Immunohistochemical demonstrations of serotonin-containing nerve fibers in the cerebellum. *Cell Tissue Res* 1982;26:1–12.

37. Wiklund L, Björklund A, Sjölund B. The indolaminergic innervation of the inferior olive: I. Convergence with direct spinal afferents in the areas projecting to the cerebellar anterior lobe. *Brain Res* 1977;131:1–21.
38. Plaitakis A, van Woert MH, Hwang EC, Berl S. The effect of acute thiamine deficiency on brain tryptophan, serotonin and 5-hydroxyindoleacetic acid. *J Neurochem* 1978;31:1087–1089.
39. Plaitakis A, Nicklas JN, Berl S. Thiamine deficiency: selective impairment of the cerebellar serotonergic system. *Neurology* 1978;28:691–698.
40. Plaitakis A, Hwang EC, van Woert MH, Szilagui PA, Berl S. Effect of thiamine deficiency on brain neurotransmitter systems. *Ann NY Acad Sci* 1982;367–381.
41. Kuhar MJ, Roth RH, Aghajanian GK. Synaptosomes from forebrains of rats with midbrain raphe lesions: selective reduction of serotonin uptake. *J Pharmacol Exp Ther* 1972;181:36–45.
42. Ghetti B, Perry KW, Fuller RW. Serotonin concentration and turnover in cerebellum and other brain regions of pcd mutant mice. *Brain Res* 1988;457:367–371.
43. Ghetti B, Perry KW, Fuller RW. Norepinephrine metabolism in the cerebellum of the Purkinje cell degeneration (pcd) mutant mouse. *Neurochem Int* 1987;10:39–47.
44. Oshugi K, Adachi K, Ando K. Serotonin metabolism in the CNS in cerebellar ataxia mice. *Experientia* 1986;42:1245–1247.
45. Kish S, Shannak KS, Hornykiewicz O. Reduction of noradrenaline in cerebellum of patients with olivo pontocerebellar atrophy. *J Neurochem* 1984;42.
46. Ichikawa N. Study on monoamine metabolite contents of cerebrospinal fluid in patients with neurodegenerative diseases. *Tohoku J Exp Med* 1986;150:435–446.
47. Baron DN, Dent CE, Harris H, Jepson JB. Hereditary pellagra like skin rash with temporary cerebellar ataxia, constant renal aminoaciduria, and other bizarre biochemical features. *Lancet* 1956;2:421–428.
48. Southren AL, Warner RRP, Christoff N, et al. An unusual neurologic syndrome associated with hyperserotoninemia. *N Eng J Med* 1959;260:1265–1268.
49. Rascol A, Clanet M, Monstastruc JL, et al. L-5-hydroxytryptophan in the cerebellar syndrome treatment. *Biomedicine* 1981;35:112–113.
50. Wessel K, Diener HC, Dichgans J. Long-loop reflexes and postural ataxia: follow-up study with and without treatment by 5-HTP in patients with Friedreich ataxia. In: Amblard V, Berthoz A, Clarac F, eds. *Posture and gait: development adaptation and modulation.* Amsterdam: Elsevier, 1988:237–244.
51. Trouillas P. L-5-Hydroxytryptophan treatment in hereditary and acquired ataxia. *Mov Disord* 1990;5(suppl 1):6.
52. Fuxe K, Agnati L. *Volume transmission in the brain. Novel mechanism for neural transmission.* New York: Raven Press, 1991.

26

L-5-Hydroxytryptophan in Cerebellar Syndrome Treatment

J. M. Senard, *W. Delage, M. Clanet, *O. Rascol, *J. L. Montastruc, and A. Rascol

*Service de Neurologie et de *Pharmacologie, CHU Toulouse, Hôpital de Purpan, 31059 Toulouse, France*

Using L-5-hydroxytryptophan (L-5-HTP), a serotonin precursor, in posthypoxic action myoclonus (3,4), and other abnormal movements (chorea, athetosis, dyskinesias), we found that this drug could be useful in the treatment of the cerebellar syndrome. We report the results of an open preliminary clinical trial performed between 1978 and 1980 already published (5). These patients were gathered because the intensity of cerebellar symptoms.

Four groups of ambulatory patients were studied: Group I included four patients presenting a chronic form of multiple sclerosis (MS) with great action tremor combined with rhythmic oscillations of head and trunk most probably owing to involvement of the upward projections of the dentatorubrothalamic fibers. Group II included 10 MS with cerebellar syndrome with either a static or kinetic component or both; some patients were in relapse, others in remission. L-5-HTP was given alone or in association with other previously prescribed drugs (steroids or immunosuppressives). Group III included four spinocerebellar degenerations (one Friedreich's disease and three heredoataxia, Pierre Marie's disease). Group IV included six patients with miscellaneous cerebellar syndromes (two cerebellar vermian atrophy, one cerebellar syndrome following cerebral thrombophlebitis, two cerebellar syndrome postcerebellar infarction, and one cerebellar and cerebral atrophy).

Treatment was discontinued in four patients (two in group II and two in group IV) owing to digestive intolerance, but tolerance was good for the other patients. Cerebellar syndrome was clearly improved in 12 patients. The beneficial effect became obvious between days 10 and 15 of treatment.

In group I, we found a good result with follow-up of 23 months and three moderate results with follow-up of 2, 4, and 6 months, respectively. In these four patients, placebo led to a recurrence of symptoms, whereas the reintroduction of L-5-HTP induced new improvement in clinical state. In group II, we observed five moderate results: however, in one case, this improvement may have been due to a spontaneous remission; in two other cases, the beneficial effect disappeared after 3 months. In four of these five patients, the efficiency of L-5-HTP was confirmed both by placebo-induced relapse and L-5-HTP-induced reimprovement. The other five patients failed to show any beneficial effect, but two patients stopped because of side effects. In group III, we noted two good results (follow-up of 33 months and 17 months) and one moderate result confirmed by use of placebo (follow-up of 6 months). In group IV there was one good result (follow-up of 12 months), two moderate results (follow-up of 2 and 6 months), two side effects, and no effect in one case.

These results showed that both static and kinetic cerebellar syndrome components were improved when the cerebral rate of serotonin was increased by L-5-HTP administration (1). The transient effect seen in four patients could be explained by a tolerance that was not noticed during posthypoxic action myoclonus or in other abnormal movements treatment (4). The pharmacological mechanism of L-5-HTP action was difficult to explain: raphe cerebellar serotoninergic pathways had been described (2).

From the results of our clinical study, it was tempting to speculate that a dysfunction of such a monoaminergic system is involved in some cerebellar syndromes. These preliminary results were rather conspicuous but had to be confirmed in controlled trials, particularly in MS cerebellar syndromes and degenerative diseases.

REFERENCES

1. Chase TN, Murphy DL. Serotonin and central nervous system function. *Annu Rev Pharmacol* 1973;13:181.
2. Fuxe H, Jonsson G. Further mapping of central 5-hydroxytryptamine neurons: studies with the neurotoxic dihydroxytryptamines. In: Costa E, Gessa GL, eds. *Serotonin: new vistas (Advances in biochemistry psychopharmacology)*. New York: Raven Press, 1974.
3. Lhermitte F, Peterfalvi M, Marteau R, Gazengel J, Serdaru M. Analyse pharmacologique d'un cas de myoclonies d'intention et d'action post-anoxique. *Rev Neurol (Paris)* 1971;124:21.
4. Rascol A, Guiraud-Chaumeil B, Laboucarié J, Montastruc JL, El-Hage W. Utilisation du L5OH tryptophane dans les myoclonies post-anoxiques. *Therapie* 1978;33:623.
5. A. Rascol, Clanet M, Montastruc JL, Delage W, Guiraud-Chaumeil B. L5OH tryptophan in the cerebellar syndrome treatment. *Biomedicine* 1981;35:112–113.

*Serotonin, the Cerebellum,
and Ataxia,* edited by
P. Trouillas and K. Fuxe.
Raven Press, Ltd., New York © 1993.

27

Treatment of Ataxia with 5-Hydroxytryptophan: Clinical Studies

K. Wessel, G. P. Huss, *K. Schimrigk, †N. Mai, and D. Kömpf

*Department of Neurology, Medical University of Lübeck, D-2400 Lübeck, Germany;
*Department of Neurology, University Homburg/Saar, D-6650 Homburg, Germany;
†Clinical Neuropsychology, Städtisches Krankenhaus München-Bogenhausen,
D-8000 Munich 50, Germany*

Modifications of serotonin (5-HT) metabolism have been shown to have an effect on experimental cerebellar (harmaline-induced tremor) symptoms (17). The application of 5-HT at the level of the inferior olive (7) or systemic administration of 5-hydroxytryptophan (5-HTP) (2) resulted in a regression of cerebellar abnormalities. A possible anatomical equivalent of these functional aspects are serotoninergic projections from raphe nuclei to the cerebellar cortex (3,8). Furthermore, in thiamine-deprived animals that exhibited ataxia, the cerebellar synaptosomal 5-HT uptake was shown to decrease (15), and a specific degeneration of the serotoninergic cerebellar raphe system was demonstrated (3). This prompted some attempts to treat patients suffering from ataxia with serotoninergic substances (5-HTP). In some of these studies the treatment with 5-HTP in doses of up to 1,000 mg per day was combined with the administration of a peripheral decarboxylase inhibitor (benserazide). In humans it has been shown that the plasma concentrations of 5-HTP were increased about 10-fold by pretreatment with decarboxylase inhibitor (10,11), and a direct proportionality between 5-HTP concentrations in plasma and in the levels of lumbar cerebrospinal fluid was found (12). On the other hand, it has been shown in pharmacological experiments that decarboxylase inhibition does not influence the 5-HT concentration and the 5-HTP uptake of the brain (1). So a combination of 5-HTP and benserazide does not seem to be indispensable. Some of the clinical studies resulted in partly positive effects of 5-HTP on ataxia (14,16,18–22) and others did not (9,26) (Table 1). Most of these clinical studies were performed with poorly defined and inhomogeneous patient groups, often including patients with multiple sclerosis. No study had a double-blind and crossover design. There is one double-blind study demonstrating a quite positive effect of 5-HTP treatment on

TABLE 1. *Positive or negative effects of 5-HTP treatment on ataxia in various clinical studies*

Study	Positive (N)	Negative (N)
van Woert and Sethy, 1975	—	2
Rascol et al., 1981	12	12
Trouillas et al., 1982, 1984	13	8
Klein et al., 1986	—	8
Wessel et al., 1985	8	5
Wessel et al., 1988	2	3
Mertens and Kohlhepp, 1987	28	32
Trouillas et al., 1988	15	—
	78	70

N, number of atactic patients treated with 5-HTP.

ataxia (20). The approach of most clinical studies was the same, assessing the patient's competence on a number of motor tasks and recording the performance in terms of the time taken to complete them. This is a valid means of assessing function because it uses tasks similar to those that the patient has to carry out daily. One particular problem with these clinical studies is the quantification and documentation of ataxia. Therefore we introduced objective measurements of atactic symptoms. As a method for quantification of postural ataxia we used posturography (4,23).

Posturography was performed while the subject stood on a force-measuring platform. Strain gauges at the four corners of the platform measured the displacement of the center-of-foot pressure (CFP) in anteroposterior and lateral directions under static conditions with the patient's eyes open or closed. The anteroposterior sway was computed from the differences between the front and back strain gauges. The lateral sway was computed in a similar manner from the two right and left force transducers. The influence of the subject's weight was electronically compensated. The anteroposterior and lateral CFP components were digitalized and on-line computations were performed with the help of a personal computer. Measurements were taken for a total of 25 sec with a sampling interval of 25 msec. The sway path (SP) traveled by the CFP on the platform and sway area (SA) covered by the SP within 25 sec were calculated with the patient's eyes open and closed. A sway direction histogram of CFP was also computed. For this purpose the full circle of possible sway directions was divided into eight intervals of 45° each. The single vectors of displacement of the CFP within each sampling interval were sorted according to their directions and summed. Straight ahead was defined as zero. SP and sway direction histograms for each subject were plotted on a digital X-Y plotter (Fig. 1). Figure 1 demonstrates an improvement in postural instability, as quantified by posturography, after 6 months treatment with 5-HTP in a dose of 1,000 mg per day in a patient with Friedreich's ataxia. This single case showing improvement in ataxia with 5-HTP treatment reflects the preliminary experience, that we have had in an open, uncontrolled trial with two of five patients with Friedreich's ataxia (22).

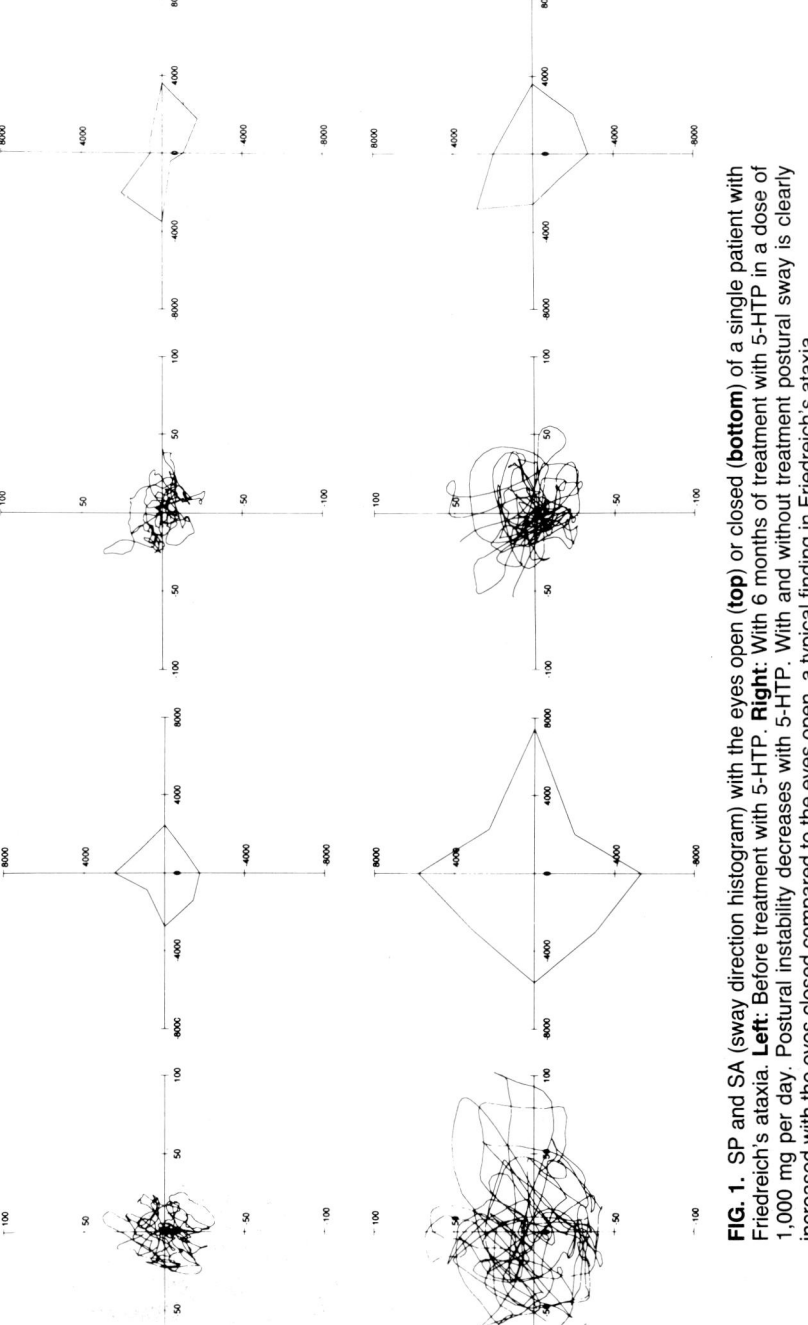

FIG. 1. SP and SA (sway direction histogram) with the eyes open (**top**) or closed (**bottom**) of a single patient with Friedreich's ataxia. **Left**: Before treatment with 5-HTP. **Right**: With 6 months of treatment with 5-HTP in a dose of 1,000 mg per day. Postural instability decreases with 5-HTP. With and without treatment postural sway is clearly increased with the eyes closed compared to the eyes open, a typical finding in Friedreich's ataxia.

Dysdiadochokinesia, dysmetria, and tremor of hand and finger movements are well-known signs of a cerebellar lesion. Using high precision force transducers and a microcomputer system, isometric finger forces were registrated. Disturbances in achieving and maintaining constant force were used to measure dysmetria and tremor. The task was to generate a prehensile force (2.5 N) and to maintain this force constant for the trial duration of 20 sec (Fig. 2). As visual feedback a vertical bar was presented on a monitor, its length corresponding to the actual force applied. A horizontal line marked the required target force. Diadochokinesia was measured in terms of fast repetitive force changes. The task was to produce, as rapidly as possible, force changes between the prescribed force levels (6.25 and 1.78 N), which were presented again as horizontal lines on the screen (Fig. 2). The actual force was displayed as a vertical bar (13). Figure 2 demonstrates improvement in dysmetria, tremor, and dysdiadochokinesia in a single patient with Friedreich's ataxia under long-term treatment with 5-HTP in a dose of 600 mg per day.

A further problem of particular clinical studies is the selection of comparable patients with ataxia to get homogeneous patient groups. On the one hand, Friedreich's ataxia represents a disease, which is relatively easy to define. The diagnostic criteria are onset usually before age of 20, progressive, unremitting ataxia of gait, dysarthria, decreased vibration and position sense in the lower limbs, deep tendon areflexia, and progressive muscle weakness in the lower extremities (5,6). An atrophy of the cranial spinal cord on midsagittal magnetic resonance imaging (MRI) planes, reflecting the main neuropathological finding of degeneration of the medulla oblongata and the spinal cord, can be used as an additional diagnostic marker (24). Patients with cerebellar atrophy, presenting a pure cerebellar syndrome after a disease duration of several years, are another relatively well-defined group to test the effect of 5-HTP on ataxia. We recommend the following diagnostic criteria: onset of the disease after the age of 30 years, progressive, unremitting or, in some cases, unchanged cerebellar symptoms and signs for several years, cerebellar atrophy on computed tomography (mostly cortical pronounced without atrophy of brain stem structures), and no signs in clinical examination and neurophysiological tests of a lesion beyond the cerebellum in terms of a multisystem disease (e.g., olivopontocerebellar atrophy) (25). In our experience, patients with olivopontocerebellar atrophy or multisystem disease do not improve with 5-HTP treatment and should be excluded from corresponding studies.

The natural history of Friedreich's ataxia and cerebellar atrophy, with which one must compare, has not been documented in detail. Therefore, it seems to be necessary that clinical studies testing the effect of 5-HTP on ataxia be designed as double-blind, crossover studies. At present we are performing such a randomized, double-blind, crossover study with 5-HTP versus placebo in 50 patients with Friedreich's ataxia or cerebellar atrophy, using the above-mentioned methods for quantification and documentation. The aim is to further test the effect of 5-HTP on ataxia using the described, well-elaborated, and comprehensive methods. The observation time of each phase (5-HTP and placebo) is 10 months. Between the two phases we introduced a washout time of 1 month; an observation time of at least 1 month after

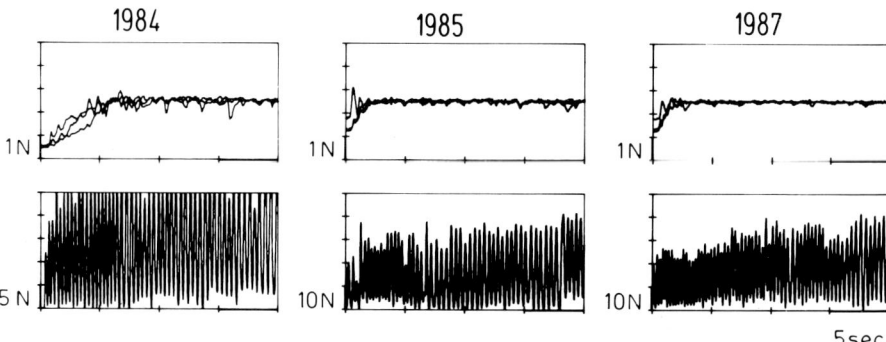

FIG. 2. Isometric finger forces of a single patient with Friedreich's ataxia before treatment (**left**), and with 5-HTP treatment in a dose of 600 mg per day (**middle** and **right**). Achieving and maintaining a constant force is displayed in *upper* panels. In the *lower* panels, the registration of fast repetitive force changes is shown. All parameters improved with long-term 5-HTP treatment.

finishing the study is included. The first phase of the study has been completed. Apart from minor gastrointestinal side effects, which did not cause real problems in the treatment, no relevant side effects were noted with long-term administration of 5-HTP in a dose of up to 1,000 mg per day.

REFERENCES

1. Bartholini. Decrease of cerebral 5-hydroxytryptamine by 3,4-dihydroxyphenylalanine after inhibition of extracerebral decarboxylase. *J Pharm Pharmacol* 1968;20:228.
2. Bowmann WC, Osuide G. Interaction between the effects of tremorine and harmine and of other drugs in chicks. *Eur J Pharmacol* 1968;3:106–111.
3. Chan-Palay V. Indoleamine neurons and their processes in the normal rat brain and in chronic diet-induced thiamine deficiency, demonstrated by 3H-serotonin. *J Comp Neurol* 1976;176:467–494.
4. Diener HC, Dichgans J, Bacher M, Gompf B. Quantification of postural sway in normals and patients with cerebellar diseases. *Electroencephalogr Clin Neurophysiol* 1984;57:134–142.
5. Geoffroy G, Barbeau A, Breton G, et al. Clinical description and roentgenologic evaluations of patients with Friedreich's ataxia. *Can J Neurol Sci* 1976;3:279–286.
6. Harding AE. Friedreich's ataxia: a clinical and genetic study of 90 families with an analysis of early diagnostic criteria and intrafamilial clustering of clinical features. *Brain* 1981;104:589–620.
7. Headley PM, Lodge D, Duggan AW. Drug-induced rhythmical activity in the inferior olivary complex of the rat. *Brain Res* 1976;101:461–478.
8. Hökfelt T, Fuxe K. Cerebellar monoamine nerve terminals, a new type of afferent fibers to the cortex cerebelli. *Exp Brain Res* 1969;9:63–72.
9. Klein P, Lees A, Stern G. Consequences of chronic 5-hydroxy-tryptophan in parkinsonian instability of gait and balance and in other neurological disorders. *Adv Neurol* 1986;45:603–604.
10. Magnussen I, Engbaek F. The effects of aromatic amino acid decarboxylase inhibitors on plasma concentrations of 5-hydroxytryptophan in man. *Acta Pharmacol Toxicol* 1978;43:36–42.
11. Magnussen I, Jensen TS, Rand JH, Van Woert MH. Plasma accumulation and metabolism of orally administered single dose L-5-hydroxytryptophan in man. *Acta Pharmacol Toxicol* 1981;49:184–189.
12. Magnussen I, Van Woert MH. Human pharmacokinetics of long term 5-hydroxytryptophan combined with decarboxylase inhibitors. *Eur J Clin Pharmacol* 1982;23:81–86.
13. Mai N, Bolsinger P, Avarello M, Diener HC, Dichgans J. Control of isometric finger force in patients with cerebellar disease. *Brain* 1988;111:973–998.

14. Mertens HG, Kohlhepp W. Spino-cerebelläre Atrophien—Diagnose und Therapie. *Verh Dtsch Ges Neurol* 1987;4:294–300.
15. Plaitakis A, Nicklas WJ, Berl S. Thiamine deficiency: selective impairment of the cerebellar serotoninergic system. *Neurology* 1978;28:691–698.
16. Rascol A, Clanet M, Montastruc JL. L-5-Hydroxytryptophan in the cerebellar syndrome treatment. *Biomedicine* 1981;35:112–113.
17. Sjölund B, Björklund A, Wiklund L. The indolaminergic innervation of the inferior olive. 2. Relation to harmaline induced tremor. *Brain Res* 1977;131:23–37.
18. Trouillas P, Garde A, Robert JM, et al. Regression du syndrome cérébelleux sous administration à long terme de 5-HTP ou de l'association 5-HTP-benserazide. *Rev Neurol (Paris)* 1982;138:415–435.
19. Trouillas P. Regression of cerebellar syndrome with long-term administration of 5-HTP or the combination 5-HTP-benserazide: 21 cases with quantified symptoms processed by computer. *Ital J Neurol Sci* 1984;5:253–266.
20. Trouillas P, Brudon F, Adeleine P. Improvement of cerebellar ataxia with levorotatory form of 5-hydroxytryptophan: a double-blind study with quantified data processing. *Arch Neurol* 1988;45:1217–1222.
21. Wessel K, Diener HC, Dichgans J. Vorläufige Therapieergebnisse mit 5-Hydroxy-Tryptophan bei Friedreich'scher Ataxie und zerebellärer Atrophie. *Psycho* 1985;11:436–437.
22. Wessel K, Diener HC, Dichgans J. Long loop reflexes and postural ataxia: follow up study with and without treatment by 5-HT in patients with Friedreich's ataxia. In: Amblard B, Berthoz A, Clarac F, eds. *Posture and gait development, adaptation and modulation*. Amsterdam: Excerpta Medica, 1988:237–244.
23. Wessel K, Diener HC, Dichgans J, Thron A. Cerebellar dysfunction in patients with bronchogenic carcinoma: clinical and posturographic findings. *J Neurol* 1988;235:290–296.
24. Wessel K, Schroth G, Diener HC, Müller-Forell W, Dichgans J. Significance of MRI-confirmed atrophy of the cranial spinal cord in Friedreich's ataxia. *Eur Arch Psychiatr Neurol Sci* 1989;238:225–230.
25. Wessel K, Huss GP, Brückmann H, Kömpf D. Follow-up of neurophysiological tests and CT in late-onset cerebellar ataxia and multiple system atrophy. *J Neurol (in press)*.
26. Woert van MH, Sethy VH. Therapy of intention myoclonus with L-5-hydroxytryptophan and a peripheral decarboxylase inhibitor, MK 486. *Neurology* 1975;25:135–140.

*Serotonin, the Cerebellum,
and Ataxia*, edited by
P. Trouillas and K. Fuxe.
Raven Press, Ltd., New York © 1993.

28

Quantitative Assessment of Postural Asynergy in Cerebellar Pathology

François Viallet, *Bernadette Bonnefoi-Kyriacou, †Jean Massion,
†Roselyne Aurenty, and *Richard Khalil

*Service de Neurologie, CHG Aix-en-Provence, 13616 Aix-en-Provence, France;
*Service de Neurologie, CHU la Timone, 13005 Marseille, France;
†CNRS LNF 3, 13402 Marseille, France*

In a general analysis of the cerebellar symptoms, asynergy was described as "the absence or disturbance of that proper synergic association in the contraction of agonists, antagonists and fixating muscles, which assures that the different components of an act follow in proper sequence, at the proper moment and are of the proper degree, so that the act is executed accurately and with the least possible expenditure of energy" (7). Nowadays, one might consider that this view of asynergy most likely corresponded to limb impairment. However, another aspect of cerebellar motor impairment, which is axial asynergy, had been previously described in cerebellar patients (1). According to that report, when the patient tried to bend the head and trunk backward, the inferior limbs stayed almost motionless; actually, flexion of the knee and hip did not take place, conversely to that observed in a normal subject. The patient had lost the capacity to control simultaneously the muscles responsible for the displacement in the opposite direction of the upper trunk, relative to lower segments, and, thus, when a backward movement had been requested, the patient fell down (Fig. 1).

Since then, impairment of this kind of postural synergy has been considered to be responsible for an imbalance while standing because the projection of the center of gravity is not maintained (9,10). In this context, it has seemed useful to develop techniques that allowed the clinician to quantify such a motor impairment. In cerebellar pathology, the main difficulty is still the evaluation of postural asynergy using a conventional examination. One way to obtain a quantitative assessment could be to use a kinematic approach: from the analogic data recorded, it would be possible to define, as a numeric variable, a true index of asynergy. This preliminary investigation was aimed specifically at patients suffering from chronic and relatively stable impairment as observed in degenerative cerebellar atrophies.

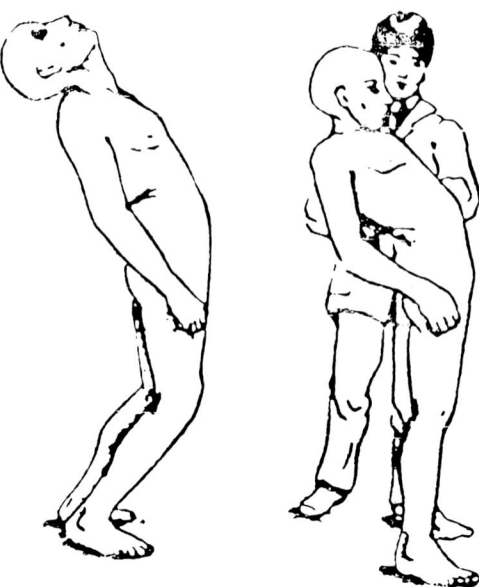

FIG. 1. Axial asynergy in backward upper trunk bending (redrawn from the original description by Babinski [1899], see ref. 1). **Left**: Normal subject performs compensatory hip and knee flexion. **right**, Cerebellar patient keeps his inferior limbs almost motionless and, if not supported, would fall down.

METHODS

Experimental Set-up

This method has been fully described in a previous paper (4). As shown in Fig. 2, the subject stood on a force platform equipped with piezoelectric transducers, giving the vertical and horizontal components of the ground reaction force. The kinematics of the movement were analyzed by means of an automatic TV image processor (ELITE system) (5). Seven hemispheral retroreflective markers (5 mm in diameter) were placed on the main reference points on the right side of the subject. Two markers were placed on the head and the remainder placed on the shoulder, anterior superior iliac crest, upper femoral trochanter, knee and ankle (Fig. 2). The ELITE system is a dedicated computer that processes TV signals in real time, recognizes all markers on the basis of their shape, and computes simultaneously the coordinates of the centroid of all the markers. The sampling rate used was 50 Hz, so that during the execution of the bending movements, the position of each marker was detected every 20 msec. Accuracy of the system was one part in 2,560. Under the present experimental condition the field explored was 2 m × 2 m, and the accuracy was thus 0.78 mm.

Experimental Paradigm

The subject was asked to stand quietly on the force platform and relax with hands on hips and eyes open. At a given signal (tone burst), the subject was asked to bend

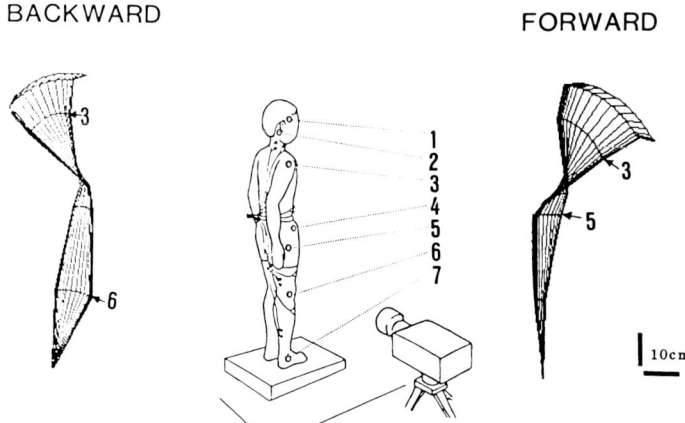

FIG. 2. The stick diagrams, obtained from a normal subject performing the movement as fast as possible, are displayed laterally (marker 3, shoulder; marker 5, hip; marker 6, knee). The experimental set-up is drawn in the middle and the numbers 1 to 7 correspond to the retroflective markers (see text for details).

both the head and trunk forward (or backward) until reaching a preestimated displacement of the head (marker 1) of about 30 cm in the sagittal plane and to keep this latter position for 3 sec. Two directions of upper trunk bending were successively studied: forward and backward bending.

For each type of axial movement, two types of instructions were given: (i) The subject was required to perform the movement from upright to maximal bending as fast as possible at the onset of a tone burst. (ii) The subject was instructed to perform the movement within 1.5 sec; the movement performed was considered to be slow and was run smoothly with the aid of a continuous tone. Five trials were conducted with each of the instructions and each type of upper trunk bending by each subject.

Patient Selection

This technique was carried out in three patients suffering from chronic cerebellar ataxia; they have given their informed consent and were not taking any active drug. Their clinical history (see appendix) was compatible with the diagnosis of progressive cerebellar ataxia of late onset (6). All these cases had been followed for more than 3 years and neither alcohol consumption nor any malignant or inflammatory pathology was found in any patient. They were two women and one man, aged 67, 40, and 48 years, respectively.

The data from the three patients were compared to those from three normal volunteers (two women, one man), aged 52, 41, and 38 years, respectively.

Variables Recorded

From the kinematic recordings (represented as stick diagrams on Fig. 2), the displacement and velocity curves for each marker as a function of time were drawn (see Fig. 3). From these analogic data, three types of numeric variables were extracted on some selected traces that corresponded to markers 3 and 5 for the forward movement and markers 3 and 6 for the backward movement (Fig. 3).

The first variable was the maximal value of the velocity (V_{max}) measured on marker 3 traces for both directions.

The second variable was termed the coordination index. It was calculated either as the ratio D5/D3 obtained from the displacement of marker 5 (D5) and that of marker 3 (D3) for the forward bending or as the ratio D6/D3 obtained from those of markers 6 (D6) and 3 (D3) for the backward bending.

The third variable was the asynergy index. It was calculated either from the absolute value of the time lag between the respective V_{max} occurrences (tV3-tV5) obtained from the velocity curves of markers 3 (tV3) and 5 (tV5) for the forward

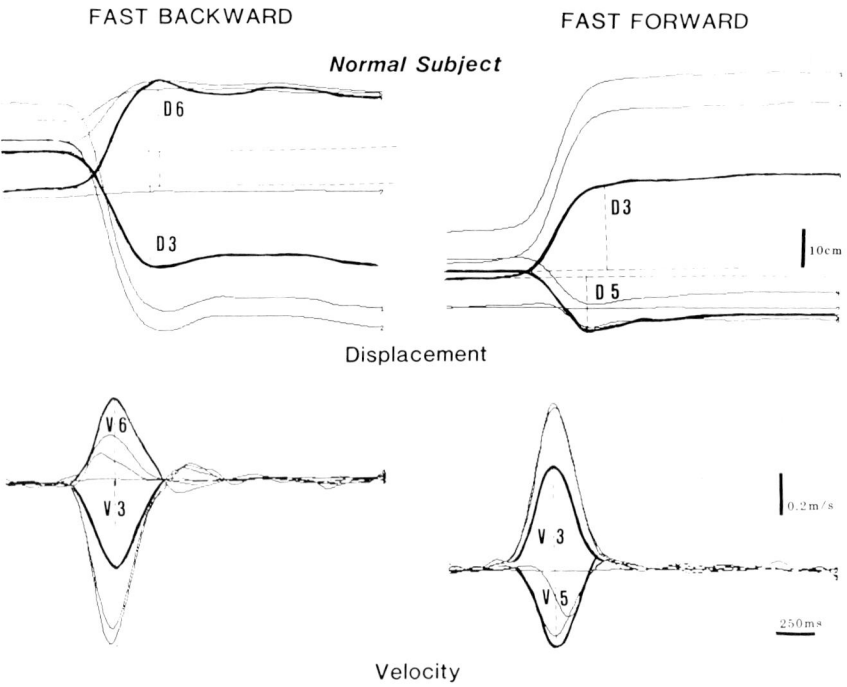

FIG. 3. Displacements and velocity curves for each marker as a function of time in a normal subject performing the movement as fast as possible. The traces corresponding to markers 3 and 5 (forward) and markers 3 and 6 (backward) are thickened and the values of the displacement (D) and maximal velocity (V) are displayed.

bending or from the absolute value of the time lag between the respective V_{max} occurrences (tV3-tV6) obtained from the velocity curves of markers 3 (tV3) and 6 (tV6) for the backward one.

The statistical analysis was made by using a nonparametric method (Mann-Whitney U) to compare the data from the patients and the normal subjects.

RESULTS

Fast Movements

Stick Diagrams (Figs. 2 and 4)

In normal subjects, as described by Crenna et al. (4), forward and backward upper trunk movements were accompanied by hip and knee displacements in the opposite direction. As illustrated in Fig. 2, it can be seen that with forward movements, the three upper markers moved forward, whereas the three lower ones moved backward. The reverse was observed with backward movements, that is, the three upper markers moved backward, whereas the three lower moved forward.

During forward bending, the excursion of the hip (markers 4 and 5) and knee (marker 6) were usually lower than that of the shoulder (marker 3). Knee displacement was comparable to that of the hip. With backward bending, the same qualitative aspects were observed. However, the excursion of the knee was always larger than that of the hips.

In cerebellar patients, the same type of axial coordination was observed, but as suggested by Fig. 4, some striking differences were observed when looking at the quantitative aspects of the movement. A marked reduction of the displacements of the lower markers was seen, particularly with backward bending.

Displacement and Velocity Curves (Figs. 3 and 5, Table 1)

In normal subjects, the range of the V_{max} (marker 3) was between 0.5 and 0.8 m/sec in the forward movement and 0.4 to 0.6 m/sec in the backward movement. In patients, the velocity curves showed many differences from the normal subjects. The main differences were the dramatic slowing of movement with a tendency toward asymmetry of the velocity curves. The range of the V_{max} was between 0.2 and 0.4 m/sec in forward bending and between 0.15 and 0.35 m/sec in backward bending. The mean values were 609 ± 100 mm/sec in forward bending and 469 ± 97 mm/sec in backward bending in normal subjects, whereas in the patients, these values were 326 ± 78 mm/sec and 205 ± 75 mm/sec, respectively. The statistical comparison showed a significant difference between normal subjects and patients in both situations: forward bending ($Z = 4.86$; $p < 0.000005$) and backward bending ($Z = 4.36$; $p < 0.00005$).

The coordination index in normal subjects had a mean value of 56.5 ± 9.6 in

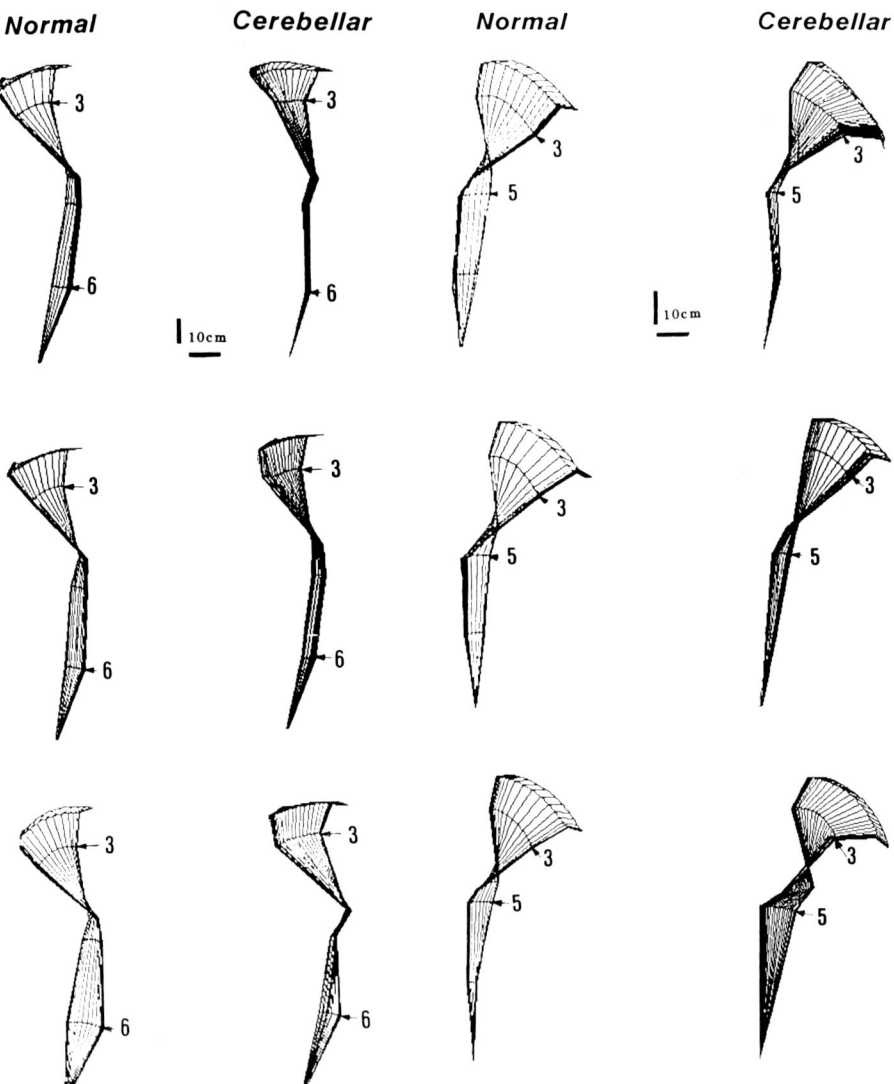

FIG. 4. Stick diagrams of normal subjects and cerebellar patients performing the movements as fast as possible. **Right**: Forward bending; **left**, backward bending (marker 3, shoulder; marker 5, hip; marker 6, knee).

forward bending and 67.8 ± 20.6 in backward bending. In patients the values were 47.4 ± 21.6 and 34.1 ± 21.1, respectively. The statistical analysis between normal subjects and patients showed a significant difference in backward bending ($Z = 3.81$; $p < 0.0005$) and in forward bending ($Z = 2.31$; $p < 0.05$).

The asynergy index showed a striking increase in patients. Actually, in normal subjects the mean values were 17 ± 19 msec in forward bending and 14 ± 22 msec in

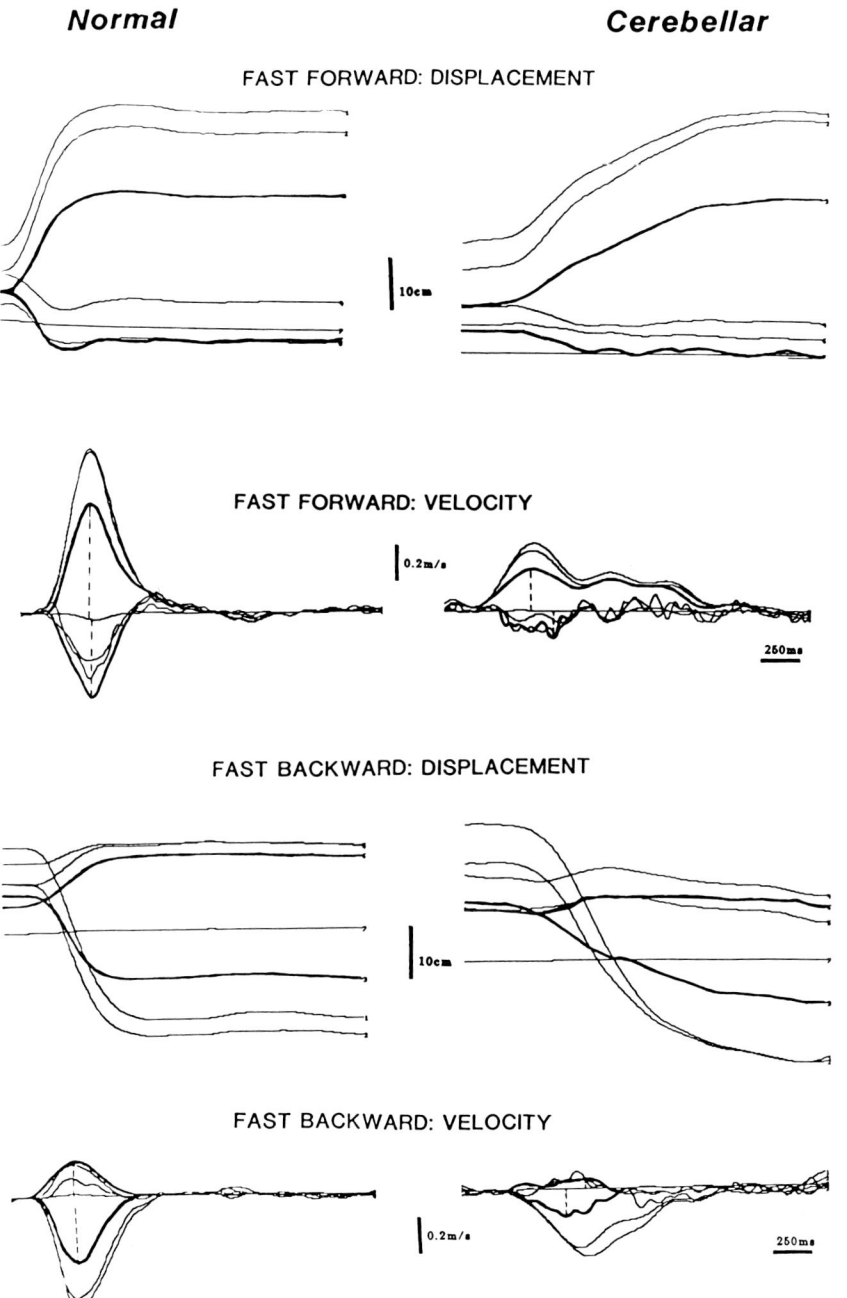

FIG. 5. Displacement and velocity curves of a normal subject and cerebellar patient performing the movement as fast as possible. The traces of markers 3 and 5 (forward) and markers 3 and 6 (backward) are thickened.

TABLE 1.

	Forward			Backward		
	V_{max} (mm/sec)	Coordination index (%)	Asynergy index (msec)	V_{max} (mm/sec)	Coordination index (%)	Asynergy index (msec)
Fast						
Controls ($N=3$)	609 ± 100	56.5 ± 9.6	17 ± 19	469 ± 97	67.8 ± 20.6	14 ± 22
Patients ($N=3$)	326 ± 78	47.4 ± 21.6	103 ± 91	205 ± 75	34.1 ± 21.0	130 ± 105
Z	4.86^a	2.31^b	3.94^a	4.36^a	3.81^a	3.93^a
Slow						
Controls ($N=3$)	244 ± 62	41.7 ± 12.3	109 ± 120	160 ± 42	42.8 ± 16.1	107 ± 94
Patients ($N=3$)	190 ± 63	42.8 ± 16.1	230 ± 154	170 ± 53	33.1 ± 22.6	307 ± 271
Z	1.15^c	0.07^c	2.21^b	0.22^c	1.30^c	2.17^b

Values are means ± SD. V_{max}, maximal velocity of marker 3. Coordination index, ratios D5/D3 (forward), D6/D3 (backward). Asynergy index, (tV3-tV5) (forward), (tV3-tV6) (backward).
$^a p<0.001$.
$^b p<0.05$.
$^c p>0.05$, no significance.

backward bending, whereas in patients these values were 103 ± 91 and 130 ± 105 msec, respectively. The statistical comparison between normal subjects and patients showed a significant difference in both situations: forward bending ($Z=3.94$; $p<0.0001$) and backward bending ($Z=3.93$; $p<0.0001$).

Slow Movements

Stick Diagrams (Fig. 6)

There were only some slight differences with respect to fast movement data. In fact, as mentioned previously (4), in normal subjects a small reduction in the compensatory displacement of the lower markers was only observed. The patients did

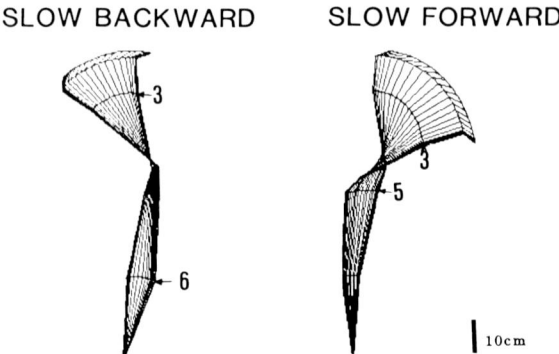

FIG. 6. Stick diagrams of a normal subject performing the movement at the slow rate (within 1.5 sec). Marker 3, shoulder; marker 5, hip; marker 6, knee).

not show any noticeable differences, probably because their velocities were grossly equivalent during the fast and slow movements.

Displacement and Velocity Curves (Fig. 7, Table 1)

The mean values of the V_{max} were 244 ± 62 mm/sec in the forward movement and 160 ± 42 mm/sec in the backward one in normal subjects, whereas these values were 190 ± 63 and 170 ± 53 mm/sec, respectively, in patients. There was no statistical difference between normal subjects and patients (forward bending: $Z = 1.15$; $p > 0.2$; backward bending: $Z = 0.22$; $p > 0.5$).

The coordination index in normal subjects had a mean value of 41.7 ± 12.3 in forward bending and 39.9 ± 18.3 in backward bending, whereas these values were 42.8 ± 16.1 and 33.1 ± 22.6, respectively, in the patients. The statistical analysis failed to show any significant difference between normal subjects and patients (forward bending: $Z = 0.07$; $p > 0.5$; backward bending: $Z = 1.30$; $p > 0.1$).

The asynergy index had, respectively, mean values of 109 ± 120 and 107 ± 94 msec in normal subjects and 230 ± 154 and 307 ± 271 msec in cerebellar patients.

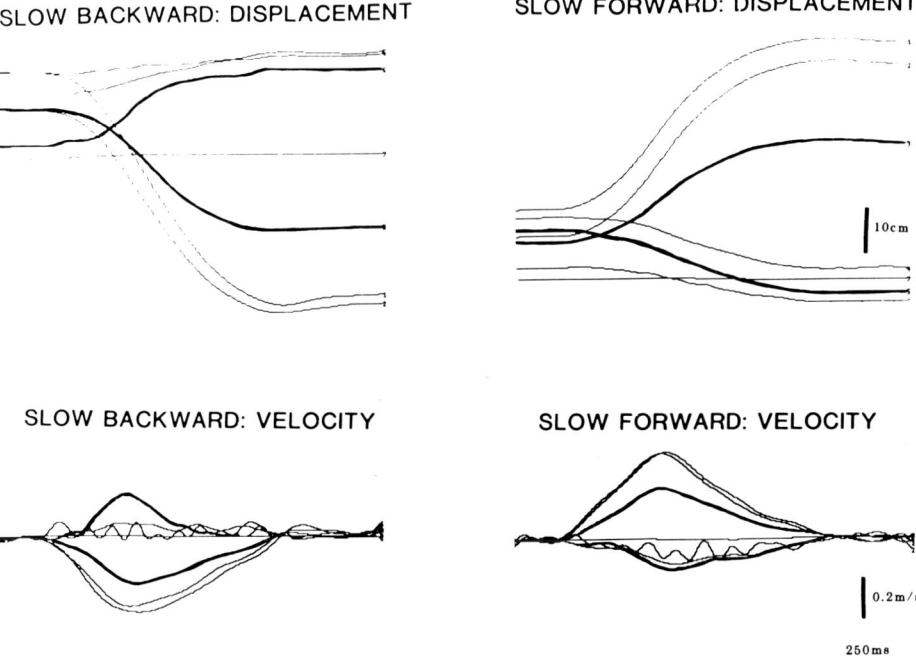

FIG. 7. Displacement and velocity curves for each marker as a function of time in a normal subject performing the movement at a slow rate (within 1.5 sec). The traces of markers 3 and 5 (forward) and 3 and 6 (backward) are thickened.

The statistical analysis showed a significant difference between normal and patients not only in forward bending ($Z=2.21$; $p<0.05$) but also in backward bending ($Z=2.17$; $p<0.05$).

DISCUSSION

The data presented here clearly show some disturbances in postural control during upper trunk bending in cerebellar patients. This impairment was assessed with the aid of three variables: the maximum value of the velocity of the shoulder (V_{max}), the coordination index (D5/D3 and D6/D3, respectively for forward and backward bending), and the asynergy index ([tV3-tV5] and [tV3-tV6], respectively, for forward and backward bending).

It should be stressed that this impairment was clearly observed when the axial upper trunk bending was performed at the fastest rate. Actually, all the patients exhibited a marked slowing of the movement when compared to controls. Despite this decrease in velocity, two of three patients failed to smoothly coordinate the displacement of their body segments and, as a consequence, showed a significant decrease in their coordination index. Finally, all the patients showed a significant increase in their asynergy index: this latter result suggests an impairment of the timing between the upper and lower parts of the body. This time lag seems to correspond to the postural asynergy previously described (1), which has been suggested to be a cardinal feature of cerebellar dysfunction (3). During the slower condition (movement performed within 1.5 msec), no significant changes were noted between patients and controls: actually, the velocity of the movement was the same in both groups, as instructed. It was interesting to note that, at this slower rate, the coordination index was not significantly modified between patients and controls, whereas the value of the asynergy index still remained significantly greater in patients than in controls. In fact, in simulation experiments of upper trunk forward bending, a displacement in the opposite direction of the hip and knee can be observed as a result of reaction forces exerted by the upper segment on the lower one; however, this mechanically induced displacement is always delayed (11).

These data suggest some comments concerning the movement disorder exhibited by the cerebellar patients. The first aspect is the slowing of movement. It might correspond to a motor strategy used by the patients according to their expectation of equilibrium control. Actually, the aim of postural coordination is to maintain the stability of the center of gravity (9). During daily life, chronic cerebellar patients can experience imbalance when walking and performing limb or trunk displacements. Consequently, they have to adapt their movement velocity to their disability. Two alternative explanations can be proposed: first, the slowing of the upper trunk movement would allow the mechanically induced opposite hip displacement (11) to take place and to prevent falling; second, the slowing of the movement would allow a kind of "discontinuous" movement to be performed, this pattern of movement corresponding to a small initial impulse that can be repeated and relies more on feedback control (2).

The second aspect is the decrease in the coordination index when compared to controls. Two patients exhibited this impairment, whereas the third did not. It would seem that, in these two patients, the slowing strategy is insufficient to keep the coordination index in the normal range, although in the third patient, this strategy is associated with a normal coordination index, which suggests a maintenance of postural coordination. However, when looking at his stick diagrams, it appears that another strategy has taken place (Fig. 8). This strategy consists of a locking of the pelvis orientation (markers 4 and 5). During forward upper trunk bending, he makes a backward translation of the axis 4-5, thus reducing the displacement of marker 3. During backward upper trunk bending, he maintains the position of the axis 4-5 without any translation or rotation. Another comment concerns the differences between the data obtained with forward versus backward bending. It would seem that, in the patients, the coordination index decreases more in backward than in forward bending. Such data confirm the importance of the motor strategy in this postural coordination. Actually, the patients expected a greater impairment in their equilibrium control during backward bending, which is unusual, than during forward bending, which is experienced daily and corresponds to a well-learned movement. As a consequence, the patients tend to increase their axial stiffness instead of coordinating the displacement of their lower body part with the upper trunk movement. This hypothesis has to be confirmed by further studies recording the ground forces during the axial bending.

The last aspect is the increase in the asynergy index. It is interesting to note that it is significantly increased in patients not only during the fast movements but also during the slow movements, whereas the two other variables (V_{max}, coordination

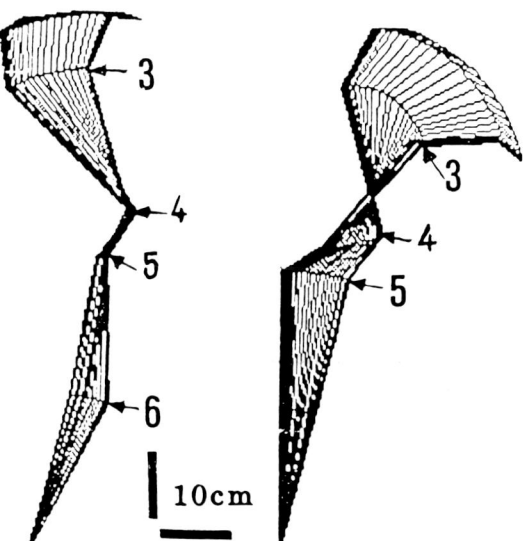

FIG. 8. Stick diagrams of the cerebellar patient having a coordination index within the normal range when performing the movement as fast as possible (see text for comments). Marker 3, shoulder; marker 4, anterior iliac crest; marker 5, trochanter; marker 6, knee.

index) become equivalent between controls and patients during the slow movements. These data suggest that the asynergy index is strongly linked to the cerebellar dysfunction since it seems to still be increased whatever the movement speed.

Beyond these phenomenological aspects of postural asynergy, the data presented here suggest that, in the future, such a quantitative study of cerebellar asynergy might be used particularly for the assessment of the effect of drugs. In cerebellar pathology, previous works have been concerned with the assessment of L-5-hydroxytryptophan (L-5-HTP): actually, some clinical investigations have shown the improvement of cerebellar ataxia by L-5-HTP (12–15), although some controversial results have been reported (8). It must be mentioned that an assessment of the effects of L-5-HTP has also been previously carried out in cerebellar patients (16) when measuring the postural sway and has shown an improvement of cerebellar ataxia with L-5-HTP. In this context, this new technique dealing with the quantitative assessment of postural coordination could become a useful tool for testing the effect of any drug, such as L-5-HTP, that is supposed to be efficient in the control of cerebellar ataxia.

APPENDIX

Case 1: M.B. was born in 1924. Her clinical history began in 1974 with gait and coordination disturbances. Her medical status in 1991 was stable and she could walk without help. Her examination showed a static cerebellar syndrome with a slight kinetic component and brisk tendon reflexes. A computed tomography (CT) scan performed in 1987 showed atrophy of the vermis, which was further confirmed on magnetic resonance imaging (MRI) in 1991. The same symptomatology was found in her older brother, whose clinical history began at the age of 60, and in her twin heterozygote sister.

Case 2: A.B. was born in 1950. In 1988 she began to complain of gait disturbance due to a static cerebellar syndrome associated with a slight kinetic component. The investigations included standard tests, electroencephalogram, lumbar puncture, evoked potentials and were normal. A CT scan and MRI performed in November 1990 showed atrophy of the vermis. No familial history was found. Her clinical status in 1991 was very stable.

Case 3: J.P.R. was born in 1943. The symptomatology began in 1977 with gait disturbances. His examination revealed an isolated static cerebellar syndrome associated with a mild kinetic component. The static cerebellar syndrome affected mainly the lower limbs. The symptomatology has progressively worsened since then. To date in 1991 he could walk without any help. In 1987 MRI had shown atrophy of the vermis. A similar history has been found in his family on his mother's side including his mother, grandmother, great aunt, and great uncle.

REFERENCES

1. Babinski J. De l'asynergie cérébelleuse. *Rev Neurol (Paris)* 1899;7:806–816.
2. Brooks VB. Motor program revisited. In: Talbott RE, Humphrey DR, eds. *Posture and movement.* New York: Raven Press, 1979:13–49.
3. Brooks VB, Thach WT. Cerebellar control of posture and movements. In: Brooks VB, ed. *Handbook of physiology: the nervous system*, vol II, part 1. Bethesda, Maryland: American Physiological Society, 1981:877–945.

4. Crenna P, Frigo C, Massion J, Pedotti A. Forward and backward axial synergies in man. *Exp Brain Res* 1987;65:538–548.
5. Ferrigno F, Pedotti A. ELITE: a digital dedicated hardware system for movement analysis via real time TV signal processor. *IEEE Trans Biomed Eng* 1985;32 (11).
6. Harding AE. *The hereditary ataxias and related disorders*. Edinburgh: Churchill Livingstone, 1984.
7. Holmes G. The symptoms of acute cerebellar injuries due to gunshot injuries. *Brain* 1917;40:461–535.
8. Klein P, Lees A, Stern G. Consequences of chronic 5-HT in parkinsonian instability of gait and balance and in other neurological disorders. In: Yahr MD, Bergmann KJ, eds. *Parkinson's disease (Advances in neurology*, vol 45). New York: Raven Press, 1987;603–604.
9. Massion J. Fonctions motrices. *Encyclopédie médicochirurgicale* (Paris), vol 1. 1984:17002 D10–11.
10. Massion J, Viallet F. Posture, coordination, mouvement. *Rev Neurol (Paris)* 1990;146:536–542.
11. Ramos CF, Stark LW. Simulation experiments can shed light on the functional aspects of postural adjustments related to voluntary movements. In: Winters JM, Woo L-Y, eds. *Multiple muscle systems: biomechanics and movement organization*. New York: Springer-Verlag, 1990:507–517.
12. Rascol A, Clanet M, Montastruc JL, Delage W, Guiraud-Chaumeil B. L-5HTP in the cerebellar syndrome treatment. *Biomedicine*, 1981;35:112–113.
13. Trouillas P, Brudon F, Adeleine P. Improvement of cerebellar ataxia with levorotatory form of 5-hydroxytryptophan: double blind study with quantified data processing. *Arch Neurol* 1988;45:1217–1222.
14. Trouillas P, Garde A, Robert JM, Adeleine P. Régression de l'ataxie cérébelleuse humaine sous administration à long terme de 5-hydroxytryptophane. *C R Acad Sci Paris* 1981;292:119–122.
15. Trouillas P, Garde A, Robert JM, et al. Régression du syndrome cérébelleux sous administration à long term de 5-HTP ou de l'association 5-HTP-bensérazide. *Rev Neurol (Paris)* 1982;138:415–435.
16. Wessel K, Diener HC, Dichgans J. Long loop reflexes and postural ataxia: follow up study with and without treatment by 5-HT in patients with Friedreich's ataxia. In: Amblard B, Berthoz A, Clarac F, eds. *Posture and gait*. Amsterdam: Elsevier, 1988:237–244.

*Serotonin, the Cerebellum,
and Ataxia*, edited by
P. Trouillas and K. Fuxe.
Raven Press, Ltd., New York © 1993.

29

Interest in L-5-HTP Administration in the Rehabilitation Course of Patients with Cerebellar Ataxia

D. Boisson, G. Rode, and C. Froment

*Service de Rééducation Fonctionnelle, Hôpital Henry Gabrielle,
69230 Saint Genis Laval, France*

Trouillas et al. (3–5) have shown that some features of human cerebellar ataxia, particularly postural equilibrium and dysarthria, can be partially regressive with long-term administration of L-5-hydroxytryptophan (L-5-HTP). This effect has been confirmed by Rascol et al. (2). In this study, patients were impaired by cerebellar ataxia mainly due to degenerative or inflammatory diseases.

In neurological rehabilitation, patients with cerebellar ataxia present a serious incapacity that can be worsened by other neurological defects (sensorimotor, visual, or cognitive). In these cases, classical rehabilitation techniques usually fail to improve the neurological state.

Thus, we have taken an interest in L-5-HTP administration to improve the functional outcome.

PATIENTS AND METHODS

Patients

Eleven patients (nine men and two women) with cerebellar ataxia were included in this study. The mean age was 43.4 ± 22.8 (20–69 years). All the patients included had a predominantly disabling cerebellar ataxia. For clinical data, see Table 1.

Parameters

For each patient, four parameters have been studied twice: before and after treatment: (i) functional ataxia score, as proposed by Trouillas et al. (5); (ii) time param-

TABLE 1. Clinical data of the population of patients

Cases	Age (years)	Delay	Static component	Kinetic component	Etiology	Other neurological disorders
R.F.	20	1 month	Absent	Bilateral	Brain stem angioma	Right hemiplegia, Foville's syndrome, internuclear ophthalomoplegia
D.N.	26	4 months	Present	Bilateral	Posttrauma brain stem injury	Tetrapyramidal syndrome
M.S.	26	10 months	Present	Bilateral	Posttrauma brain stem injury	Right hemiplegia, left III palsy
D.G.	65	2 months	Present	Right	Right ischemic cerebellar lesion	
S.R.	50	3 months	Present	Absent	Brain stem ischemic stroke	Complete Wallenberg's syndrome
T.P.	62	1.5 years	Present	Bilateral	Brain stem ischemic stroke	Right hemiplegia
D.S.	42	2.5 years	Present	Right	Brain stem ischemic stroke	Incomplete Wallenberg's syndrome
A.R.	69	4 years	Present	Right	Brain stem ischemic stroke	Incomplete Wallenberg's syndrome
G.M.	50	1 year	Present	Absent	Brain stem ischemic stroke	Complete Wallenberg syndrome
F.A.	68	1 month	Present	Right	Hypertensive brain stem hematoma	Right hemiplegia
W.M.	52	1 year	Present	Absent	Hypertensive brain stem hematoma	Right hemiplegia, left V palsy

eters including time to walk a distance of 12 m, time to stand up, and time to speak the classical French phrase *l'espieglerie du spectacle tchécoslovaque*; (iii) posturography with a statokinesimeter (1); subjective evaluation. Six measurements were performed for every test.

Treatment

Each patient had 10 mg/kg per day of the levorotatory form of 5-HT with 150 mg of a peripheral 5-hydroxycarboxylase inhibitor (benserazide) for 2 months.

Method

This study was prospective but without a control group. All patients were examined by the same observer before and after treatment. The means of pre- and post-therapeutic measures were compared by t test for eight patients. Three patients were excluded due to other pathological events.

RESULTS

Functional Ataxia Score

A significant difference was observed only for the static score ($p<0.05$). The improvement concerned mainly the patients with severe initial score (see Fig. 1).

Time Parameters

Statistical analysis showed a significant reduction of time parameters following treatment for the time of standing ($p<0.05$) and the time of speech ($p<0.0001$). No difference was observed for the time of walking (see Table 2).

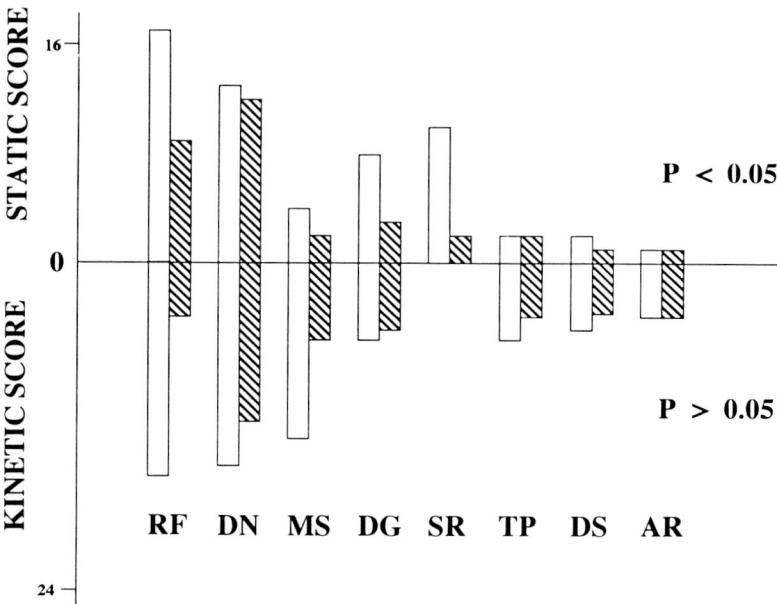

FIG. 1. Functional ataxia scores from eight patients before (*open columns*) and after (*hatched columns*) L-5-HTP–benserazide administration. The results of the comparison of the means of the scores before and after treatment of these eight patients are given on the right.

TABLE 2. *Comparison of the means of time parameters of eight patients before and after L-5-HTP–benserazide administration*

Task	Before treatment	After treatment
Time to walk[a]	37.7 ± 12.8	32 ± 7.2
Time to stand up[a]	4.2 ± 2.2	2.6 ± 1.1
Time to pronounce standard sentence[a]	4.4 ± 1.5	3.6 ± 1.1

[a] In seconds.

Posturography

In spite of an interesting improvement in posturographs, the comparison of the means of the sway area, which account for the pressure changes (Kg) before and after trial, was not significant.

Subjective Analysis

Improvement was observed for two patients in drawing Archimedes' spiral and writing a sentence (see Fig. 2).

DISCUSSION

Our results are not strong enough to conclude that administration of L-5-HTP–benserazide significantly improves the functional outcome of patients with cerebellar ataxia. However, several results deserve to be emphasized:

1. A dramatic improvement was reported for two patients (R.F. and M.S.). For patient M.S. (posttraumatic brain stem injury), the treatment was given a long time after the trauma. The interruption of treatment was immediately followed by an increase in ataxia. These two patients (R.F. and M.S.) chose to continue the treatment.

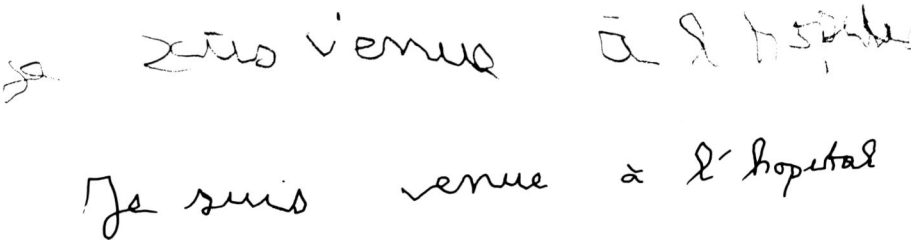

FIG. 2. Improvement in writing a sentence in a patient (M.S.) with L-5-HTP–benserazide administration.

2. Improvement was more significant in static components and dysarthria than kinetic components. However, this effect, in our small population, has not been confirmed by posturography data.

3. Five patients presented some gastrointestinal side effects (mild enough to allow the treatment). Surprisingly the most atactic patients had the best tolerance of the treatment.

Although the number of patients was too small for the results to be conclusive, we think that L-5-HTP–benserazide could have a use in the rehabilitation of patients with severe cerebellar ataxia.

REFERENCES

1. Crosbie WJ, Nimmo MA, Banks MA, et al. Standing balance responses in two populations of ederly women: a pilot study. *Arch Phys Med Rehab* 1989;70:751–754.
2. Rascol A, Clanet M, Montastruc JL, et al. L-5-Hydroxytryptophan in the cerebellar syndrome treatment. *Biomedecine* 1981;35:112–113.
3. Trouillas P, Garde A, Robert JM, et al. Régression du syndrome cérébelleux sous administration à long terme du L-5HTP ou de l'association 5-HTP-bensérazide: vingt-cinq observations quantifiées et traitées par ordinateur. *Rev Neurol (Paris)* 1980;12:891.
4. Trouillas P, Garde A, Robert JM, et al. Régression de l'ataxie cérébelleuse humaine sous administration à long terme de 5-hydrotryptophane. *C R Acad Sci* 1981;292:119–122.
5. Trouillas P, Brudon F, Adeleine P. Improvement of cerebellar ataxia with levorotatory form of 5-hydroxytryptophan. *Arch Neurol* 1988;45:1217–1222.

30

Continuous Subcutaneous Lisuride Infusion in Olivopontocerebellar Atrophies

L. Schöls, A. Heinz, M. Langkafel, J. Wöhrle, and H. Przuntek

Neurologische Universitätsklinik im St. Josef Hospital, D-4630 Bochum, Germany

The olivopontocerebellar atrophies (OPCA) are a heterogeneous group of degenerative diseases involving atrophy of the cerebellar cortex, a loss of cells in the inferior olives, and a shrinkage of the ventral parts of the pons (1). Apart from these regularly affected structures, many other systems like the cerebellar vermis and nuclei, the long tracts of the spinal cord, the peripheral nerves, and the cerebral cortex are involved to some extent. The frequency of extrapyramidal system involvement differs a lot depending on the kind of the investigation. Pathological studies find degenerative changes of the substantia nigra in about 80% of cases (2). From the clinical point of view rigidity and akinesia are obvious in about 10% to 20% (2–4). In a small number of patients parkinsonism is the major symptom.

In patients suffering from both cerebellar and nigrostriatal degeneration, the combination of ataxia with rigidity and akinesia causes a potentiation of disability. This is the reason for the poor prognosis of the disease if not treated. Treatment with levodopa (5), amantadine, and dopaminergic drugs (6) has been shown to be helpful. Nevertheless they are often not sufficient.

We examined the effect of continuous subcutaneous application of the ergot derivate lisuride hydrogen maleate by a small external pump. We used MRS 2 pumps (Disetronic AG, Burgdorf, Switzerland), which are comparable to the insulin infusion pumps used in diabetes. The subcutaneous lisuride infusion combines the advantages of parenteral medication with the advantages of permanent monoaminergic stimulation. It minimizes fluctuations in motility during the day and allows a more intense monoaminergic stimulation compared to oral treatment: Much higher daily doses are tolerated before side effects arise when lisuride is given in a continuous subcutaneous manner. When comparing oral with subcutaneous doses, one has to take into account that 1 mg of subcutaneous lisuride has a comparable effect to 3 to 10 mg of the oral preparation.

Treatment with subcutaneous lisuride is possible even if patients have severe difficulties in swallowing, and it is independent from changes in bowel motility and intestinal absorption.

Lisuride influences a broad spectrum of monoaminergic receptors (Table 1). In the dopaminergic system it acts as a D_2 agonist and a partial D_1 antagonist with agonistic elements (7,8). In the serotonergic system there are hints of a $5-HT_{1A}$ agonistic effect (9), at least in the raphe (10), hippocampus, and cortex (11). Apart from that, it works as an antagonist at the $5-HT_2$ receptor, as demonstrated by the stimulation of male rat sexual behavior in the animal model (12). At the $5-HT_3$ receptor lisuride shows a high affinity, but its function is still not known. At adrenoceptors it has the role of a partially selective α_2 receptor antagonist. But in high concentrations it is an antagonist at α_1 and even at β receptors as well (13).

In comparison to other dopamine agonists, like bromocriptine, lisuride differs principally by its serotonergic component. As the serotonergic system is thought to be irritated in OPCA (14), lisuride is an especially interesting drug to be tested in this disease.

We treated four patients with OPCA with severe symptoms of parkinsonism. Table 2 shows the clinical data of our four patients: There were three female and one male patients. No patient had a family history of OPCA, and in no case had a primary cause of the multisystem degeneration been found. In all patients diagnosis was confirmed by computed tomography and magnetic resonance imaging findings.

All four patients had the late-onset type of OPCA. Symptoms started between the ages of 44 and 61. The initial signs varied: In the patients E.A. and K.B., an akinetic, rigid Parkinson's syndrome was diagnosed in the beginning, while patient M.B. presented first with tremor of the hands, followed soon by gait ataxia and dysphagia. Patient B.F. initially showed typical signs of a system-overlapping cerebellar degeneration like ataxia of gait and stance, cerebellar dysarthria, and hyperactive tendon reflexes.

During the course of the disease the involvement of several neural systems became obvious in all patients. Some of the symptoms are listed in the last column of Table 2. There were signs of extrapyramidal and cerebellar damage in all four

TABLE 1. *Effects of lisuride at monoaminergic receptors*

Dopaminergic receptors (high affinity)
  D_1 receptor: partial antagonist/partial agonist
  D_2 receptor: agonist
Serotonergic receptors
  $5-HT_{1A}$ receptor: strong agonist
  $5-HT_2$ receptor: strong antagonist
  $5-HT_3$ receptor: high affinity; effect not known
Adrenoceptors
  α_1 receptor: antagonist
  α_2 receptor: antagonist
  Potency of α_2 antagonism $\gg$ α_1 antagonism
  β receptors: antagonist in high concentrations

TABLE 2. *Patients*

Patient	Sex	Age at baseline (years)	Disease duration	Clinical signs	Main problems at baseline	Improvement	Side effects at overdose
E.A.	F	58	5	Initially: akinesia, rigor; later: gait ataxia, hypotension, incontinence	Rigor + akinesia → anarthria; wheelchair bound; unable to look after herself	Speech partially comprehensible; walks with help; improved manual skills	Dysphagia → aspiration + pneumonia; dizziness
M.B.	F	56	10	Initially: tremor; later: gait ataxia, dysarthria	Rigor, akinesia + ataxia → anarthria; wheelchair bound; dependent on help; severe dysphagia	Speech partially comprehensible; rigor decreased; improved manual skills	Deterioration of dysarthria + dysphagia; hyperkinesia
K.B.	M	69	8	Initially: akinesia, rigor; later: cerebellar ataxia and dysarthria	Permanent "off"; anarthria; wheelchair bound	5 hr "on"; speech partially comprehensible; walks with small steps; participates in family life	Dysphagia; increase in libido; psychosis
B.F.	F	60	7	Initially: gait and stance ataxia; dysarthria; later: parkinsonism	Akinesia, rigor → wheelchair bound; speech partially incomprehensible; hygiene with help;	Walks with small steps; speech monotoneous but comprehensible; hygiene alone	

patients. Apart from that, pyramidal signs have been seen in three patients and orthostatic dysregulation and incontinence in two patients.

At the time lisuride application by pump was started, rigidity and akinesia had become the most disabling problems in all four patients. At that time they all were wheelchair bound. Three patients had completely incomprehensible speech, and the speech of B.F. was partially incomprehensible. M.B. and B.F. were dependent on some help for activities of daily living like hygiene, dressing, and feeding, while E.A. and K.B. were completely unable to look after themselves.

Before the trial with the lisuride infusion pumps was started, all patients had been treated with oral antiparkinsonian drugs for several years. The medication is shown in Table 3. All patients received levodopa and selegeline, a monoamine oxidase B inhibitor, in almost constant doses during the whole time of the trial. Two patients took bromocriptine in a daily dose of 25 mg, and one patient received 1.0 mg of oral lisuride in the beginning. This oral dopamine agonist medication was stopped when lisuride infusion was started.

Subcutaneous lisuride was given in a continuous regimen. Most patients had a step-like pump profile with maximum dosage during the day and a reduced flow over night.

All patients benefited from the continuous subcutaneous application of lisuride. We tried to estimate the changes with the King's College Hospital Parkinson's Disease Rating Scale (KCH-PDRS). This score mainly concerns symptoms of parkinsonism like facial expression, seborrhea, salivation, posture, tremor, and rigidity. Nevertheless, it is a quite useful score for OPCA because it assesses disability as a whole with parameters like speech, writing, hygiene, feeding, dressing, and going to bed.

Figure 1 gives a graphic impression of the improvement. The patients were scored three times: First at baseline, before the lisuride infusion started, a second time after dose titration at the time of hospital discharge, and a third time after 6 months at home, when all the hospital specific effects could be expected to have disappeared.

In all four patients score values improved remarkably. Looking at the mean value of the four patients, the score dropped from 85.25 before lisuride infusion to 74.5 at discharge from the hospital. This is a significant improvement (Wilcoxon test: $p = 0.03$). After 6 months of treatment two patients had improved even a little more; M.B. kept stable and E.A. worsened minimally. The mean value improved a little more to 70.25.

In practical terms this improvement in the score manifested as follows (Table 2): E.A.'s speech became comprehensible, although with some remaining difficulties. She was able to walk with help on the ward. The manual skills improved greatly, e.g., washing was possible with little help. Posture, stability, rigidity, and salivation improved partially.

M.B.'s speech also became partially comprehensible so that communication became possible again. The finger skills became good enough to take a bath and get herself dressed with some help, although this took her a long time in the morning.

TABLE 3. *Medication and Parkinson score*

Patient	Medication at baseline	Score	Medication when side effects increased intolerably	Score	Medication at hospital discharge	Score	Medication after 6 months of treatment	Score
E.A.	Levodopa 600 mg; selegiline 10 mg; lisuride oral 1 mg	80	Levodopa 600 mg; selegiline 10 mg; lisuride s.c. 1.0 mg	67	Levodopa 600 mg; selegiline 5 mg; lisuride s.c. 0.6 mg	67	Levodopa 600 mg; selegiline 5 mg; lisuride s.c. 0.6 mg	69
M.B.	Levodopa 350 mg; selegiline 5 mg; amantadine 300 mg; bromocriptine 20 mg	82	Levodopa 350 mg; selegiline 5 mg; amantadine 300 mg; lisuride s.c. 1.1 mg		Levodopa 350 mg; selegiline 5 mg; amantadine 300 mg; lisuride s.c. 0.8 mg	64	Levodopa 350 mg; selegiline 5 mg; amantadine 300 mg; lisuride s.c. 0.8 mg	64
K.B.	Levodopa 650 mg; selegiline 7.5 mg; bromocriptine 22.5 mg	90	Levodopa 650 mg; selegiline 7.5 mg; lisuride s.c. 1.2 mg		Levodopa 650 mg; selegiline 7.5 mg; lisuride s.c. 0.6 mg	84	Levodopa 400 mg; selegiline 7.5 mg; lisuride s.c. 0.5 mg	72
B.F.	Levodopa 475 mg; selegiline 5 mg	89	—		Levodopa 475 mg; selegiline 5 mg; lisuride s.c. 0.5 mg	83	Levodopa 475 mg; selegiline 5 mg; lisuride s.c. 0.5 mg	76

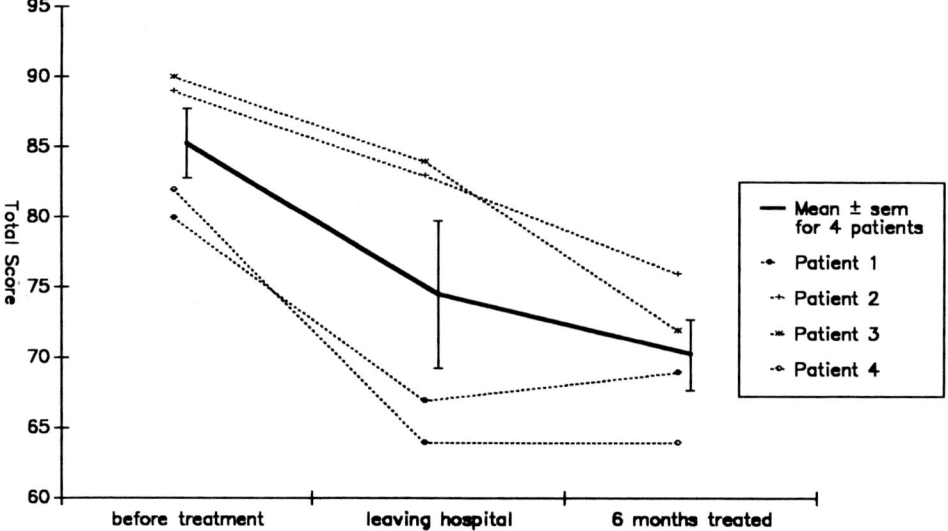

FIG. 1. Improvement of parkinsonian disability in four patients with OPCA under continuous lisuride infusion scored with King's College Hospital's Parkinson's Disease Rating Scale.

K.B. was in a permanent off-period before lisuride infusion. Afterward he experienced on-periods of up to 5 hr per day. During this time he was able to walk with small steps, and his speech became partially comprehensible. Due to the lisuride pump he was able to participate in family life much better than before.

B.F.'s speech also improved and she was able to walk with small steps. She now managed to take care of her own hygiene.

Overall, quality of life of the patients improved remarkably. Lisuride dosage was limited by the side effects listed in Table 2. Some are strikingly different from those seen in classic parkinsonian patients. In three patients severe problems with dysphagia arose. The remarkable point is that swallowing improved first when lisuride dosage was increased slowly. But when a critical dose of 1.0 to 1.2 mg/day was reached, oropharyngeal dystonia developed and swallowing deteriorated suddenly and dramatically. We saw severe complications like pneumonia from aspiration. For that reason we had to reduce lisuride doses significantly to 0.6 to 0.8 mg/day.

In one patient (K.B.) mild nocturnal psychotic episodes had existed for years before the lisuride pump was given. He decompensated completely with a productive psychosis when lisuride was increased to 1.2 mg/day subcutaneously. Dose reduction to 0.6 mg/day diminished the problem; only vivid dreams remained.

K.B. also had signs of increased libido with exhibitionistic tendencies under high-dose treatment. This problem was again resolved by dose reduction.

Another tolerable side effect in all patients was the development of small subcutaneous nodules at the infusion sites.

We assume that the specific effects and side effects of lisuride in OPCA with parkinsonism are caused by the diverse modulations of monoaminergic receptors demonstrated before. The dopaminergic effects of lisuride explain the improvement in parkinsonism.

The increase in libido of patient K.B. is likely to be of serotonergic origin. It resembles the 5-HT_2-mediated effect of lisuride seen in the animal model.

Although lisuride has a chemical structure very similar to the hallucinogen LSD, we saw drug-induced psychosis in just one of four patients. The psychosis of patient K.B. is likely to be of dopaminergic, and not serotonergic, origin because it had existed before therapy with lisuride was started, while the patient was taking only dopaminergic drugs.

The influence of lisuride on the serotonergic system, especially in the brain stem nuclei, may play an important role for its striking effect on the ability to swallow, even more so if one considers that these effects were not seen with other dopaminergic drugs lacking a serotonergic component.

CONCLUSIONS

1. Continuous subcutaneous pump application of lisuride improves akinesia, rigidity, dysarthria, and dysphagia in OPCA better than oral dopaminergic treatment.
2. Drug-induced oropharyngeal dystonia limits clinical results.
3. We assume that lisuride is superior to other dopaminergic drugs because of its influence on the serotonergic system, which seems to be especially helpful in OPCA patients.

REFERENCES

1. Konigsmark BC, Weiner LP. The olivopontocerebellar atrophies: a review. *Medicine* 1970;227–241.
2. Jellinger K, Tarnowska-Dziduszko E. Die ZNS-Veränderungen bei den olivo-ponto-cerebellären Atrophien. *Z Neurol* 1971;199:192–214.
3. Harding AE. Idiopathic late onset cerebellar ataxia. *J Neurol Sci* 1981;51:259–271.
4. Harding AE. The clinical features and classification of the late onset autosomal dominant cerebellar ataxias. *Brain* 1981;105:1–28.
5. Klawans HL, Zeitlin E. Levodopa on parkinsonism associated with cerebellar dysfunction (probable olivopontocerebellar degeneration). *J Neurol Neurosurg Psychiatry* 1971;34:14–19.
6. Goetz CG, Tanner CM, Klawans HL. The pharmacology of OPCA. In: Duvoisin RC, Plaitakis A, eds. *The olivopontocerebellar atrophies*. New York: Raven Press, 1984:143–148.
7. Horowski R, Obeso JA. Lisuride: a direct dopamine agonist in the treatment of Parkinson's disease. In: Koller WC, Paulson G, eds. *Therapy in Parkinson's disease*. New York: Marcel Dekker, 1990: 269–309.
8. Palacios JM, Camps M, Cortes R, Charuchinda C. Characterisation and distribution of brain dopamine receptors. In: Jankovic J, Tolosa E, eds. *Parkinson's disease and movement disorders*. Baltimore: Urban and Schwarzenberg, 1988:27–36.
9. Kehr W. Effect of lisuride and ergot derivates on monoaminergic mechanism in rat brain. *Eur J Pharmacol* 1977;41:261–263.
10. Walters JR, Baring MD, Lakosi JM. Effects of ergolines on dopaminergic and serotonergic single

unit activity. In: Fuxe K, Calne DB. *Dopaminergic ergot derivates and motor function.* New York: Pergamon Press, 1979:207–221.
11. Rosenfeld MR, Makman MH. The interaction of lisuride, an ergot derivate, with serotonergic and dopaminergic receptors in rabbit brain. *J Pharmacol Exp Ther* 1981;216:526–531.
12. Ahlenius S, Larsson K. Antagonism by lisuride and 8-OH-DPAT of 5-HTP-induced prolongation of the performance of male rat sexual behavior. *Eur J Pharmacol* 1985;110:379–381.
13. McPherson GA. In vitro selectivity of lisuride and other ergot derivates for alpha$_1$-adrenoceptors. *Eur J Pharmacol* 1984;97:151–155.
14. Trouillas P. Improvement of cerebellar ataxia with levorotatory form of 5-hydroxytryptophan. *Arch Neurol* 1988;45:1217–1222.

Subject Index

A

Abducens nucleus, 45
Acetylcholine
  biological effect, 245–247
  in thiamine deficiency, 281
3-Acetylpyridine, neurotoxicity, 187–188, 270–276, 291–292
Adenylate cyclase, regulation, 205, 206
β-Adrenergic antagonist binding, 25
Adrenoceptors, lisuride effects, 364
Alcoholic ataxia, 314, 317–318, 320–321, 327
Alzheimer's disease
  5-HT in, 37, 74
  raphe nuclei in, 74
D-(−)-2-Amino-5-phosphonopentanoic acid, 159, 161
2-Amino-5-phosphonovalerate, 229–230
Amino acids, 5-HT interactions, 102–103, 104, 105, 109, 155–165
Amitriptyline, 197–198
Amyotrophic lateral sclerosis, 273
Angiotensin II IR, 29–31, 32
Angiotensinogen IR, 29
Angiotensin peptides, therapeutic uses, 30–31
Antidepressants, 191–192, 196, 198–199
Antiobsessional drugs, 198–199
Anxiolytics, 198–199
Aspartate
  5-HT interactions, 102–103, 105, 109, 155, 230–232
  Purkinje cell effects, 226–227
  in thiamine deficiency, 280, 282
Asynergy, defined, 343
Asynergy index, 346–347, 348, 350
Ataxia, cerebellar,
  3-acetylpyridine model, 270–274
  animal models, 270, 326–327
  cerebrospinal fluid abnormalities, 311–321, 327
  characterization, 323
  climbing fibers in, 296
  deficiency induced, 269–286
  5-HT mechanisms, 251, 282–286, 323–332,
  human models, 327–328
  monoaminergic paradigm, 316–318
  pathophysiology, 269–286
  pharmacological data, 328–332
  symptom assessment, 338–340, 343–354
  therapy, 29, 31, 33, 165, 209, 335–336, 337–341, 357–361
  thiamine-deficient model, 276–286
  tryptophan metabolism in, 328

B

B9 serotoninergic cell group, 239, 240
Baclofen, 214
Basic fibroblast growth factor IR, 29–31
Basket cells, immunoreactivity, 131, 132
Benserazide, 331, 337, 358–361
BMY-7378, 260, 262, 263
Bolton-Hunter-8-methoxy-2-(N-propyl-N-propyl-amino)tetralin, 180–183, 185–187
Brachium conjunctivum, 142
Brain
  amino acid levels, 280–283
  developmental disturbances, 74
  5-HT content, 241, 242
  5-HT systems, anatomy, 63–74
  protein synthesis, 307–309
Brain stem
  anatomy, human, 63–74
  5-HT content, 137–152
  5-HT receptors, 167–176
  MAO immunoreactive areas, human, 42–46
  neurons, 56–59
  PH8 immunoreactivity, 37–47
  raphe neurons, human, 37–47
Bromocriptine, 366, 367
Bulbar reticular neurons, 255–257
Buspirone, 246, 249, 257

C

Calbindin D-28k, 131, 132
Calcium conductance, 116–117
Calcium spikes, 214–216
Carbamazepine, 198
5-Carboxamidotryptamine, 213
Catecholamine nerve terminal networks, 10, 16, 19, 23
Caudal dorsal accessory nucleus, innervation, 113–115
Caudal medial accessory olivary nucleus, innervation, 113–115
Caudal mesencephalon, 70, 73
Caudal pons, 68–69
Caudal raphe nuclei, 5-HT neurons, 107–108
Caudal raphe subnuclei, 42
Caudate-putamen, 208
Central nervous system
  communication modes, 5–13
  computational mechanisms, 13
  dysfunction, neuronal loss, 297–298
  modulatory mechanisms, 225

Central nervous system (*contd.*)
  oscillation, 221–222
  resonance, 221–222
Cerebellar ataxia. *See* Ataxia, cerebellar
Cerebellar atrophy, therapy, 328–330, 340–341
Cerebellar cortex
  GAD immunoreactivity, 131, 132
  5-HT$_{1A}$ receptors, 188
  5-HT innervation, 59
  5-HT IR fiber distribution, 140
  5-HT neurons, 59–60
  5-HT source, 107–108
  5-HT uptake sites, 170
  innervation, 12, 59, 129–134, 298
  monoaminergic innervation, 298
  morphological alterations, 26
  noradrenergic fibers, 123–124
  pcd mutant mice, 301–303
  raphe nuclei and, 51–52
Cerebellar nuclear neurons, 5-HT
  effects, 225–234
Cerebellar nuclei
  5-HT fiber distribution, 140, 143
  5-HT in, species differences, 150–151
  5-HT uptake sites, 175
Cerebellar syndrome, therapy, 335–336
Cerebellar vermis
  autoradiograms, 180–181, 182, 186
  histology, 461, 462
Cerebellum
  development, opossum, 137–152
  diseases
    animal models, 297–305
    historical aspects, 269
    therapy, 155
  glutamatergic systems, 155–165
  histology, 141–146, 169–176
  5-HT afferents, 92
  5-HT development, opossum, 137–152
  5-HT innervation, 51–60
  5-HT receptors, 205, 207
    development, 179–189
    distribution, 169–176
  5-HT system, 1–33, 91–110
  intercellular communication, 5–13
  lesions, 27–29, 340
Cerebrospinal fluid, 7
  abnormalities, 311–321, 327
Chlorimipramine, 241
p-Chlorophenylalanine, 307–309
Cholera toxin, beta subunit, 238–239
Choline, in thiamine deficiency, 281
Citalopram, 163, 165, 168, 170, 171, 173, 175,
    191–192, 194–198
Climbing fibers, 59, 167, 175, 226
  activation, 102, 104
  in ataxias, 296
  characterization, 291, 292
  collateral sprouting, 291–296
  as neurotransmitters, 110
  pathways, 255, 256
  spikes induced by, 212
Climbing fiber system, olivocerebellar, 113–117
Climbing fiber terminals, 5-HT$_{1A}$ receptors, 187
Clonidine, 251
Colloidal gold/apo horseradish peroxidase, as tracer,
    52–54, 56

Compensation responses, neural, 28–29
Computers, 3D reconstruction by, 124–125
Coordination disorders, assessment, 338–340,
    343–354
Coordination index, 346, 347–348
Cortical cerebellar atrophy, 312–318, 327
Corticosterone
  5-HT system effects, 23–26
  neonatal effects, 23–26
Corticosterone-releasing factor IR fibers, 17–18
Cuneate nuclei, 171
6-Cyano-7-nitroquinoxaline-2,3-dione, 229, 230

D
DARPP-32, 10, 13, 14
DARPP-32 IR, 18, 19, 22
Deep cerebellar nuclear neurons
  discharge rate, 230–234
  excitatory amino acid receptors, 226–230
Deficiency, thiamine. *See* Thiamine deficiency
Deficiency induced ataxias, 269–286
  deficiency-alcoholic ataxia, 314, 317–318,
    320–321, 327
Degenerative disorders, glutamate dehydrogenase-
    induced, 270–276
Dementia
  5-HT in, 37
  studies, 37–47, 130–131
Dendrites, 5-HT$_{1A}$ receptors, 188
Dentate nucleus, 143, 145
Depression
  5-HT and, 37, 74, 251
  raphe nuclei and, 74
Dihydroergocristine, 192
5,6-Dihydroxytryptamine, 241, 243
1-(2,5-Dimethoxy-4-iodophenyl)-2-aminopropane
    hydrochloride, 105, 106, 156–162, 165,
    213, 246
Diphenylhydantoin, 328
Displacement curves, 346, 347–350, 351–354
Dopamine-β-hydroxylase, 241
Dopamine nerve terminal networks, 9, 10, 31–32
Dopaminergic receptors, lisuride effects, 364
Dopaminergic system, in ataxias, 319
Dorsal column nuclei, 171
Dorsal hippocampus pyramidal neurons, firing,
    258–262
Dorsal motor vagal nucleus, 45
Dorsal raphe neurons, 40–41
  firing, 257, 260, 262
Dorsal raphe nucleus, 5-HT neurons in, 147, 149,
    151
Dysdiadochokinesia, 340
Dysmetria, 340
Dystonic rats, genetic, 188

E
ELITE system, 344
Endothelin-1, lesions caused by, 4–5, 27–29
Excitatory amino acid receptors
  characterization, 227–230
  deep cerebellar nuclear neurons, 226–230
  Purkinje cells, 226–230
Excitatory amino acids, 5-HT interactions, 155–165,
    214, 225–234

External granule layer
  development, 142, 146

F

Fascicularis longitudinalis medialis, 239
Fastigial neuron activity, 255–257
Fastigial nucleus, 143
(+)Fenfluramine, 163, 165
d-Fenfluramine, 250–251
Fixation procedures, 64–65
Flesinoxan, 257, 260
Fluorescent microspheres, 138
Fluoxetine, 250
Friedreich's ataxia, 312, 315–319, 320–321, 327
  monoaminergic disturbances, 320
  therapy, 316, 319, 320, 328, 330, 335–336, 338–341

G

Galanin receptors, 13–16
Gamma-aminobutyric acid
  biological effect, 214, 245
  5-HT interaction, 103, 109
  in thiamine deficiency, 281
Gamma-aminobutyric acid$_A$-benzodiazepine receptors, 264
Gamma-aminobutyric acid$_A$ receptor, immunoreactivity, 131–132
Gamma-aminobutyric acid neurons, 129–134
Gene expression
  postnatal influences, 19
  tryptophan hydroxylase, 88
Gepirone, 257, 260
GFAP IR, 27
Gigantocellular nucleus, 171, 173
Glial cells, 5-HT$_{1A}$ receptors, 185, 188
Globus pallidus, 208
Glucocorticoid receptor IR, 18–19
Glutamate
  5-HT interactions, 59, 102–105, 109, 155–165, 230–233, 245–249
  locus coeruleus excitation, 245–249
  as mossy fiber transmitter, 158
  Purkinje cell effects, 226–227
  in thiamine deficiency, 280, 282
Glutamate decarboxylase
  immunoreactivity, 131, 132
Glutamate dehydrogenase, 84
  characterization, 272–273
  cloning of cDNA, 273–274
  deficiency, 270–276
Glutamatergic systems, 274–276
  5-HT control, 155–165
Glycine, biological effect, 245
cGMP system
  regulation, 159, 161, 162, 163–164
  in thiamine deficiency, 281
Golgi cells, immunoreactivity, 131, 132
G protein-coupled receptors, 204–205
G proteins, 13, 14
Granular cell islands, 16–18, 19–20
  innervation, 23
Granular cell layer
  development, 142, 146
  5-HT IR fibers, 140–141

5-HT IR profiles, 94–98, 107
5-HT terminals, 11, 59
5-HT uptake sites, 175
Granular cell-Purkinje cell interface, 140–141
Granular cells
  immunoreactivity, 131, 132
  inhibition, 16–17
  innervation, 17–18
  regulation, 23, 26

H

Hallucinogenic 5-HT agonists, 244–245
Harmaline
  characterization, 255
  GABA$_A$-benzodiazepine receptor interactions, 264
  5-HT interactions, 255–265, 324
  in 5-HT receptor activation, 258–262
  Purkinje cell firing effects, 264–265
  tremogenic action, 113–117, 188, 324
Homovanillic acid, in ataxias, 311–321, 327
Horseradish peroxidase-peroxidase-antiperoxidase
  method, 138–139
5-HT
  adenylate cyclase interactions, 205, 206
  agonists, hallucinogenic, 244–245
  amino acid interactions, 102–103, 104, 105, 109, 155–165, 214, 225–234
  aspartate interactions, 102–103, 105, 109, 155, 230–232
  in ataxias, 251, 282–286, 311–321, 323–332
  autoregulation, 191–199
  binding sites, 9, 13
  brain development role, 108
  brain stem origin, 107–108, 137–152
  cerebellar nuclei, species differences, 150–151
  characterization, 37, 91, 109–110, 137, 234
  decoding system, 13–16
  deficiency, in ataxias, 328
  developmental expression, 137–152
    species differences, 152
  distribution, species differences, 147–150
  excitatory amino acid interactions, 155–165, 214, 225–234
  GABA interactions, 103, 109
  glutamate interactions, 59, 102–105, 109, 155–165, 230–232, 245–249
  harmaline interactions, 255–265, 324
  5-HT$_{1A}$ autoreceptor effects, 198
  innervation by, 51–60, 113–117
    relation to harmaline innervation, 114–115
    species differences, 150
  intercellular communication and, 5–13
  inward rectifier current and, 216–218, 220, 221
  locus coeruleus discharge and, 245–249
  metabolism, 277–280
    in ataxias, 319, 320
    regulation, 191–199
  motor activity regulation, 110
  as neurohormone at 5-HT$_{1A}$ receptors, 188
  in neurologic disorders, 74, 251, 282–286, 311–321, 323–332
  neuromodulatory role, 110, 201–209, 222, 225–234, 324–325
  neurotransmission, harmaline effects, 255–265
  noradrenergic system control, 175–176
  olivary neurons and, 113–117

5-HT (contd.)
  physiological effects, 93–94, 108–109
  in protein synthesis, 307–309
  in Purkinje cell polarization, 214–216, 218–223
  in Purkinje cell regulation, 102, 104–106, 108, 110, 211–223, 225–234, 324
    quasisteady-state current and, 216, 218–219
    release studies, 194–196
    steady-state holding current and, 216–218, 221
    thiamine deficiency and, 326–327
    transient outward current and, 216, 219, 223
  tremogenic action, 113–117
  uptake inhibition
    antidepressant effects, 191–192
    and 5-HT autoregulation, 191–199
  as VT transmitter, 7
5-HT afferents
  characterization, 92, 155
  distribution, 94–99, 325–326
    species differences, 147–150
  in locus coeruleus modulation, 237–251
  origin, 94–102, 103
  raphe nuclei and, 100, 102
  ultrastructure, 94–99
5-HT fibers
  distribution, 140–147
  in glutamate release, 59
5-HT IR, morphology, 2–5, 8, 11, 13, 19–22
5-HT IR fibers
  analysis, 92, 93
  development, 137–152
  distribution, 94–98, 140–147
  pcd mutant mice, 300–301
5-HT IR neurons
  distribution, 52–60, 97, 100–102
  projecting to cerebellar cortex, 56, 59
5-HT IR profiles
  granule cell layer, 94–98, 107
  Purkinje cell layer, 94–97
5-HT IR terminals, 1–5, 7–8, 9, 11, 13, 28, 31–32.
    See also 5-HT terminals
5-HT neurons. See also 5-HT IR neurons
  distribution
    animal models, 238–240
    humans, 63–74
    morphology, 1–4
    projecting to cerebellar cortex, 59–60
  in raphe nuclei, 51, 107–108
  role, 60
  TpOH protein synthesis regulation, 81–88
5-HTP, 193, 195–197
  D-L-5-HTP, therapeutic uses, 328
  L-5-HTP
    in protein synthesis, 307–309
    therapeutic uses, 29, 33, 309, 319, 320, 328–331, 335–336, 354, 357–361
  therapeutic uses, 226, 316, 319, 320, 337–341
5-HT projections, organization, 94–102, 103
5-HT receptors
  activation, 158–159, 161, 163–164, 258–262
  autoreceptors, 191–192, 196–199, 264
  cAMP assays, 202, 204
  characterization, 103–107, 324–325
  classes, 156, 167–168
  cloning, 201, 202
  EAA release regulation, 156–157

and effects of 5-HT on Purkinje cells, 213–214
feedback mechanisms, 15–16
genomic clones, 202
in glutamate release, 158–160, 161–164
5-HT$_{1A}$ autoreceptor, 191, 198
5-HT$_{1A}$-like receptor, 325
5-HT$_{1A}$ receptor, 13–16
  activation, 258, 265
  binding sites, 13, 16, 180–186
  characterization, 7, 103–107, 201
  on climbing fiber terminals, 187
  in control of motor behavior, 188
  distribution, 169–176, 182–185, 188
  5-HT nerve fiber growth and, 188
  as mediator, 108–109
  in molecular layer, 182
  and norepinephrine receptors, 16, 24, 26, 31–32
  olivocerebellar, 179–189
  potassium channel activation, 109
  in Purkinje cell layer, 182
  visualization, 181, 186, 187
5-HT$_{1B/1D}$ sites, 208
5-HT$_{1B}$-like receptor, 207
5-HT$_{1B}$ receptor
  activation, 264
  binding sites, 208–209
  characterization, 201–209
  distribution, 169–176, 324–325
  drug implications, 209
  expression, 202, 204, 205, 207, 208–209
  genomic clone, 201–209, 202
  5-HT$_{1B}$ mRNA, 205, 207–208
  nucleotide sequences, 203
5-HT$_{1C/2}$ receptor, 105
5-HT$_{1C}$ receptor, 105, 107, 201
  distribution, 169–176, 324
5-HT$_{1D}$-like receptor, 167
5-HT$_{1D}$ receptor, 7, 201
5-HT$_1$-like receptor, 158
5-HT$_1$ receptor, 7, 245, 246
5-HT$_{2/1C}$ receptor, 105
5-HT$_2$ receptor, 7, 105–107, 158, 201, 213, 244–245, 246
  distribution, 169–176, 324
5-HT$_3$ receptor, 106, 107, 167, 168, 169
5-HT$_4$ receptor, 167
hybridization, 204
identification, 103–107
labeling, 168–169
lisuride effects, 364
pharmacological profiles, 205, 206
in Purkinje cell regulation, 234
receptor-receptor interactions, 16, 24, 26, 31–32
RNA analysis, 204
visualization, 167–176, 181, 186, 187
5-HT systems,
  in ataxias, 251, 282–286, 311–321, 323–332
  basic fibroblast growth factor in, 29
  cerebellum, 91–110
  corticosterone effects, 23–26
  development, human, 73
  distribution in human brain, 37–47
  endothelin-1 effects, 27–29
  lisuride effects, 369
  6-OHDA effects, 16–23
  pcd mutant mice, 300–301, 304–305, 327

Purkinje cells in, 326
   regulation, 81–88
   as repair mechanisms, 33
5-HT terminals, 12, 13, 23, 26, 60. *See also* 5-HT IR terminals
   in granule cell layer, 59
   in locus coeruleus area, 238
   neurotoxin effects on, 241, 243
   sprouting, 21
Huntington's chorea, 208, 209
Hybridization histochemistry, 168–169
8-Hydroxy-2-(di-n-propylamino)tetralin, 14, 16, 17, 21–22, 24, 26, 103–107, 156–162, 165, 168, 183–184, 188, 205, 213, 216, 217, 246, 249
m-Hydroxybenzylhydrazine, 193
6-Hydroxydopamine, biological effects, 16–23, 25, 26, 27
5-Hydroxyindoleacetic acid, 21, 278–280
   in ataxias, 311–321, 326, 327
5-Hydroxytryptamine. *See* 5-HT
5-Hydroxytryptophan (5-HTP). *See* 5-HTP
Hyperserotoninemia, 328

I

Imipramine, 198
Immunohistochemistry, methodology, 81–82, 92, 130–131, 138, 168–169
Immunoreactivity, human, 65
Indolpyruvate, therapeutic uses, 29, 33
Inferior olive
   histology, 52–60
   5-HT_{1A} binding sites, 187–188
   5-HT uptake sites, 171, 173
   innervation, 12, 59, 113–117
   lesions, 291–296
   neurons, 59, 147, 148, 151
Internal granule layer, 5-HT IR fibers in, 140–141
Interpeduncular region, 44
Interpositus anterior, 142, 143
Interpositus posterior, 142, 143, 145
Inward rectifier current, 216–218, 220, 221
Iodocyanopindolol, 168, 171, 173
Ipsapirone, 103, 106–107, 213
Ischemia, cerebral, 282
Ischemia, induced, 27–29

K

Kainate, 227
Ketanserin, 156–157, 160, 161–163, 168, 205, 213, 246, 249
King's College Hospital Parkinson's Disease Rating Scale, 366–368
Korsakoff's psychosis, 276
Krebs cycle, 281–282
Kynurenate, 250–251

L

Labeling techniques, 121–126, 138–139, 168–169
Lateral reticular nuclei, 171, 174
Levodopa, 366, 367
Lisuride, therapeutic uses, 363–369

Locus coeruleus
   electrophysiology, 244–251
   5-HT effects, 237–251
   5-HT fiber origin, 238–240
Locus coeruleus neurons, 44
   activation, 246, 248, 250–251
   firing, 245–246
   5-HT neurons, 147–149, 150, 151
   noradrenergic neurons, 237–251
Lysergic acid diethylamide, 191, 193, 194–197, 205, 257

M

Machado-Joseph disease, therapy, 329, 330
Marinesco-Sjögren syndrome, therapy, 329, 330
Medial vestibular nucleus, 171
Median raphe, 239, 240
Median raphe neurons, 40–42
Medullary reticular formation, 45, 173
   5-HT neurons in, 147, 151
Memory function, 5-HT neurons in, 286
Mesencephalic nucleus, 173
Mesencephalon, 70–73, 74–75
Mesulergine, 168
Metergoline, 213, 243, 244
Methionine, interaction with L-5-HTP, 308
Methiothepin, 156–157, 161–163, 191, 197–198, 243, 244, 246, 248
8-Methoxy-2-(*N*-propyl-*N*-propyl-amino)tetralin, 180–183, 185–187
5-Methoxy-N,N-dimethyltryptamine, 116
5-Methoxytryptamine, 192
1-Methyl-4-phenyl-1,2,3,6-tetrahydropyridine, 270
Methyl-5-HT, 106, 107
N-Methyl-D-aspartate, 227–233
Methysergide, 213, 246, 248
Molecular layer, 5-HT IR fibers, 94–95
Monoamine oxidase A
   antibodies, 38
   function, 47
   immunoreactivity, 42–46
Monoamine oxidase B
   antibodies, 38
   immunoreactivity, 42–46, 129–134
Monoamine oxidase inhibitor, 116, 257
Monoamine oxidase IR structures, 42–46
Monoaminergic nerve terminals, *pcd* mutant mice, 301–303
Monoaminergic receptors, lisuride effects, 364
Monoaminergic systems, in degenerative disorders, 297–305
Monosodium glutamate, 274
Mossy fibers, 58, 59, 110, 158, 167, 172, 173, 175, 226
Motor control centers, 5-HT receptors, 201–209
Motor skills, neonatal influences, 26
Movement disorders, assessment, 338–340, 343–354
Multiple sclerosis, therapy, 329, 335–336
Muscimol, 214

N

Naloxone, 250–251
Neonatal period, effect of stress, 26
Nerve terminals, *pcd* mutant mice, 301–303

Neurological mutant mice, 297–305
Neuromodulators, see also 5-HT biological effect, 211–212
Neurons. See also specific types of neurons
 histology, 52–60
 morphology, 1–4, 39–42
Neurotoxins, effects on 5-HT terminals, 241, 243
Neurotransmitters
 biological effect, 211–212
 characterization, 225
Noradrenergic fibers, in cerebellar cortex, 123–124
Noradrenergic system, 5-HT control, 175–176
Norepinephrine
 biological effect, 17, 21–22, 211–212, 245, 247
 regulation, 240, 241, 243
Norepinephrine nerve terminal networks, 9, 10, 16, 31–32
Norepinephrine receptors, 16, 24, 26
 and 5-HT$_{1A}$ receptors, 16, 24, 26, 31–32
Norepinephrine system, pcd mutant mice, 300, 301, 304
Nucleus caudal linear, 76
Nucleus centralis superior, 44
Nucleus paragigantocellularis lateralis, 238
Nucleus prepositus hypoglossi, 238
Nucleus raphe dorsalis
 anatomy, 70–71, 73, 74–75
 enzymes, 81–88
 histology, 83
 5-HT neurons, 239, 240
 TpOH cell distribution, 82–84
 TpOH proteins, 84–88
Nucleus raphe dorsalis dorsomedialis, 82
Nucleus raphe dorsalis lateralis, 82
Nucleus raphe dorsalis ventromedialis, 82
Nucleus raphe magnus, 68, 69
Nucleus raphe medialis, 68–72
Nucleus raphe obscurus, 65, 67, 68
Nucleus raphe pallidus, 65, 67
Nucleus reticularis gigantocellularis, 5-HT neurons in, 147, 148

O

Oculomotor nuclei, 45
Olivary neurons,
 5-HT$_{1A}$ receptors, 188
 innervation, 113–117, 255–257
Olivary nuclei, 46
Olivocerebellar projection, organization, 113
Olivocerebellar system, 325–326
 climbing fiber system, 113–117, 255, 256, 291–296
 5-HT$_{1A}$ receptors, 179–189
Olivocerebellofastigiobulbar system, 255, 256
Olivopontocerebellar atrophy, 270–276, 327
 therapy, 328–330, 332, 340, 363–369
Opiate withdrawal, and hyperactivity of locus coeruleus neurons, 246, 248, 250–251
Ornithine decarboxylase IR, 19–20, 24

P

Parachlorophenylalanine, 86–88, 241, 242, 244
Paragigantocellular nucleus, 175–176
Parallel fibers, 212, 226
Paramedian lobule, 94–95
Paramedian reticular nucleus, 173
Paranigral nucleus, 44
Pargyline, 264
Parkinson's disease, 273
 5-HT in, 37, 74
 models, 270
 raphe nuclei in, 74
 rating scales, 366–368
 therapy, 47
Pars reticulata, 44
Parvalbumin, 131
Parvocellular reticular nucleus, 171, 173–175
pcd mutant mice, 327
Periaqueductal gray, 46
Perikarya, tyrosine hydroxylase distribution, 86
Periolivary neurons, innervation by, 59
PH8 antibody, 39–42, 130–134
Pierre Marie's disease, therapy, 335–336
Pons, anatomy, 66–70
Pontine nuclei, 171, 174, 240
Posterior vermis
 5-HT uptake sites, 175
 Purkinje cells, 121–126
Postnatal period, gene expression in, 19
Postural asynergy, assessment, 343–354
Posturography, 338, 339
Potassium, in glutamate release, 155–165
Potassium channels, regulation, 109, 110
Potassium spikes, 212
Precerebellar nuclei, 5-HT terminals, 175
Probenecid, 312, 327
Purkinje cell degeneration mutant mice, 297–305
Purkinje cell-granule cell interface, 140–141
Purkinje cell layer
 development, 142, 144, 146
 5-HT$_{1A}$ receptors, 182, 185
 5-HT IR profiles, 94–97
Purkinje cell/molecular layer, 5-HT$_{1A}$ binding sites, 182, 185–186
Purkinje cells
 aspartate effects, 226–227
 calcium spikes, 214–216
 characterization, 121–126, 291
 current clamp studies, 214–216
 degeneration, animal models, 297–305
 electrophysiology, 211–223
 excitatory amino acid receptors, 226–230
 firing, 30–31, 33, 110, 212, 220–222, 255–257
 5-HT effects, 102, 104–106, 110, 213–214, 230–234
 glutamate effects, 226–227
 in granule cell innervation, 17–18
 harmaline effects, 264–265
 5-HT$_{1A}$ receptors, 188
 5-HT$_{1B}$ receptors, 207–208, 209
 5-HT$_{1B}$ receptor sites, 175
 5-HT$_1$ receptors, 7, 10
 5-HT effects, 108, 110, 211–223, 225–234, 326
 5-HT IR fibers, 94–97
 5-HT polarization, 214–216, 218–223
 immunoreactivity, 131, 132
 innervation, 292–295
 as integrator of WT and VT signals, 10, 12, 33
 ionic conductance, 212, 214–223
 labeling, 121–126

malfunctioning, 28
morphology, 122–125
NMDA receptors, 230
oscillation, 220–222
potassium spikes, 212
regulation, 16, 33
renin IR in, 29
sodium spikes, 212, 214–216
voltage clamp studies, 214–216, 216–220
Pyramidal bundle, 5–HT neurons in, 148
Pyrithiamine, 277

Q

Quasisteady-state current, 216, 218–219
Quipazine, 116, 244
Quisqualate, 227–228, 230–233

R

Raphe dorsalis, enzymes, 81–88
Raphe magnus nucleus, 40–41
Raphe neurons
  cerebellar projection, 51–60
  5-HT neurons, 37–47, 51, 107–108, 326
  immunoreactivity, 134
Raphe nuclei
  axon branching, 56
  cerebellar cortex connection, 51–52
  distribution, 73
  histology, 52–60
  5-HT afferents, 100, 102, 238
  5-HT innervation of cerebellar cortex, 51–60
  5-HT origin, 134
  immunoreactive areas, 44–45
  role in diseases, 74
Raphe obscurus nucleus, 40–41
Raphe-olivocerebellar system, 325–326
Raphe pallidus nucleus, 40–41
Raphe projection, function, 213
Raphe system, electrolytic lesions, 240
RDC4 receptor, 207
Red nucleus, 173
Renin-angiotensin system, 29–31
Renin IR, 29–31
Reserpine, 328
Reticular formation
  5-HT receptors, 173
  as source of 5–HT, 107–108
Reticulotegmental nucleus, 171
Ritanserin, 105, 107
Rostral medulla, 65, 67
Rostral mesencephalon, 71–72, 76
Rostral pons, 68–72
RU24969, 246

S

Schut-Haymaker olivopontocerebellar atrophy, 273
Selegeline, 366, 367
Serotonergic drugs, biological effect, 198–199
Serotonergic motor syndrome, tremor component, 115–117
Serotonin. See 5-HT
Sertraline, 244, 250
Sodium conductance, 116–117
Sodium spikes, 212, 214–216
Solitary nucleus, 45
Spinal vestibular nucleus, 171

Spiperone, 104–106, 168, 213
Steady-state holding current, 216–218, 221
Stellate cells, immunoreactivity, 131, 132
Stick diagrams, 345, 347, 348, 350–354
Striatum, 5-HT receptors, 205, 207–208
Substance P receptors, 13
Substantia nigra, 44, 208, 209
Suicide
  5-HT and, 74
  raphe nuclei and, 74
Synaptosomes, 158–159, 161
  5-HT uptake, 277–278

T

Tandospirone, 257, 260
Thalamic nuclei, 173
Thiamine deficiency, 276–286
  amino acid levels in, 280–283
  biochemical lesion, 283–284
  5-HIAA in, 320
  5-HT in, 278–280, 283, 284–285, 326–327
  neurologic manifestations, 284–286
  neurotransmitters in, 281–283
  sleep disturbances in, 286
  in synaptic transmission, 277
Transient outward current, 216, 219, 223
Tremogenic substances, 113–117, 188, 255–265, 324
Tremor
  in climbing fiber system, 113–117
  measurement, 340
  pathological, 117
m-Trifluoromethylphenylpiperazine, 213, 246
Trochlear nucleus, 45
Tryptophan
  L-tryptophan, 116
  metabolism, in ataxias, 328
Tryptophan hydroxylase
  antibodies, 64
  gene expression, 88
  innervation by, 129–134
  regulation, 81–88, 193–194
Tryptophan hydroxylase IR cell bodies, distribution, 65–74
Tryptophan hydroxylase IR neurons, distribution, 63–74
Tryptophan hydroxylase positive cell bodies, measurement, 82–84
Tryptophan hydroxylase protein
  measurement, 84–86
  synthesis, 86–88
Tyrosine hydroxylase
  antibodies, 38, 42, 121–126
  distribution, 86
  regulation, 240–244
Tyrosine hydroxylase IR, 14
Tyrosine hydroxylase IR nerve terminals, 10, 21, 23
Tyrosine hydroxylase IR neurons, 42

V

Velocity curves, 346, 347–350, 351–354
Vestibular nuclei, 173
Voltage-dependent currents, modulation, 212
Volume transmission, 5–13, 150, 225, 279–280
  morphological indications, 7, 9–10, 12

Volume transmission (*contd.*)
　in plasticity responses, 29–31
　Purkinje cells in, 10, 12, 33

W

Wernicke-Korsakoff syndrome, 282, 286
Wernicke's encephalopathy, 276

Wiring transmission, 5–13, 225, 279–280
　Purkinje cells in, 10, 12, 33

Z

Zacopride, 168
Zimelidine, 198